The blood–brain barrier is a vital yet all too frequently misunderstood biological membrane, which serves to protect the brain from toxic substances whilst simultaneously allowing access to essential nutrients and chemical signals. In its protective role, of course, it also functions to hinder the supply of many important medicines to the brain. At the interface between brain and body, adequate knowledge of the blood–brain barrier forms an essential component in the complete understanding of a large proportion of medical disciplines. Nevertheless, it seems that ignorance of both the biology of this important membrane and the methodology suitable for its investigation still remains an impediment to progress in many fields, including, for example, the development of new and efficacious neuropharmaceuticals, cerebrovascular disease, Alzheimer's disease, cerebral AIDS and brain tumors.

This introduction to the topic for both researchers and clinicians across the medical sciences is intended to aid both those beginning work directly in this area and those wishing simply to be better informed when interpreting information where the blood–brain barrier may be involved. Recent advances in both methodology and biology are detailed in 50 state-of-the-art chapters from international authorities.

Introduction to the Blood–Brain Barrier

Methodology, biology and pathology

Introduction to the Blood–Brain Barrier

Methodology, biology and pathology

WILLIAM M. PARDRIDGE, MD

Professor of Medicine, UCLA School of Medicine, USA

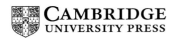

CAMBRIDGE
UNIVERSITY PRESS

PUBLISHED BY THE PRESS SYNDICATE OF THE UNIVERSITY OF CAMBRIDGE
The Pitt Building, Trumpington Street, Cambridge CB2 1RP, United Kingdom

CAMBRIDGE UNIVERSITY PRESS
The Edinburgh Building, Cambridge CB2 2RU, United Kingdom
40 West 20th Street, New York, NY 10011-4211, USA
10 Stamford Road, Oakleigh, Melbourne 3166, Australia

First published 1998

Printed in the United Kingdom at the University Press, Cambridge

Typeset in Monotype Baskerville 10/12pt

A catalogue record for this book is available from the British Library

Library of Congress Cataloguing in Publication data

An introduction to the blood–brain barrier : methodology, biology and
  pathology / [edited by] William M. Pardridge.
       p.   cm.
    ISBN 0 521 58124 9 (hb)
    1. Blood–brain barrier.   2. Blood–brain barrier disorders.
  I. Pardridge, William M.
    [DNLM: 1. Blood–Brain Barrier – physiology.   2. Brain – pathology.
  3. Brain – drug effects.   4. Drug Delivery Systems.
  5. Neurophysiology – methods.   6. Neuropharmacology – methods. WL
  200 I614 1998]
  QP375.5.I63 1998
  612.8'24 – dc21   97-26483 CIP
  DNLM/DLC
  for Library of Congress

ISBN 0 521 58124 9 hardback

Every effort has been made in preparing this book to provide accurate and up-to-date
information which is in accord with accepted standards and practice at the time of publication.
Nevertheless, the authors, editors and publisher can make no warranties that the information
contained herein is totally free from error, not least because clinical standards are constantly
changing through research and regulation. The authors, editors and publisher therefore
disclaim all liability for direct or consequential damages resulting from the use of material
contained in this book. The reader is strongly advised to pay careful attention to information
provided by the manufacturer of any drugs or equipment that they plan to use.

Contents

Part II   **Transport biology**

Part III   **General aspects of CNS transport**

Part IV   **Signal transduction/biochemical aspects**

Contributors

N. JOAN ABBOTT
Physiology Group
Biomedical Sciences Division
King's College London
Strand
London WC2R 2LS
UK

MARIO ALBERGHINA
Institute of Biological Chemistry
University of Catania
Viale Andrea Doria 6
95125 Catania
Italy

KENNETH L. AUDUS
Department of Pharmaceutical
Chemistry
The University of Kansas
2095 Constant Avenue
Lawrence, Kansas 66047-2504
USA

ROUMEN BALABANOV
Department of Neurology
Wayne State University School of
Medicine
421 E Canfield Ave, 3124 Elliman
Building
Detroit, MI 48021
USA

JORGE R. BARRIO
Department of Molecular and Medical
Pharmacology
UCLA School of Medicine
10833 Le Conte Ave
Los Angeles, CA 90095-6948
USA

HANNELORE BAUER
Institute of Molecular Biology
Austrian Academy of Sciences
Billrothstr 11
A-5020 Salzburg
Austria

E. BEAULIEU
Université du Québec à Montréal
Département de chimie et de biochimie
CP 8888, succursale Centre-ville
Montréal, Québec H3C 3P8
Canada

DAVID J. BEGLEY
Biomedical Sciences Division
Physiology Group
King's College London
Strand
London WC2R 2LS
UK

RICHARD BÉLIVEAU
Université du Québec à Montréal
Département de chimie et de biochimie
CP 8888, succursale Centre-ville
Montréal, Québec H3C 3P8
Canada

A. LORRIS BETZ
Departments of Surgery, University of
Michigan
5605 Kresge I, Box 0532
1500 East Medical Center Drive
Ann Arbor, MI 48109-0532
USA.

CARSTEN T. BEUKMANN
Institut für Biochemie
Westfälische Wilhelms-Universität
Münster
Wilhelm-Klemm Str. 2
D-48149 Münster
Germany

ULRICH BICKEL
Institute of Physiology
Deutschhausstr 2
35037 Marburg
Germany

RUBEN J. BOADO
Department of Medicine
UCLA School of Medicine
C-Lot RM 112
Los Angeles, CA 90095
USA

RONALD T. BORCHARDT
Department of Pharmaceutical
Chemistry
The University of Kansas
2095 Constant Avenue
Lawrence, Kansas 66047-2504
USA

P. BORST
The Netherlands Cancer Institute
Department of Molecular Biology
Plesmanlaan 121
1066 CX Amsterdam
The Netherlands

JEAN-MARIE BOURRE
INSERM U 26
Hôpital Fernand Widal
200 rue du Faubourg Saint Denis
75475 Paris cedex 10
France

DOUWE D. BREIMER
Sylvius Laboratories
Leiden/Amsterdam Center for Drug
Research
PO Box 9503, Wassenaarseweg 72
2300 RA Leiden
The Netherlands

MILTON W. BRIGHTMAN
Laboratory of Neurobiology
NINDS, Bld. 36, Rm 2A-21
National Institutes of Health
Bethesda, MD, 20892-4062
USA

CELIA F. BROSNAN
Departments of Pathology and
Neuroscience
Albert Einstein College of Medicine
1300 Morris Park Ave
New York, NY 10461
USA

R. E. CATALÁN
Departamento de Biología Molecular
Centro 'Severo Ochoa' (CSIC-UAM)
Universidad Autónoma de Madrid
E-28049 Madrid
Spain

SYLVIE M. CAZAUBON
CNRS UPR 415
Institut Cochin de Génétique
Moléculaire
22 rue Méchain
75014 Paris
France

ROMÉO CECHELLI
INSERM U325
Institut Pasteur de Lille
59019 Lille Cedex
France

LUZ CLAUDIO
Department of Environmental Medicine
The Mount Sinai School of Medicine
One Gustave Levy Place
New York, NY 10029-6574
USA

EAIN M. CORNFORD
W127B Southwest Regional VA
Epilepsy Center
Veterans Affairs West LA Medical
Center
11301 Wilshire Boulevard
Los Angeles, CA 90073
USA

PIERRE OLIVIER COURAUD
CNRS UPR 415
Institut Cochin de Génétique
Moléculaire
22 rue Méchain
75014 Paris
France

ALBERTUS G. DE BOER
Sylvius Laboratories
Leiden/Amsterdam Center for Drug
Research
PO Box 9503, Wassenaarseweg 72
2300 RA Leiden
The Netherlands

ELIZABETH C. M. DE LANGE
Sylvius Laboratories
Leiden/Amsterdam Center for Drug
Research
PO Box 9503, Wassenaarseweg 72
2300 RA Leiden
The Netherlands

BÉNÉDICTE DEHOUCK
INSERM U325
Institut Pasteur de Lille
59019 Lille Cedex
France

MARIE-PIERRE DEHOUCK
INSERM U325
Institut Pasteur de Lille
59019 Lille Cedex
France

M. DEMEULE
Université du Québec à Montréal
Département de chimie et de biochimie
CP 8888, succursale Centre-ville
Montréal, Québec H3C 3P8
Canada

PAULA DORE-DUffY
Department of Neurology
Wayne State University School of
Medicine
421 E Canfield Ave, 3124 Elliman
Building
Detroit, MI 48021
USA

LESTER R. DREWES
Department of Biochemistry and
Molecular Biology
University of Minnesota School of
Medicine
10 University Drive
Duluth, MN 55812
USA

K. M. DZIEGIELEWSKA
Department of Anatomy and Physiology
University of Tasmania
GPO Box 252-24
Hobart, Tasmania 7001
Australia

STEVEN R. ENNIS
Departments of Surgery, University of
Michigan
5605 Kresge I, Box 0532
1500 East Medical Center Drive
Ann Arbor, MI 48109-0532
USA.

LAURENCE FENART
INSERM U325
Institut Pasteur de Lille
59019 Lille Cedex
France

JOSEPH D. FENSTERMACHER
Department of Anesthesiology, CFP-1
Henry Ford Hospital
2799 West Grand Boulevard
Detroit, MI 48202-2689
USA

MARK FISHER
Director, Stroke Research Program
USC School of Medicine
1333 San Pablo Street MCH 246
Los Angeles, CA 90033
USA

CHRISTIAN FRELIN
Institut de Pharmacologie Moléculaire
et Cellulaire du CNRS
Sophia Antipolis
660 route des Lucioles
06560 Valbonne
France

MIKIO FURUSE
Department of Cell Biology
Kyoto University
Konoe-Yoshida
Sakyo-ku, Kyoto 606
Japan

HANS-JOACHIM GALLA
Institut für Biochemie
Westfälische Wilhelms-Universität
Münster
Wilhelm-Klemm Str 2
D-48149 Münster
Germany

HEINZ GÖGELEIN
Hoechst AG
Cardiovascular Agents, H 821
D-65926 Frankfurt/Main
Germany

CLIVE P. HAWKINS
Department of Neurology
North Staffs Royal Infirmary
Princes Road
Stoke on Trent
ST4 7LN
UK

RICHARD A. HAWKINS
The Chicago Medical School
3333 Green Bay Road
North Chicago, IL 60064
USA

CARL HOH
Department of Molecular and Medical
Pharmacology
UCLA School of Medicine
10833 Le Conte Ave
Los Angeles, CA 90095-6948
USA

JOACHIM HOYER
Universitätsklinikum Benjamin Franklin
Hindenburgdamm 30
D-12200 Berlin
Germany

SUNG-CHENG HUANG
Department of Molecular and Medical
Pharmacology
UCLA School of Medicine
10833 Le Conte Ave
Los Angeles, CA 90095-6948
USA

MASAHIKO ITOH
Department of Cell Biology
Kyoto University
Konoe-Yoshida
Sakyo-ku, Kyoto 606
Japan

L. JETTÉ
Université du Québec à Montréal
Département de chimie et de biochimie
CP 8888, succursale Centre-ville
Montréal, Québec H3C 3P8
Canada

CONRAD E. JOHANSON
Department of Clinical Neurosciences
Rhode Island Hospital
593 Eddy Street
Providence, RI 02903
USA

BARBRO B. JOHANSSON
Department of Neurology
Lund University Hospital
S-22185 Lund
Sweden

RICHARD F. KEEP
Departments of Surgery, University of
Michigan
5605 Kresge I, Box 0532
1500 East Medical Center Drive
Ann Arbor, MI 48109-0532
USA.

GITTE MOOS KNUDSEN
Dept of Neurology N2082
Rigshospitalet
9 Blegdamsvej
DK-2100 Copenhagen
Denmark

ALBERT S. LOSSINSKY
NYS Institute for Basic Research in
Developmental Disabilities
1050 Forest Hill Road
Staten Island, NY 10314
USA

RICHARD M. MCCARRON
Department of Pathology
Uniformed Services University of the
Health Sciences
Bethseda, Maryland 20814-4799
USA

D. MIKULIS
Department of Medical Imaging
University of Toronto
Toronto, Ontario M5S 1A8
Canada

LOUISE MORGAN
Eisai London Laboratories
University College London
Gower Street
London WC1E 6BT
UK

SUKRITI NAG
The Toronto Hospital, Western
Division
399 Bathurst Street
Toronto, Ontario M5T 2S8
Canada

WILLIAM M. PARDRIDGE
Department of Medicine
UCLA School of Medicine
Los Angeles, CA 90095-1682

JAAKKO PARKKINEN
Finnish Red Cross
Blood Transfusion Service
Kivihaantie 7
FIN-00310 Helsinki
Finland

OLAF B. PAULSON
Department of Neurology N2082
Rigshospitalet
9 Blegdamsvej
DK-2100 Copenhagen
Denmark

DARRYL R. PETERSON
Professor of Physiology and Biophysics
The Chicago Medical School
3333 Green Bay Road
North Chicago, IL 60064
USA

CAROL K. PETITO
Department of Pathology
University of Miami School of Medicine
1550 N W 10th Avenue
Papanicolaou Building, Room 417
Miami, FL 33136
USA

MICHAEL E. PHELPS
Department of Molecular and Medical
Pharmacology
UCLA School of Medicine
10833 Le Conte Ave
Los Angeles, CA 90095-6948
USA

RÜDIGER POPP
Johann Wolfgang Goethe-Universität
Zentrum der Physiologie
Theodor-Stern-Kai 7
D-60590 Frankfurt/Main
Germany

Contributors

JOHN T. POVLISHOCK
Medical College of Virginia
Virginia Commonwealth University
1101 E Marshall Street
Richmond, VA 23298-0709
USA

LISE PRESCOTT
3919 Boulevard LaSalle
Verdun, Quebec
QC H4G 2A1
Canada

JAYNA M. ROSE
Department of Pharmaceutical
Chemistry
The University of Kansas
2095 Constant Avenue
Lawrence, Kansas 66047-2504
USA

LEE L. RUBIN
Eisai London Laboratories
University College London
Gower Street
London WC1E 6BT
UK

N. R. SAUNDERS
Department of Anatomy and Physiology
University of Tasmania
GPO Box 252-24
Hobart, Tasmania 7001
Australia

A. H. SCHINKEL
The Netherlands Cancer Institute
Department of Molecular Biology
Plesmanlaan 121
1066 CX Amsterdam
The Netherlands

BÜRKHARD SCHLOSSHAUER
NMI
Universität Tübingen in Reutlingen
Markwiesenstr 55
D-72770 Reutlingen
Germany

MALCOLM SEGAL
Sherrington School of Physiology
UMDS
St Thomas's Hospital
Lambeth Palace Road
London SE1 7EH
UK

QUENTIN SMITH
Chief, Neurochemistry and Brain
Transport Section
Laboratory of Neurosciences
National Institute on Aging
NIH Bldg 10 Room 6C-103
Bethesda, MD 20892-1582
USA

MARIA SPATZ
Stroke Branch, NINDS
Bldg 36 Room 4A03
36 Convent Drive, MSC 4128
Bethesda, Maryland 20892-4128
USA

JAMES M. STADDON
Eisai London Laboratories
University College London
Gower Street
London WC1E 6BT
UK

P. A. STEWART
Departments of Anatomy and Cell
Biology
University of Toronto
Toronto, Ontario M5S 1A8
Canada

JAMES STOLL
Laboratory of Neurosciences
National Institute on Aging
NIH Bldg 10 Room 6C-103
Bethseda, MD 20892-1582
USA

IKUMI TAMAI
Department of Pharmaceutics
Faculty of Pharmaceutical Sciences
Kanazawa University
Takara-machi, Kanazawa 920
Japan

TETSUYA TERASAKI
Department of Pharmaceutics
Faculty of Pharmaceutical Sciences
Tohoku University
Aoba-ku, Sendai 981
Japan

GÉRARD TORPIER
INSERM U325
Institut Pasteur de Lille
59019 Lille Cedex
France

AKIRA TSUJI
Department of Pharmaceutics
Faculty of Pharmaceutical Sciences
Kanazawa University
Takara-machi, Kanazawa 920
Japan

SHOICHIRO TSUKITA
Department of Cell Biology
Kyoto University
Konoe-Yoshida
Sakyo-ku, Kyoto 606
Japan

GARETH TURNER
University Department of Cellular
Science,
Level 5 Laboratory, R5501
The John Radcliffe Hospital,
Oxford OX3 9DU
UK

PAUL VIGNE
Institut de Pharmacologie Moléculaire
et Cellulaire du CNRS
Sophia Antipolis
660 route des Lucioles
06560 Valbonne
France

HARRY V. VINTERS
Chief, Section of Neuropathology
UCLA Medical Center, CHS 18-170
Los Angeles, CA 90095-1732
USA

WEN WANG
Department of Pharmaceutical
Chemistry
The University of Kansas
2095 Constant Avenue
Lawrence, Kansas 66047-2504
USA

LING WEI
Department of Anesthesiology, CFP-1
Henry Ford Hospital
2799 West Grand Boulevard
Detroit, MI 48202-2689
USA

HENRYK M. WISNIEWSKI
NYS Institute for Basic Research in
Developmental Disabilities
1050 Forest Hill Road
Staten Island, NY 10314
USA

1 Blood–brain barrier methodology and biology

WILLIAM M. PARDRIDGE

- Introduction
- Blood–brain barrier methodologies and the evolution of multi-disciplinary research approaches
- Dialectics in blood–brain barrier research
- Role of blood–brain barrier research within the neurosciences

Introduction

The blood–brain barrier (BBB) is formed by the brain capillary endothelial cell. In addition to brain endothelial transport processes, BBB research encompasses all of brain microvascular biology. The latter involves the interaction of the capillary endothelium with microvascular pericytes, neuronal inputs, astrocyte foot processes, perivascular microglial cells, and circulating leukocytes. Since the BBB forms the interface between blood and brain, the biology of the BBB plays a role in multiple disciplines other than the neurosciences, including pharmacology, physiology, pathology, and internal medicine. Despite the important role played by the BBB in so many fields, the number of laboratories worldwide engaged in BBB research is comparatively small. The relative underdevelopment of BBB research has important implications for the practical application of advances in the neurosciences (see last section of this chapter). However, this underdevelopment provides opportunities for young scientists to enter into a new area of neuroscience research.

The proposition that BBB research is still markedly underdeveloped, compared to other sectors of the neurosciences, may be examined from the perspective of the large number of areas in

Table 1.1. *A partial list of important yet underdeveloped problems in blood–brain barrier biology*

1. Cloning of cDNAs for BBB transport systems.
2. Cell biology and signal transduction of brain capillary endothelial transcytosis.
3. Molecular characterization of 'induction factors' that are secreted by the brain and induce gene expression in brain capillary endothelial cells.
4. Signal transduction mechanisms and tight junction function.
5. Bidirectional paracrine interactions between brain endothelial cells and astrocytes or neurons.
6. Isolation and characterization of brain endothelial tight junction proteins.
7. Cytokines and the brain microvasculature.
8. Molecular mechanisms underlying hemostasis and leukocyte migration at the BBB.
9. Molecular basis of microbe interaction with brain endothelial cells.
10. Enzymatic barrier mechanisms.

BBB biology that have both great significance for understanding how the brain functions and a relatively thin or nonexistent knowledge base. Table 1.1 lists ten such problems. Cloning of brain capillary

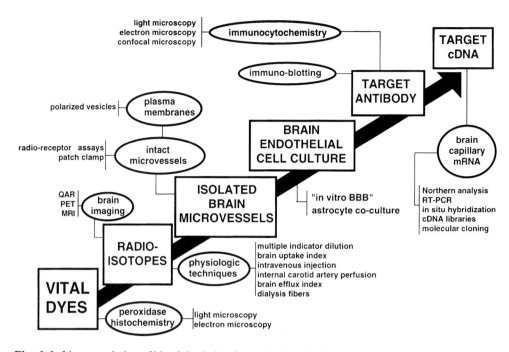

Fig. 1.1. Linear evolution of blood–brain barrier methodologies from vital dyes to molecular biology.

endothelial transporter genes has not been widely performed, despite the availability of methodologies for isolation of brain capillary-derived mRNA molecules. Little is known about the cell biology of brain capillary endothelial transcytosis pathways, particularly at the ultrastructural and cell biological levels. There is evidence that the brain, perhaps astrocyte foot processes, secretes inductive factors that are sequestered by the capillary endothelium to cause tissue-specific gene expression within the cell (Stewart and Wiley, 1981). However, to date no such putative brain-derived inductive factors have been purified. The capillary endothelium and the astrocyte foot process are separated by a basement membrane filled space that is only 20 nm in length; however, there is very little information on the bi-directional paracrine interactions between the endothelium and the astrocyte. The brain capillary endothelial cells produce tight junctions with electrical resistance as high as 8000 ohm-cm^2 (Smith and Rapoport, 1986). Tight junction proteins have been isolated and characterized in peripheral tissues, but to date, no unique tight junction proteins have been purified from brain capillary endothelial cells. The effects of cytokines on the brain microvasculature is only recently being investigated, and there is no information on

putative cytokines that are secreted to the brain by the capillary endothelium. Progress in understanding the biochemistry and cell biology of CNS hemostasis lags behind that in heart and peripheral tissues. Other important areas in need of molecular and cellular-based investigations are the mechanisms of microbial interactions at the brain capillary endothelium, and brain microvascular enzymatic barriers (Table 1.1).

Blood–brain barrier methodologies and the evolution of multi-disciplinary research approaches

Much of BBB investigation is rooted in a single-methodology approach. For example, a given laboratory may investigate BBB transport with either peroxidase histochemistry, intravenous injection techniques using radioisotopes, intracerebral dialysis fibers, in vitro BBB models using cultured endothelium, or quantitative autoradiography (QAR). There are multiple methodologies available for studying BBB transport processes, and these methodologies have generally evolved over time as depicted in Fig. 1.1. Vital dyes were initially used to investigate the BBB in the nineteenth century, and this experimental approach is still used today. In the 1960s and 1970s, peroxidase histochemistry at either the light microscopic or electron microscopic level was introduced. Also at this time, the use of radioisotopes was developed (Fig. 1.1), as were different physiologic techniques applied to anesthetized or conscious laboratory animals, including intracarotid arterial injection techniques such as the multiple indicator dilution (MID) technique, or the brain uptake index (BUI) method, and the intravenous single injection technique. More recently, internal carotid artery perfusion techniques and the brain efflux index (BEI) method have been used. The application of intracerebral dialysis fibers has been introduced, which allows for direct sampling of brain interstitial fluid (ISF). The use of radioisotopes also led to the development of radioimaging techniques such as QAR in laboratory animals, or positron emission tomography (PET) in humans. Magnetic resonance imaging (MRI) allows for functional brain imaging in humans without the use of radioisotopes.

In the mid-1970s, techniques for the isolation of brain microvessels became available, and intact microvessels have been used to investigate the brain microvasculature with radioreceptor assays, immunocytochemistry, or patch clamp techniques. Isolated microvessels also allowed for the isolation of microvascular plasma membranes, which may be used to obtain enriched preparations of lumenal or ablumenal endothelial membrane vesicles. In the early 1980s, it was recognized that isolated brain microvessels are metabolically impaired and fail to exclude vital dyes such as Trypan Blue (Lasbennes and Gayet, 1983). This property and the desire to establish endothelium/astrocyte co-culture techniques led to the development of methods for primary cultivation of brain capillary endothelial cells. When these cultured cells are grown on a filter that may be placed inside side-to-side diffusion chambers, transport across the endothelial monolayer may be investigated, which is a kind of 'in vitro BBB' model system. Finally, in the 1980s and 1990s, immunochemical and molecular biology techniques were introduced to BBB research. The availability of a target antibody allows for the evaluation of brain microvascular-specific proteins using biochemical-based electrophoretic techniques such as Western blotting, or cell biology-based techniques such as immunocy-

tochemistry using either light microscopy, electron microscopy, or confocal fluorescence microscopy. The availability of target cDNAs allows for the investigation of brain microvascular transcripts at the morphological level using in situ hybridization (ISH). These cDNAs may be used in conjunction with the isolation of brain capillary-derived mRNA to study BBB-specific transcripts using either Northern analysis or reverse transcriptase-polymerase chain reaction (RT-PCR). The availability of capillary-specific mRNA preparations also allows for the production of brain capillary-specific cDNA libraries, and for the molecular cloning of brain microvascular-specific genes (Fig. 1.1).

Blood–brain barrier research problems have been traditionally investigated with one of the single methodologies outlined in Fig. 1.1. However, complex biological problems invariably require a multi-disciplinary or team approach. Team approaches may be at specific institutions, but more likely in the future will evolve as the cooperation between different laboratories throughout the world is fostered by Internet-based electronic media and newsgroups. In this regard, Dr. Joerg Huwyler has designed a Blood–Brain Barrier web site at http://www.med.ucla.edu/divisions/endo/homepage.html.

Apart from the complexity of many BBB research problems, another reason for taking a multi-disciplinary approach to BBB research is that each individual methodology has its own inherent limitations. The failure to recognize these limitations gives rise to differences in interpretation of experimental data and occasionally to profound differences in models describing BBB biology. Some of these dialectics are illustrated below.

Dialectics in blood–brain barrier research

(1) The blood–brain barrier in newborns is said to be leaky compared to the adult

Measurements of the total protein content in CSF in newborns shows that the CSF protein is elevated in the developing stage. As reviewed in Chapter 30 of this volume, there has been a historical tendency to refer to the brain barriers as if they comprised a single entity, and to lump the blood–brain barrier (which segregates blood and ISF), with the choroid plexus, i.e. the blood–CSF barrier (which segregates blood from CSF). A corollary of this view is that BBB permeability may be inferred from CSF sampling. However, protein content in CSF is a function of (i) the rate of protein influx into that compartment via transport across the blood–CSF barrier, and (ii) the rate of protein egress from that compartment via absorption of CSF into the superior sagittal sinus across the arachnoid villi. The maturation of the latter process is delayed in newborns, and this is the principal reason for the increased protein content in the CSF of newborns. In fact, the BBB of newborns is as highly developed as is the BBB in adults. The tight junctions cementing brain capillary endothelium are laid down within the first trimester of human fetal life (Mollgard and Saunders, 1975).

(2) Azidothymidine (AZT) is believed to cross the BBB readily because it rapidly distributes into the CSF from plasma

Drugs such as AZT or foscarnet are said to penetrate the BBB readily, because the CSF/plasma ratio of these drugs is high in humans. Both of these are highly charged drugs, and it would be expected that both drugs undergo negligible transport through the BBB in the absence of specific carrier-mediated transport systems. Such transport systems are localized at the choroid plexus and the blood–CSF barrier, but are absent at the BBB. Indeed these drugs may actually undergo active efflux from brain ISF to plasma across the brain capillary endothelium. The rapid distribution of these drugs into CSF is a good predictor of possible transport systems at the blood–CSF barrier, but not necessarily the BBB.

(3) Morphine 6-glucuronide (M6G) is said to have special transport properties at the BBB because, despite the high polarity of this compound compared to morphine, the two molecules enter into brain interstitial fluid (ISF) at identical rates based on dialysis fiber measurements.

The 1-octanol partition coefficient (P) of morphine is more than a hundred-fold greater than that of M6G. Therefore, in the absence of a special transport system for M6G, the BBB penetration of morphine should be at least a log order greater than that of M6G. However, when the drug penetration into brain ISF is measured with intracerebral dialysis fibers, both drugs are found to cross the BBB at comparable rates (Aasmundstad et al., 1995). When BBB permeability to the two drugs is measured with either an internal carotid artery perfusion or an intravenous single injection technique, the BBB permeability-surface area (PS) product for morphine is more than tenfold greater than the PS product of M6G (Bickel et al., 1996; Wu et al., 1997). The measurement of comparable BBB permeability coefficients for the two drugs with intracerebral dialysis fibers is an artefact. The artefact arises because there is BBB disruption in the dialysis fiber model system; the implantation of an intracerebral dialysis fiber causes brain injury, which leads to BBB disruption as reflected by albumin immunocytochemistry (Westergren et al., 1995). The pore in the BBB created by the implantation of the dialysis fiber is relatively small, and selectively affects the estimation of the BBB permeability for poorly diffusible molecules (Morgan et al., 1996), such as M6G, which has a BBB PS product comparable to that of sucrose, as opposed to moderately diffusible molecules such as morphine, which has a BBB permeability comparable to that of urea. The artefact pertaining to M6G permeability at the BBB can be avoided if dialysis fiber measurements are made in conjunction with direct estimation of BBB permeability using either the internal carotid artery perfusion or intravenous single injection technique.

(4) Brain endothelial cells are posited to present antigen to circulating leukocytes at the luminal membrane, because brain capillary endothelium expresses class II histocompatibility (DR) antigen based on immunocytochemistry of either brain tissue sections or isolated brain capillaries

Isolated brain microvessels are comprised of endothelial cells, pericytes, arteriolar smooth muscle cells, and astrocyte foot processes that remain attached to the abluminal pole of the microvessel. Therefore, the finding of immunoreactivity in an isolated microvessel preparation does not necessarily represent an endothelial cellular origin for the antigen. In tissue sections of brain, it is generally not possible to differentiate endothelial cells and pericytes at the light microscopic level. However, examination of cytospun isolated human brain capillary specimens does allow for differentiation of brain capillary endothelial cells and pericytes. The brain microvascular DR antigen immunoreactivity in diseases such as multiple sclerosis is confined to the pericyte rather than to the endothelium (Pardridge *et al.*, 1989). Antigen presentation at the pericyte means that circulating leukocytes must first undergo transcytosis through the BBB and enter brain ISF prior to antigen presentation in brain.

(5) P-glycoprotein is hypothesized to limit drug transport across the BBB, because immunoreactive P-glycoprotein is found in brain capillary endothelium in either brain sections or isolated capillaries

Isolated brain capillary preparations contain abundant astrocyte foot processes that remain adhered to the abluminal pole of the microvessel following the homogenization of brain (White *et al.*, 1981). Therefore, the finding of P-glycoprotein immunoreactivity in isolated brain microvessels is not direct evidence for an endothelial origin of this protein. Indeed, when confocal fluorescent microscopy is used with isolated human brain capillaries and the MRK16 murine monoclonal antibody to human P-glycoprotein, the P-glycoprotein immunoreactivity in this preparation is found to localize nearly exactly with astrocyte foot processes that are immunoreactive for glial fibrillary acidic protein (GFAP) (Pardridge *et al.*, 1997). Moreover, when isolated brain capillaries are immunostained with an antibody to GFAP, these structures are brightly illuminated owing to the astrocyte foot process remnants that remain attached to the microvessels. GFAP is an astrocyte marker yet its immunoreactivity in isolated microvessel preparations is abundant. Similarly, it is often times not possible to differentiate an endothelial versus an astrocyte foot process origin of the antigen in tissue sections and light microscopy. The principle distribution of P-glycoprotein at the astrocyte foot process in brain

is not incompatible with the observation that the distribution in brain of P-glycoprotein substrates is increased in the mdr1a (P-glycoprotein) knockout mouse (Chapter 21). Loss of active efflux of drug at the astrocyte membrane will also lead to enhanced distribution of drug in brain.

(6) Pericytes are said to have a contractile function, because immunoreactive α-actin is abundant in pericytes in tissue culture

If the brain microvascular pericyte has a contractile function at the microvasculature *in vivo*, then this cell should also express the smooth muscle α-actin isoform, which is produced by brain microvascular pericytes in tissue culture. However, immunocytochemistry of CNS microvessels in either retina (Nehls and Drenckhahn, 1991) or brain (Boado and Pardridge, 1994) shows that brain capillary pericytes *in vivo* do not express immunoreactive α-actin protein. The gene for α-actin may be expressed in brain microvascular pericytes in pathophysiologic states. However, under control conditions, these cells appear to lack a contractile function *in vivo*. These findings illustrate the limitations of performing an experiment solely in a tissue culture system, and extrapolating to the *in vivo* state without parallel experiments using *in vivo* models.

(7) Transferrin is said to undergo an obligatory retroendocytosis at the brain capillary endothelium because transferrin receptor is not detectable at the abluminal endothelial membrane based on pre-embedding electron microscopic immunogold studies

The brain microvascular endothelium has abundant transferrin receptor, which allows for receptor-mediated endocytosis of transferrin at the luminal membrane of the brain capillary endothelium. One model posits that the iron is released from the transferrin within the brain capillary endothelium and the apotransferrin undergoes retroendocytosis back to blood. This model, however, does not explain how iron undergoes exocytosis from the brain capillary endothelium, much less endocytosis into brain cells following the separation of the metal from circulating transferrin. The retroendocytosis model is based on the failure to observe immunoreactive transferrin receptor at the abluminal membrane using pre-embedding electron microscopic immunogold studies (Roberts et al., 1993). However, the studies of Vorbrodt (1989) show clearly that abluminal membrane receptors are not detectable with pre-embedding immunolabeling procedures, because only the luminal endothelial membrane is exposed to the antibodies with a pre-embedding protocol. It is necessary to perform post-embedding immunolabeling methods to visualize abluminal endothelial receptors. When transferrin transport across the brain microvascular endothelium is measured with internal carotid artery perfusion/capillary depletion methods or thaw mount autoradiography in the absence of the high concentrations of unlabeled transferrin in the circulation, then radiolabeled transferrin is observed to undergo rapid transport through the brain microvascular endothelium and to distribute into brain interstitial fluid in vivo (Fishman et al., 1987; Skarlatos et al., 1995).

(8) Neuropeptides are said to undergo transport through the BBB in vivo, because the brain volume distribution (V_D) exceeds the plasma space in brain (V_O) using internal carotid artery perfusion methods.

The brain V_D may exceed the brain V_O following carotid artery perfusion if the peptide is sequestered within the capillary endothelium. For example, the V_D of acetylated low density lipoprotein (LDL) exceeds the V_O in brain following a ten minute internal carotid artery perfusion, owing to receptor-mediated endocytosis of this ligand by the brain capillary endothelial scavenger receptor (Triguero et al., 1990). However, capillary depletion analysis shows that the acetylated LDL does not undergo exocytosis from the endothelium and does not enter into brain ISF.

The capillary depletion technique can only be used for ligands that are tightly bound by the brain microvasculature, which prevents dissociation of the ligand from the microvessels during the homogenization involved in the capillary depletion procedure. For example, the BBB penetration of an opioid peptide, which nonspecifically absorbs to the capillary vasculature following internal carotid artery perfusion, is overestimated with the capillary depletion technique owing to nonspecific dissociation from the microvessels during the homogenization (Samii et al. 1994). However, a post-perfusion wash procedure demonstrates the nonspecific absorption of the neuropeptide during carotid artery perfusion. In this case, the BBB permeability of the neuropeptide is greatly overestimated with the internal carotid artery perfusion technique compared to the permeability value measured with the single intravenous injection method.

(9) Neuropeptides are said to undergo transport through the BBB, because $V_D > V_O$ as measured with the single intravenous injection technique.

The intravenous injection of radiolabeled peptides leads in most cases to the rapid appearance in the circulation of radiolabeled amino acids, e.g. iodotyrosine, owing to the rapid peripheral degradation of the neuropeptide. The radiolabeled amino acid may then undergo carrier-mediated transport through the BBB and create a situation where the $V_D > V_O$. However, this does not mean there is effective transport of the peptide through the BBB, but rather the $V_D > V_O$ observation arises from peripheral metabolism. When the peripheral metabolism is blocked by attachment of polyethylene glycol (PEG) strands to the peptide, then the experimentally observed V_D in brain is not significantly different from the plasma volume (Sakane and Pardridge, 1997). In this setting, there has been no transport of the non-pegylated peptide across the BBB, and the brain V_D exceeds the brain V_O, owing to peripheral conversion of the radiolabeled peptide into radiolabeled amino acids.

(10) Blood–brain barrier transport may be studied in tissue culture using an 'in vitro BBB' model, because the brain capillary endothelial cells in culture form a tight barrier compared to cultured human umbilical vein endothelial cells

The electrical resistance in in vitro BBB models ranges from 50 to 500 Ω cm^2, and sometimes as high as 1000 Ω cm^2. However, this electrical resistance is still small compared to the electrical resistance across intra-parenchymal brain capillaries. The resistance across pial vessels, which are only partially supported by a glial limitans and which lack a fully developed BBB, is approximately $3000 \, \Omega \, cm^2$ (Butt and Jones, 1992). The resistance across intra-parenchymal brain capillaries is estimated to be of the order of $8000 \, \Omega \, cm^2$ (Smith and Rapoport, 1986). In addition to the loss in electrical resistance, there is a profound downregulation of gene expression of BBB nutrient transporters in capillary endothelial cells during primary culture. This leads to a marked underestimation of BBB permeability for those molecules or drugs that undergo carrier-mediated transport across the BBB *in vivo*. In addition, there is a substantial increase in the nonspecific paracellular and transcellular flux of solute across brain capillary endothelial cells grown in tissue culture. This leads to an overestimation of BBB permeability to drugs that undergo transport across the BBB via lipid-mediated transport *in vivo*. For example, octreotide undergoes negligible transport across the BBB *in vivo* (Pardridge *et al.*, 1990), but is relatively rapidly transported across the capillary endothelium in tissue culture. Confocal microscopy studies show that this transport of octreotide across the *in vitro* BBB is nonsaturable, and occurs only via the paracellular route (Jaehde *et al.*, 1994).

The above dialectics in BBB research illustrate the need for recognition of the advantages and disadvantages of different methodologies and techniques for studying the blood–brain barrier. Differences in interpretation can often times be avoided by a multidisciplinary approach, as opposed to reliance on single methodologies. A multidisciplinary approach can be constructed from the parallel use of the different methods shown in Fig. 1.1 and reviewed in the chapters of this book.

Role of blood–brain barrier research within the neurosciences

A puzzling phenomenon is that despite the importance of blood–brain barrier research to the overall neuroscience mission, there has been little integration of blood–brain barrier or brain microvascular research within the fundamental neuro-

sciences. This problem is visible from several vantage points. (i) The Introduction of a neuroscience treatise indicates the brain is comprised of two cells (neurons and glia) and the endothelium is only informally discussed in an appendix to this textbook (Kandel, *et al.*, 1991). (ii) The majority of neuroscience graduate students study doctorate courses with barely a single lecture on the BBB. (iii) Less than 0.5% of Society for Neuroscience abstracts are devoted to the BBB.

The causes for the relative underdevelopment of BBB research within the neurosciences are multiple but two factors seem primary. First, many neuroscientists maintain a persistent indifference to this area of the brain. This could ultimately have a negative impact on societal funding of molecular neuroscience research. The latter provides the platform for CNS new drug discovery, which is intended to yield societal benefit through alleviation of neurologic and mental disorders. However, few of the new drugs that emanate from the molecular neurosciences will undergo significant transport through the BBB, in the absence of a brain drug delivery strategy. Fundamental research in BBB transport processes provides the platform for CNS drug delivery and CNS drug targeting. It is no coincidence that >99% of worldwide CNS drug development is devoted solely to CNS drug discovery, and <1% is directed to CNS drug delivery. This imbalance between CNS drug discovery and CNS drug delivery can be directly linked to the imbalance in BBB research in the fundamental neurosciences. The second possible explanation for the relatively poor penetration of the neurosciences by BBB research is that the latter has been historically 'technique oriented'. Laboratories specialize in a single technique and fit multiple biological problems to this technique, as opposed to bringing multiple methodologies to bear on a single biological problem. The important questions pertaining to BBB biology (a partial list is given in Table 1.1) are too difficult to address with a single technique, but rather require a multidisciplinary approach that employs parallel use of several of the methodologies shown in Fig. 1.1.

The methodologies needed for examining almost any problem of BBB biology are presently available, and most of these are reviewed in this book. There has been much progress in recent years towards defining cellular and molecular paradigms of BBB transport processes, many of which are reviewed in the second half of this book. In any given problem, however, one senses that 'only the surface has been scratched'. This underdevelopment in many aspects of BBB research provides opportunities for young investigators in the neurosciences, and in pharmacology, physiology, or pathology. Young scientists in these fields may direct their efforts to BBB research and find an abundance of biological problems that both are crucial to the neuroscience mission and are historically underdeveloped.

Acknowledgments

This work was supported by NIH Grant NS-25554.

References

Aasmundstad, T. A., Morg, J. and Paulsen, R. E. (1995). Distribution of morphine 6-glucoronide and morphine across the blood–brain barrier in awake, freely moving rats investigated by in vivo microdialysis sampling. *J. Pharmacol. Exp. Ther.*, **275**, 435–41.

Bickel, U., Schumacher, O., Kang, Y. -S. and Voigt, K. (1996). Poor permeability of morphine-3-glucuronide and morphine-6-glucuronide through the blood–brain barrier in the rat. *J. Pharmacol. Exp. Ther.*, **278**, 107–13.

Boado, R. J. and Pardridge, W. M. (1994). Differential expression of α-actin mRNA and immunoreactive protein in brain microvascular pericytes and smooth muscle cells. *J. Neurosci. Res.*, **39**, 430–5.

Butt, A. M. and Jones, H. C. (1992). Effect of histamine and antagonists on electrical resistance across the blood–brain barrier in rat brain-surface microvessels. *Brain Res.*, **569**, 100–5.

Fishman, J. B., Rubin, J. B., Handrahan, J. V. *et al.* (1987). Receptor mediated transcytosis of transferrin across the blood–brain barrier. *J. Neurosci. Res.*, **18**, 299–304.

Jaehde, U., Masereeuw, R., De Boer, A. G. *et al.* (1994). Quantification and visualization of the transport of octreotide, a somatostatin analogue, across monolayers of cerebrovascular endothelial cells. *Pharmaceut. Res.*, **11**, 442–8.

Kandel, E. R. (1991). Brain and behavior. In *Principles of Neural Science*, 3rd edn, ed. E. R. Kandel, J. J. Schwartz, and T. M. Jessell, pp 5–17. NewYork: Elsevier.

Lasbennes, R. and Gayet, J. (1983). Capacity for energy metabolism in microvessels isolated from rat brain. *Neurochem. Res.*, **9**, 1–9.

Mollgard, K. and Saunders, N. R. (1975). Complex tight junctions of epithelial and of endothelial cells in early foetal brain. *J. Neurocytol.*, **4**, 453–68.

Morgan, M. E., Singhal, D. and Anderson, B. D. (1996). Quantitative assessment of blood–brain barrier damage during microdialysis. *J. Pharmacol. Exp. Ther.*, **277**, 1167–76.

Nehls, V. and Drenckhahn, D. (1991). Heterogeneity of microvascular pericytes for smooth muscle type alpha-actin. *J. Cell Biol.*, **113**, 147–54.

Pardridge, W. M., Yang, J., Buciak, J. and Tourtellotte, W. W. (1989). Human brain microvascular DR antigen. *J. Neurosci. Res.*, **23**, 337–41.

Pardridge, W. M., Triguero, D., Yang, J. and Cancilla, P. A. (1990). Comparison of *in vitro* and *in vivo* models of drug transcytosis through the blood–brain barrier. *J. Pharmacol. Exp. Ther.*, **253**, 884–91.

Pardridge, W. M., Golden, P. L., Kang, Y. -S. and Bickel, U. (1997). Brain microvascular and astrocyte localization of P-glycoprotein. *J. Neurochem.*, **68**, 1278–85.

Roberts, R. L., Fine, R. E. and Sandra, A. (1993). Receptor mediated endocytosis of transferrin at the blood–brain barrier. *J. Cell Sci.*, **104**, 521–32.

Sakane, T. and Pardridge, W. M. (1997). Carboxyl-directed pegylation of brain-derived neurotrophic factor markedly reduces systematic clearance with minimal loss of biological activity. *Pharamacol. Res.*, **14**, 1085–91.

Samii, A., Bickel, U., Stroth, U. and Pardridge, W. M. (1994). Blood–brain barrier transport of neuropeptides: analysis with a metabolically stable dermorphine analogue. *American Journal of Physiology*, **267**, E124–E131.

Skarlatos, S., Yoshikawa, T. and Pardridge, W. M. (1995). Transport of [125I] transferrin through the rat blood–brain barrier in vivo. *Brain Res.*, **683**, 164–71.

Smith, Q. R. and Rapoport, S. I. (1986). Cerebrovascular permeability coefficients to sodium, potassium and chloride. *J. Neurochem.*, **46**, 1732–42.

Stewart, P. A. and Wiley, M. J. (1981). Developing nervous tissue induces formation of blood–brain barrier characteristics in invading endothelial cells: a study using quail-chick transplantation chimera. *Dev. Biol.*, **84**, 183–92.

Triguero, D., Buciak, J. B. and Pardridge, W. M. (1990). Capillary depletion method for quantifying blood–brain barrier transcytosis of circulating peptides and plasma proteins. *J. Neurochem.*, **54**, 1882–8.

Vorbrodt, A. W. (1989). Ultracytochemical characterization of anionic sites in the wall of brain capillaries. *J. Neurocytol.*, **18**, 359–68.

Westergren, I., Nystrom, B., Hamberger, A. and Johansson, B. B. (1995). Intracerebral dialysis and the blood–brain barrier. *J. Neurochem.*, **64**, 229–34.

White, F. P., Dutton, G. R. and Norenberg, M. D. (1981). Microvessels isolated from rat brain: localization of astrocyte processes by immnohistochemical techniques. *J. Neurochem.*, **36**, 328–32.

Wu, D., Kang, Y. -S., Bickel, U. and Pardridge, W. M. (1997). Blood–brain barrier permeability to morphine-6-glucuronide is markedly reduced compared to morphine. *Drug Metab. Dirp.*, **25**, 768–71.

PART I
Methodology

2   The carotid artery single injection technique

EAIN M. CORNFORD

- Introduction
- Injection method
- ^{113m}Indium and its use in membrane transport studies
- ^{3}H-water and other reference isotopes
- Potential pitfalls in quantitation
- Substitute reference isotopic compounds
- Calculation of brain extraction
- Plasma-borne compounds as modifiers of BBB transport
- Contributions of BUI transport studies to the human
- Conclusions

Introduction

The most widely used single-arterial injection technique used for analysis of blood–brain barrier function is without doubt the Brain Uptake Index (BUI) method. This is a tissue-sampling, multiple isotope technique that was first described by Oldendorf (1970). Although widely applied to animal studies, the origins of the method may lie in the training that Bill Oldendorf received as a neurology resident at the University of Minnesota. A case of status epilepticus was not responding to even vigorous treatment and the serious consequences of this situation were being discussed. Dr Juhn Wada, a fellow resident, indicated that he could stop the seizures. Bill Oldendorf related that Dr Wada simply proceeded to inject barbiturate directly into the common carotid artery, and the seizures were arrested. Neurologists and neurosurgeons all know Juhn Wada for the test that bears his name, wherein a short-acting barbiturate is injected into the carotid artery of a conscious patient to determine the dominant cerebral hemi-

sphere. In current clinical practice, the intracarotid injection is achieved via a femoral catheter rather than direct needle puncture of the carotid artery. In the 1950s, neurology residents at Minnesota were trained in intracarotid angiography, and Bill Oldendorf had 15 years of clinical experience with this method and had performed the procedure more than 600 times without incident prior to the time the brain uptake index was developed for experimental studies in rats.

It is also appropriate to point out that the double-indicator method of Chinard *et al.* (1955) measured tissue extraction in an organ after intraarterial injection of a test substance together with a non-diffusible reference (such as Evans Blue or radiolabeled serum albumin). This indicator diffusion technique (Crone, 1963, 1965) was applied to brain in a series of studies, and the advantages of carotid arterial presentation had been previously recognized. Bill Oldendorf's personal interests in radiology and nuclear medicine, together with a sabbatical year with the late Dr Hugh Davson, no doubt were also contributing influences on the

Table 2.1. *Selected examples of the development, and some applications and adaptations of the brain uptake index method*

Date	Observation	Reference
1970	BBB uptake using ^3H water internal standard, intracarotid injection	Oldendorf, 1970
1970	Beta counting of ^{113m}In conversion electrons with ^3H and ^{14}C	Sisson *et al.*, 1970
1971	Se–methionine uptake in brain is studied in phenylketonurics	Oldendorf *et al.*, 1971
1971	Pulse-labeling brain lipids after intracarotid ^{14}C acetate	Dhopeshwarkar *et al.*, 1971
1972	↑ carbon atoms in monocarboxylic acids increases brain uptake	Oldendorf, 1972a
1972	BUIs of morphine, codeine, heroin and methadone show lipid solubility is a major determinant of brain uptake	Oldendorf *et al.*, 1972
1973	'Brain Uptake Index' (BUI%) is coined: uptake of ^{14}C-test substance is expressed relative to tritiated water	Oldendorf, 1973; 1974
1975	When CBF is known, BUI data provide BBB permeability (= *PS*) surface area measurements; *PS* is recognized as V_m/K_m ratio, and kinetic characterization of BBB nutrient transporters becomes routine.	Pardridge and Oldendorf, 1975
1975	Increased BBB uptake of ketone bodies in fasting	Gjedde and Crone, 1975
1975	Brain efflux measured after intracarotid injection	Bradbury *et al.*, 1975
1975	Adaptation to hepatic study, Liver Uptake Index (LUI)	Pardridge and Jefferson, 1975
1976	Brain Uptake Index with ^{113m}In-EDTA to correct for incomplete vascular washout of ^{14}C test	Oldendorf and Szabo, 1976
1976	Developmental changes in BUI	Cremer *et al.*, 1976
1976	Simultaneous dual carotid BUI injections for regional analyses	Pollay, 1976
1977	Albumin-bound tryptophan uptake via neutral amino acid carrier	Yuwiler *et al.*, 1977
1978	BUI performed in conscious, cannulated rats	Cornford *et al.*, 1978
1978	↑ BBB neutral amino acid uptake in experimental liver disease	James *et al.*, 1978
1979	Placental Transfer Uptake Index (PTUI) is developed	Bissonette *et al.*, 1979
1979	BBB thyroid hormone transporter is kinetically characterized	Pardridge, 1979
1979	Simultaneous blood flow (^{131}I-iodoantipyrine) and BUIs	Pollay and Stevens, 1979
1980	Liver Uptake Index nutrient transporters kinetically characterized	Cornford *et al.*, 1980
1980	BUI measurements in newborn BBB	Braun *et al.*, 1980
1981	Triple-isotope Tissue Uptake Index measures transfer *in vitro*	Cornford and Huot, 1981
1982	Brain glucose utilization rates measured after carotid injection	Oldendorf *et al.*, 1982
1982	Reduced testosterone transport to brain in cirrhotic serum is attributed to increased plasma SHBG levels	Sakiyama *et al.*, 1982
1983	Uterine Uptake Index (UUI)	Laufer *et al.*, 1983
1983	Enhanced dissociation and transport of orosomucoid-bound drugs	Pardridge *et al.*, 1983
1984	Albumin-bound ligand (testosterone) is shown to dissociate and be transported in a single transcapillary passage; enhanced dissociation mechanism of plasma-protein mediated transport	Pardridge and Landaw, 1984
1985	Demonstration of < 5% mixing of plasma with BUI bolus injection	Pardridge *et al.*, 1985
1985	Erythrocyte-borne drug dissociates and is transported at the BBB	Cornford and Landon, 1985
1985	*N*-isopropyl-*p*^{125}I-iodoamphetamine internal reference	Pardridge and Fierer, 1985
1985	Abluminal BBB active efflux mechanism shown by washout of ^{14}C valproate relative to tritiated water	Cornford *et al.*, 1985
1986	Intra-arterial measurements of salivary gland uptake index (SUI)	Cefalu *et al.*, 1986
1986	Globulin (CBG) does not restrict BBB corticosterone transport	Pardridge *et al.*, 1986
1986	Salivary and brain uptake of orosomucoid-borne drug compared	Terasaki *et al.*, 1986
1987	Intra-arterial measurements of Kidney Uptake Index (KUI)	Chaudhuri *et al.*, 1987

Table 2.1. (*cont.*)

Date	Observation	Reference
1987	Lymph Node Uptake Index (NUI)	Cefalu and Pardridge, 1987
1988	Testis Uptake Index (TUI) and Prostate Gland Uptake Index (PUI)	Sakiyama *et al.*, 1988
1990	Intra-arterial measurements of prostate gland metabolism	Ellison and Pardridge, 1990
1991	BUI adapted to cuttlefish and dogfish for analyses of glial barriers	Abbott, 1991
1992	Blood–tumor barrier and BBB transport compared in brain tumors	Cornford *et al.*, 1992
1995	BUI adapted to mouse for study of genetic models of disease	Cornford *et al.*, 1995

development of the brain uptake index technique for studying BBB transport phenomena. But Bill alone is responsible for the synthesis and development of the method (Oldendorf, 1970; 1972*a*, 1976, 1977, 1981) which has arguably contributed more to contemporary understanding of BBB nutrient transporters and brain capillary transfer phenomena than any other single technique. Development of the method is itemized in Table 2.1, along with some selected examples of its adaptations to illustrate the rich diversity in application of the technique.

Injection method

For the study of BBB transfer, a rat is rendered unresponsive with an anesthetic (such as intraperitoneal sodium pentobarbital, or ketamine and xylazine). It is placed in a supine position, the neck is shaved, and a small incision is made in the skin. The animal is positioned on a surgical board with traction hooks on all four extremities and the incisors, with the placement of the head in the opening of a Harvard Apparatus (Millus, MA) rat guillotine. The right common carotid artery is isolated by blunt dissection, and its sheath freed from the vagosympathetic trunk using a small length of #1 suture. The carotid artery is punctured with a sharp 27 gauge needle. The needle may be bent to an angle of 40–50° at a point 3–5 mm behind the sharp bevelled point. (This is easily accomplished with a small hemostat, but care must be exercised to avoid touching the sharpened bevel since the procedure is more difficult with a dull needle.) For washout studies (Bradbury *et al.*, 1975), where there may be an extended time period between

injection and decapitation, the carotid artery is usually punctured for injection directly through the carotid sheath; this requires greater surgical dexterity because the sheath may slip and move on the artery, but typically results in minimal bleeding through the injection puncture. Because the artery stretches slightly just before it is punctured, there is a tendency for the stretched vessel to recoil, and care must be taken to avoid having the needle point go rapidly through the arterial lumen and puncture the opposite wall. When the bent needle tip is placed parallel to the vessel lumen, the puncture of the arterial wall can be accomplished by picking up the edge of the vessel with the needle tip and moving it gently forward. Puncture of the arterial wall is rapid, and the vessel recoils backward resulting in the puncture point ending up at the bend of the needle, and the tip resting within the vessel lumen. It is also possible to inject both carotids simultaneously, for analyses of midbrain and cortical regions (Pollay, 1976) or tumor-implanted and control hemispheres (Cornford *et al.*, 1992), and BUIs have been performed in hamsters, mice, jirds, and even frogs.

The essence of the technique is outlined in Fig. 2.1. A mixture of radioisotopes is prepared in saline containing 10 mM HEPES buffer, tritiated water, a ^{14}C test substance, with or without ^{113m}In chelated to EDTA. The buffered saline injection solution typically contained 0.1–0.25 µCi of ^{14}C test isotope, about 1.0 µCi of ^{3}H-water and 5–20 µCi of ^{113m}In in a total volume of 1.0 ml. This isotopic mixture is divided into 3–4 different 1 cm^3 syringes, one syringe for each replicate animal studied. 0.2 ml of this mixture is rapidly injected (in about 0.25 s) into the carotid artery. The artery blanches momentarily as the injection

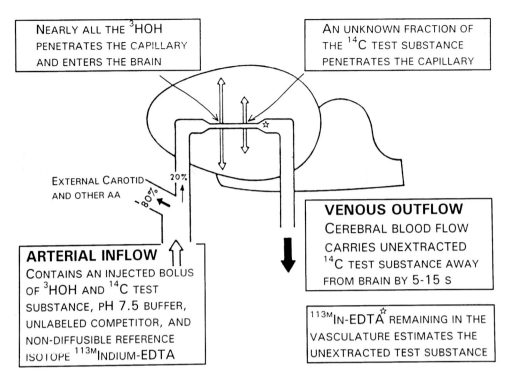

Fig. 2.1. The Brain Uptake Index method. Adapted from Oldendorf, 1976, 1977, 1981.

is made, and the needle is held in place in such a way as to permit carotid blood flow to continue past the puncture site unimpeded; this permits washout of unextracted isotopes from the brain vasculature.

Depending on the volume injected into the carotid, and the rate of the injection, a variable quantity of the isotopic mixture may reflux back down the artery. If this happens, some of the isotopic solution will be delivered down the right brachial artery, and the aortic arch (Oldendorf, 1981). The clearance of ^{35}S-selenomethionine did not differ significantly when variable injection volumes (0.05–5.0 ml) were employed, but studies with ^{141}Ce-labeled spheres indicate that relatively more of the injected bolus refluxes back to the aorta with larger injection volumes (Oldendorf, 1981). When intracarotid injections have been performed during carotid arterial blood flow monitoring (with an electromagnetic flow meter), we have observed that there is only a transient alteration in flow, and restoration to normal rates coincides with emptying the syringe. It has been shown that there is less than 5% mixing of the traditional

0.2 ml injected bolus with the plasma (Pardridge *et al.*, 1985). When the test isotope is a plasma component and its concentration is significantly lower than plasma, this mixing can produce a lowered estimate of brain uptake.

As the mixture traverses the capillary bed, the ^3HOH is highly extracted by the brain, and an unknown fraction of the ^{14}C test substance is extracted. When ^{113m}In is added to the injection mixture, it is chelated to EDTA (or it may be bound to plasma transferrin), and this isotope does not cross intact membranes. It has been shown that the transferrin-bound $^{113m}Indium$ macromolecule displays a penetrance and distribution similar to that of radio-iodinated serum albumin (Oldendorf, 1972). In the intracarotid injection method, this isotope is used to identify that fraction of the injected test isotope that remains in the vascular space. Although this is typically a very small quantity, it is measurably higher (and much more variable) in certain pathophysiological conditions. The developing rabbit brain has been shown to have a larger and more variable vascular space (Cornford *et al.*, 1982a), and indium correction was found to provide an added measure of precision in measuring penetration of low uptake compounds (Cornford and Oldendorf, 1975; Oldendorf and Szabo, 1976), in neonates (Braun *et al.*, 1980) and in analyses of experimental brain tumors (Cornford *et al.*, 1992).

Five seconds after the arterial injection, the rat is decapitated. In the original studies, this interval was 15 s, selected on the basis of clearance studies of ^{14}C-sucrose in conjunction with ^{3}H-water (Oldendorf, 1970). Subsequent analyses using indium-EDTA with ^{14}C-butanol indicated that reducing the interval from 15 to 5 s resulted in a reduced washout of test and reference substances. Passage of the injection bolus is essentially completed in 1–2 s, and arterial washout of the radiolabels from brain parenchyma begins (Oldendorf and Braun, 1976).

The brain is dissected free from the skull and the right cerebral hemisphere prepared for liquid scintillation counting. Dissection of different brain regions may be performed at this time, if desired. More rapid solubilization of the hemisphere can be effected by extruding the brain tissue through a 20-gauge needle into duplicate 1–2 ml aliquots of commercial solubilizer (Soluene, Packard Instruments, Downers Grove, IL). Tightly capped vials are then gently shaken for about 1 hour at about 55 °C, and when digestion is complete the vials are cooled to room temperature (to minimize possible evaporative loss of radiolabel), scintillation fluid is added, and the indium counting is performed without delay.

[113m]Indium and its use in membrane transport studies

Indium is a transition metal which, like iron, occurs in both divalent and trivalent forms. For many years this isotope was produced commercially and tin–indium generators were used clinically in pancreatic scanning. The [113]Sn parent isotope is absorbed onto a zirconium oxide matrix, and when a small volume of dilute HCl is passed over this matrix, the metastable [113m]In is eluted for laboratory use. Gamma rays produced by the indium nucleus account for about 65% of the radioactivity. The remainder of the activity

(~35%) comes from internal conversion electrons produced by the interaction of gamma rays with electrons in the k, l, and m shells. These high energy (365–392 Kev) internal conversion electrons are readily distinguishable from ^{3}H and ^{14}C beta emissions (<100 Kev), and so the activity of all three of these isotopes can be measured in a beta counter (Sisson *et al.*, 1970). Indium activity can be measured with nearly equal efficiency in a gamma or beta (scintillation) counter; the 65% gamma emissions are quantitated with 50% efficiency in a gamma counter, or the 35% conversion electrons are counted with almost 100% efficiency in a scintillation counter (Sisson *et al.*, 1970). Because [113m]In has a short half-life (~100 min), activity of this isotope must be determined without delay. [113m]In gamma activity in a brain sample can be measured prior to digestion (solubilization) of the tissue, if necessary. Routine ^{3}H and ^{14}C liquid scintillation spectrometry are typically performed 2–3 days later, after all of the indium activity has decayed (Oldendorf and Szabo, 1976).

Other workers have used a different indium chelate, [113m]In-DPTA, in intracarotid injection studies, and observed a similarity in vascular space identification (Pollay and Stevens, 1980). Alternatively, the vascular space volume may be measured using other non-penetrating isotopes such as sucrose, mannitol or dextran. Indium can be easily chelated by mixing 0.5 ml of the eluate from the generator with 1.0 mg of ethylene diamine tetracetic acid (EDTA), then neutralized with sodium bicarbonate for inclusion in the injection mixture. Alternatively, we have mixed 0.1 ml of the In–HCl eluate with 0.05 ml of human transferrin (100 mg/ml; Sigma Chemical, St Louis MO) and neutralized the mixture with 10 mM HEPES buffer. In our laboratory, *in vitro* column chromatography (Sephadex G-25–150) indicated that 93% of the radioactivity eluted in the transferrin-bound saline peak, with the remaining (background) radioactivity evenly distributed in the other 14 fractions. In the rat brain, EDTA-chelated indium uptake was $1.2 \pm 0.2\%$ ($n = 48$) compared to $0.9 \pm 0.1\%$ ($n = 20$) for transferrin bound indium. We have observed in other tissues the same molecular-weight dependent, reduced distribution of transferrin bound versus EDTA-chelated indium.

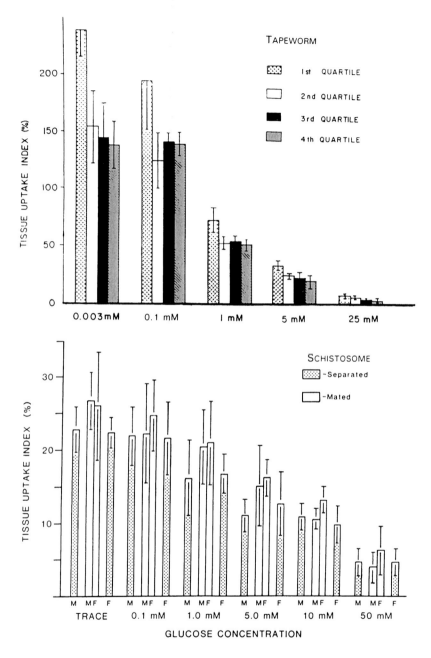

Fig. 2.2. Application of the Oldendorf triple isotope technique to *in vitro* analyses of glucose transport in parasitic helminths. In these invertebrates, the penetration of the tritiated-water-diffusible reference isotope is directly proportional to their mass. They also have amplified brush-border-like surface membranes through which nutrients are transported, and the inclusion of [113m]In-EDTA as a non-diffusible reference isotope estimates the proportion of nonextracted test (^{14}C-glucose) that passively adheres to the helminth surface membranes. Glucose transport in the blood-dwelling schistosome is via a GLUT1-like transporter, but the intestinal-dwelling tapeworm possesses an active, SGLT1-like transporter. Note that at low glucose concentrations, where incorporation of ^{14}C-glucose is maximal, the Tissue Uptake Indices are of the order of 30% in the schistosome; i.e. 30% of the rate of water diffusion, and similar to the glucose BUI at tracer concentrations (Oldendorf, 1981). In contrast, in

³H-water and other reference isotopes

Tritiated water has several advantages as a highly diffusible reference isotope. It is inexpensive, and not subject to radiolysis. Water is the biologically universal solute, ubiquitous and represents ~70% of the the total mass of most living cells and tissues. The original selection of ³H-water as a diffusible reference was supported by the report of Yudilevich and De Rose (1971) indicating that it was nearly completely cleared after a single transcapillary transit. Another advantage of the use of tritiated water as a high uptake reference isotope is that it readily identifies the so-called active transporters, as demonstrated in Fig. 2.2. In these *in vitro* Tissue Uptake Index studies, the schistosome parasite, which has a facilitative GLUT1-like glucose transporter (Skelly *et al.*, 1994) is shown to take up glucose maximally at about 30% of the rate at which water is taken up. In contrast, the intestinal-dwelling tapeworm must compete for glucose with the sodium-dependent, SGLT1 transporter of the intestinal epithelium; both intestine and tapeworm possess concentrative, or active glucose transporters. Note that at high glucose specific activity (low glucose concentrations) the uptake of glucose is 1–2 fold greater than that of water, as indicated by the Tissue Uptake Indices, which are in excess of 100%. This same concept was utilized to demonstrate active efflux of valproic acid in the rat blood–brain barrier abluminal surface (Cornford *et al.*, 1985), and this phenomenon has been recently confirmed using alternate methods (Adkinson *et al.*, 1994).

Potential pitfalls in quantitation

The brain extraction of water is reduced in non-anesthetized rat ($E = \sim 0.65$; and in the barbiturate-anesthetized mouse $E = \sim 0.73$), where higher cerebral blood flow rates are known. This means that brain water extraction (and CBF) must be defined for any altered physiological condition [such as fasting (Cornford *et al.*, 1993) or experimental diabetes (Cornford *et al.*, 1995)]. Brain Uptake Index measurements for non-electrolytes are highly correlated with lipid solubility, as shown in Fig. 2.3. Changes in the BUI of many of these compounds were seen in the neonatal blood–brain barrier. However, when the data are converted to estimates of permeability (changes that recognize the effects of altered cerebral blood flow and water extraction), the similarity in neonatal and adult lipid-mediated BBB transport is apparent (Cornford *et al.*, 1982*b*).

Other factors may also modify water transport, and their potential to influence BUI measurements must be recognized. Vasopressin activity is known to regulate water transport through the distal nephron (Gottschalk and Lassiter, 1979), and hormonal and noradrenergic effects on BBB water transport have been reported (Grubb *et al.*, 1978; Raichle and Grubb, 1978). Reid *et al.* (1983) have also demonstrated that dexamethasone decreases BBB water permeability and that estradiol increases barrier water transport.

Water transport through tissue capillaries occurs via two mechanisms: (a) filtration through large pores, and (b) diffusion through endothelial membranes. In erythrocytes, it is known that small, specific water pores exist for the (water diffusion) transport function (Solomon, 1968; Sha'afi and Feinstein, 1977). It has been postulated that a similar water pore may be found in BBB capillaries, and experimental data suggest that this putative specific water pore would have a radius of about 6 Å. The possibility that this pore could be subject to more subtle alterations in certain forms of brain injury has also been raised (Pardridge, 1983*b*).

Caption for Fig. 2.2 (*cont.*)
the tapeworm, the rate of ¹⁴C-glucose incorporation is two-fold greater than that of water (TUI ~200% at low substrate concentrations), indicating the presence of active concentration of glucose against a concentration gradient (from Cornford *et al.*, 1988 and Cornford, 1991). This concept was employed to demonstrate active efflux of valproic acid at the abluminal BBB capillary membrane (Cornford *et al.*, 1985), a phenomenon that was recently confirmed using other methods (Adkinson *et al.*, 1994).

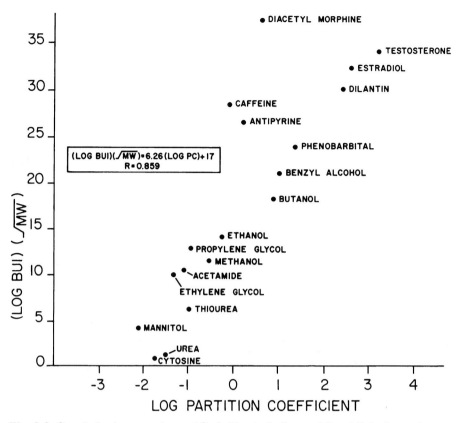

Fig. 2.3. Correlation between observed Brain Uptake Indices and lipophilicity (octanol:water partition coefficient) in the adult rat blood–brain barrier, from Cornford *et al.* (1982*b*). In a comparison of neonatal and adult brain transfer, it was demonstrated that some quantitative differences in BUI were attributable to changes in blood flow rates and differential extraction of the tritiated water reference compound in the neonate. There was no change in neonatal versus adult BBB lipid-mediated permeability.

Substitute reference isotopic compounds

Alternate diffusible reference compounds that have been employed in intra-arterial, single-injection brain uptake studies include ^{14}C-butanol (Oldendorf, 1981), iodinated amphetamine (Pardridge and Fierer, 1985), and diazepam (which is commercially available as either a ^{3}H or ^{14}C labeled product). Butanol is a useful diffusible reference when the only available test isotope is tritium-labeled. A disadvantage, however, is that it is not completely cleared (E = ~ 0.85 in the ketamine-anesthetized rat) and care must be observed to ensure that butanol is not lost to evaporation during heat-solubilization of brain tissue. Iodoamphet-

amine and diazepam offer the distinct advantage that they are both 100% extracted in a single brain capillary transit. These isotopes are thus not subject to altered extraction when pathophysiological events may induce marked changes in cerebral blood flow rates, or regional flow changes, which may occur in certain conditions. Iodoamphetamine has the disadvantage that the ^{125}I-iodinated isotopes have relatively short half-lives, and so there is a distinct cost disadvantage if these isotopes are to be used over an extended time period.

Diazepam is also completely extracted in the course of a single transit through brain capillaries (Takasato *et al.*, 1984), and for this reason it has become one of the more frequently used diffusible reference isotopes. The only disadvantage to using this compound is that it binds tenaciously to glass and plastic syringes, needles, tubing and containers. It is essential to ensure that binding is accounted for and that the concentration of isotopic diazepam reaching the brain vasculature is precisely determined, to ensure the precision of brain uptake and extraction measurements.

Oldendorf (1981) has also pointed out that for a more precise estimation of low-uptake test compounds, low-uptake diffusible reference materials present certain advantages. For example, comparisons of the extraction of a highly cleared diffusible reference and a low-extraction test compound are subject to experimental errors in regions of the brain that have markedly different blood flow rates. To measure low-uptake test compounds ^{14}C-thiourea (Cornford *et al.*, 1978*b*) and ^{3}H-tryptamine (Oldendorf and Braun, 1976) have been shown to provide relatively precise estimates of low-extraction test compounds. A disadvantage of tryptamine is that this basic compound is subject to pH-dependent changes in brain extraction.

Calculation of brain extraction

As originally described, the brain uptake index of a test compound was simply determined as the ratio of ^{14}C test compound/^{3}H reference in the brain, divided by the ^{14}C/^{3}H ratio in the injection mixture:

$$\text{Brain Uptake Index} = \text{BUI} = \frac{\left[\dfrac{\text{brain}^{14}\text{C}}{\text{brain}^3\text{H}}\right]}{\left[\dfrac{\text{injected}^{14}\text{C}}{\text{injected}^3\text{H}}\right]} \times 100\%$$

When indium correction was introduced, to quantitatively estimate the fraction of isotopic mixture that remained in the vascular compartment, the Brain Uptake Index was modified as follows:

$$\text{BUI} = \left\{ \frac{\dfrac{\text{brain}[^{14}\text{C}]}{\text{brain}[^3\text{H}]}}{\dfrac{\text{injected}[^{14}\text{C}]}{\text{injected}[^3\text{H}]}} - \frac{\dfrac{\text{brain}[^{113m}\text{In}]}{\text{brain}[^3\text{H}]}}{\dfrac{\text{injected}[^{113m}\text{In}]}{\text{injected}[^3\text{H}]}} \right\} \times 100\%$$

More simply, the BUI = $\{[E^{\text{test}} - E^{\text{Indium}}]/E^{\text{reference}}\}$ $\times 100\%$, where the test isotope is ^{14}C-labeled, and the reference isotope is ^{3}H-labeled.

Plasma-borne compounds as modifiers of BBB transport

The single arterial injection technique has been instrumental in providing estimates of the *in vivo* dissociation constant of a variety of plasma-protein bound ligands. These estimates are obtained from a comparison of the brain extractions of saline-borne versus albumin-borne ligands (Pardridge and Landaw, 1984). The *in vitro* dissociation constants are determined from *in vitro* dialysis determinations. For example, the anticonvulsant drug phenytoin is 90% bound to serum albumin in *in vitro* dialysis studies. If only the freely dialyzable fraction (10%) was available for BBB transport, then one would expect a 90% reduction of brain phenytoin extraction in the presence of serum versus saline. However saline borne phenytoin $E = 23\%$, and in the presence of serum one would predict $E = 2.3\%$, but the measured $E = 11\%$ for serum borne phenytoin (Cornford, 1984). Similar observations have been made for BBB transport of testosterone, where this steroid is 80–95% bound (measured by *in vitro* dialysis), but brain extraction of this steroid drops from only 85% (in saline) to (albumin-borne) $E = 75\%$ (Pardridge and Landaw, 1984). These results are attributed to predicted conformational changes in the albumin molecule during its transcapillary passage, which in turn result in enhanced dissociation of protein-bound ligands in the capillary milieu (Pardridge and Landaw, 1984; Pardridge, 1987). The fact that there is no albumin receptor present on BBB capillaries (Pardridge *et al.*, 1985*a*) further supports the concept of enhanced dissociation in the microvasculature. This tissue-mediated, enhanced dissociation of ligands from plasma proteins has been termed Protein Mediated Transport (Pardridge, 1987). It has been demonstrated for a large number of ligands, and it has recently been reviewed in detail (Pardridge, 1997).

Contributions of BUI transport studies to the human

It has been shown that the kinetic parameters derived for the rat BBB *in vivo* (Pardridge, 1983*a*) are consistent with neutral amino acid transporter characteristics determined in isolated human brain capillaries (Pardridge and Choi, 1986), and glucose transporter characteristics available from positron emission tomographic analyses of the half-saturation constant (Brooks *et al.*, 1986) and transporter maximal velocity (Feinendegen *et al.*, 1986). Furthermore, other analyses where serum from various clinical states is presented to the rat BBB *in vivo* (Fig. 2.4) provide compelling evidence that BBB transport of testosterone and estradiol is inversely related to steroid hormone binding globulin concentrations, which fluctuate in the various clinical conditions shown (Pardridge *et al.*, 1980), and in diseases such as cirrhosis (Sakiyama *et al.*, 1982).

Conclusions

The brain uptake index method is ideal for screening relative BBB permeabilities of different compounds. Optimal conditions for these studies are present when CBF is measured, the diffusible reference is completely (100%) extracted, and mixing of the bolus is controlled. Other advantages are that regional studies can be performed in a brain of any size; typically, no weighing is required; isotope usage is more efficient than in traditional intravenous studies; and the procedure is easy to perform and calculate (Oldendorf, 1981). The simplicity of this method has also contributed to its versatility. It has been successfully applied in tissues, organs and membrane systems (both *in vivo* and *in vitro*) far beyond the blood–brain barrier (Table 2.1), and these applications and uses will no doubt extend beyond the present decade of the brain.

Acknowledgments

I thank Leon Braun, Shigeyo Hyman, the late Bill Oldendorf, and Bill Pardridge for contributions to my understanding of blood–brain barrier permeability studies. Supported in part by NIH grant NS 25554.

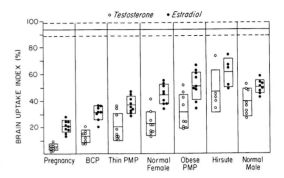

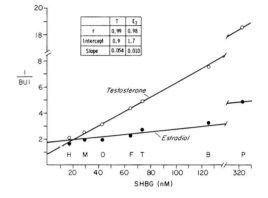

Fig. 2.4. Examples of the addition of human serum from different clinical states to the (rat) BUI injectate, as a predictor of altered human BBB steroid transport. Upper panel: the brain uptake index (BUI) for [^{3}H]-testosterone and [^{3}H]-estradiol relative to [^{14}C]-butanol is measured in the presence of serum (from 5–9 patients) in seven clinical conditions. Vertical rectangles describe mean ±SD, horizontal line depicts the mean BUI of saline-borne testosterone or estradiol. BCP, birth control pill-treated women; PMP, postmenopausal women.

Lower panel: the reciprocal of the testosterone (T) or estradiol (E$_2$) BUI is plotted as a function of the level of sex hormone binding globulin (SHBG) in the same human serum samples represented in the upper panel. P, pregnancy; B, birth control pills; T, thin postmenopausal female; F, normal follicular phase female; O, obese postmenopausal female; M, normal male; H, hirsute female. Linear regression data are shown in inset for both plots. Reproduced from Pardridge *et al.*, 1980; with permission.

References

Abbott, N. J. (1991). Permeability and transport of glial blood–brain barriers. *Ann. Acad. Sci.*, **633**, 378–94.

Adkinson, K. D., Artu, A. A., Powers, K. M. and Shen, D. D. (1994). Contribution of probenecid-sensitive anion transporters at the brain capillary endothelium and choroid plexus to the efficient efflux of valproic acid from the central nervous system. *J. Pharmacol. Exp. Ther.*, **268**, 797–805.

Bissonette, J. M., Cronan, J. Z., Richards, L. L. and Wickham, W. K. (1979). Placental transfer of water and nonelectrolytes during a single circulatory passage. *Am. J. Physiol.*, **236**, C47–C52.

Bradbury, M., Patlak, C. S. and Oldendorf, W. H. (1975). Analysis of brain uptake and loss of radiotracers after intracarotid injection. *Am. J. Physiol.*, **230**, 94–8.

Braun, L. D., Cornford, E. M. and Oldendorf, W. H. (1980). Newborn rabbit blood–brain barrier is selectively permeable and differs substantially from the adult. *J. Neurochem.*, **34**, 147–52.

Brooks, D. J., Gibbs, J. S. R., Sharp, P. *et al.* (1986). Regional cerebral glucose transport in insulin-dependent diabetic patients studies using [¹¹C]3-*O*-methyl-D-glucose and positron emission tomography. *J. Cereb. Blood Flow Metab.*, **6**, 240–4.

Cefalu, W. T. and Pardridge, W. M. (1987). Augmented transport and metabolism of sex steroids in lymphoid neoplasia in the rat. *Endocrinology*, **120**, 1000–9.

Cefalu, W. T., Pardridge, W. M., Chaudhuri, G. and Judd, H. L. (1986). Serum bioavailability and tissue metabolism of testosterone and estradiol in rat salivary gland. *J. Clin. Endocrinol. Metab.*, **63**, 20–8.

Chaudhuri, G., Verheugen, C., Pardridge, W. M. and Judd, H. L. (1987) Selective availability of estrogen and estrogen conjugates to the rat kidney. *J. Endocrinol. Invest.*, **10**, 283–90.

Chinard F. P., Vosburgh, C. J. and Enns, T. (1955). Transcapillary exchange of water and other substances in certain organs of the dog. *Am. J. Physiol.*, **183**, 221–34.

Cornford, E. M. (1984). Blood brain barrier permeability to anticonvulsant drugs. In *Workshop on the Metabolism of Antiepileptic Drugs*, ed R. H. Levy, pp. 129–42. New York: Raven Press.

Cornford, E. M. (1991). Regional modulations in glucose transporter kinetics in the rat tapeworm. *Exp. Parasitol.*, **73**, 489–99.

Cornford, E. M. and Huot, M. E. (1981). Glucose transfer from male to female schistosomes. *Science*, **213**, 1269–71.

Cornford, E. M. and Landon, K. P. (1985). Blood–brain barrier transport of CI-912: single passage equilibration of erythrocyte-borne drug. *Ther. Drug Monit.*, **7**, 247–54.

Cornford, E. M. and Oldendorf, W. H. (1975). Independent blood–brain barrier transport systems for nucleic acid precursors. *Biochim. et Biophys. Acta*, **394**, 211–19.

Cornford, E. M., Braun L. D. and Oldendorf, W. H. (1978*a*). Carrier mediated blood–brain barrier transport of choline and certain choline analogs. *J. Neurochem.*, **30**, 299–308.

Cornford, E. M., Braun L. D. and Oldendorf, W. H. (1978*b*). Blood–brain barrier restriction of peptides and the low uptake of enkephalins. *Endocrinology*, **103**, 1297–303.

Cornford, E. M., Braun, L. D., Pardridge, W. M. and Oldendorf, W. H. (1980). Blood flow rate and cellular influx of glucose and arginine in mouse liver in vivo. *Am. J. Physiol.*, **238**, H553–H560.

Cornford, E. M., Braun, L. D. and Oldendorf, W. H. (1982*a*). Developmental modulations of blood–brain barrier permeability as an indicator of changing nutritional requirements in the brain. *Ped. Res.*, **16**, 324–8.

Cornford, E. M., Braun, L. D., Oldendorf, W. H. and Hill, M. A. (1982*b*). Comparison of lipid-mediated blood–brain barrier penetrability in neonates and adults. *Am. J. Physiol.*, **243**, C161–C168.

Cornford, E. M., Diep, C. P. and Pardridge, W. M. (1985). Blood–brain barrier transport of valproic acid. *J. Neurochem.*, **44**, 1541–50.

Cornford, E. M., Fitzpatrick, A. M., Quirk, T. L. *et al.* (1988). Tegumental glucose permeability in male and female *Schistosoma mansoni*. *J. Parasitol.*, **74**, 116–28.

Cornford, E. M., Young, D., Paxton, J. W. *et al.* (1992). Melphalan penetration of the blood–brain barrier via the neutral amino acid transporter in tumor bearing brain. *Cancer Res.*, **52**, 138–43.

Cornford, E. M., Young, D., Paxton, J. W. *et al.* (1993). Characterization of blood–brain barrier glucose transport in the fasting mouse. *Neurochem. Res.*, **18**, 591–7.

Cornford, E. M., Hyman, S., Cornford, M. E. and Clare-Salzler, M. (1995). Down-regulation of blood–brain glucose transport in the hyperglycemic nonobese diabetic mouse. *Neurochem. Res.*, **20**(7), 869–73.

Cremer, J. E., Braun, L. D. and Oldendorf, W. H. (1976). Changes during development in transport processes of the blood–brain barrier. *Biochim. Biophys. Acta*, **488**, 633–7.

Crone, C. (1963). The permeability of capillaries in various organs as determined by the use of the 'Indicator diffusion' method. *Acta Physiol. Scand.*, **58**, 292–305.

Crone, C. (1965). Facilitated transfer of glucose from blood into brain tissue. *J. Physiol. (Lond.)*, **181**, 103–13.

Dhopeshwarkar, G. A., Subramanian, C. and Mead J. F. (1971). Rapid uptake of [1-¹⁴C] acetate by the rat brain 15 seconds after carotid injection. *Biochim. Biophys. Acta*, **248**, 41–7.

Ellison, S. A. and Pardridge, W. M. (1990). Reduction of testosterone availability to 5α-reductase by human sex hormone-binding globulin in the rat ventral prostate gland in vivo. *The Prostate*, **17**, 281–91.

Feinendegen, L. E., Herzog, H., Wieler, H. *et al.* (1986). Glucose transport in the human brain: model using carbon-11 methylglucose and positron emission tomography. *J. Nucl. Med.*, **27**, 1867–77.

Gjedde, A. and Crone, C. (1975). Induction processes in blood–brain transfer of ketone bodies during starvation. *Am. J. Physiol.*, **225**, 1165–9.

Gottschalk C. W. and Lassiter, W. E. (1979). Transport of water: renal concentrating mechanism. In *Membrane transport and biology*, ed. G. Giebisch, D. C. Tosteson and H. Hussing, Vol. IVA, pp. 449–71. New York: Springer-Verlag.

Grubb, R. L., Raichle, M. E. and Eichling, J. O. (1978). Peripheral sympathetic regulation of brain water permeability. *Brain Res.*, **144**, 204–7.

James, J. H., Escourrou, J. and Fischer, J. E. (1978). Blood–brain neutral amino acid transport activity is increased after portacaval anastomosis. *Science*, **200**, 1395–8.

Laufer, L. R., Gambone, J. C., Chaudhuri, G. *et al.* (1983). The effect of membrane permeability and binding by human serum proteins on sex steroid influx into the uterus. *J. Clin. Endocrinol. Metabol.*, **57**, 160–5.

Oldendorf, W. H. (1970). Measurement of brain uptake of radiolabeled substances using a tritiated water internal standard. *Brain Res.*, **24**, 372–6.

Oldendorf, W. H. (1972a). Blood–brain barrier permeability to lactate. *Eur. Neurol.*, **6**, 49–55.

Oldendorf, W. H. (1972b). Distribution of various classes of radiolabeled tracers in plasma, scalp, and brain. *J. Nucl. Med.*, **13**, 681–5.

Oldendorf, W. H. (1973). Stereo-specificity of blood–brain barrier permeability of amino acids. *Am. J. Physiol.*, **224**, 967–9.

Oldendorf, W. H. (1974). Lipid solubility and drug penetration of the blood brain barrier. *Proc. Soc. Exp. Biol. Med.*, **147**, 813–16.

Oldendorf, W. H. (1976). The blood–brain barrier. In *Brain Metabolism and Clinical Disorders*, 2nd edn, ed. H. E. Himwich, pp. 163–80. New York: Spectrum Publications.

Oldendorf, W. H. (1977). The blood–brain barrier. In *The Ocular and Cerebral Spinal Fluids*, ed. L. Z. Bito, H. Davson and J. D. Fenstermacher. *Experimental Eye Research (Suppl.)*, pp. 177–90.

Oldendorf, W. H. (1981). Clearance of radiolabeled substances by brain after arterial injection using a diffusible internal standard. In *Research Methods in Neurochemistry*, ed N. Marks and R. Rodnight, pp. 91–112. New York: Plenum Publishing.

Oldendorf, W. H. and Braun, L. D. (1976). [^{3}H]-Tryptamine and [^{3}H]-water as diffusible internal standards for measuring brain extraction of radiolabeled substances following carotid injection. *Brain Res.*, **113**, 218–24.

Oldendorf, W. H. and Szabo, J. (1976). Amino acid assignment to one of three blood–brain barrier amino acid carriers. *Am. J. Physiol.*, **230**, 94–8.

Oldendorf, W. H., Sisson, W. B. and Silverstein, A. (1971). Reduced brain uptake of selenomethionine Se-75 in phenylketonuria. *Arch. Neurol.*, **24**, 524–8.

Oldendorf, W. H., Hyman, S. H., Braun, L. D. and Oldendorf, S. Z. (1972). Blood–brain barrier: penetration of morphine, codeine, heroin and methadone after intracarotid injection. *Science*, **178**, 984–6.

Oldendorf, W. H., Pardridge, W. M., Braun, L. D. and Crane P. D. (1982). Measurement of cerebral glucose utilization using washout after intracarotid injection. *J. Neurochem.*, **38**, 1413–18.

Pardridge, W. M. (1979). Carrier mediated transport of thyroid hormones through the rat blood–brain barrier: primary role of albumin bound hormone. *Endocrinology*, **105**, 605–12.

Pardridge, W. M. (1983a). Brain metabolism: A perspective from the blood–brain barrier. *Physiol. Rev.*, **63**, 1481–535.

Pardridge, W. M. (1983b). Cerebral vascular permeability status in brain injury. In *Central Nervous System Trauma Status Report*, pp. 503–12.

Pardridge, W. M. (1987). Plasma protein mediated transport of steroid and thyroid hormones. *Am. J. Physiol.*, **252**, E157–E164.

Pardridge, W. M. (1998). Targeted delivery of hormones to tissues by plasma proteins. In *Handbook of Physiology*, vol. I, ed. P. M. Conn. New York: Oxford University Press.

Pardridge, W. M. and Choi, T. B. (1986). Neutral amino acid transport at the human blood–brain barrier. *Fed. Proc.*, **45**, 2073–8.

Pardridge, W. M. and Fierer, G. (1985). Blood–brain barrier transport of butanol and water relative to *N*-isopropyl-p-[^{125}I]iodoamphetamine as the internal reference. *J. Cereb. Blood Flow Metab.*, **5**, 275–81.

Pardridge, W. M. and Jefferson (1975). Liver uptake of amino acids and carbohydrates during a single circulatory passage. *Am. J. Physiol.*, **228**, 1155–61.

Pardridge, W. M. and Landaw, E. M. (1984). Tracer kinetic model of blood–brain barrier transport of plasma protein bound ligands. *J. Clin. Invest.*, **74**, 745–52.

Pardridge, W. M., and Oldendorf, W. H. (1975). Kinetics of blood–brain barrier transport of hexoses. *Biochim. Biophys. Acta*, **382**, 377–92.

Pardridge, W. M., Mietus, L. J., Frumar, A. M. *et al.* (1980). Effects of human serum on transport of testosterone and estradiol in rat brain. *Am. J. Physiol.*, **239**, E103–E108.

Pardridge, W. M., Sakiyama, R. and Fierer, G. (1983). Transport of propranolol and lidocaine through the rat blood–brain barrier. *J. Clin. Invest.*, **71**, 900–8.

Pardridge, W. M., Eisenberg, J., and Cefalu, W. T. (1985a). Absence of albumin receptor on brain capillaries in vivo or in vitro. *Am. J. Physiol.*, **249**, E264–E267.

Pardridge, W. M., Landaw, E. M., Miller, L. P. *et al.* (1985b). Carotid artery injection technique: Bounds for mixing by plasma and by brain. *J. Cereb. Blood Flow Metab.*, **5**, 576–83.

Pardridge, W. M., Eisenberg, J., Fierer, G. and Kuhn R. W. (1986). CBG does not restrict blood–brain barrier corticosterone transport in rabbits. *Am. J. Physiol.*, **251**, E204–E208.

Pollay, M. (1976). Regional transport of phenylalanine across the blood–brain barrier. *J. Neurosci. Res.*, **2**, 11–19.

Pollay, M. and Stevens, A. (1979). Simultaneous measurement of regional blood flow and glucose extraction in rat brain. *Neurochem. Res.*, **4**, 109–23.

Pollay, M. and Stevens, A. (1980). Blood–brain barrier restoration following cold injury. *Neurol. Res.*, **1**, 239–45.

Raichle, M. E. and Grubb, R. L. (1978). Regulation of brain water permeability by centrally-released vasopressin. *Brain Res.*, **143**, 191–4.

Reid, A. C., Teasdale, G. M. and McCullough, J. (1983). The effects of dexamethasone administration and withdrawal on water permeability across the blood–brain barrier. *Ann. Neurol.*, **13**, 28–31.

Sakiyama, R., Pardridge, W. M. and Judd, H. L. (1982). Effects of human cirrhotic serum on estradiol and testosterone transport into rat brain. *J. Clin. Endocrinol. and Metab.*, **54**, 1140–4.

Sakiyama, R., Pardridge, W. M. and Musto, N. A. (1988). Influx of testosterone-binding globulin (TeBG) and TeBG-bound sex steroid hormones into rat testis and prostate. *J. Clin. Endocrinol. and Metab.*, **67**, 98–103.

Sha'afi, R. I. and Feinstein M. B. (1977). Membrane water channels and SH-groups. *Adv. Exp. Biol. Med.*, **84**, 67–83.

Skelly, P. J., Kim, J. W., Cunningham, J. and Shoemaker, C. B. (1994). Cloning, characterization and functional expression of cDNAs encoding glucose transporter proteins from the human parasite *Schistosoma mansoni*. *J. Biol. Chem.*, **269**, 4247–93.

Sisson, W. B., Oldendorf, W. H. and Cassen, B. (1970). Liquid scintillation counting of ^{113m}In conversion electrons in the presence of ^{3}H and ^{14}C. *J. Nucl. Med.*, **11**, 749–52.

Solomon, A. K. (1968). Characterization of biological membranes by equivalent pores. *J. Gen. Physiol.*, **51**, 335–64.

Takasato, Y., Rapoport, S. I. and Smith, Q. R. (1984). An in situ brain perfusion technique to study cerebrovascular transport in the rat. *Am. J. Physiol.*, **247**, H484–H493.

Terasaki, T., Pardridge, W. M. and Denson, D. D. (1986). Differential effect of plasma protein binding of bupivacaine on its *in vivo* transfer into brain and salivary gland of rats. *J. Pharmacol. Exp. Ther.*, **239**, 724–9.

Yudilevich, D. L. and De Rose, N. (1971). Blood–brain transfer of glucose and other molecules measured by rapid indicator dilution. *Am. J. Physiol.*, **220**, 841–6.

Yuwiler, A., Oldendorf, W. H., Geller, E. and Braun, L. (1977). Effect of albumin binding and amino acid competition on tryptophan uptake into brain. *J. Neurochem.*, **28**, 1015–23.

3 Development of Brain Efflux Index (BEI) method and its application to the blood–brain barrier efflux transport study

TETSUYA TERASAKI

- Introduction
- Theory
- Methods
- Development
- BBB efflux transport system

Introduction

Brain interstitial fluid concentration of drugs and/or nutrients, a significantly important value for the central nervous system (CNS) effects and/or the cerebral functions, is believed to be mainly governed by the net flux between the brain interstitial fluid and the circulating blood in the brain capillaries across the blood–brain barrier (BBB). Although several influx transport systems at the BBB have been characterized (Pardridge and Oldendorf, 1977; Pardridge, 1983; Smith *et al.*, 1987; Terasaki *et al.*, 1991), only a limited amount of information appears to be available on the transport process from the brain interstitial fluid to the circulating blood at the BBB (Betz and Goldstein, 1978; Oldendorf *et al.*, 1982; Barrera *et al.*, 1991; Banks *et al.*, 1993), i.e. the BBB efflux transport process. For an understanding of the physiological function of the BBB, presumably as a regulating machinery of brain interstitial fluid constituents balance including nutrients, neurotransmitters and its metabolites, it is significantly important to clarify the efflux transport process across the BBB. Moreover, it would also be helpful for the development of the CNS-acting drugs to characterize the drug efflux transport process from the brain, while most studies have been focused on the influx process from the circu-

lating blood to the brain. The purpose of this chapter is to describe the Brain Efflux Index (BEI) method, a newly developed method to determine the *in vivo* efflux transport clearance across the BBB (Kakee *et al.*, 1996). Moreover, employing the BEI method, several new findings for the BBB efflux transport systems have been obtained and are also described in this chapter (Kakee, *et al.* 1995, Takasawa *et al.*, 1997, Kitazawa *et al.*, 1996).

Theory

Definition of the Brain Efflux Index (BEI)

Figure 3.1 represents the principle of the Brain Efflux Index (BEI) method. The BEI value was defined as the relative percentage of test compound effluxed from the ipsilateral cerebrum to the circulating blood across the BBB compared with the amount of test compound injected into the cerebrum, i.e.

$$BEI(\%) = \frac{\text{Amount of test compound effluxed at the BBB}}{\text{Amount of test compound injected into the brain}} \times 100 \quad (3.1)$$

As the amount of test compound effluxed from

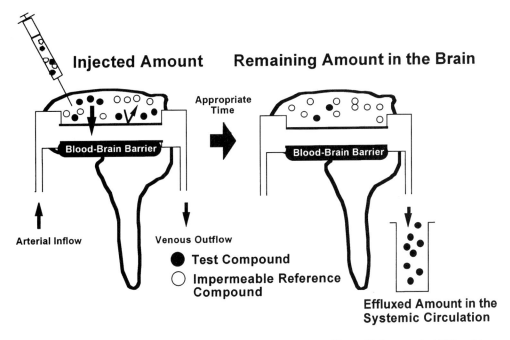

Fig. 3.1. Schematic diagram of brain efflux index (BEI) method. (From Kakee *et al.*, 1996, with permission.)

the brain is equal to the amount of injected test compound minus the test compound remaining in the ipsilateral cerebrum, Eqn (3.1) can be rearranged to,

$$\text{BEI(\%)} = \frac{\begin{array}{c}\text{Amount of}\\ \text{test compound}\\ \text{injected into}\\ \text{the brain}\end{array} - \begin{array}{c}\text{Amount of}\\ \text{test compound}\\ \text{remaining}\\ \text{in the brain}\end{array}}{\begin{array}{c}\text{Amount of test compound}\\ \text{injected into the brain}\end{array}} \times 100 \quad (3.2)$$

To determine the amount of test compound injected, a reference compound that does not cross the BBB was simultaneously administered into the cerebrum. Hence, the BEI value of test compound was obtained from the following equation.

$$\text{BEI(\%)} = \left(1 - \frac{\begin{array}{c}\text{Remaining}\\ \text{amount}\\ \text{of test}\\ \text{compound}\\ \text{in the brain}\end{array} \Big/ \begin{array}{c}\text{Remaining}\\ \text{amount of}\\ \text{reference}\\ \text{compound}\\ \text{in the brain}\end{array}}{\begin{array}{c}\text{Injected}\\ \text{amount}\\ \text{of test}\\ \text{compound}\end{array} \Big/ \begin{array}{c}\text{Injected}\\ \text{amount of}\\ \text{reference}\\ \text{compound}\end{array}}\right) \times 100 \quad (3.3)$$

Apparent efflux rate constant (K_{eff}) and the apparent efflux clearance ($CL_{\text{eff,BBB}}$) at the BBB

As the percentage test compound remaining $(100 - \text{BEI})$ in the ipsilateral cerebrum is described as

$$100 - \text{BEI(\%)} = \frac{\begin{array}{c}\text{Remaining}\\ \text{amount}\\ \text{of test}\\ \text{compound}\\ \text{in the brain}\end{array} \Big/ \begin{array}{c}\text{Remaining}\\ \text{amount of}\\ \text{reference}\\ \text{compound}\\ \text{in the brain}\end{array}}{\begin{array}{c}\text{Concentration}\\ \text{of test}\\ \text{compound in}\\ \text{injectate}\end{array} \Big/ \begin{array}{c}\text{Concentration}\\ \text{of reference}\\ \text{compound in}\\ \text{injectate}\end{array}} \times 100 \quad (3.4)$$

the apparent efflux rate constant of test compound from the brain, K_{eff}, can be obtained by the nonlinear regression analysis of a semilogarithmic plot of the percentage test compound remaining, i.e. $(100 - \text{BEI})$, versus time. Multiplying the apparent efflux rate constant, K_{eff}, by the distribution volume of the test compound in the brain, V_{br}, the apparent efflux clearance at the BBB, $CL_{\text{eff,BBB}}$, is obtained as follows;

$$CL_{\text{eff,BBB}} = K_{\text{eff}} V_{\text{br}} \quad (3.5)$$

25

Methods

Intracerebral microinjection

A mixture of test and reference compounds was injected into the brain as follows. Rats were anesthetized and placed in a stereotaxic frame. A small hole was drilled at the targeted region of the left cerebrum to allow entry of an injection needle and then an aliquiot of 0.2 or 0.5 µl of the ECF buffer (122 mM NaCl, 25 mM NaHCO$_3$, 10 mM D-glucose, 3 mM KCl, 1.4 mM CaCl$_2$, 1.2 mM MgSO$_4$, 0.4 mM K$_2$HPO$_4$ and 10 mM HEPES, pH 7.4) containing both the test and reference compounds was injected for 1 s via a 5 µl microsyringe fitted with a needle 330 mm in diameter. The craniometric data and the precise localization of the regions to be injected were determined with a stereotaxic atlas (Paxinos and Watson, 1986). The cerebral regions examined were as follows: 0.2 mm anterior and 5.5 mm lateral to the bregma and 4.5 mm deep as measured from the surface of the skull, called the parietal cortex area2 (Par2), 3.3 mm posterior and 2.0 mm lateral to the bregma and 1.5 mm deep, called the frontal cortex area1 (Fr1), 3.3 mm posterior and 2.0 mm lateral to the bregma and 3.0 mm deep, called the hippocampal fissure (HiF), 5.6 mm posterior and 5.0 mm lateral to the bregma and 2.5 mm deep, called the entorhinal cortex (Ent), 5.6 mm posterior and 5.0 mm lateral to the bregma and 5.0 mm deep, called the Field CA2 of Ammon's horn (CA2). After microinjection into the cerebrum, the remaining amount of test and reference compounds in the ipsilateral and contralateral cerebrum and cerebellum and CSF were determined.

Distribution volume in the brain (V_{br})

The distribution volume in the brain, V_{br}, was determined by *in vitro* brain slice uptake experiments. Brain slices were prepared as reported previously with minor modification (Newman *et al.*, 1991). After pre-incubation of a hypothalamic slice 300 µm thick of rat cerebrum for 5 min at 37 °C, the brain slice was transferred to oxygenated incubation medium containing test compound or [^{14}C]inulin as an adsorbed water volume marker. The apparent steady-state slice to medium concentration ratio of test compound was determined and

the apparent zero-time intercept of the [^{14}C]inulin uptake time-profile, i.e. 0.125±0.013 ml/g slice (the mean±S.E., $n=9$) was subtracted as an adsorbed water volume.

Development

In order to validate the BEI method, the following criteria have been assessed: (1) apparent efflux clearance of test compound selectively reflects the efflux transport process across the BBB, but not via a blood–cerebrospinal fluid barrier (BCSFB); (2) reference compound is not eliminated from the brain for a certain period of time examined; (3) intracerebral microinjection causes only slight disruption to the BBB; (4) maximum apparent efflux rate can be predicted for the substrate to be transported by the blood flow limited process; (5) apparent efflux process characterized for the substrate that is transported by the facilitated transport system reflects that predicted from the influx process at the BBB, i.e. a positive control study as a symmetrical and carrier-mediated transport process across the BBB.

The recovery of [^{14}C]inulin, a reference compound for the BEI method, was determined for the ipsilateral cerebrum, contralateral cerebrum, cerebellum and CSF after 0.2 µl microinjection into Par2, Fr1, HiF, Ent and CA2. Only 1.9% of the [^{14}C]inulin was found in the CSF at 20 min after microinjection into the Par2 region, whereas 12 to 57% was found in the CSF after microinjection into the CA2, Ent, HiF and Fr1 regions. Moreover, less than 1% was found in the contralateral cerebrum and cerebellum in the case of the Par2 region, which was significantly lower than for the CA2, Ent, HiF and Fr1 regions. No significant decrease was observed for the recovery of [^{14}C]-inulin in the ipsilateral cerebrum with increasing time up to 20 min after microinjection into Par2. These results demonstrate that microinjection of [^{14}C]inulin into Par2 meets the above criteria of (1) and (2).

Moreover, no significant difference between the ipsilateral and contralateral cerebrum was observed for the apparent influx clearance of [^{14}C]inulin across the BBB and its apparent zero time distribution volume after microinjection into Par2, indicating that the BEI method also meets the criterion of (3).

In the case of substrates that exhibit extensive permeability through the BBB, the efflux from the brain to the systemic circulation is considered to follow cerebral blood flow rate-limited elimination. As the extraction ratio of $[^3H]H_2O$ from the circulating blood to the brain was reported to be 55% (Pardridge and Fierer, 1985), the efflux process of $[^3H]H_2O$ from the brain was also analyzed employing the BEI method. Constructing a physiological pharmacokinetic model in the brain and assuming that the intrinsic BBB efflux clearance is the same as that of the influx process, the time course of the remaining percentage of $[^3H]H_2O$ in the ipsilateral cerebrum following a microinjection into Par2 was predicted. As shown in Fig. 3.2, there was significant coincidence between the observed and predicted values. However, no significant elimination of $[^3H]H_2O$ was observed for the ipsilateral cerebrum after microinjection into a hemisphere in the sacrificed rats, i.e. when the cerebral blood flow rate is zero. These results demonstrate that the BEI method meets the criterion (4).

The hexose transport system is known to exhibit the greatest V_{max} value among nutrient transport systems located at the BBB (Pardridge, 1983), and has been demonstrated as Na^+-independent GLUT-1 (Takakura *et al.*, 1991; Boado and Pardridge, 1993, 1994; Boado *et al.*, 1994). Moreover, employing a brain washout method, the hexose transport system has been suggested to exhibit symmetrical transport (Oldendorf *et al.*, 1982). Figure 3.3 shows the time-profile of the remaining percentage of $[^3H]3OMG$ (^3H-3-*O*-methyl-D-glucose) in the ipsilateral cerebrum. Apparent efflux rate constant of $[^3H]3OMG$, K_{eff}, was found to be 0.129 ± 0.014 min^{-1}. Performing the brain slice uptake study, the cerebral distribution volume of 3OMG was determined to be 0.788 ± 0.008 ml/g brain, indicating no significant binding of 3OMG in the brain parenchymal tissues. No significant difference was observed between the apparent efflux clearance of 3OMG (101.7 ± 16.0 μl/min/g brain) and the influx clearance determined by the Brain Uptake Index (BUI) method (Oldendorf, 1970 and also see Chapter 2) (92.6 ± 13.6 μl/min/g brain). Moreover, no significant efflux was observed for $[^3H]$L-glucose, a stereoisomer of D-glucose, in

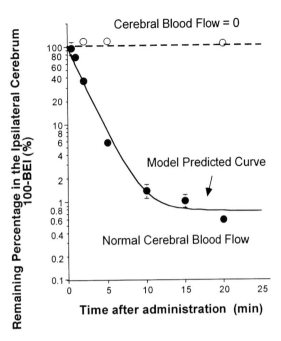

Fig. 3.2. Time-courses of $[^3H]H_2O$ in the ipsilateral cerebrum after intracerebral microinjection in normal or sacrificed rats in the presence of $[^{14}C]$inulin as an internal reference. $[^3H]H_2O$ (2 μCi) and $[^{14}C]$inulin (0.1 μCi) dissolved in 0.2 μl ECF buffer were injected intracerebrally to normal male or sacrificed Sprague-Dawley rats. Rats were decapitated at 0.5, 1, 2, 5, 10, 15 and 20 min after administration. The radioactivity of the ipsilateral cerebrum was measured using a scintillation counter. Closed and open circles represent the time-courses of (100-BEI) values for $[^3H]H_2O$ in normal ($n=4$–7) and sacrificed rats ($n=4$), respectively. The solid line represents the efflux curve of $[^3H]H_2O$ in normal rats predicted by the physiological pharmacokinetic model. The dashed line represents the assumption that the intrinsic efflux clearance, PS_{eff}, equals zero. (From Kakee *et al.*, 1996, with permission.)

the ipsilateral cerebrum, demonstrating a significant stereospecific efflux of hexose from the cerebrum across the BBB (Fig. 3.3). These results coincide well with those of reported characteristics for the uptake process of hexose (Pardridge and Oldendorf, 1977; Cornford, 1985), demonstrating that the presently developed BEI method also meets criterion (5).

As the injectate will be diluted in the ipsilateral cerebrum following microinjection, the dilution factor was evaluated by the injection of Trypan Blue solution. The dilution factors determined at 2 min and 20 min were 39.9 ± 2.2% and 42.4 ± 5.7%

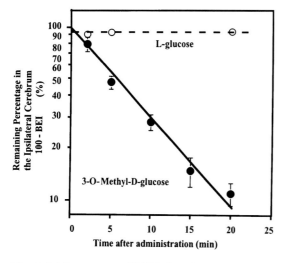

Fig. 3.3. Time-courses of [³H]3-O-methyl-D-glucose and [³H]L-glucose in the ipsilateral cerebrum after intracerebral microinjection into the normal male Sprague-Dawley rats in the presence of [¹⁴C]carboxyl-inulin as an internal reference. [³H]3-O-methyl-D-glucose or [³H]L-glucose (10 µCi/ml) and [¹⁴C]inulin (1 µCi/ml) dissolved in 0.5 µl ECF buffer were injected intracerebrally to the rats. Rats were decapitated at 2, 5, 10, 15 and 20 min after administration. The radioactivity in the ipsilateral cerebrum was measured using a scintillation counter. Closed and open circles represent the time-courses of (100 − BEI) values for [³H]3-O-methyl-D-glucose (n = 4) and [³H]L-glucose (n = 4), respectively. Solid and dashed lines represent the regression line for 3OMG and L-glucose, respectively. (From Kakee et al., 1996, with permission.)

for 0.2 µl of microinjection and 30.3 ± 4.4% and 46.2 ± 1.1% for 0.5 µl of microinjection, respectively. Assuming the dilution factor is the same as that of Trypan Blue, the cerebral concentration of test compound was obtained for the kinetic analysis of saturable and inhibitable efflux transport process at the BBB.

BBB efflux transport system

As a transendothelial exchange between the circulating blood and the interstitial fluid of the liver or the kidney is significantly rapid, these two disposing organs are well known to act as efficient detoxicating organs for the whole body. However, a substrate exchange between the brain interstitial fluid and the circulating blood is strictly regulated by the

transport functions of the BBB. Hence, it would be possible to assume that the BBB acts as a brain selective detoxicating system by pumping out substrates from the brain interstitial fluid to the circulating blood not only for hydrophilic substrates such as neurotransmitters or their metabolites released but also hydrophobic xenobiotics that may cause significant toxic effects on the CNS. In the previous studies, it has been revealed that MDR1, a P-glycoprotein, acts as an efflux transport system at the BBB, restricting the cerebral distribution of vincristine and cyclosporin A (Tatsuta et al., 1992; Tsuji et al., 1992, 1993) using cultured brain capillary endothelial cells. Moreover, several studies have also suggested that there are some efflux transport systems different from P-glycoprotein at the BBB to explain the mechanism of restricted distribution in the brain (Cornford et al., 1985; Emanuelsson et al., 1987; Wong et al., 1993; Adkison et al., 1994).

As para-aminohippuric acid (PAH) is a well-known substrate for the organic anion transport systems in the kidney (Pritchard, 1988; Hori et al., 1993) and also at the BCSFB (Holloway and Cassin, 1972; Domer, 1973), it would be of importance to examine whether the BBB has a similar efflux transport system or not. Employing the BEI method, the apparent efflux rate constant of [³H]PAH has been determined to be $5.87 \times 10^{-2} \pm 0.65 \times 10^{-2}$ min⁻¹ (Kakee et al., 1995). The apparent efflux clearance of PAH across the BBB was found to be 46.9 ± 3.8 µl/min/g brain incorporating the K_{eff} and the determined V_{br} (0.800 ± 0.051 ml/g brain) into Eqn (3.5). No significant metabolism in the ipsilateral cerebrum was demonstrated in the brain for at least 20 min. The apparent elimination rate constant was decreased in a saturable manner, showing that the Michaelis constant, K_{m}, and the maximum velocity, V_{max}, for the PAH efflux were 396 ± 73 (µM) and 23.4 ± 2.7 (nmol/min/g brain). Interestingly, no significant influx rate of PAH at the BBB was obtained, supporting the hypothesis that the BBB transports PAH selectively from the brain to the circulating blood via a carrier-mediated system (Kakee et al., 1995).

There have been several reports that 3′-azido-3′-deoxythymidine (AZT) and 2′,3′-dideoxyinosine (DDI) and related nucleotide derivatives, as anti-HIV drugs for the treatment of the AIDS demen-

Table 3.1 *Effect of AZT, DDI, thymidine, probenecid, PAH, PCG and DIDS on the efflux of [³H]AZT from rat brain*

Inhibitor	Concentration in the brain[a] (mM)	n	Percentage remaining in the brain[b]
Control	3.3×10^{-5} of AZT	15	53.8 ± 1.8
AZT	3.3×10^{-3}	3	56.4 ± 4.9
	1.7×10^{-2}	4	63.1 ± 8.5
	3.3×10^{-2}	4	68.7 ± 3.4**
	0.17	4	67.0 ± 5.0*
	1.7	8	65.0 ± 3.8**
DDI	1.7	4	64.3 ± 3.9 *
Thymidine	1.7	4	58.0 ± 2.9
	3.3	4	55.4 ± 1.9
Probenecid	3.3×10^{-3}	4	55.1 ± 3.1
	6.6×10^{-3}	4	55.7 ± 4.4
	3.3×10^{-2}	4	65.9 ± 4.1**
	0.33	3	69.3 ± 6.0**
	1.7	6	66.7 ± 2.6**
PAH	3.3	8	67.6 ± 3.3**
PCG	3.3	10	66.9 ± 2.2**
DIDS	3.3×10^{-2}	7	64.2 ± 3.5**

[a] The brain concentration was estimated from the injectate concentration divided by the dilution factor, i.e. 30.3, which has been reported previously (Kakee *et al.*, 1996).

[b] The values were determined 20 min after intracerebral microinjection. *$P < 0.05$, **$P < 0.01$

(From Takasawa *et al.*, 1997)

tia complex (ADC) or AIDS encephalopathy, distribute in the CNS in a strictly restricted manner (Doshi *et al.*, 1989; Wang and Sawchuk, 1995). Although AZT exhibited significantly low apparent influx rate at the BBB (Terasaki and Pardridge, 1988), recent studies also suggested that efficient efflux transport across the BBB may also contribute to the apparent restricted distribution of AZT in the CNS (Wang and Sawchuk, 1995). Following an intracerebral microinjection of [³H]AZT, the K_{eff} value of AZT was determined as $3.17 \times 10^{-2} \pm 0.68 \times 10^{-2}$ (min⁻¹) (Takasawa, *et al.*,

1997). As summarized in Table 3.1, significant increasing effects of unlabeled AZT, DDI, PAH, probenecid, benzylpenicillin (PCG), and 4,4′-diisothiocyanostilbene-2,2′-disulfonic acid (DIDS) were demonstrated for the remaining percentage of [³H]AZT in the brain 20 min following microinjection (Table 3.1). No significant effect of thymidine was observed for the efflux process of [³H]AZT (Table 3.1). Intracerebroventricular injection of probenecid had no effect on the apparent efflux of [³H]AZT after intracerebral microinjection, suggesting that the efflux transport system of the BCSFB is not responsible for the apparent efflux from the cerebral cortex, Par2. These results suggest that the PAH-sensitive organic anion efflux transport system at the BBB is responsible for the efficient efflux of AZT from the brain to the circulating blood (Takasawa *et al.*, 1997)

As a model substrate to examine whether the BBB has an efflux transport system similar to that of liver or not, taurocholic acid (TCA) has been chosen for the BEI study (Kitazawa *et al.*, 1996). The apparent efflux rate constant of [³H]TCA was obtained to $2.33 \times 10^{-2} \pm 0.25 \times 10^{-2}$ (min⁻¹). The efflux rate constant of [³H]TCA decreased with increasing concentration of unlabeled TCA and cholic acid. Moreover, the apparent efflux of [³H]TCA was inhibited by BQ-123, a cyclo-octapeptide antagonist of the endothelin receptor. An efflux transport of [³H]BQ-123 across the BBB was also shown to be saturable and inhibited by taurocholic acid, however, the results of kinetic analysis of mutual inhibition studies suggest that BQ-123 is effluxed across the BBB via a carrier-mediated system different from that of TCA (Kitazawa *et al.*, 1996).

The present studies demonstrate that the Brain Efflux Index (BEI) method is a useful technique to characterize the efflux transport system across the BBB, while it is difficult to identify whether the efflux transport system is located at the luminal membrane or abluminal membrane of brain capillary endothelial cells. Employing the BEI method, several unidentified transport systems across the BBB could be elucidated in the future and those new findings might lead to better understanding of the physiological role of the BBB as a detoxifying system that maintains cerebral function.

References

Adkison, K. D. K., Artru, A. A., Powers, K. M. and Shen, D. D. (1994). Contribution of probenecid-sensitive anion transport processes at the brain capillary endothelium and choroid plexus to the efficient efflux of valproic acid from the central nervous system. *J. Pharmacol. Exp. Ther.*, **268**, 797–805.

Banks, W. A., Kastin, A. J. and Ehrensing, C. A. (1993). Endogenous peptide Tyr-Pro-Trp-Gly-NH$_2$ (Tyr-W-MIF-1) is transported from the brain to the blood by peptide transport system-1. *J. Neurosci. Res.*, **35**, 690–5.

Barrera, C. M., Kastin, A. J., Fasold, M. B. and Banks, W. A. (1991). Bidirectional saturable transport of LHRH across the blood–brain barrier. *Am. J. Physiol.*, **261** (Endocrinol. Metab. **24**), E312–E318.

Betz, A. L. and Goldstein, G. W. (1978). Polarity of the blood–brain barrier: Neutral amino acid transport into isolated brain capillaries. *Science*, **202**, 225–7.

Boado, R. J. and Pardridge, W. M. (1993). Glucose deprivation causes posttranscriptional enhancement of brain capillary endothelial glucose transporter gene expression via GLUT1 mRNA stabilization. *J. Neurochem.*, **60**, 2290–6.

Boado, R. J. and Pardridge, W. M. (1994). Measurement of blood–brain barrier GLUT1 glucose transporter and actin mRNA by a quantitative polymerase chain reaction assay. *J. Neurochem.*, **62**, 2085–90.

Boado, R. J., Wang, L. and Pardridge, W. M. (1994). Enhanced expression of the blood–brain barrier GLUT1 glucose transporter gene by brain-derived factors. *Mol. Brain Res.*, **22**, 259–67.

Cornford, E. M. (1985). The blood–brain barrier, a dynamic regulatory interface. *Mol. Physiol.*, **7**, 219–60.

Cornford, E. M., Diep, C. P. and Pardridge, W. M. (1985). Blood–brain barrier transport of valproic acid. *J. Neurochem.*, **44**, 1541–50.

Domer, F. R. (1973). Drug inhibition of PAH transport from cerebrospinal fluid in rabbits. *Exp. Neurol.*, **40**, 414–23.

Doshi, K. J., Gallo, J. M., Boudinot, F. D et al. (1989). Comparative pharmacokinetics of 3′-azido-3′-deoxythymidine (AZT) and 3′-azido-2′,3′-dideoxyuridine (AZddU) in mice. *Drug Metab. Dispos.*, **17**, 590–4.

Emanuelsson, B. -M., Paalzow, L. and Sunzel, M. (1987). Probenecid-induced accumulation of 5-hydroxyindoleacetic acid and homovanillic acid in rat brain. *J. Pharm. Pharmacol.*, **39**, 705–10.

Holloway, L. S. and Cassin, S. (1972). In vitro uptake of PAH-^{3}H by choroid plexus from dogs of various ages. *Am. J. Physiol.*, **223**, 507–9.

Hori, R., Okamura, M., Takayama, A. et al. (1993). Transport of organic anion in the OK kidney epithelial cell line. *Am. J. Physiol.*, **264**, F975–F980.

Kakee, A., Terasaki, T. and Sugiyama, Y. (1995). Organic anion transport system acting as an efflux pump at the blood–brain barrier: demonstration by a newly developed brain efflux index (BEI) method. *Proc. 22nd Intl. Symp. Contrl. Release Bioact. Mater.*, pp. 15–16.

Kakee, A., Terasaki, T. and Sugiyama, Y. (1996). Brain efflux index as a novel method of analyzing efflux transport at the blood–brain barrier. *J. Pharmacol. Exp. Ther.*, **277**, 1550–9.

Kitazawa, T., Terasaki, T., Kakee, A., and Sugiyama, Y. (1996). Bile acid efflux transport system at the blood–brain barrier: demonstration by the brain efflux index (BEI) method. *Proc. 23rd Intl. Symp. Contrl. Release Bioact. Mater.*, pp. 433–4.

Newman, G. C., Hospod, F. E. and Schissel, S. L. (1991). Ischemic brain slice glucose utilization: effects of slice thickness, acidosis, and K$^+$. *J. Cereb. Blood Flow Metabol.*, **11**, 398–406.

Oldendorf, W. H. (1970). Measurement of brain uptake of radiolabeled substances using a tritiated water internal standard. *Brain Res.*, **24**, 372–6.

Oldendorf, W. H., Pardridge, W. M., Braun, L. D. and Crane, P. D. (1982). Measurement of cerebral glucose utilization using washout after carotid injection in the rat. *J. Neurochem.*, **38**, 1413–18.

Pardridge, W. M. (1983). Brain metabolism: a perspective from the blood–brain barrier. *Physiol. Rev.*, **63**, 1481–535.

Pardridge, W. M. and Fierer, G. (1985). Blood–brain barrier transport of butanol and water relative to N-isopropyl-p-iodoamphetamine as the internal reference. *J. Cereb. Blood Flow Metabol.*, **5**, 275–81.

Pardridge, W. M. and Oldendorf, W. H. (1977). Transport of metabolic substrates through the blood–brain barrier. *J. Neurochem.*, **28**, 5–12.

Paxinos, G. and Watson, C. (1986). *The Rat Brain in Stereotaxic Coordinates.* New York: Academic Press.

Pritchard, J. B. (1988). Coupled transport of p-aminohippurate by rat kidney basolateral membrane vesicles. *Am. J. Physiol.*, **255**, F597–F604.

Smith, Q. R., Momma, S., Aoyagi, M. and Rapoport, S. I. (1987). Kinetics of neutral amino acid transport across the blood–brain barrier. *J. Neurochem.*, **49**, 1651–8.

Takakura, Y., Kuentzel, S. L., Raub, T. J. et al. (1991). Hexose uptake in primary cultures of bovine brain microvessel endothelial cells. I. Basic characteristics and effects of D-glucose and insulin. *Biochim. Biophys. Acta*, **1070**, 1–10.

Takasawa, K., Terasaki, T., Suzuki, H. and Sugiyama, Y. (1997). In vivo evidence for carrier-mediated efflux transport of 3′-azido-3′-deoxythymidine and 2′-3′-dideoxyinosine across the blood–brain barrier via a probenecid-sensitive transport. *J. Pharmacol. Exp. Ther.*, **281**, 369–75.

Tatsuta, T., Naito, M., Oh-Hara, T. et al. (1992). Functional involvement of P-glycoprotein in blood–brain barrier. *J. Biol. Chem.*, **267**, 20383–91.

Terasaki, T. and Pardridge, W. M. (1988). Restricted transport of 3′-azido-3′-deoxythymidine and dideoxynucleosides through the blood–brain barrier. *J. Infect. Dis.*, **158**, 630–2.

Terasaki, T., Takakuwa, S., Moritani, S. and Tsuji, A. (1991). Transport of monocarboxylic acids at the blood–brain barrier: studies with monolayers of primary cultured bovine brain capillary endothelial cells. *J. Pharmacol. Exp. Ther.*, **258**, 932–7.

Tsuji, A., Terasaki, T., Takabatake, Y. *et al.* (1992). P-glycoprotein as the drug efflux pump in primary cultured bovine brain capillary endothelial cells. *Life Sci.*, **51**, 1427–37.

Tsuji, A., Tamai, I., Sakata, A. *et al.* (1993). Restricted transport of cyclosporin A across the blood–brain barrier by a multidrug transporter, P-glycoprotein. *Biochem. Pharmacol.*, **46**, 1096–9.

Wang, Y. and Sawchuk, R. J. (1995). Zidovudine transport in the rabbit brain during intravenous and intracerebroventricular infusion. *J. Pharm. Sci.*, **84**, 871–6.

Wong, S. L., Van Belle, K. and Sawchuk, R. J. (1993). Distributional transport kinetics of zidovudine between plasma and brain extracellular fluid/cerebrospinal fluid in the rabbit: investigation of the inhibitory effect of probenecid utilizing microdialysis. *J. Pharmacol. Exp. Ther.*, **264**, 899–909.

4 *In situ* brain perfusion

DAVID J. BEGLEY

- Introduction
- Methods
- Presentation and analysis of data
- Conclusions

Introduction

For many applications, *in situ* brain perfusion offers a number of advantages over other methods when studying the penetration of solutes into brain. The technique is particularly suited to solutes that penetrate into brain slowly as it allows for an extended exposure of the solute of interest to the cerebral vascular endothelium that forms the blood–brain barrier. In addition, the composition of the perfusing medium can be precisely manipulated, thus allowing the inclusion of competitive and non-competitive inhibitors of transport in the perfusate and so allowing kinetic studies to be performed. When investigating kinetics and rates of uptake with brain perfusion methods the technique is essentially revealing events at the luminal plasma membrane of the cerebral vasculature, which for most solutes will be the rate-limiting step.

If a saline-based perfusate is used, the exclusion of plasma enzymes allows the brain-uptake of solutes that are unstable in the general circulation to be determined in an intact form. A saline-based perfusion fluid also allows the role of specific ecto-enzymes to be studied where these are relevant, for example peptidases embedded in the luminal plasma membrane of the endothelial cells forming the blood–brain barrier, (Zlokovic *et al.*, 1988*a*; Begley, 1996).

Usually radiolabelled tracers are included in the perfusate and are subsequently quantified in brain tissue by scintillation counting or autoradiography. By employing manual dissection of the brain after perfusion, or by quantitative autoradiographic methods, regional brain-uptake and permeabilities for individual brain structures can be computed (Groothuis *et al.*, 1984; Gjedde and Diemer, 1985; Smith, 1989, 1992). Autoradiography has the advantage of a high resolution and the possibility of quantifying uptake in a large number of brain areas. Also brain areas of interest can be selected visually after development of the autoradiograph. Manual dissection is limited to a smaller number of predetermined brain regions but has the advantage of being a more rapid method. With both methods it is essential to subtract the tracer radioactivity trapped in the intravascular compartment of the tissue when computing brain-uptake.

It is important to appreciate that it is uptake of radiolabel that is being determined under the experimental conditions and, as a result of metabolic conversion after transport, the chemical form of the labelled material within the brain may be very different from that added to the perfusate. In this context HPLC or mass spectrographic analysis of tissue after perfusion may be useful in confirming the integrity of the labeled tracer.

The technique of post-perfusion capillary depletion is a useful indicator to determine whether tracer has crossed the cerebral endothelium and entered brain extracellular fluid. After intravascular perfusion a tissue sample can be gently homogenized and centrifuged to provide a vascular pellet and a post-vascular supernatant. After the application of suitable controls the presence of intact radiolabelled tracer in the supernatant is indicative of the transcytosis of tracer into brain extracellular fluid (Triguero *et al.*, 1990).

Examples of the successful application of *in situ* brain perfusion techniques to studies of the brain-uptake of various solutes are ions (Deane and Bradbury, 1990; Rabin *et al.*, 1993; Buxani-Rice *et al.*, 1994; Ennis *et al.*, 1996); bilirubin (Ives and Gardiner, 1990); glucose (Betz *et al.*, 1973, 1974; Suzuki, *et al.* 1994); amino acids and related compounds (Betz *et al.*, 1975; Takasato *et al.*, 1983, 1985; Smith *et al.* 1984, 1985, 1987; Smith and Takasato, 1986; Zlokovic *et al.*, 1986; Momma *et al.*, 1987; Greenwood *et al.*, 1988; Greig *et al.*, 1988; Takada *et al.*, 1991, 1992; Stoll *et al.*, 1993; Ennis et al, 1994; Al-Sarraf *et al.* 1995; Benrabh *et al.*, 1995); thyroid hormones (Hokari and Smith, 1994); adenosine (Pardridge *et al.*, 1994): drugs (Greig *et al.*, 1988, 1990; Takada *et al.*, 1992; Chikhale *et al.*, 1995*a*); peptides (Zlokovic *et al.*, 1987, 1988*a,b*, 1989*a,b*, 1990*a*, 1994; Begley, 1992*a*; Samii *et al.*, 1994; Chikhale *et al.*, 1994, 1995*b*; Begley, 1996: and proteins (Triguero *et al.*, 1990; Zlokovic *et al.* 1990*b*; Bickel *et al.*, 1994; Skarlatos *et al.*, 1995).

Methods

The experimental technique of perfusing the cerebral vasculature with an artificial medium has regularly appeared in the literature in recent years. Broman and Lindeberg-Broman (1945), Andjus *et al.*, (1967), Thompson *et al.*, (1968) and Zivin and Snarr (1972) have all described successful cerebral perfusions of the isolated brain of the rat. The technique of cerebral perfusion was further refined by Takasato *et al.* (1982, 1983, 1984, 1985) in the rat and Zlokovic *et al.* (1986, 1987, 1988*a*, 1989*a,b*) in the guinea pig. In addition, Betz *et al.* (1973, 1974, 1975) have successfully used an isolated dog-brain preparation to study glucose and amino acid uptake. Generally the larger mammalian species

have not been regularly used because the large volumes of perfusate required to ensure adequate cerebral flow rates over a sufficient experimental time period become a limiting factor. Many of the early brain perfusion techniques were elaborate and required extensive and often damaging surgery to remove and isolate the brain from the head. The pioneering experiments were often conducted with single-pass techniques which are relatively insensitive for slowly penetrating solutes. More recently it has been realized that leaving the brain *in situ* offers considerable advantages, despite that fact that tissues in the head other than the brain are being perfused during the experimental period.

By sampling brain tissue at the end of a perfusion period, brain-uptake over time can be established, even for slowly penetrating compounds. Perfusion time may range from a few seconds (Takasato *et al.*, 1982, 1984) to several hours (Richerson and Getting, 1990), with indices of brain function, for example EEG and blood–brain barrier integrity, determined with an impermeant tracer such as mannitol, remaining normal (Zlokovic *et al.*, 1986). Brain ATP content, energy charge potential (ECP), water, Na^+/K^+ ratio and mannitol space all remain within normal limits during perfusion, (Zlokovic *et al.*, 1986; Preston *et al.*, 1995). In addition perfusion pressure, perfusion rate, and brain blood flow can all be maintained within the physiological range (Zlokovic *et al.*, 1986; Preston *et al.*, 1995).

Regional blood flow under the conditions of perfusion can be determined by the inclusion of a radiolabelled flow-dependent marker in the perfusate such as butanol (Gjedde, *et al.*, 1980), diazepam (Gratton *et al.*, 1993), and antipyrine (Bradbury *et al.*, 1984, Ennis, *et al.*, 1996). Cerebral tissue flow under perfusion conditions using these markers may be determined using the algorithm developed by Sakurada *et al.* (1978).

Access to the cerebral circulation varies from insertion of the perfusing cannula into the ascending aorta, resulting in the head and the upper thorax being perfused (Greenwood *et al.*, 1985, 1988), to placement of the cannula retrogradely into the external carotid and ligating the common carotid and the pterygopalatine artery (Takasato *et al.*, 1984), thus directing the perfusate almost exclusively to the ipsilateral side of the circle of Willis.

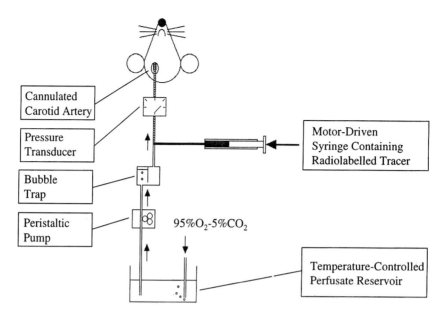

Fig. 4.1. A generalized perfusion system. The precise arrangement will vary from laboratory to laboratory according to the requirements of the perfusion. The perfusion cannula may be placed in the common carotid, the internal carotid or the external carotid artery. For bilateral carotid perfusions the system is duplicated for each carotid artery with a two-channel peristaltic pump feeding both perfusion lines at the same flow rate and two motor-drive syringes calibrated to give identical rates of delivery.

Surgical techniques are generally directed at preserving the natural blood flow to the brain until the last moment before perfusion begins.

During perfusion it is highly desirable to prevent significant mixing of perfusate with the animal's own blood. Some techniques simply rely on the perfusion pressure exceeding the animal's endogenous blood pressure to prevent a mixture of perfusate with the animal's blood occurring. In other the experimental animals, circulation may be arrested by opening the left ventricle of the heart at the start of perfusion. The intracarotid techniques of Takasato *et al.* (1984) and Zlokovic *et al.* (1986), adequately perfuse the ipsilateral hemisphere of the brain.

A further improvement to the *in situ* perfusion technique is a bilateral carotid perfusion that has been employed by Preston *et al.* (1995) and Al-Sarraf *et al.* (1995). Simultaneous perfusion of both carotids ensures that the entire fore-brain is well perfused and therefore bilateral tissue samples can be taken thus reducing the number of animals required. Also, because the choroid plexuses are adequately perfused, at the termination of the per-

fusion a CSF sample may be obtained by cisternal puncture and the kinetics of penetration into the CSF compartment may be quantified.

A generalized perfusion system is illustrated in Fig. 4.1. Most perfusion systems use a saline-based perfusate or plasma diluted with saline as the perfusate. A typical saline-based perfusate would have the following composition: (mmol l^{-1}) NaCl 123, KCl 4.7, CaCl$_2$ 2.5, MgCl$_2$ 1.2, NaHCO$_3$ 24.8, KH$_2$PO$_4$ 1.2, glucose 10.0 (Preston *et al.*, 1995). Colloid osmotic pressure may be provided by adding 60–70 000 M_r dextran 48 g l^{-1} (Zlokovic *et al.*, 1986) or with bovine serum albumin 40 g l^{-1} (Preston *et al.*, 1995). The addition of erythrocytes, protein or dextran to the perfusate increases viscosity and thus the perfusion pressure required for a given tissue flow rate is increased.

Increased oxygen carriage may be provided by adding washed erythrocytes to the perfusate (Zlokovic *et al.*, 1986) or by the addition of perfluoro-chemicals (Bradbury *et al.*, 1984). Simply gassing a saline-based perfusate with a 95%O$_2$–5%CO$_2$ gas mixture appears to provide adequate tissue oxygenation with the preservation of blood–brain barrier integrity and normal biochemical indices of brain function (Al-Sarraf *et al.*, 1995; Preston *et al.*, 1995). Indeed, the addition of the metabolic inhibitor 2, 4-dinitrophenol (DNP) 2 mmol, to a saline-based perfusate appears to have no effect on the integrity of the blood–brain barrier to mannitol for at least the first 10 minutes of perfusion (Greenwood *et al.*, 1988). The control of pH in saline-based perfusates may be achieved by the addition of bicarbonate to the perfusate, and by careful gassing with 95%O_2–5%CO_2 or by the addition of 15–20 mmol HEPES (Gratton *et al.*, 1993).

Radiolabelled tracer may be added, either directly to the perfusate reservoir, or via a side-arm just before the perfusate enters the carotid. In this case tracer can be introduced at a controlled rate by means of a motor-driven syringe. The advantage of using a motor-driven syringe is that the entire perfusion can be stabilized for flow and pressure before radiolabelled tracer is added. However, any adjustment to flow rate during the period of perfusion will result in a change in the concentration of tracer in the perfusate. If a coloured marker, for example Evans Blue, is added to the tracer in the syringe, zero-time when the tracer first enters the perfusate can easily be established. In this experimental situation the radioactive concentration of tracer must be established in the perfusate at the end of the experiment by careful decapitation of the animal, without disturbing the flow rate and the collection of an aliquot of perfusate from the cannula.

Presentation and analysis of data

Volume of distribution

The uptake of radiolabelled tracer into brain may be most simply expressed as a distribution volume (V_d) and is defined as the ratio of the radioactive concentration per unit weight of tissue (C_{br}) and the radioactive concentration of tracer per unit volume of perfusate (C_{pf}).

Hence:

$$V_d = \frac{C_{br}}{C_{pf}} \qquad (4.1)$$

Units are usually $\mu l\ g^{-1}$ of brain. Direct comparison of volumes of distribution can only be made if the duration of perfusion is constant for each experimental animal.

Unidirectional influx constant (single-time-point)

If a time dimension is added to Eqn (1), for example:

$$K_{in} = \frac{C_{br}}{C_{pf}(T)} \qquad (4.2)$$

where T is the duration of the perfusion, a single-time-point unidirectional influx constant (K_{in}), sometimes referred to as the unidirectional transfer constant, may be derived with the dimensions $\mu l\ g^{-1}\ min^{-1}$

Also if a blood–brain barrier impermeant marker such as inulin or polyethyleneglycol-4000 is added to the perfusate, the extracellular intravascular volume and thus the tracer trapped within this space (C_{iv}), can be calculated and subtracted from the true CNS distribution volume or K_{in} as:

$$V_d = \frac{C_{br} - C_{iv}}{C_{pf}} \qquad (4.3)$$

or

$$K_{in} = \frac{C_{br} - C_{iv}}{C_{pf}(T)} \qquad (4.4)$$

Where C_{iv} is the calculated radioactive intravascular concentration tracer per unit weight of brain, (Blasberg *et al.*, 1983, Smith, 1989, Begley, 1992*b*).

Unidirectional influx constant (multiple-time-point)

The unidirectional influx constant (K_{in}), may be determined most accurately from multiple-time-point regression analysis which offers a greater precision of measurement of K_{in} than other methods but requires a larger number of experimental animals.

The following equation describes K_{in}:

$$\frac{C_{tr}(T)}{C_{pf}(T)} = K_{in} \frac{\int_0^T C_{pf}(t)dt}{C_{pf}(T)} + V_i \qquad (4.5)$$

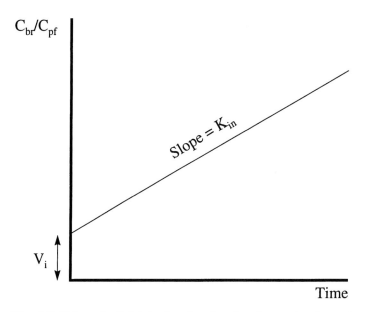

Fig. 4.2. If the ratio C_{br}/C_{pf} is plotted against time for a series of experimental animals perfused for various experimental times, Eqn (4.7) can be solved graphically. The inititial volume of distribution or rapidly equilibrating space (V_i) is represented by the ordinate intercept and the slope of the plot is the unidirectional influx constant (K_{in}).

Where $C_{br}(T)$ and $C_{pl}(T)$ are the radioactive concentrations per unit mass of brain at time T, when T is the duration of perfusion. V_i is the initial volume of distribution or the rapidly equilibrating space within the brain. Under the conditions of perfusion the concentration of radioactive tracer is constant and equal to $C_{pf}(T)$. Thus the ratio

$$\frac{\int_0^T C_{pf}(t)\mathrm{d}t}{C_{pf}(T)} \qquad (4.6)$$

becomes unity and Eqn (4.3) simplifies to:

$$\frac{C_{tr}(T)}{C_{pf}(T)} = K_{in}T + V_i \qquad (4.7)$$

Eqn (4.7) describes a straight line with a slope K_{in} which is the unidirectional influx constant. The ordinate intercept V_i represents the initial volume of distribution for the tracer under study. The V_i varies with the tracer employed and in practice is usually larger than the vascular space determined in the intact animal by intravenous injection of an impermeant marker (Smith, 1992). Eqn (4.7) may be solved graphically by plotting the ratio C_{br}/C_{pf} against experimental time T, for a series of animals

perfused for increasing experimental times (Fig. 4.2). The slope of the line can then be determined by the least squares method and the K_{in} with a standard error estimated as the slope of the plot. The units for K_{in} are usually quoted as $\mu l\ g^{-1}\ min^{-1}$. A departure from a straight line with the plot flattening out would indicate a backflux from the brain, either of intact tracer or of a smaller or more diffusible metabolite. Unidirectional influx constants determined from multiple time point regression analysis are not influenced by tracer remaining trapped in the vasculature.

Permeability coefficient

The influx constant may be transformed into a permeability coefficient if the surface area of the blood–brain barrier can be estimated per unit weight of brain. An average estimate for the surface area of the blood–brain barrier is $100\ cm^2\ g^{-1}$ of brain, (Bradbury, 1979). Thus the permeability coefficient P is given by:

$$P = \frac{K_{in}}{S} \qquad (4.8)$$

Where S is blood–brain barrier surface area in $cm^2 g^{-1}$ of brain. Units are $cm s^{-1}$. However the blood–brain barrier surface area per unit weight or volume of brain varies in different brain regions (Fenstermacher *et al.*, 1981) and if regional permeability coefficients are to be calculated the appropriate surface area for the selected region should be used.

Kinetics of transport

For substances that cross the blood–brain barrier by a carrier-mediated process Michaelis–Menten kinetics may be derived. Under conditions of perfusion where flow substantially exceeds the influx constant, $(F >> K_{in})$, the unidirectional influx constant K_{in} is equivalent to the permeability surface area product PA (or PS), (Fenstermacher *et al.*, 1981; Takasato *et al.*, 1985; Gjedde 1988; Zlokovic *et al.*, 1988; Ennis *et al.*, 1996) and has the same dimensions of $\mu l min^{-1} g^{-1}$. Thus under perfusion conditions:

$$K_{in} = \frac{V_{max}}{(K_m + C_{pf})} + K_d \qquad (4.9)$$

Where V_{max} is the maximum velocity of transport, K_m is the Michaelis–Menten constant (affinity) and K_d is the diffusion constant. By adding increasing amounts of non-radioactive tracer to the perfusate, saturation kinetics may be demonstrated for the tracer. A curve may be fitted to a plot of brain-uptake, K_{in}, against the concentration of tracer in the perfusate and the K_m and V_{max} determined.

This form of kinetic analysis employing *in situ* brain perfusion has been successfully applied to amino acids (Smith *et al.*, 1984, 1987), peptides (Zlokovic *et al.*, 1989*b*; 1990*a*), drugs (Takada *et al.*, 1992) and sodium (Ennis *et al.*, 1996).

Conclusions

The technique of *in situ* brain perfusion has proved especially useful in determining the true permeability of the blood–brain barrier to solutes, both passive and carrier-mediated, in the absence of competing endogenous compounds and complications caused by metabolism of the solute of interest in the circulation. The ability to manipulate and control the composition of the perfusate accurately enables precise kinetic and mechanistic studies of transport to be carried out and the effects of plasma protein binding on transport to be determined. In addition, comparisons of brain-uptake data determined by brain perfusion with brain-uptakes computed in intact animals after intravenous infusion or injection, allows the importance of pharmacokinetic and metabolic influences on brain-uptake to be determined.

Thus *in situ* brain perfusion techniques allow transport phenomena in the undisturbed blood–brain barrier to be directly investigated free of any complicating influences. The method provides a means whereby the properties of the intact vascular endothelium forming the blood–brain barrier can be evaluated and directly compared with those of *in vitro* models of the blood–brain barrier.

References

Al-Sarraf, H., Preston, J. E. and Segal, M. B. (1995). The entry of acidic amino acids into brain and CSF during development, using *in situ* perfusion in the rat. *Dev. Brain Res.*, **90**, 151–8.

Andjus, R. K., Suhara, K. and Sloviter, H. A. (1967). An isolated, perfused rat brain preparation, its spontaneous and stimulated activity. *J. Appl. Physiol.*, **22**, 1033–9.

Begley, D. J. (1992*a*). Peptides and the blood–brain barrier. In *Handbook of Experimental Pharmacology, Vol 103. Physiology and Pharmacology of the Blood–Brain Barrier.*, ed. M. W. Bradbury, pp. 151–203. Berlin: Springer-Verlag.

Begley, D. J. (1992*b*). The interaction of some centrally active drugs with the blood–brain barrier and circumventricular organs. In *Circumventricular Organs and Brain Fluid Environment*, ed. A. Ermisch, R. Landgraf and H.-J. Rühle. *Progress in Brain Research*, **91**, 163–9. Amsterdam: Elsevier.

Begley, D. J. (1996). The blood–brain barrier: Principles for targeting peptides and drugs to the central nervous system. *J. Pharm. Pharmacol.*, **48**, 136–46.

Benrabh, H., Bourre, J. M. and Lefauconnier. J. M. (1995). Taurine transport at the blood–brain barrier: An in vivo brain perfusion study. *Brain Res.*, **692**, 57–65.

Betz, A. L., Gilboe, D. D., Yudilevich, D. L. and Drewes, L. R. (1973). Kinetics of unidirectional glucose transport into the isolated dog brain. *Am. J. Physiol.*, **225**, 586–92.

Betz, A. L., Gilboe, D. D. and Drewes, L. R. (1974). Effects of anoxia on net uptake and unidirectional transport of glucose into the isolated dog brain. *Brain Res.*, **67**, 307–16.

Betz, A. L., Gilboe, D. D. and Drewes, L. R. (1975). Kinetics of unidirectional leucine transport into brain: effects of isoleucine, valine and anoxia. *Am. J. Physiol.*, **228**, 895–900.

Bickel, U., Kang, Y. S., Yoshikawa, T. and Pardridge, W. M. (1994). In vivo demonstration of subcellular localization of anti-transferrin receptor monoclonal antibody-colloidal gold conjugate in brain capillary endothelium. *J. Histochem. Cytochem.*, **42**, 1493–7.

Blasberg, R. G., Fenstermacher, J. F. and Patlak, C. S. (1983). Transport of α-aminoisobutyric acid across the brain capillary and cellular membranes. *J. Cereb. Blood Flow Metab.*, **3**, 8–32.

Bradbury, M. W. B (1979). *The Concept of a Blood–Brain Barrier*, pp. 137–40. Chichester: Wiley.

Bradbury, M. W., Deane, R. and Rosenberg, G. (1984). Regional blood flow, EEG and electrolytes in mouse brain perfused with perfluorchemical, FC-43. *J. Physiol.* **355**, 31P.

Broman, T. and Lindeberg-Broman, A. M. (1945). An experimental study of disorders in the permeability of the cerebral vessels ('the blood–brain barrier') produced by chemical and physico-chemical agents. *Acta Physiol. Scand.*, **10**, 102–25.

Buxani-Rice, S., Ueda, F. and Bradbury, M. W. B. (1994). Transport of zinc-65 at the blood–brain barrier during short cerebrovascular perfusion in the rat: Its enhancement by histidine. *J. Neurochem.*, **62**, 665–72.

Chikhale, E. G., Ng, K., Burton, P. S. and Borchardt, R. T. (1994). Hydrogen bonding potential as a determinant of the in vitro and in situ blood–brain barrier permeability of peptides. *Pharmacol. Res.*, **11**, 412–19.

Chikhale, E. G., Chikhale, P. J. and Borchardt, R. T. (1995a). Carrier-mediated transport of the antitumour agent acivicin across the blood–brain barrier. *Biochem. Pharmacol.*, **49**, 941–5.

Chikhale, E. G., Burton, P. S. and Borchardt, R. T. (1995b). The effect of verapamil on the transport of peptides across the blood–brain barrier in rats: Kinetic evidence for an apically polarised efflux mechanism. *J. Pharm. Exp. Ther.*, **273**, 298–303.

Deane, R. and Bradbury, M. W. B. (1990). Transport of Lead-203 at the blood–brain barrier during short cerebrovascular perfusion with saline in the rat. *J. Neurochem.*, **54**, 905–14.

Ennis, S. R., Ren, X. D. and Betz, A. L. (1994). Transport of alpha-aminoisobutyric acid across the blood–brain barrier studied with an in situ perfusion of the rat brain. *Brain Res.*, **643**, 100–7.

Ennis, S. R., Ren, X. D. and Betz, A. L. (1996). Mechanisms of sodium transport at the blood–brain barrier studied with in situ perfusion of rat brain. *J. Neurochem.*, **66**, 756–63.

Fenstermacher, J., Blasberg, R. and Patlak, C. (1981). Methods for quantifying the transport of drugs across the brain barrier systems. *Pharmacol. Ther.*, **14**, 217–48.

Gjedde, A. (1988). Exchange diffusion of large neutral amino acids between blood and brain. In *Peptide and Amino Acid Transport Mechanisms in the Central Nervous System*, ed. Lj. Rakic, D. J. Begley, H. Davson and B. V. Zlokovic, pp. 209–17. Basingstoke, London and New York: Macmillan.

Gjedde, A. and Diemer, N. H. (1985). Double-tracer study of the fine regional blood–brain glucose transfer in the rat by computer assisted autoradiography. *J. Cereb. Blood Flow Metab.*, **5**, 282–9.

Gjedde, A., Hansen A. J. and Siemkovicz, E. (1980). Rapid simultaneous determination of regional blood flow and blood–brain barrier glucose transfer into brain of rat. *Acta Physiol. Scand.*, **108**, 321–30.

Gratton, J. A., Lightman, S. L. and Bradbury, M. W. (1993). Transport into retina measured by short vascular perfusion in the rat. *J. Physiol.*, **470**, 651–63.

Greenwood, J., Luthert, P. J., Pratt, O. and Lantos, P. L. (1985). Maintenance of the integrity of the blood–brain barrier in the rat during an in situ saline-based perfusion. *Neurosci. Lett.*, **56**, 223–7.

Greenwood, J., Luthert, P. J., Pratt, O. E. et al. (1988). A supravital brain perfusion technique for the study of the blood–brain barrier: with special reference to leucine transport. In *Peptide and Amino Acid Transport Mechanisms in the Central Nervous System*, ed. Lj. Rakic, D. J. Begley, H. Davson and B. V. Zlokovic, pp. 317–31. Basingstoke, London and New York: Macmillan.

Greig, N. H., Momma, S., Sweeney, D. J. and Rapoport, S. I. (1988). Facilitated transport of melphalan at the rat blood–brain barrier by the large neutral amino acid carrier system. *Cancer Res.*, **47**, 1541.

Greig, N. H. Soncrant, T. T., Shetty, H. V. et al. (1990). Brain uptake and anticancer activity of vincristine and vinblastine are restricted by their low cerebrovascular permeability and binding to plasma constituents in the rat. *Cancer Chemother. Pharmacol.*, **26**, 263–8.

Groothuis, D. R., Molnar, P. and Blasberg, R. G. (1984). Regional blood flow and blood-to-tissue transport in five brain tumour models. *Prog. Exp. Tumour Res.*, **27**, 132–53.

Hokari, M. and Smith, Q. R. (1994). Thyroid hormones express high affinity for both the thyroid hormone and large neutral amino acid transporters of the blood brain barrier. *Soc. Neurosci. Abst.*, **20**, 1335.

Ives, N. K. and Gardiner, R. M. (1990). Blood–brain barrier permeability to bilirubin in the rat studied using intracarotid bolus injection and in situ brain perfusion techniques. *Pediatric Res.*, **27**, 436–41.

Momma, S., Aoyagi, M., Rapoport, S. I. and Smith, Q. R. (1987). Phenylalanine transport across the blood–brain barrier as studied with the in situ brain perfusion technique. *J. Neurochem.*, **48**, 1291–300.

Pardridge, W. M., Yoshikawa, T., Kang, Y. S. and Miller, L. P. (1994). Blood–brain barrier transport and brain metabolism of adenosine and adenosine analogs. *J. Pharmacol. Exp. Ther.*, **268**, 14–18.

Preston, J. E., Al-Sarraf, H. and Segal, M. B. (1995). Permeability of the developing blood–brain barrier to ^{14}C-mannitol using the rat in situ brain perfusion technique. *Dev. Brain Res.*, **87**, 69–76.

Rabin, O., Hegedus, L., Bourre, J. M. and Smith, Q. R. (1993). Rapid brain uptake of manganese (II) across the blood–brain barrier. *J. Neurochem.*, **61**, 509–17.

Richerson, G. B. and Getting, P. A. (1990). Preservation of integrative function in a perfused guinea pig brain. *Brain Res.*, **517**, 7–18.

Sakurada, O., Kennedy, C., Jehle, J. *et al.* (1978). Measurement of local cerebral blood flow with iodo[14]C]-antipyrine. *Am. J. Physiol.*, **234**, H59–66.

Samii, A., Bickel, U., Stroth, U. and Pardridge, W. M. (1994). Blood–brain barrier transport of neuropeptides: analysis with a metabolically stable dermorphin analogue. *Am. J. Physiol.*, **276**, E124–E131.

Skarlatos, S., Yoshikawa, T and Pardridge, W. M. (1995). Transport of ^{125}I]-transferrin through the rat blood–brain barrier. *Brain Res.*, **683**, 164–71.

Smith, Q. R. (1989). Quantitation of blood–brain barrier permeability. In *Implications of the Blood-Brain Barrier and its Manipulation*, Vol. 1, ed. E. A. Neuwalt, pp. 85–118. New York and London: Plenum Medical.

Smith, Q. R. (1992). Methods of study. In *Handbook of Experimental Pharmacology, Vol 103, Physiology and Pharmacology of the Blood-Brain Barrier*, ed. M. W. Bradbury, pp. 23–52. Berlin: Springer-Verlag.

Smith, Q. R. and Takasato, Y. (1986). Kinetics of amino acid transport at the blood–brain barrier studied using an in situ brain perfusion technique. *Ann. N. Y. Acad. Sci.*, **481**, 186–201.

Smith, Q. R., Takasato, Y. and Rapoport, S. I. (1984). Kinetic analysis of L-leucine transport across the blood–brain barrier. *Brain Res.*, **311**, 167–70.

Smith, Q. R., Takasato, Y., Sweeney, D. J. and Rapoport, S. I. (1985). Regional cerebrovascular transport of leucine as measured by the in-situ brain perfusion technique. *J. Cereb. Blood Flow Metab.*, **5**, 300–11.

Smith, Q. R., Momma, S., Aoyagi, M and Rapoport, S. I. (1987). Kinetics of neutral amino acid transport across the blood–brain barrier. *J. Neurochem.*, **49**, 1651–8.

Stoll, J., Wadwani, K. C. and Smith, Q. R. (1993). Identification of the cationic amino acid transporter (system y⁺). of the rat blood–brain barrier. *J. Neurochem.*, **60**, 1956–9.

Suzuki, H., Nagashiwa,T., Fujita, K. *et al.* (1994). Cerebral ischaemia alters glucose transporter kinetics across rat brain microvascular endothelium: quantitative analysis by an in situ brain perfusion method. *J. Auton. Nerv. Syst.*, **49**, S173–S176.

Takada, Y., Greig , N. H., Vistica, D. T. *et al.* (1991). Affinity of antineoplastic amino acid drugs for the large amino acid transporter of the blood–brain barrier. *Cancer Chemother. Pharmacol.*, **29**, 89.

Takada, Y., Vistica, D. T., Greig, N. H. *et al.* (1992). Rapid high-affinity transport of a chemotherapeutic amino acid across the blood–brain barrier. *Cancer Res.*, **52**, 2191–6.

Takasato, Y., Rapoport, S. I. and Smith, Q. R. (1982). A new method to determine cerebrovascular permeability in the anaesthetised rat. *Soc. Neurosci. Abstr.*, **8**, 850.

Takasato, Y., Smith, Q. R. and Rapoport, S. I. (1983). Transport kinetics of large neutral amino acids across the blood–brain barrier. *Soc. Neurosci. Abstr.*, **9**, 889.

Takasato, Y., Rapoport, S. I. and Smith, Q. R. (1984). An in situ brain perfusion technique to study cerebrovascular transport in the rat. *Am. J. Physiol.*, **247**, H484–H493.

Takasato, Y., Momma, S. and Smith, Q. R. (1985). Kinetic analysis of cerebrovascular isoleucine transport from saline and plasma. *J. Neurochem.*, **45**, 1013–20.

Thompson, A. M., Robertson, R. C. and Baum, Th. A. (1968). A rat head perfusion technique for the study of brain uptake of materials. *J. Appl. Physiol.*, **24**, 407–11.

Triguero, D., Buciak, J. and Pardridge, W. M. (1990). Capillary depletion method for the quantification of blood–brain barrier transport of circulating peptides and plasma proteins. *J. Neurochem.*, **54**, 1882–8.

Zivin, J. A. and Snarr, J. F. (1972). A stable preparation for rat brain perfusion, effect of flow rate on glucose uptake. *J. Appl. Physiol.*, **32**, 658–63.

Zlokovic, B. V., Begley, D. J., Duricic, B. M. and Mitrovic, D. M. (1986). Measurement of solute transport across the blood–brain barrier in the perfused guinea pig brain: method and application to N-methyl-α-aminoisobu-tyric acid. *J. Neurochem.*, **46**, 1444–51.

Zlokovic, B. V., Lipovac, M. N., Begley, D. J. *et al.* (1987). Transport of leucine enkephalin across the blood–brain barrier in the perfused guinea pig brain. *J. Neurochem.*, **49**, 310–15.

Zlokovic, B. V., Lipovac, M. N., Begley, D. J. *et al.* (1988*a*). Slow penetration of thyrotropin-releasing hormone across the blood–brain barrier of an in situ perfused guinea pig brain. *J. Neurochem.*, **51**, 252–7.

Zlokovic, B. V., Begley, D. J., Segal, M. B. *et al.* (1988*b*). Neuropeptide transport mechanisms in the central nervous system. In *Peptide and Amino Acid Transport Mechanisms in the Central Nervous System*, ed. Lj. Rakic, D. J. Begley, H. Davson and B. V. Zlokovic, pp. 3–19. Basingstoke, London and New York: Macmillan.

Zlokovic, B. V., Susic, V. T., Davson, H. *et al.* (1989*a*). Saturable mechanism for delta sleep-inducing peptide (DSIP) at the blood–brain barrier of the vascularly perfused guinea pig brain. *Peptides*, **10**, 249–54.

Zlokovic, B. V., Mackic, J. B., Duricic, B. M. and Davson, H. (1989*b*). Kinetic analysis of leucine enkephalin cellular uptake at the luminal side of the blood–brain barrier of an in situ perfused guinea pig brain. *J. Neurochem.*, **53**, 1333–40.

Zlokovic, B. V., Hyman, S., McComb, J. G. *et al.* (1990*a*). Kinetics of arginine vasopressin uptake at the blood–brain barrier. *Biochem. Biophys. Acta.*, **1025**, 191–8.

Zlokovic, B. V., Skundric, D. S., Segal, M. B. *et al.* (1990*b*). A saturable mechanism for transport of immunoglobulin G across the blood–brain barrier of the guinea pig. *Exp. Neurol.*, **107**, 263–70.

Zlokovic, B. V., Mackic, J. B., McComb, J. G. *et al.* (1994). Evidence for transcapillary transport of reduced glutathione in vascular perfused guinea pig brain. *Biochem. Biophys. Res. Comm.*, **201**, 402–8.

5 Intravenous injection/pharmacokinetics

ULRICH BICKEL

- Introduction
- Evaluation of initial rate experiments
- Detection and treatment of saturable transport
- Evaluation in the presence of efflux
- Characteristics of the intravenous approach compared to other techniques

Introduction

Measurement of brain uptake rates after intravenous (i.v.) administration of a test substance followed by sampling of brain tissue has been the most widely used approach compared to other techniques for measuring the permeability of the blood–brain barrier (BBB). In contrast to single-passage methods such as the brain uptake index (BUI) and to the indicator dilution technique, brain uptake in i.v. experiments is measured after multiple passages through the capillary bed and offers the highest potential sensitivity of the available techniques. However, the apparent experimental simplicity may mislead the investigator about the fact that the obtained data are readily misinterpreted. Awareness of potential pitfalls associated with the method is required to avoid mistakes in the experimental protocol and evaluation that could distort the results. The purpose of this chapter is to briefly introduce aspects of pharmacokinetic evaluations and highlight specific advantages and disadvantages of the intravenous approach, with examples.

Technically, measurement of brain uptake typically involves injection of the test compound as a radiolabeled tracer in physiological solution as an i.v. bolus. Radiolabeling is not required if suf-

ficiently sensitive analytical methods are available for measuring the substance under investigation in plasma and tissue. Corresponding to the species in which the study is performed, the injected volume should be sufficiently small compared to the total intravascular volume not to introduce a systematic error. With compounds that are poorly soluble in aqueous solution, this may occasionally present a practical problem. If solution enhancers are necessary, care should be taken not to use amounts of vehicles that could alter the integrity of the BBB. For example, low doses in the mg/kg range of the solvents ethanol and DMSO (dimethylsulfoxide) have both been shown to compromise the integrity of the BBB after systemic administration (Brink and Stein, 1967; Hanig *et al.*, 1972).

In the evaluation of BBB permeability following systemic drug administration two situations can be distinguished: (i) unidirectional uptake from plasma into brain tissue, or (ii) reversible uptake, i.e. influx and efflux are present simultaneously. Which of these cases apply is a function of the compound under study and of the time frame within which the experiment is performed. Unless there is - irreversible binding of the test substance in brain tissue and no formation of metabolites that leave the organ, case (ii) will eventually apply to any compound. The majority of studies are 'initial rate' experiments performed in the unidirectional influx phase, because no assumptions are required on the events taking place after a substance has entered brain tissue. Those events are often not directly accessible to experimental quantification and include, in addition to efflux, cellular binding, cellular uptake, and metabolic degradation. In long-term experiments the sink action of cerebrospinal fluid for brain tissue concentrations has to be taken into account, too (Collins and Dedrick, 1983).

Evaluation of initial rate experiments

Two pharmacokinetic approaches are commonly used for the analysis of 'initial rate' brain uptake after i.v. bolus injections: single time point analysis (Ohno *et al.*, 1978) and analysis of multiple-time uptake data (Patlak *et al.*, 1983).

Single time point analysis

Following the injection of the test substance into a peripheral vein, arterial blood samples are taken from a catheterized artery at appropriate intervals to allow for a precise analysis of the plasma concentration time curve. After the final blood sample is taken, the animal is sacrificed and brain tissue is taken. The concentrations of the test substance in brain, C_{br}, and in the plasma samples, C_p, are determined by measuring activity of the isotopes when radiolabeled tracers are used or by quantitative chromatography. It is essential to correct the total brain concentration for the fraction trapped in the intravascular volume of the tissue, V_0, to measure true tissue uptake with that method. In order to minimize errors due to different states of vasodilation, which would affect V_0, a simultaneous measurement of V_0 in the same animals is preferred to a correction with V_0 determined in a separate series of experiments. Experimentally this is most often accomplished by the co-administration of a vascular marker that does not undergo significant accumulation in brain tissue during the time course of the experiment, e.g. radiolabeled serum albumin, inulin, or sucrose. For poorly permeable solutes corrections of intravascular content have been applied where the test compound labeled by a different isotope is injected a second time briefly prior to collecting the final plasma sample and tissue (Go and Pratt, 1975).

V_0 is then used for the calculation of the corrected brain concentration, $C_{br(corr)}$, according to

$$C_{br(corr)} = (V_D - V_0)C_p \qquad (5.1)$$

where V_D represents the apparent volume of distribution of the test substance in brain, i.e. C_{br}/C_p.

If the condition of unidirectional influx applies, two parameters determine the tissue concentration accumulated in brain at time T according to the pharmacokinetic relation

$$C_{br(corr)} = K_{in} \times \text{AUC} \big|_0^T \qquad (5.2)$$

where K_{in} is the unidirectional influx constant from plasma to brain and $\text{AUC}\big|_0^T$ (area under the curve) is the integral of plasma concentrations from time $= 0$ to time $= T$. The AUC in plasma or blood is calculated after fitting by least squares nonlinear regression the concentration–time points to an appropriate exponential disposition function of the form

$$C = \sum_{i=1}^{n} C_i e^{-\lambda_i t} \qquad (5.3)$$

where λ_i is a rate constant and C_i is the initial concentration ($t=0$) associated with that rate constant. K_{in} is the parameter of brain uptake derived from the measured quantities in the experiment,

$$K_{in} = \frac{(V_D - V_0)C_p(T)}{\text{AUC}\big|_0^T} \qquad (5.4)$$

It has the dimensions of a clearance [volume mass^{-1} time^{-1}] from blood into brain and may also be expressed as a function of cerebral plasma flow, F, and extraction fraction during a single pass through the capillary bed, E:

$$K_{in} = v_f FE \qquad (5.5)$$

where v_f is the fractional volume of blood that contributes to brain uptake. $v_f F$ equals plasma flow if no binding to blood cells or plasma proteins is present. The Kety–Renkin–Crone Eqn of capillary transport (Kety, 1951; Renkin, 1959; Crone, 1963) provides the relation between E, $v_f F$ and the product of permeability, P, and capillary surface area, S:

$$E = 1 - e^{PS/v_f F} \qquad (5.6)$$

Combining Eqn (5.5) and (5.6) gives the relation of unidirectional influx K_{in} and PS product:

$$K_{in} = v_f F (1 - e^{PS/v_f F}) \qquad (5.7)$$

from where it can be derived that K_{in} values will lie between two boundaries. K_{in} will be equivalent to PS (error $\leq 10\%$) if BBB permeability is low ($PS \leq 0.2\, v_f F$), (Fenstermacher *et al.*, 1981). On the other hand, Eqn (5.7) implies that a simultaneous knowledge of cerebral blood flow is required for the correct estimation of $PS > 0.2\, v_f F$ from experimentally determined K_{in} values. In the case of high PS products ($PS \geq 2.3\, v_f F$), K_{in} will approach cerebral blood flow (with an error $\leq 10\%$). Experimental conditions such as vasoactive effects of the drug studied and the type of anesthesia, can profoundly influence cerebral blood flow. Measurement in the same experimental animal is therefore required. A method developed for cerebral blood flow determination (van Uitert *et al.*, 1981) can be applied that also offers an alternative approach to K_{in} measurements in short term experiments up to a few minutes duration. The direct experimental determination of the plasma concentration–time integral is here achieved by the withdrawal of an arterial blood sample into a syringe at a constant rate after an i.v. bolus injection of tracer, thus replacing the mathematical fitting of the plasma disposition curve. In this way an external organ is created, and the K_{in} for brain tissue can be calculated from the ratio of concentrations of the test substance in brain (after correction for intravascular volume) and in the blood sample.

The morphine metabolite morphine-6-glucuronide may serve as an example of a small-molecule drug with low and apparently unidirectional uptake over an experimental period of up to 60 min (Bickel *et al.*, 1996). The PS-values as determined according to Eqn (5.4) after 30 and 60 min were 0.13 ± 0.03 and 0.11 ± 0.01 µl min^{-1} g^{-1} and were not significantly different.

Multiple-time uptake data

In this approach animals are sacrificed at various time points T after injection of the test substance. While the underlying pharmacokinetic principles correspond to the approach outlined above, a method has been formulated to estimate K_{in} from a graphical representation of the data (Patlak *et al.*, 1983). V_D is plotted versus the ratio AUC $|_0^T / C_p(T)$, also called the 'exposure time'. The plot yields a straight line for the period of unidirectional uptake and linear regression analysis is applied. A fit of the data to the Eqn used in this approach:

$$\frac{C_{br}(T)}{C_p(T)} = K_{in} \frac{AUC\,|_0^T}{C_p(T)} + V_i \qquad (5.8)$$

where the concentration ratio $C_{br}(T)/C_p(T)$ is the distribution volume in brain at sampling time T, provides K_{in} as the slope of the regression line. V_i is the ordinate and is called the initial volume of distribution. That quantitity comprises plasma space and any brain compartments in rapid equilibration with plasma (Blasberg *et al.*, 1983). In contrast to the single time point analysis, total brain concentrations are evaluated and no vascular marker is used. An interpretation of V_i values, however, is difficult in a physiological sense.

Detection and treatment of saturable transport It follows from Eqn (5.2) that the plasma concentration time integral contributes equally to brain uptake as K_{in}. A substance that is rapidly cleared from the systemic circulation (high total clearance, CL) yields a low AUC, since AUC and CL are inversely correlated (AUC = D/CL, where D = dose). The evaluations discussed above assumed linear pharmacokinetics, where K_{in} or PS values are constants and systemic clearance is independent of dose. The latter implies that plasma concentrations and AUC, when standardized by the injected dose, will also be constant. If saturable processes are involved, the analysis as outlined will reveal dose dependence of these parameters. An example where saturable components are involved both in the systemic clearance and in brain uptake is demonstrated in Figs. 5.1 and 5.2. The effect of co-injection of different doses of a monoclonal antibody on the receptor-mediated brain uptake of a labeled form of the same antibody (Kang *et al.*, 1994) was investigated. With increasing dose there was an increase in standardized plasma AUC, which is apparently due to saturation of systemic clearance (Fig. 5.1). However, brain concentrations expressed as the percentage of injected dose per gram (%ID/g) did

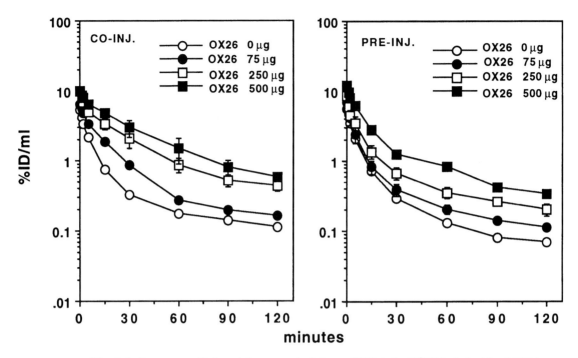

Fig. 5.1. Percentage of injected dose per ml of plasma (%ID/ml) of [³H]biotin/avidin-OX26 is plotted versus the time after intravenous injection of the conjugate in the presence of 0, 75, 250, or 500 μg of OX26 in a co-loading experiment (left). In other experiments, the [³H]biotin/avidin-OX26 was injected 60 min following a pre-injection of either 0, 75, 250, or 500 μg of OX26 (right). [³H]biotin/avidin-OX26 is a 1:1 conjugate of the anti-transferrin receptor antibody OX26 and avidin and is radiolabeled by [³H]biotin. The tracer dose of [³H]biotin/avidin-OX26 corresponded in both experiments to 15 μg of the OX26 antibody. From Kang *et al.*, 1994.

not rise proportionately, but remained at the same level over the examined range. Calculation of the apparent BBB *PS* products at the various doses resulted in a more than 4-fold decrease with increasing dose (Fig. 5.2) that has to be attributed to a partial saturation of the brain uptake mechanism.

The quantitative analysis of saturable processes involved in brain uptake, such as the facilitated transport of nutrients (see Chapters 18–20), requires the incorporation of Michaelis–Menten kinetics (Pardridge, 1983). *PS* is treated as a function of V_{max}, the maximal rate of the saturable component of transport, K_m, the arterial plasma concentration at which half maximal transport occurs, and K_d, the nonsaturable, diffusion mediated component of brain uptake in the form:

$$PS = \frac{V_{max}}{K_m + C_a} + K_d \qquad (5.9)$$

A plot of the BBB *PS* products versus the corresponding arterial plasma concentrations (C_a) is then subjected to nonlinear regression fitting. Although it is much easier to manipulate vascular concentrations in methods such as the brain uptake index or brain perfusion, this type of analysis from i.v. data is possible when brain uptake is studied at different constant plasma concentrations covering the desired range (Murphy *et al.*, 1991), which may be achieved for the experimental period by programmed infusions (Patlak and Pettigrew, 1976). The infusion rates are based on the parameters for disposition from plasma obtained in a pilot study with i.v. bolus injection.

Evaluation in the presence of efflux

Figure 5.3 demonstrates an experimental situation where efflux from brain of the test substance

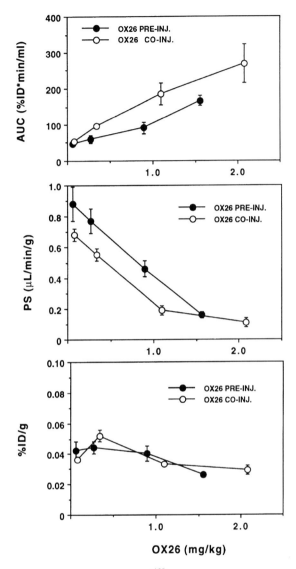

Fig. 5.2. The plasma AUC $|_0^{120}$ (top panel), determined from the data in Fig. 5.1, the BBB *PS* product (middle panel) and the %ID/g brain (bottom panel) of [^{3}H]biotin/avidin-OX26 is plotted versus the dose of OX26 preload or co-load. From Kang *et al.*, 1994.

galanthamine, an alkaloid, was significant at early sampling times. The apparent K_{in} values as calculated according to Eqn (5.4) would decrease with increasing time. Plotting the data as described for the graphical analysis would result in a deviation from linearity. When efflux is significant, even at short experimental times, the kinetic analysis of brain tissue concentrations by unidirectional uptake

analysis is not feasible. In the absence of direct experimental measurement of efflux (see Chapter 3) compartmental models may be used for the evaluation of brain tissue concentrations (Rapoport *et al.*, 1982). Alternatively, a system analytical approach was applied for the evaluations of the galanthamine data. Brain concentrations could be adequately described by convolution of function with a monoexponential elimination from brain tissue (k_{out} = elimination rate constant of brain tissue) and an input rate $CL_{in} C_p(t)$ to brain tissue from plasma (CL_{in} is the product of K_{in} and brain weight, m_{br}). Fitting the measured brain concentrations to the resulting Eqn describing the brain concentration–time course

$$C_{br}(t) = \frac{CL_{in}}{m_{br}} \sum_{i=1}^{n} C_i \frac{e^{-k_{out}t} - e^{-\lambda_i t}}{\lambda_i - k_{out}} \quad (5.10)$$

where C_i and λ_i are the parameters of elimination from plasma (Eqn 5.3), provided the parameters CL_{in} and k_{out}. Eqn (5.10) is equivalent to Eqn (5.2) for the case $k_{out} = 0$ (no efflux).

Characteristics of the intravenous approach compared to other techniques

Simple technical requirements and the low level of manipulations of the physiological state are points in favour of the intravenous technique. Since brain uptake from the circulation is measured in the presence of blood (cellular elements and plasma), the impact of plasma protein binding and distribution between blood cells and plasma is implicitly included in K_{in} as determined according to Eqn (5.4). With the additional measurement of blood flow and of the degree of protein binding, K_{in} may then be converted to the *PS* product using the relation given in Eqn (5.7). Of all the methods applied to determine BBB permeability, only the i.v. technique simultaneously provides information about systemic pharmacokinetics of a compound and its accumulation in brain.

Experiments with i.v. administration can reveal artifacts in vascular perfusion methods where buffer solutions are used as the perfusion fluid. This was demonstrated in a study with the opioid peptide

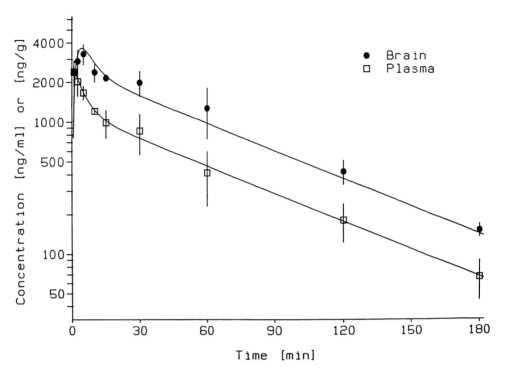

Fig. 5.3. Time course of concentrations of galanthamine in plasma and brain after intravenous bolus injection of 4 mg/kg in mice. Concentrations in brain and plasma were measured by reverse phase HPLC. From Bickel *et al.*, 1991.

DALDA (Tyr-D-Arg-Phe-Lys-NH₂). The *PS* product determined by the intravenous method was 5 to 50 times lower than the apparent *PS* from brain perfusion experiments under various conditions (Samii *et al.*, 1994) and was attributed to nonspecific binding to the vascular bed in the perfusion experiments. The discrimination between mere binding to the vascular elements and complete penetration through the BBB represents a problem for all *in vivo* techniques. The capillary depletion method (Triguero *et al.*, 1990), which involves a density centrifugation step to separate capillaries from the rest of the brain tissue, has been shown to give reliable results if the transport process involves specific binding as in the case of receptor-mediated transcytosis of macromolecules. Capillary depletion is applicable after i.v. injection, too (Pardridge *et al.*, 1995). The method is prone to produce artifacts if low affinity nonspecific binding to the endothelial cell plasma membrane occurs, as observed with DALDA. As an alternative, autoradiography of tissue sections can be performed to quantify the

tissue distribution of tracers at the cellular level (Duffy and Pardridge, 1987).

The presence of plasma constituents can also present a problem in the measurement of saturable uptake at the BBB. This may be exemplified by the difficulty to demonstrate brain uptake of transferrin using the i.v. technique (Morris *et al.*, 1992). Under physiological conditions transferrin concentrations in plasma are 5000-fold higher than the affinity constant of the endothelial transferrin receptor. Therefore it can be predicted that the i.v. administration of a trace amount of labeled transferrin cannot result in measurable brain uptake even at long experimental periods of 24 h, as the receptor is saturated by non-labeled endogenous transferrin. In this case perfusion techniques are the preferred alternative because serum-free conditions can be used to reveal significant brain uptake (Fishman *et al.*, 1987, Skarlatos *et al.*, 1995).

Another main limiting factor of the i.v. approach is rapid metabolism of the test compound either in the periphery or in the brain. Valid measurements may be performed with test substances that are taken up by brain and converted to a metabolite trapped in brain tissue. An example are the deoxyglucose methods for measurement of glucose uptake (Gjedde, 1992). However, i.v. techniques are frequently used for the measurement of brain uptake of labile tracers such as peptides or oligonucleotides, where the metabolic breakdown can occur at multiple locations (plasma, peripheral organs, brain endothelial cells, brain tissue) and during sample processing. Analytical methods to determine the fraction of intact tracer in plasma and tissue are obligatory. For macromolecular compounds (proteins, oligonucleotides) the precipitability by trichloroacetic acid (TCA) can be used as a rapid screening method to discriminate the quantity of small molecular weight degradation products such as free radionuclides (^{125}I) or labeled amino acids (Tyr, Lys) that are the common targets of radiolabeling procedures. The latter may even show enhanced brain uptake due to facilitated transport at the blood–brain barrier. The TCA precipitation method should be confirmed by suitable chromatographic or electrophoresis methods to permit identification of undegraded tracer. It may occur that radiolabeled metabolites are incorporated in brain into TCA precipitable products (Pardridge *et al.*, 1990).

Whatever analytical technique is used, it cannot be determined whether metabolites found in brain are the result of local breakdown after uptake or reflect uptake of degraded material from the circulation. Linear uptake in the graphical method may also be unable to discriminate metabolite uptake. For example, in a study with tumor necrosis factor apparent brain V_D plotted versus exposure time increased apparently linearly up to late sampling times of 90 min, although HPLC analysis revealed degradation of at least 20% of the tracer in plasma and brain after 30 min (Gutierrez *et al.*, 1993). Similarly, ^{125}I-leptin V_D in brain showed a linear increase for at least 20 min after injection in mice

(Banks *et al.*, 1996). During that period, the fraction of intact peptide in brain and serum already had decreased to 60% and 72%, respectively, as determined by HPLC analysis.

Binding to capillary endothelial cells and rapid metabolic degradation of injected tracer in the circulation may occur simultaneously. The problem to interpret K_{in} values derived from the brain uptake analysis in such a case was illustrated in a study with brain-derived neurotrophic factor (BDNF) (Pardridge *et al.*, 1994). One hour after i.v. injection the fraction of tracer that was precipitable by TCA had decreased to 20% from an initial value of 93%. By the same method, the fraction of intact tracer in brain tissue at 60 min was estimated 35%. After correction for metabolic degradation, a low but significant K_{in} at the BBB of 0.67 µl/min/g was calculated. Additional binding experiments with isolated brain capillaries and the application of brain perfusion and capillary depletion then revealed strong binding and internalization of the tracer by capillaries, but no significant transport into brain tissue beyond the BBB.

The interference of metabolic breakdown products in studies of brain uptake is not restricted to macromolecules of peptide character but also applies to other chemical structures such as oligonucleotides. It has been shown that the TCA-precipitable fraction in plasma of a 36-mer phosphodiester oligonucleotide decreased to less than 60% within 15 min after injection (Kang *et al.*, 1995).

In conclusion, whether the measurement of brain uptake after i.v. injection allows us to take advantage of the potential sensitivity of the method is critically dependent on the physico-chemical properties of a given test substance, which determine its metabolic and pharmacokinetic fate. Proper analytical methods are crucial to detect artifactual uptake. In the case of brain uptake of labile test substances, a countercheck of results from i.v. experiments with brain perfusion methods is advisable.

References

Banks, W. A., Kastin, A. J., Huang, W, Jaspan, J. B. and Maness, L. B. (1996). Leptin enters the brain by a saturable system independent of insulin. *Peptides*, **17**, 305–11.

Bickel, U., Thomsen, T., Fischer, J. P., Weber, W. and Kewitz, H. (1991). Galanthamine: pharmacokinetics, tissue distribution and cholinesterase inhibition in brain of mice. *Neuropharmacology*, **30**, 447–54.

Bickel, U., Schumacher, O. P., Kang, Y. S. and Voigt, K. (1996). Poor permeability of morphine 3-glucuronide and morphine 6-glucuronide through the blood–brain barrier in the rat. *J. Pharmacol. Exp. Ther.*, **278**, 107–13.

Blasberg, R. G., Fenstermacher, J. D. and Patlak, C. S. (1983). Transport of α-aminoisobutyric acid across brain capillary and cellular membranes. *J. Cereb. Blood Flow Metab.*, **3**, 8–32.

Brink, J. J. and Stein, D. G. (1967). Pemoline levels in brain: enhancement by dimethyl sulfoxide. *Science*, **158**, 1479–80.

Collins, J. M. and Dedrick, R. L. (1983). Distributed model for drug delivery to CSF and brain tissue. *Am. J. Physiol.*, **245**, R303–R310.

Crone, C. (1963). Permeability of capillaries in various organs as determined by use of the 'indicator diffusion' method. *Acta Physiol. Scand.*, **58**, 292–305.

Duffy, K. R. and Pardridge, W. M. (1987). Blood brain barrier transcytosis of human insulin in developing rabbits. *Brain Res.*, **420**, 32–8.

Fenstermacher, J. D., Blasberg, R. G. and Patlak, C. S. (1981). Methods for quantifying the transport of drugs across brain barrier systems. *Pharmacol. Ther.*, **14**, 217–48.

Fishman, J. B., Rubin, J. B., Handrahan, J. V., Connor, J. R. and Fine, R. E. (1987). Receptor mediated transcytosis of transferrin across the blood–brain barrier. *J. Neurosci. Res.*, **18**, 299–304

Gjedde, A., (1992) Blood brain glucose transfer. In *Physiology and Pharmacology of the Blood-Brain Barrier*, ed. M. W. B. Bradbury, pp. 65–115. Berlin: Springer.

Go, K. G. and Pratt, J. J. (1975). The dependence of the blood to brain passage of radioactive sodium on blood pressure and temperature. *Brain Res.*, **93**, 329–36.

Gutierrez, E. G., Banks, W. A. and Kastin, A. J. (1993). Murine tumor necrosis factor alpha is transported from blood to brain in the mouse. *J. Neuroimmunol.*, **47**, 169–76.

Hanig, J. P., Morrison, J. M. and Krop, S. (1972). Ethanol enhancement of blood–brain barrier permeability to catecholamines in chicks. *Eur. J. Pharmacol.*, **18**, 79–82.

Kang, Y. S., Bickel, U. and Pardridge, W. M. (1994). Pharmacokinetics and saturable blood–brain barrier transport of biotin bound to a conjugate of avidin and a monoclonal antibody to the transferrin receptor. *Drug Metab. Disp.*, **22**, 99–105.

Kang, Y. S., Boado, R. J. and Pardridge, W. M. (1995). Pharmacokinetics and organ clearance of a 3′-biotinylated, internally labeled phosphodiester oligodeoxynucleotide coupled to a neutral avidin/monoclonal antibody conjugate. *Drug Metab. Disp.*, **23**, 55–9.

Kety, S. S. (1951). The theory and applications of the exchange in inert gas at the lungs and tissues. *Pharmacol. Rev.*, **3**, 1–41.

Morris, C. M., Keith, A. B., Edwardson, J. A. and Pullen, R. G. L. (1992). Uptake and distribution of iron and transferrin in the adult rat brain. *J. Neurochem.*, **59**, 300–6.

Murphy, V. A., Wadhwani, K. C., Smith, Q. R. and Rapoport, S. I. (1991). Saturable transport of manganese(II) across the rat blood–brain barrier. *J. Neurochem.*, **57**, 948–54.

Ohno, K., Pettigrew, K. D. and Rapoport, S. I. (1978). Lower limits of cerebrovascular permeability to nonelectrolytes in the conscious rat. *Am. J. Physiol.*, **235**, H299–H307.

Pardridge, W. M. (1983). Brain metabolism: a perspective from the blood–brain barrier. *Physiol. Rev.*, **63**, 1481–535.

Pardridge, W. M., Triguero, D. and Buciak, J. L. (1990). β-endorphin chimeric peptides: transport through the blood–brain barrier *in vivo* and cleavage of disulfide linkage by brain. *Endocrinology*, **126**, 977–84.

Pardridge, W. M., Kang, Y. S. and Buciak, J. L. (1994). Transport of human recombinant brain-derived neurotrophic factor (BDNF) through the rat blood–brain barrier *in vivo* using vector-mediated peptide drug delivery. *Pharmaceut. Res.*, **11**, 738–45.

Pardridge, W. M., Kang, Y. S., Buciak, J. L. and Yang, J. (1995). Human insulin receptor monoclonal antibody undergoes high affinity binding to human brain capillaries in vitro and rapid transcytosis through the blood–brain barrier *in vivo* in the primate. *Pharmaceut. Res.*, **12**, 807–16.

Patlak, C. S. and Pettigrew, K. D. (1976). A method to obtain infusion schedules for prescribed blood concentration time courses. *J. Appl. Physiol.*, **40**, 458–63.

Patlak, C. S., Blasberg, R. G. and Fenstermacher, J. D. (1983). Graphical evaluation of blood-to-brain transfer constants from multiple-time uptake data. *J. Cereb. Blood Flow Metab.*, **3**, 1–7.

Rapoport, S. I., Fitzhugh, R., Pettigrew, K. D., Sundaram, U. and Ohno, K (1982). Drug entry into and distribution within brain and cerebrospinal fluid: [^{14}C]urea pharmacokinetics. *Am. J. Physiol.*, **242**, R339–R348.

Renkin, E. M. (1959). Transport of potassium-42 from blood to tissue in isolated mammalian skeletal muscles. *Am. J. Physiol.*, **197**, 1205–10.

Samii, A., Bickel, U., Stroth, U. and Pardridge, W. M. (1994). Blood–brain barrier transport of neuropeptides: analysis with a metabolically stable dermorphin analogue. *Am. J. Physiol.*, **267**, E124–E131.

Skarlatos, S., Yoshikawa, T. and Pardridge, W. M. (1995). Transport of [^{125}I]transferrin through the rat blood brain barrier. *Brain Res.*, **683**, 164–71.

Triguero, D., Buciak, J. L. and Pardridge, W. M. (1990) Capillary depletion method for quantification of blood–brain barrier transport of circulating peptides and plasma proteins. *J. Neurochem.*, **54**, 1882–8.

van Uitert, R. L., Sage, J. I., Levy, D. E. and Duffy, T. E. (1981). Comparison of radio-labeled butanol and iodoantipyrine as cerebral blood-flow markers. *Brain Res.*, **222**, 365–72.

6 Isolated brain capillaries: an *in vitro* model of blood–brain barrier research

WILLIAM M. PARDRIDGE

- Introduction
- Blood–brain barrier peptide receptors
- Blood–brain barrier nutrient transporters
- Pericyte-specific proteins
- Neurologic disorders and isolated human brain capillaries
- Brain capillary-specific proteins (BSPs)
- Summary

Introduction

The development of techniques for isolation of capillaries from either laboratory animal brain or human autopsy brain was an important event in the evolution of blood–brain barrier (BBB) methodologies. It was the availability of isolated capillaries that allowed BBB research to evolve from organ physiology to the cellular and molecular level. Bovine and human brain capillaries were initially isolated by Siakatos *et al.* (1969) and by several groups in the early and mid-1970s (Joo and Karnushina, 1973; Brendel *et al.*, 1974; Goldstein *et al.*, 1975). These methodologies uniformly used mechanical homogenization techniques and subsequent studies showed that capillaries isolated with mechanical homogenization methods did not exclude Trypan Blue and were metabolically leaky (Williams *et al.*, 1980). Although microvessels isolated with an enzymatic homogenization technique and which are not mechanically disturbed do generally exclude Trypan Blue, these microvessels are also metabolically impaired. The adenosine triphosphate (ATP) concentration in capillaries isolated from brain with either a mechanical or an enzymatic homogenization technique is decreased

more than 90% (Lasbennes and Gayet, 1984). The serious depletion of ATP in brain microvessels isolated with an enzymatic homogenization technique is a puzzling phenomenon since, in general, cells that are isolated with an enzymatic homogenization technique have normal ATP supplies (Kilberg, 1982). The reason for the ATP depletion in isolated brain capillaries is at present unknown and may be related to the abrupt physical separation between the endothelial cells and astrocytes that takes place when brain is homogenized.

Isolated brain capillaries are metabolically active. The microvessels concentrate potassium cations (Eisenberg and Suddith, 1979), and oxidize glucose (Goldstein *et al.*, 1977), and may be studied acutely for a variety of metabolic events, albeit with the caveat that these cells are ATP-depleted. As reviewed by Balabanov and Dore-Duffy (Chapter 39 in this volume), isolated microvessels may be incubated for periods up to 36 hours in tissue culture medium for the study of cytokine action. Isolated microvessels may be enzymatically disrupted into isolated endothelial cells and pericytes for growth in tissue culture (DeBault *et al.*, 1979; Bowman *et al.*, 1981). However, many BBB characteristics are lost in tissue culture, even in primary

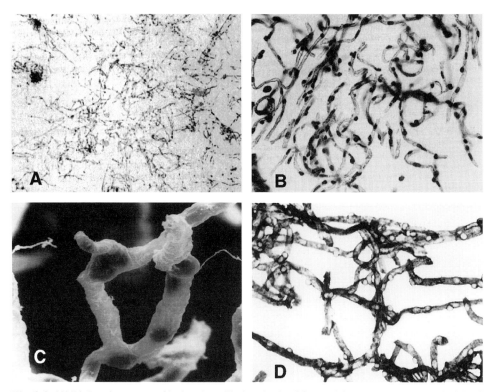

Fig 6.1. (A) Light microscopy of isolated capillaries obtained from 42 hour post-mortem rabbit brain. The capillaries are isolated in high yield as shown by this low-power magnification. (B) Light microscopy of isolated capillaries obtained from human autopsy brain. The capillaries are isolated in high yield (approximately 2 mg protein/10 g brain) and grossly free of adjoining brain tissue. The microvessels are comprised of endothelial cells, which line the interior lumen, and pericytes at an approximate 3:1 ratio. The cells are stained with *o*-Toluidine Blue. (C) Scanning electron micrograph of isolated bovine brain capillaries showing the vessels grossly free of adjoining brain tissue except an occasional nerve ending. (D) Human brain capillaries were cytospun to a glass slide and immuno-stained with an antibody to glial fibrillary acidic protein (GFAP). This pattern of immunostaining, which could be confused with immunostaining of an endothelial antigen, illustrates that microscopic remnants of astrocyte foot processes remain attached to the brain surface of the isolated brain microvessels. From Choi and Pardridge, 1986, with permission.

tissue culture, as the endothelial cells have lost the close intimate physical contact with astrocyte foot processes. The distance separating the astrocyte foot process and the ablumenal surface of the endothelial cell *in vivo* is only approximately 20 nm or 200 Å (Paulson and Newman, 1987), a space filled with the microvascular basement membrane.

Isolated brain capillaries are also referred to as isolated brain microvessels because these preparations invariably contain pre-capillary arterioles, which are comprised of endothelial cells and smooth muscle cells. In addition, the capillaries are comprised of pericytes, which have an abundance of approximately one-third that of the capillary endothelial cells. The ablumenal surface of isolated brain capillaries is also richly studded with remnants of astrocyte foot processes that remain adhered to the basement membrane of the capillary subsequent to the shear forces generated by the homogenization (White *et al.*, 1981). As shown in Fig. 6.1, isolated brain capillaries are immuno-stained with an antibody to glial fibrillary acidic protein (GFAP), which is due to the extensive astrocyte foot processes that remain attached to the capillary basement membrane surface. These astrocyte foot processes are not directly visible when the microvessels are stained with violet dyes and viewed with light microscopy. Isolated microvessels may also contain an occasional nerve ending that remains attached to the basement membrane surface of the capillary following the mechanical homogenization (Fig. 6.1). The measurement of cerebroside has been used as a biochemical measurement of possible neuronal contamination of isolated capillaries (Tsuji *et al.*, 1987).

Despite the reservations regarding the metabolic viability of freshly isolated brain capillaries, these structures may be regarded as intact membrane preparation and may be used for the biochemical analysis of a variety of BBB functions. Many of these biochemical functions remain intact in the isolated brain capillary preparation despite a period of up to 42 hours between death and isolation of the capillaries (Choi and Pardridge, 1986). In this regard, one of the most important applications of the isolated brain capillary is the biochemical analysis of the human BBB using capillaries isolated from human autopsy brain obtained from a variety of neurologic disorders, including Alzheimer's disease, multiple sclerosis, brain tumors, and other diseases.

Blood–brain barrier peptide receptors

Receptors may exist on the lumenal and ablumenal membranes of the brain capillary endothelial cells for the purposes of mediating signal transduction phenomena induced by either blood-borne or brain-derived peptides, or for the purposes of mediating the receptor-mediated transcytosis of circulating peptides through the BBB. Saturable binding to isolated human brain capillaries has been demonstrated for insulin, insulin-like growth factor (IGF)-1, IGF-2, transferrin, and leptin (Table 6.1). Affinity cross-linking studies have been used to demonstrate the molecular weight of the peptide binding receptor protein in human brain capillary plasma membranes (Pardridge *et al.*, 1985; Frank *et al.*, 1986*a*). Isolated human brain capillaries have also been used to characterize the binding of receptor-specific monoclonal antibodies (MAb) at the human BBB. MAb83-14 and MAb83-7, which are murine MAbs specific for the α-receptor

Table 6.1. *Peptide dissociation constant (K_D) and receptor binding capacity (B_{max}) for human brain capillary peptide receptors*

Peptide	K_D (nM)	B_{max} (pmol/mg$_p$)
Leptin	5.1±2.8	0.34±0.16
IGF-2	1.1±0.1	0.21±0.01
IGF-1	2.1±0.4	0.17±0.02
Insulin	1.2±0.5	0.17±0.08
Transferrin	5.6±1.4	0.10±0.02

From Pardridge *et al.*, 1985, 1987*a*; Duffy *et al.*, 1988; Golden *et al.*, 1997.
mg$_p$ is mg of protein.

of the human insulin receptor (Soos *et al.*, 1989), avidly bind to isolated human brain capillaries *in vitro* and undergo receptor-mediated transcytosis through the primate BBB *in vivo* (Pardridge *et al.*, 1995). Since receptor-mediated endocytosis is the first step in transcytosis through the BBB, the investigation of receptor-mediated endocytosis of peptides or receptor-specific MAbs with isolated human brain capillaries are viewed as a first step towards characterization of peptide or MAb transport systems at the BBB. Capillaries have also been isolated from brain of laboratory animals under pathophysiologic conditions. Streptozotocin-induced diabetes mellitus is associated with a downregulation of the rat brain capillary insulin receptor (Frank *et al.*, 1986*b*). If the BBB insulin receptor is a transport system, and if brain does not produce insulin, then one would predict a decrease in the brain/plasma ratio of insulin in streptozotocin diabetes mellitus and this observation has, in fact, been experimentally recorded (Frank *et al.*, 1986). Conversely, the BBB insulin receptor is upregulated in developing rabbits and the brain/plasma insulin ratio in this condition is proportionally increased (Frank *et al.*, 1985).

Polycationic proteins undergo absorptive-mediated endocytosis into isolated brain capillaries and this preparation has been used to quantify the absorptive-mediated endocytosis of cationized albumin, histone, cationized antibodies, and avidin (Kumagai *et al.*, 1987; Triguero *et al.*, 1989; Pardridge *et al.*, 1989*b*; Pardridge and Boado, 1991). In the case of protamine, isolated brain capillaries were used to demonstrate vectorial-mediated up-take of plasma proteins (albumin, globulins) by protamine owing to plasma protein binding to the polycationic protein, protamine (Pardridge *et al.*, 1993).

Blood–brain barrier nutrient transporters

Isolated brain capillaries have been used to characterize glucose transport into the endothelial cell. When glucose uptake is measured (Goldstein *et al.*, 1977), the determining uptake parameters are the combined actions of the plasma membrane glucose transporter and the intracellular phosphorylation mediated by hexokinase. When glucose uptake is limited by phosphorylation, as is the case with isolated brain capillaries, then the saturable binding kinetics of glucose uptake will appear as high affinity owing to the low K_M for the hexokinase reaction (Betz *et al.*, 1979). Therefore, when measuring transport of metabolic nutrients into isolated brain capillaries, it is essential to experimentally differentiate membrane transport from intracellular metabolism.

More than 90% of BBB glucose transport is mediated via the GLUT1 isoform of the sodium-independent glucose transporter gene superfamily and Western blotting with GLUT1-specific antibodies and isolated brain capillaries may be used to examine the biochemistry of the BBB GLUT1 glucose transporter (Fig. 6.2). Given the availability of human erythrocyte-purified GLUT1 protein as an assay standard, a quantitative Western blot may be established to determine the pmol/mg protein of immunoreactive GLUT1 in isolated brain capillaries (Fig. 6.2). Isolated brain capillaries may also be used in [^{3}H]-cytochalasin B radioreceptor assays to quantify the total number of glucose binding sites in plasma membranes of isolated brain capillaries (Fig. 6.2). These studies show there is no statistical difference between the total number of glucose transporters and the concentration of immunoreactive GLUT1 glucose transporter in isolated brain capillaries from either bovine or rabbit brain (Pardridge *et al.*, 1990*a*; Dwyer and Pardridge, 1993). Although these studies do not rule out the presence of other glucose

transporters in isolated brain capillaries, the studies in Fig. 6.2 do indicate that more than 90% of BBB glucose transport under normal conditions is mediated via the GLUT1 isoform. Isolated brain capillaries may also be used for purification of poly(A) mRNA from these structures and Northern blotting for quantification of the GLUT1 glucose transporter mRNA (Boado and Pardridge, 1990). Initial studies showed that the concentration of the GLUT1 mRNA was enriched in isolated brain capillaries as compared to whole brain (Flier *et al.*, 1987). However, subsequent quantitative studies showed that essentially all of the brain GLUT1 mRNA could be traced to a brain capillary origin (Pardridge *et al.*, 1990*a*; Boado and Pardridge, 1990). For example, the GLUT1/actin ratio in isolated brain capillaries is 20 times greater than the corresponding ratio in total brain homogenate (Boado and Pardridge, 1990; Dwyer and Pardridge, 1993), suggesting that more than 95% of brain GLUT1 mRNA is derived from the capillaries. Brain homogenate may be depleted of brain capillaries and when Northern blotting studies are performed on RNA derived from the post-capillary supernatant, no detectable GLUT1 transcript is experimentally observed (Boado and Pardridge, 1990; Dwyer and Pardridge, 1993). *In situ* hybridization studies also fail to document in normal brain GLUT1 mRNA in parenchymal areas of brain other than the capillary structures (Pardridge *et al.*, 1990). Although the GLUT1 isoform was originally termed the rat brain glucose transporter (Birnbaum *et al.*, 1986), these studies demonstrate that the GLUT1 isoform is confined to the capillary endothelium in brain. The GLUT3 isoform mediates glucose transport into neurons (Nagamatsu *et al.*, 1992), and the glucose transporter isoform mediating sugar uptake into glial cells *in vivo* is not clearly defined.

Isolated brain capillaries have also been used to characterize amino acid transport at the BBB *in vitro*. These studies show there is no statistical difference in the kinetic parameters of phenylalanine transport in isolated brain capillaries obtained from rabbits following either 0 or 42 post-mortem hours between expiration and isolation of the capillaries (Choi and Pardridge, 1986). There was also no discernible difference between the molecular sizes of proteins comprising rabbit brain capillaries

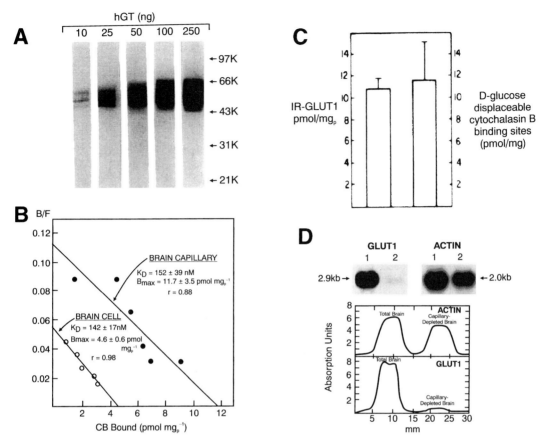

Fig 6.2. (A) Purified human erythrocyte glucose transporter (hGT) was applied to SDS-PAGE wells in amounts of 10–250 ng/well and the blotted membranes were reacted with a 1:500 dilution of rabbit polyclonal antiserum directed against a synthetic peptide encoding the 13 amino acids of the carboxyl terminus of the GLUT1 protein, which migrates with an average molecular weight of 52 kDa. These data establish a standard curve for quantitative Western blotting and for determination of the concentration of the immunoreactive GLUT1 in bovine brain capillary plasma membranes. (B) [³H]-cytochalasin B (CB) Scatchard plot is graphed by plotting the bound/free (B/F) ratio versus the amount of D-glucose-displaceable [³H]-cytochalasin B-bound when either capillary-depleted brain cell or brain capillary membranes are incubated with varying concentrations of unlabeled cytochalasin B. The dissociation constant (K_D) and the number of binding sites (B_{max}) were computed by nonlinear regression analysis. (C) The concentration of immunoreactive GLUT1 and the total concentration of D-glucose transporter sites in bovine brain microvessel membranes is not significantly different. (D) Removal of GLUT1 poly(A)⁺ mRNA transcript from rabbit brain homogenate by capillary depletion: 10 μg per lane of RNA from total brain (lane 1) and from capillary-depleted brain (lane 2) were probed with GLUT1 and actin cDNAs labeled with ³²P. The data show greater than 95% depletion of the GLUT1 transcript in the capillary-depleted brain, which still gives a normal signal for actin. (From Pardridge *et al.*, 1990a; Dwyer and Pardridge, 1993; with permission from The American Society for Biochemistry & Molecular Biology and the Endocrine Society, respectively.)

isolated from brain subjected to either 0 or 42 hours of post-mortem autolysis time (4 °C). Given the preservation of the amino acid transport characteristics with isolated brain capillaries despite autolysis time up to 42 hours, subsequent studies were performed with capillaries isolated from human autopsy brain with autolysis times ranging from 28 to 45 hours (Choi and Pardridge, 1986;

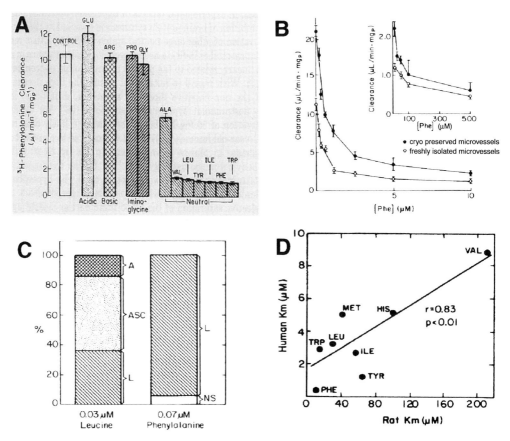

Fig. 6.3. Neutral amino acid transport into isolated human brain capillaries. (A) Competition of [³H]-phenylalanine uptake by human brain capillaries is marked for large neutral amino acids, minimal for small neutral amino acids (alanine), and immeasurable for iminoglycine (proline, glycine), acidic (glutamate), or basic (arginine) amino acids (Choi and Pardridge, 1986). Amino acids were present individually at concentrations of 50 μM. Abbreviations used: GLU, glutamate; ARG, arginine; PRO, proline; GLY, glycine; ALA, alanine; VAL, valine; LEU, leucine; TYR, tyrosine; ILE, isoleucine; PHE, phenylalanine; TRP, tryptophan. (B) Clearance of phenylalanine in freshly isolated and cryo-preserved human brain microvessels isolated from the same brain. Incubations were performed at room temperature for 2 mins in the presence of 0.4 μCi/ml [¹⁴C]-sucrose and 2.0 μCi/ml of [³H]-phenylalanine. Each point represents the mean ± SE (of three replicates). The data show saturation through both a high affinity and low affinity component. (C) Characterization of leucine and phenylalanine transport by different amino acid transporters in isolated human brain capillaries. Clearance data are expressed as percentage of total transport by the A (alanine)-preferring system, ASC (alanine, serine, cysteine)-preferring system, and the L(leucine)-preferring system. Nonsaturable transporter is designated as NS. The A-system is sodium-dependent and NMAIB-sensitive; the ASC-system is sodium dependent and NMAIB-insensitive; the L-system is sodium independent and BCH-sensitive, where BCH is 2-aminobicyclo[2.2.1] heptane-2-carboxylic acid, and NMAIB is ɴ-methylaminoisobutaric acid. (D) Comparison of human brain capillary K_m measured *in vitro* (Hargreaves and Pardridge, 1988) and rat brain capillary K_m measured *in vivo* (Smith *et al.*, 1987).

Hargreaves and Pardridge, 1988). The uptake of phenylalanine by isolated human brain capillaries was not inhibited by acidic amino acids (glutamate), basic amino acids (arginine), iminoglycine amino acids (proline, glycine), but was inhibited modestly by small neutral amino acids (alanine), and greatly by large neutral amino acids (Fig. 6.3). The effects of sodium depletion or transporter isoform-specific inhibitors was tested for leucine and phenylalanine with isolated human brain capillaries, and these studies demonstrate that virtually all of phenylalanine transport was mediated via the leucine (L)-preferring system, whereas leucine uptake in isolated human brain capillaries was mediated via the L-system, the A-system, and the ASC-system, where A is alanine-preferring system, and ASC is alanine/serine/cysteine-preferring systems (Fig. 6.3). The A- and ASC-systems are concentrative amino acid transport systems and are presumably localized on the ablumenal membrane of the brain capillary endothelial cell (Betz and Goldstein, 1978), whereas the L-system is an equilibrative transport system that is presumably expressed on both lumenal and ablumenal membranes. The K_M of amino acid transport into isolated human brain capillaries *in vitro* correlates with the K_M of amino acid transport through the rat BBB *in vivo* (Fig. 6.3). However, the *in vitro* K_M is 8- to 40-fold lower than the corresponding K_M value for the rat BBB *in vivo*. The finding that the affinity of the transporter for the large neutral amino acids *in vitro* in isolated brain capillaries is much higher (lower K_M) than that found *in vivo* is a puzzling observation that has thus far not been explained. Amino acid transport into isolated brain capillaries reflects the simultaneous action of transporters at both the lumenal and ablumenal membranes. This is because the capillaries are patent, and there is rapid equilibration of medium solute with the lumenal compartment in *in vitro* incubations. Thus, the complexity of amino acid transport through the BBB *in vivo* may be much greater than that represented by a single membrane model traditionally used in *in vivo* studies.

Pericyte-specific proteins

The permeability barrier, *per se*, is comprised of the brain capillary endothelium. However, the brain capillary is comprised of two cells, the endothelial cell and the pericyte, which share a common basement membrane. The pericyte sits across the ablumenal membrane of the endothelial cell and sends out finger-like cytoplasmic projections that form circumferential belts around the microvessel (Inokuchi *et al.*, 1989). In light microscopic examination of isolated brain capillaries, one sees a pericyte nucleus between every three to four endothelial nuclei. The pericyte has been described to have either a contractile function (Joyce *et al.*, 1984) or a phagocytic function (van Deurs, 1976). If the pericyte has a contractile function and is indeed the smooth muscle analogue of the capillary, then this cell should normally express α-actin, the smooth muscle-specific actin isoform. Pericytes grown in tissue culture express α-actin (Herman and D'Amore, 1985). However, to date, there is no evidence that pericytes in brain *in vivo* express α-actin. This can be shown using isolated brain capillaries cytospun to a glass slide and immunostained with α-actin-specific antibodies (Fig. 6.4). These studies show the actin MAb avidly decorates pre-arteriole smooth muscle cells, but does not stain capillary pericytes (Boado and Pardridge, 1994). Although capillary pericyte α-actin may be induced in pathophysiologic states, this has to date not been demonstrated *in vivo*.

Pericytes have also been regarded as phagocytic cells and are a potential site of antigen presentation in brain. Antigen presentation is mediated by the class II histocompatability antigen, also termed the DR-antigen. Immunocytochemical studies of brain sections with antibodies specific for the DR-antigen have localized DR-immunoreactivity to brain microvessels (Kohsaka *et al.*, 1989). On this basis, it has been assumed that antigen presentation may occur at the lumenal surface of the endothelial cell in brain *in vivo*. However, using immunocytochemistry and tissue sections of brain, it is not possible to differentiate microvascular endothelial cells from pericytes. Conversely, the differentiation of these two cells is easily made using isolated brain capillaries and immunocytochemistry. As shown in Fig. 6.4, there is abundant expression of immunoreactive DR-antigen in smooth muscle cells of pre-capillary arterioles in control brain and no immunoreactive DR-antigen is identifiable at the capillary pericyte level (Pardridge *et al.*, 1989c). Conversely, in microvessels isolated from multiple sclerosis (MS) brain, immunoreactive DR-antigen is abundant in pericytes (Fig. 6.4). These studies showing DR-antigen on smooth muscle cells and pericytes indicate antigen presentation in brain occurs largely on the brain side of the BBB.

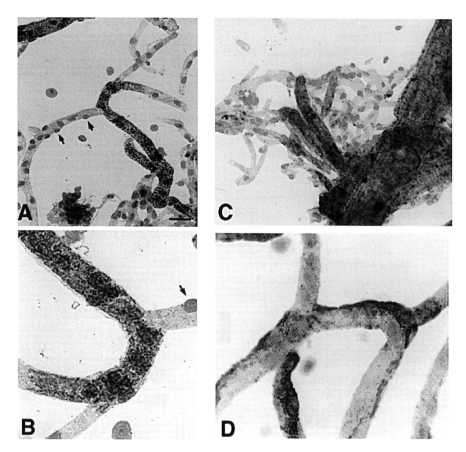

Fig. 6.4. Avidin–biotin immunoperoxidase histochemistry showing immunostaining of actin (A,B) and DR-antigen (C,D) in isolated bovine brain and human brain capillaries, respectively. In panels A and B, bovine brain capillaries were reacted with a mouse monoclonal antibody directed against smooth muscle α-actin. No immunoreactive smooth muscle α-actin is detected in either endothelial cells or capillary pericytes but immunoreactive α-actin is abundant in precapillary arteriolar smooth muscle cells. From Boado and Pardridge (1994). Human brain microvessels were immunostained with a mouse monoclonal antibody to the human DR-antigen and these studies show abundant DR-immunoreactivity in precapillary arteriolar smooth muscle cells in capillaries isolated from control brain (C) and in capillary pericytes in microvessels isolated from multiple sclerosis brain (D). From Pardridge *et al.* (1989c), reprinted by permission of Wiley-Liss, Inc., a subsidiary of John Wiley & Sons, Inc.

Neurologic disorders and isolated human brain capillaries

The capillary vascular interface of brain is the site of pathogenesis of many neurologic diseases, including Alzheimer's disease, MS, infectious diseases, brain tumors, and multiple other conditions. A puzzling phenomenon in neurologic research is that the isolated human brain capillary has not

been used as a model system to an extent greater than what has heretofore taken place. The studies in Fig. 6.4 show that the isolation of microvessels from MS plaque tissue leads to the unequivocal localization of DR-antigen immunoreactivity to pericytes of capillaries in this condition (Pardridge *et al.*, 1989c). This suggests that antigen presentation occurs distal to the BBB in MS and that activated lymphocytes must first undergo transport through the endothelial cell in order to present

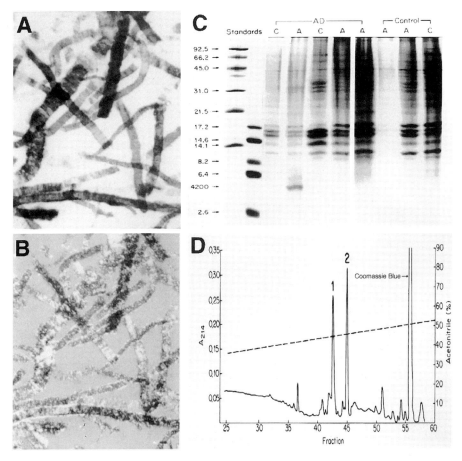

Fig. 6.5. Cerebrocortical arterioles were isolated from a patient with Alzheimer's disease and amyloid angiopathy, fixed to a glass slide, and stained with 0.05% Congo Red (A), and viewed under polarized light. Apple-green birefringence characteristic of amyloid is found (B). The microvessels were solubilized in formic acid and subjected to urea/SDS-PAGE and the gel was stained (C). The arterioles shown in panel A contained a 4200 Da peptide that was detected in lane 4 by Coomassie Blue staining and this peptide was eluted from the gel and subjected to reverse phase HPLC purification (D). The HPLC analysis showed the 4200 Da peptide eluted as two peaks and both peaks had identical amino acid composition analysis. From Pardridge *et al.* (1987*b*), with permission.

antigen in brain. Another important neurologic condition is Alzheimer's disease and this disorder is associated with the deposition of amyloid in brain comprising vascular amyloid plaques and neuritic (senile) plaques. Electron microscopic studies suggest that this amyloid is produced at the capillary level by pericytes and/or smooth muscle cells (Wisniewski *et al.*, 1992). Thus, the cells comprising the important loci of amyloid production in human brain (i.e., microvascular smooth muscle cells and pericytes) are directly amenable to experimental isolation by initially isolating capillaries

from human Alzheimer's disease (AD) brain. AD brain microvessels may be easily isolated and demonstrate apple green birefringence when stained with Congo Red and visualized under polarized light (Fig. 6.5). The microvessels may be subsequently solubilized in formic acid, and separated on urea–sodium dodecyl sulfate polyacrylamide gel electrophoresis (SDS-PAGE). This approach allows for the isolation of the 4200 dalton Aβ-amyloidotic peptide of Alzheimer's disease (Fig. 6.5). Following elution from the urea/SDS-PAGE gel and HPLC purification (Fig. 6.5), the Aβ-peptide may be subjected to microsequence analysis and amino acid composition analysis (Pardridge *et al.*, 1987*b*). The Aβ-amyloid isolated from cortical microvessels, from meningeal microvessels, and from neuritic plaque all contain one threonine residue, indicating the Aβ-peptide comprising amyloid is composed of 43 amino acids, since the lone threonine residue in the Aβ-peptide is at the 43 position.

Brain capillary-specific proteins (BSPs)

Isolated capillaries may also be used to identify proteins that are specific for the brain capillary endothelium that are not produced in other cells in brain. Isolated bovine brain capillaries were converted to a plasma membrane preparation using the method of Lidinsky and Drewes (1983), and these plasma membranes were injected into rabbits for the production of polyclonal antisera (Pardridge *et al.*, 1986). These antisera react with multiple organs in immunocytochemistry. However, when the anti-brain capillary antiserum is pre-absorbed with acetone powders of rat liver and rat kidney, the multi-organ immunoreactivity is removed and the absorbed antiserum reacts only with brain capillary endothelial cells in brain and also reacts with the basolateral membrane of choroid plexus epithelium (Fig. 6.6). Western analyses show the anti-BSP antiserum reacts with a triplet of proteins with molecular weight of 200, 53, and 45 kDa (Pardridge *et al.*, 1990*b*). Although the 200 kDa protein is detected on Western immunoblot analysis in bovine choroid plexus, the 53 and 45 kDa proteins are specific to brain microvessels (Pardridge *et al.*, 1990*b*). Electron microscopic immunogold analysis of the BSP localization in the brain capillary endothelium shows the antigen is distributed to both lumenal and ablumenal membranes in the endothelial cell (Fig. 6.6). The 53 and 45 kDa proteins identified on Western immunoblot analysis are visualized as a single protein with molecular weight of 46 kDa when isolated brain capillary plasma membranes are iodinated and immunoprecipitated with anti-BSP antiserum (Pardridge *et al.*, 1986). A major protein identified on Coomassie Blue staining of isolated brain capillary plasma membranes also

has a molecular weight of 45 to 46 kDa and microsequence analysis demonstrated this protein is actin (Pardridge *et al.*, 1989*a*), an abundant protein found in all cells. However, the immunoreactive 46 kDa BSP is distinct from actin. The anti-BSP antiserum does not stain cells other than brain capillary endothelium or choroid plexus, although these cells are abundant in actin and the actin-BSP antiserum does not label actin on Western blotting (Pardridge *et al.*, 1990*b*). The specificity of the anti-BSP antiserum is demonstrated by the fact that capillary depleted brain cell membranes are not immunoreactive with this antiserum (Pardridge *et al.*, 1986). The function of BSPs, such as the 45 and 53 kDa proteins is at present not known, but may be elucidated with subsequent molecular cloning studies of the cDNAs encoding these proteins. Other examples of brain capillary-specific surface antigens are reviewed by Schlosshauer in this volume (Chapter 34).

Summary

In conclusion, the isolation of capillaries from brains of either experimental animals or human autopsy or neurosurgical specimens is a powerful approach to extending BBB research to the molecular and cellular level. Isolated capillaries may be cryo-preserved for subsequent studies; may be cytospun to glass slides for immunocytochemistry of the capillary endothelial cells, smooth muscle cells and pericytes; may be disrupted for the purposes of preparing BBB plasma membrane fractions; may be enzymatically disrupted into isolated endothelial cells and pericytes for growth in primary tissue culture; or may be injected into rabbits or mice for preparation of anti-BBB antisera. In particular, capillaries may be isolated from human autopsy brain in a variety of neuropathologic conditions and this approach has thus far been under-utilized in the neurosciences.

Acknowledgments

Emily Yu skillfully prepared the manuscript. This research was supported by NIH grant P01-NS25554.

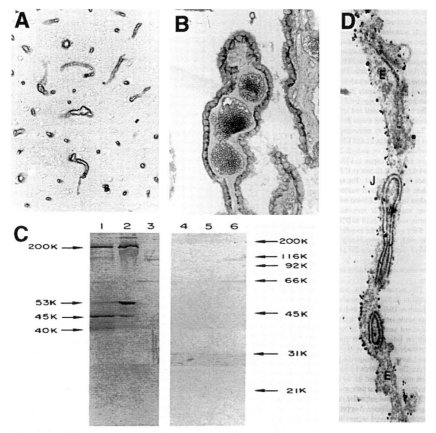

Fig. 6.6. (A) Light microscopic immunoperoxidase studies showing reactivity of the anti-BSP antiserum with brain microvasculature but no reaction with neuropil (BSP is brain capillary specific protein). (B) The anti-BSP antiserum does not react with choroid plexus microvasculature but does react with the basolateral membrane of choroid plexus epithelium (Pardridge *et al.*, 1990*b*). (C) Western immunoblotting with a 1 : 2000 dilution of anti-BSP antiserum (lanes 1–3) and pre-immune serum (lanes 4–6). The antigen sources in these blots are cryopreserved isolated bovine brain capillaries (lanes 1,4), freshly isolated bovine brain capillaries (lanes 2,5), and capillary-depleted bovine brain cell membranes (lanes 3,6). Although the 200 kDa protein is preserved in cultured bovine brain capillary endothelium, there is minimal expression of the immunoreactive 45- and 53-kDa proteins in tissue culture. (D) Electron microscopic immunogold silver staining (IGSS) is performed on isolated bovine brain microvessels with the anti-BSP antiserum. The secondary antibody used in these studies is a 1 : 50 dilution of a goat anti-rabbit antiserum conjugated with 1 nm gold particles, which were subsequently enhanced with silver staining. The study shows immunostaining of both lumenal and ablumenal surfaces as well as the tight junctional (J) region between endothelial (E) cells. Light aldehyde fixation was used to preserve immunogenicity. From Farrell and Pardridge (1991), with kind permission of Elsevier Science – NL, Sara Burgerhartstraat 25, 1055 KV Amsterdam, The Netherlands.

References

Betz, A. L. and Goldstein, G. W. (1978). Polarity of the blood–brain barrier: neutral amino acid transport into isolated brain capillaries. *Science*, **202**, 225–7.

Betz, A. L., Csejtey, J. and Goldstein, G. W. (1979). Hexose transport and phosphorylation by capillaries isolated from rat brain. *Am. J. Physiol.*, **236**, C96–C102.

Birnbaum, M. J., Haspel, H. C. and Rosen, O. M. (1986). Cloning and characterization of a cDNA encoding the rat brain glucose-transporter protein. *Proc. Natl. Acad. Sci. USA*, **83**, 5784–8.

Boado, R. J. and Pardridge, W. M. (1990). The brain-type glucose transporter mRNA is specifically expressed at the blood–brain barrier. *Biochem. Biophys. Res. Comm.*, **166**, 174–9.

Boado, R. J. and Pardridge, W. M. (1994). Differential expression of α-actin mRNA and immunoreactive protein in brain microvascular pericytes and smooth muscle cells. *J. Neurosci. Res.*, **39**, 430–5.

Bowman, P. D., Betz, A. L., Ar, D., Wolinsky, J. S., Penney, J. B., Shivers, R. R. and Goldstein, G. W. (1981). Primary culture of capillary endothelium from rat brain. *In Vitro*, **17**, 353–62.

Brendel, K., Meezan, E. and Carlson, E. C. (1974). Isolated brain microvessels: a purified, metabolically active preparation from bovine cerebral cortex. *Science*, **185**, 953–5.

Choi, T. and Pardridge, W. M. (1986). Phenylalanine transport at the human blood–brain barrier. Studies in isolated human brain capillaries. *J. Biol. Chem.*, **261**, 6536–41.

DeBault, L. E., Kahn, L. E., Frommes, S. P. and Cancilla, P. A. (1979). Cerebral microvessels and derived cells in tissue culture: isolation and preliminary characterization. *In Vitro*, **7**, 473–87.

Duffy, K. R., Pardridge, W. M. and Rosenfeld, R. G. (1988). Human blood–brain barrier insulin-like growth factor receptor. *Metabolism*, **37**, 136–40.

Dwyer, K. J. and Pardridge, W. M. (1993). Developmental modulation of blood–brain barrier and choroid plexus GLUT1 glucose transporter mRNA and immunoreactive protein in rabbits. *Endocrinology*, **132**, 558–65.

Eisenberg, H. M. and Suddith, R. L. (1979). Cerebral vessels have the capacity to transport sodium and potassium. *Science*, **206**, 1083–5.

Farrell, C. L. and Pardridge, W. M. (1991). Ultrastructural localization of blood–brain barrier-specific antibodies using immunogold-silver enhancement techniques. *J. Neurosci. Meth.*, **37**,103–10.

Flier, J. S., Mueckler, M., McCall, A. L. and Lodish, H. F. (1987). Distribution of glucose transporter messenger RNA transcripts in tissues of rat and man. *J. Clin. Invest.*, **79**, 657–61.

Frank, H. J. L., Jankovic-Vokes, T., Pardridge, W. M. and Morris, W. L. (1985). Enhanced insulin binding to blood–brain barrier in vivo and to brain microvessels in vitro in newborn rabbits. *Diabetes*, **34**, 728–33.

Frank, H. J. L., Pardridge, W. M., Morris, W. L., Rosenfeld, R. G. and Choi, T. B. (1986*a*). Binding and internalization of insulin and insulin-like growth factors by isolated brain microvessels. *Diabetes*, **35**, 654–61.

Frank, H. J. L., Pardridge, W. M., Jankovic-Vokes, T., Vinters, H. V. and Morris, W. L. (1986*b*). Insulin binding to the blood–brain barrier in the streptozotocin diabetic rat. *J. Neurochem.*, **47**, 405–11.

Golden, P. L., Maccagnan, T. J. and Pardridge, W. M. (1997). Human blood–brain barrier leptin receptor. Binding and endocytosis in isolated human brain microvessels. *J. Clin. Invest.*, **99**, 14–18.

Goldstein, G. W., Wolinsky, J. S., Csejtey, J. and Diamond, I. (1975). Short communication: isolation of metabolically active capillaries from rat brain. *J. Neurochem.*, **25**, 715–17.

Goldstein, G. W., Csejtey, J. and Diamond, I. (1977). Carrier mediated glucose transport in capillaries isolated from rat brain. *J. Neurochem.*, **28**, 725–8.

Hargreaves, K. M. and Pardridge, W. M. (1988). Neutral amino acid transport at the human blood–brain barrier. *J. Biol. Chem.*, **263**, 19392–7.

Herman, I. M. and D'Amore, P. A. (1985). Microvascular pericytes contain muscle and nonmuscle actins. *J. Cell Biol.*, **101**, 43–52.

Inokuchi, T., Yokoyama, R., Satoh, H., Hamasaki, M. and Higashi, R. (1989). Scanning electron microscopic study of periendothelial cells of the rat cerebral vessels revealed by a combined method of corrosion casting and KOH digestion. *J. Elect. Microsc.*, **38**, 201–13.

Joo, F. and Karnushina, I. (1973). A procedure for the isolation of capillaries from rat brain. *Cytobios*, **8**, 41–8.

Joyce, N. C., DeCamilli, P. and Boyles, J. (1984). Pericytes, like vascular smooth muscle cells, are immunocytochemically positive for cyclic GMP-dependent protein kinase. *Microvasc. Res.*, **28**, 206–19.

Kilberg, M. S. (1982). Amino acid transport in isolated rat hepatocytes. *J. Memb. Biol.*, **69**, 1–12.

Kohsaka, S., Shinozaki, T., Nakano, Y., Takei, K., Toya, S. and Tsukada, Y. (1989). Expression of Ia antigen on vascular endothelial cells in mouse cerebral tissue grafted into the third ventricle of rat brain. *Brain Res.*, **484**, 340–7.

Kumagai, A. K., Eisenberg, J. and Pardridge, W. M. (1987). Absorptive-mediated endocytosis of cationized albumin and a β-endorphin-cationized albumin chimeric peptide by isolated brain capillaries. Model system of blood–brain barrier transport. *J. Biol. Chem.*, **262**, 15214–19.

Lasbennes, F. and Gayet, J. (1984). Capacity for energy metabolism in microvessels isolated from rat brain. *Neurochem. Res.*, **9**, 1–9.

Lidinsky, W. A. and Drewes, L. R. (1983). Characterization of the blood–brain barrier: protein composition of the capillary endothelial cell membrane. *J. Neurochem.*, **41**, 1341–8.

Nagamatsu, S., Kornhauser, J. M., Burant, C. F., Seino, S., Mayo, K. E. and Bell, G. I. (1992). Glucose transporter expression in brain. *J. Biol. Chem.*, **267**, 467–72.

Pardridge, W. M. and Boado, R. J. (1991). Enhanced cellular uptake of biotinylated antisense oligonucleotide or peptide mediated by avidin, a cationic protein. *FEBS Lett.*, **288**, 30–2.

Pardridge, W. M., Eisenberg, J. and Yang, J. (1985). Human blood–brain barrier insulin receptor. *J. Neurochem.*, **44**, 1771–8.

Pardridge, W. M., Yang, J., Eisenberg, J. and Mietus, L. J. (1986). Antibodies to blood–brain barrier bind selectively to brain capillary endothelial lateral membranes and to a 46 K protein. *J. Cereb. Blood Flow Metab.*, **6**, 203–11.

Pardridge, W. M., Eisenberg, J. and Yang, J. (1987*a*). Human blood–brain barrier transferrin receptor. *Metabolism*, **36**, 892–5.

Pardridge, W. M., Vinters, H. V., Yang, J., Eisenberg, J., Choi, T., Tourtellotte, W. W., Huebner, V. and Shively, J. E. (1987*b*). Amyloid angiopathy of Alzheimer's disease: amino acid composition and partial sequence of a 4200 dalton peptide isolated from cortical microvessels. *J. Neurochem.*, **49**, 1394–401.

Pardridge, W. M., Nowlin, D. M., Choi, T. B., Yang, J., Calaycay, J. and Shively, J. E. (1989*a*). Brain capillary 46 K protein is cytoplasmic actin and is localized to endothelial plasma membrane. *J. Cereb. Blood Flow Metab.*, **9**, 675–80.

Pardridge, W. M., Triguero, D. and Buciak, J. B. (1989*b*). Transport of histone through the blood–brain barrier. *J. Pharmacol. Exp. Ther.*, **251**, 821–26.

Pardridge, W. M., Yang, J., Buciak, J. and Tourtellotte, W. W. (1989*c*). Human brain microvascular DR antigen. *J. Neurosci. Res.*, **23**, 337–41.

Pardridge, W. M., Boado, R. J. and Farrell, C. R. (1990*a*). Brain-type glucose transporter (GLUT-1) is selectively localized to the blood–brain barrier. Studies with quantitative Western blotting and in situ hybridization. *J. Biol. Chem.*, **265**, 18035–40.

Pardridge, W. M., Yang, J., Buciak, J. L. and Boado, R. J. (1990*b*). Differential expression of 53 kDa and 45 kDa brain capillary-specific proteins by brain capillary endothelium and choroid plexus in vivo and by brain capillary endothelium in tissue culture. *Molec. Cell Neurosci.*, **1**, 20–8.

Pardridge, W. M., Buciak, J. L., Kang, Y.-S. and Boado, R. J. (1993). Protamine-mediated transport of albumin into brain and other organs in the rat. Binding and endocytosis of protamine-albumin complex by microvascular endothelium. *J. Clin. Invest.*, **92**, 2224–9.

Pardridge, W. M., Kang, Y. -S., Buciak, J. L. and Yang, J. (1995). Human insulin receptor monoclonal antibody undergoes high affinity binding to human brain capillaries in vitro and rapid transcytosis through the blood–brain barrier in vivo in the primate. *Pharmaceut. Res.*, **12**, 807–16.

Paulson, O. B and Newman, E. A. (1987). Does the release of potassium from astrocyte endfeet regulate cerebral blood flow? *Science*, **237**, 896–8.

Siakotos, A. N., Rouser, G. and Fleischer, S. (1969). Isolation of highly purified human and bovine brain endothelial cells and nuclei and their phospholipid composition. *Lipids*, **4**, 234–42.

Smith, Q. R., Momma, S., Aoyagi, M. and Rapoport, S. I. (1987). Kinetics of neutral amino acid transport across the blood–brain barrier. *J. Neurochem.*, **49**, 1651–8.

Soos, M. A., O'Brien, R. M., Brindle, N. P., Stigter, J. M., Okamoto, A. K., Whittaker, J. and Siddle, K. (1989). Monoclonal antibodies to the insulin receptor mimic metabolic effects of insulin but do not stimulate receptor autophosphorylation in transfected NIH 3T3 fibroblasts. *Proc. Natl. Acad. Sci. USA*, **86**, 5217–21.

Triguero, D., Buciak, J. B., Yang, J. and Pardridge, W. M. (1989). Blood–brain barrier transport of cationized immunoglobulin G. Enhanced delivery compared to native protein. *Proc. Natl. Acad. Sci. USA*, **86**, 4761–5.

Tsuji, T., Mimori, Y., Nakamura, S. and Kameyama, M. (1987). A micromethod of the isolation of large and small microvessels from frozen autopsied human brain. *J. Neurochem.*, **49**, 1796–800.

Van Deurs, B. (1976). Observations on the blood–brain barrier in hypertensive rats, with particular reference to phagocytic pericytes. *J. Ultrastruc. Res.*, **56**, 65–77.

White, F. P., Dutton, G. R. and Norenberg, M. D. (1981). Microvessels isolated from rat brain: localization of astrocyte processes by immunohisto-chemical techniques. *J. Neurochem.*, **36**, 328–32.

Williams, S. K., Gillis, J. F., Matthews, M. A., Wager, R. C. and Bitensky, M. W. (1980). Isolation and characteri-zation of brain endothelial cells: morphology and enzyme activity. *J. Neurochem.*, **35**, 374–81.

Wisniewski, H. M., Wegiel, J., Wang, K. C. and Lach, B. (1992). Ultra-structural studies of the cells forming amyloid in the cortical vessel wall in Alzheimer's disease. *Acta Neuropathol.*, **83**, 117–27.

7

Isolation and behavior of plasma membrane vesicles made from cerebral capillary endothelial cells

DARRYL R. PETERSON and RICHARD A. HAWKINS

- Introduction
- Isolation of luminal and abluminal plasma membrane vesicles from the blood–brain barrier
- Markers to identify luminal and abluminal membrane domains
- Measuring transport and enzymatic activities in luminal and abluminal membrane vesicles
- Transport studies
- Concluding remarks

Introduction

The endothelial cells of cerebral capillaries are joined by tight junctions that impede paracellular movement of solutes. Therefore, nutrients and ions must be transported across the respective luminal (blood-facing) and abluminal (brain-facing) plasma membranes (Brightman and Reese, 1969; Pardridge, 1983). These membranes are structurally and functionally different, resulting in a polarized configuration typical of epithelial cells (Betz and Goldstein, 1978; Betz et al., 1980). Such an arrangement favors net unidirectional transport of certain solutes across the barrier, and implies that transendothelial flux is a balance of events occurring at each membrane domain (Ennis et al., 1996). Clearly, the properties of both membranes must be defined and distinguished to characterize the blood–brain barrier properly. A technique is herein described for the isolation of enriched luminal and abluminal plasma membranes. Because these membranes spontaneously form tightly sealed vesicles, they can be used to study the transport and enzymatic properties of each side of the blood–brain barrier separately.

Isolation of luminal and abluminal plasma membrane vesicles from the blood–brain barrier

Plasma membrane vesicles from bovine cerebral capillary endothelial cells are isolated in two stages. During the first phase, brain microvessels are isolated as described by Pardridge in Chapter 6. In the second phase, the endothelial cells are broken by further homogenization, and the individual membrane domains are separated on a discontinuous Ficoll gradient. The luminal and abluminal membrane vesicles are identified by assaying for specific markers.

Luminal and abluminal plasma membrane vesicles are derived from the brain microvessels by homogenizing them and separating the freed membranes on a discontinuous Ficoll gradient. The steps are shown in Fig. 7.1. Approximately 18–24 g of frozen microvessels are thawed at room temperature. The thawed microvessels are centrifuged at $2000 \times g$ for 4 min (4 °C), after which the pellets are resuspended in cold TSEM buffer (10 mM Tris–HCl, pH 7.4, 250 mM sucrose, 0.1 mM EGTA, 0.5 mM $MgCl_2$) and recentrifuged.

Brain Capillaries (18–24 g)

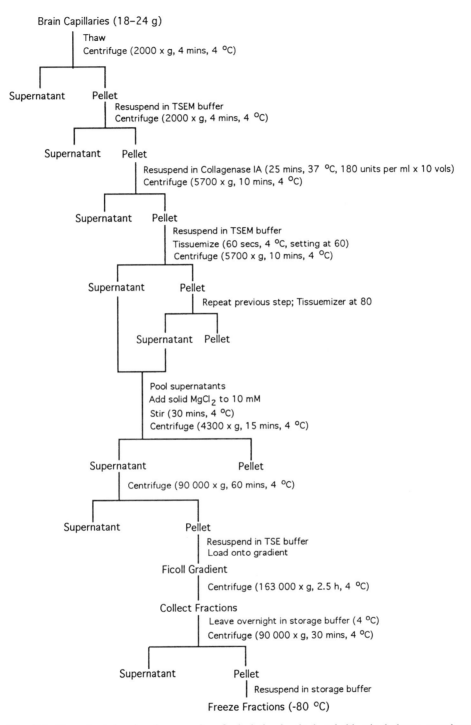

Fig. 7.1. Flow-chart showing the procedure for isolating luminal and abluminal plasma membrane vesicles from bovine capillary endothelial cells forming the blood–brain barrier.

The basement membrane, astrocytic end-feet, pericytes and other cellular contaminants that may be associated with microvessels are removed by treatment with collagenase (Sanchez del Pino *et al.*, 1995*a*). This is accomplished by suspending the pelleted microvessels in a solution (1 g/10 ml) containing 1800 units of collagenase type 1A, 101 mM NaCl, 4.6 mM KCl, 2.5 mM $CaCl_2 \cdot 2H_2O$, 1.2 mM KH_2PO_4, 1.2 mM $MgSO_4$, 7.0 mM NaOH and 14.5 mM HEPES, pH 7.4. The resuspended microvessels are incubated in a shaking water bath for 25 min at 37 °C. Following digestion, the microvessels are centrifuged at $5700 \times g$ for 10 min at 4 °C, after which they are resuspended in cold TSEM buffer and placed on ice. All subsequent steps in the preparation of membranes are conducted at 4 °C unless otherwise stated.

To fracture the capillary endothelial cells and free the plasma membranes, the resuspended microvessels are disrupted using a Polytron Tissuemizer (Tekmar) at setting 60 for 60 s. The suspension is centrifuged at $5700 \times g$ for 10 min, and the supernatants containing the membranes are pooled. The pellets are resuspended in nine volumes of cold TSEM buffer and rehomogenized for 60 s at a setting of 80 to retrieve additional membranes not released during the previous homogenization. After centrifugation at $5700 \times g$ for 10 min, the supernatants are pooled with those from the previous step. Sufficient $MgSO_4$ is added to the pooled supernatant to reach a concentration of 10 mM. The mixture is stirred for 30 minutes, and then centrifuged at $4300 \times g$ for 15 min to remove additional debris. To collect the membranes, the supernatants are transferred to polycarbonate ultracentrifuge tubes (Beckman, size 25×89 mm, 26.3 ml) and centrifuged at $90\,000 \times g$ for 1 h in a Beckman L-60 Ultracentrifuge (70Ti rotor). Following centrifugation, the membranes are suspended in 20–25 ml of TSE buffer (TSEM without $MgCl_2$). The membranes are dissociated by passage through a syringe first with a 20 gauge needle, and subsequently with a 26 or 27 gauge needle. The dissociated membrane suspension is now ready for fractionation.

A discontinuous Ficoll (Sigma) gradient is used to separate the luminal and abluminal membranes. Eight gradients are prepared using four concentrations of Ficoll in TSE buffer (20%, 15%,

10%, 5%) and layering the following volumes in each of eight Beckman Quick-Seal centrifuge tubes (25×89 mm): 7 ml of 20%, 9 ml of 15%, 8 ml of 10%, and 10 ml of 5%. Equal aliquots of the dissociated membrane suspension are applied to the top of the gradients. The tubes are filled completely with TSE buffer, sealed, and centrifuged at $163\,000 \times g$ (70Ti rotor) for 2.5 h. After opening the seal at the top of each tube with a razor blade, the interfaces are collected in descending order by placing the tip of a 15 gauge stainless steel needle at each interface, and drawing the suspension into a 10 ml syringe until tissue localized there is removed (4–9 ml). The fractions are designated as follows: F1 is the 0/5% interface, F2 is the 5/10% interface, F3 is the 10/15% interface, F4 is the 15/20% interface, and F5 is the pellet plus what remains of the gradient (i.e. the pooled regions between the interfaces). Each of the fractions is diluted with storage buffer (290 mM mannitol, 10 mM Tris–HCl, pH 7.4), and left on ice overnight. The fractions are then centrifuged at $90\,000 \times g$ (4 °C) for 30 min in the ultracentrifuge (Beckman Type 35 rotor), and the pellets are resuspended in 1–2 ml of storage buffer. Aliquots (200–800 µl) are

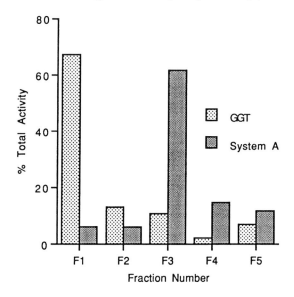

Fig. 7.2. Distribution of luminal (GGT) and abluminal (System A transport activity) membrane markers in a discontinuous Ficoll gradient. Luminal and abluminal membranes are enriched in fraction F1 and F3, respectively.

stored at −80 °C for future use. The total yield of membrane protein is approximately 8 mg from 20 g of capillaries.

Markers to identify luminal and abluminal membrane domains

Gamma-glutamyl transpeptidase (GGT) and the System-A amino acid transporter are plasma membrane proteins (Novogrodsky *et al.*, 1976; Betz and Goldstein, 1978; Betz *et al.*, 1980; Ghandour *et al.*, 1980; Tayarani *et al.*, 1987; Bradbury, 1989; Knudsen *et al.*, 1990) that serve as specific markers for the respective luminal and abluminal membrane domains of the blood–brain barrier (Sanchez del Pino *et al.*, 1995*a*). System A transport activity is

measured by quantifying the initial rate of sodium-dependent ^{14}C-labeled *N*-(methylamino)-isobutyric acid (MeAIB) uptake (Sanchez del Pino *et al.*, 1995*b*). These markers distribute into two distinct fractions of the Ficoll gradient (Sanchez del Pino *et al.*, 1995*a*; Lee *et al.*, 1996), with GGT localizing in fraction F1, and System-A transport activity appearing primarily in fraction F3 (Figs. 7.2 and 7.3).

To provide a more accurate measure of fractionation, a mathematical model was constructed to quantify the distribution of these and other markers between the luminal and abluminal membrane domains (Sanchez del Pino *et al.*, 1995*a*). This procedure generates an *f*-value, which by definition assigns a marker with a value of 1.0 solely to the luminal plasma membrane, and a value of 0 to the abluminal membrane. Values in

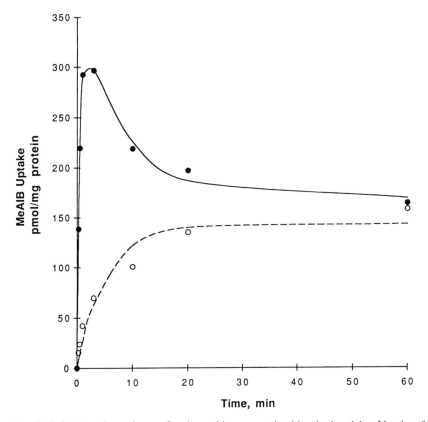

Fig. 7.3. Sodium dependence of amino acid transport in abluminal vesicles. Uptake of a tracer concentration of MeAIB by abluminal vesicles was measured in the presence of 50 mM external KCl (open symbols) and 50 mM external NaCl (filled symbols). The ability of an inwardly directed sodium gradient to increase initial rate of uptake and cause the transient concentration of MeAIB, over the equilibrium value, is a consequence of the sodium-dependent transport System A located in the abluminal membrane.

between signify a distribution of activities between both membrane domains. Using this analysis, GGT and the System-A transporter were confirmed as markers of the luminal and abluminal membranes, respectively (Sanchez del Pino *et al.*, 1995*a*).

Measuring transport and enzymatic activities in luminal and abluminal membrane vesicles

The membranes isolated in fractions F1 and F3 may be used to measure transport and enzymatic activities associated with the luminal and abluminal plasma membranes of the blood–brain barrier. As indicated above, these two fractions are enriched in the markers for the respective membrane domains. During isolation, the membranes form sealed vesicles that are relatively impermeable to the passive diffusion of sucrose (Sanchez del Pino *et al.*, 1995*a*), and that seal primarily right-side-out (Sanchez del Pino *et al.*, 1992). They are reasonably free of contamination by subcellular membranes (Sanchez del Pino *et al.*, 1992, 1995*a*), and have been used successfully in transport studies, and in assigning the distribution of various membrane-associated enzymes (Lee *et al.*, 1996; Sanchez del Pino *et al*, 1992, 1995*a,b*).

Transport of radiolabeled substrates is easily measured by using a rapid filtration technique (Skopicki *et al.*, 1989; Sanchez del Pino *et al.*, 1992). Frozen membrane vesicles are thawed, centrifuged at $37\,500 \times \boldsymbol{g}$ for 25 min (4 °C), and resuspended in storage buffer to a concentration of 2.5–5.0 mg/ml. Uptake is initiated by adding 10 µl of a solution containing a substrate (uptake solution) to 10 µl of the membrane preparation, and incubating at 37 °C for a specific period of time. The uptake solution comprises radiolabeled substrate placed in storage buffer, and additional co-factors that may be required by the experimental protocol. This solution is usually hyperosmotic compared to the intravesicular solution, to counteract osmotic effects associated with uptake of a permeant substrate (Hopfer, 1989; Sanchez del Pino *et al.*, 1995*b*). Thus, 50–100 mM (final concentration) NaCl, KCl, or choline chloride may be added to the incubation medium. The reaction is stopped by

adding 1 ml of an ice-cold stopping-solution containing 145 mM NaCl and 10 mM HEPES-Tris, pH 7.4, and immediately filtering through a 0.45 µm Gelman Metricel filter. The filter is washed four times with 1 ml aliquots of cold stopping solution, and the radioactive material associated with the retained membrane vesicles is measured.

Measurements of membrane-associated enzyme activities are made by standard biochemical methods (Sanchez del Pino *et al.*, 1992., 1995*a*). If the substrates used in the assays do not penetrate the membranes, and the active site of the enzyme is on the inside surface, detergents may be required to open the vesicles. We have found that Triton X-100 (0.1%, v/v) and deoxycholate (0.06%, w/v) are useful to make permeable the luminal and abluminal membranes, respectively (Sanchez del Pino *et al.*, 1992).

The distribution of functional transporters or enzymes between the luminal and abluminal membrane domains may be calculated using isolated membrane vesicles (Sanchez del Pino *et al.*, 1995*a*). To make this calculation, it is necessary to know the percentage of luminal and abluminal membrane in each of two fractions, and the total units of transporter or enzyme activity in each fraction. Thus, the following equation is used:

$$f = 1/1 + R$$

where $R = (U_i L_j - U_j L_i)/(U_j A_i - U_i A_j)$, U is total units of activity, L and A are the percentages of luminal and abluminal membrane, and i and j refer to the two fractions. L and A are determined by assaying for the respective GGT and System-A marker activities in each of the fractions within the gradient, and expressing total activity (specific activity $\times$ mg of protein) in each of the two fractions as a percentage of total activity for the entire gradient. This equation is a derivation of the mathematical model referred to above, which is described in detail elsewhere (Sanchez del Pino *et al.*, 1995*a*). As previously explained, an *f*-value of 1.0 indicates that the transporter or enzyme in question is located only on the luminal membrane of the blood–brain barrier. A value of 0 implies an abluminal position, and numbers in between describe the relative distribution between both membranes.

BLOOD

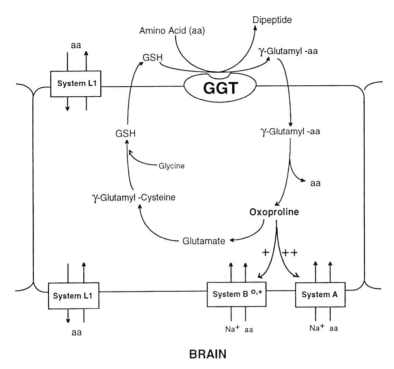

BRAIN

Fig. 7.4. A schematic representation of amino acid transport by the blood–brain barrier. The System L1 carrier protein is equally distributed between both membrane domains, and mediates facilitative transport of predominantly large neutral amino acids from the blood to the brain. Systems A and $B^{o,+}$ are present only in the abluminal membrane, and serve to remove amino acids from the brain extracellular fluid by a secondary active transport mechanism requiring sodium. These abluminal amino acid transporters are stimulated by oxoproline, suggesting that the γ-glutamyl cycle may serve to sense the status of amino acid delivery to the brain and regulate net transport of certain amino acids. Reproduced with permission from Lee *et al.*, 1996.

Transport studies

Figure 7.4 summarizes the results from several of our studies using isolated membrane vesicles to characterize neutral amino acid transport (Lee *et al.*, 1996; Sanchez del Pino *et al.*, 1992, 1995a,b). The L1 facilitative carrier, which favors large neutral amino acids, was found to be equally distributed between the luminal and abluminal membrane domains of the bovine blood–brain barrier (Sanchez del Pino *et al.*, 1992, 1995a). Transport of L-phenylalanine was characterized by an apparent K_m of 11 μM, which confirms the affinity that others have reported for phenyl-

alanine uptake by this carrier system (Smith *et al.*, 1987). As anticipated from the literature (Betz and Goldstein, 1978; Betz *et al.*, 1980; Tayarani *et al.*, 1987; Bradbury, 1989; Knudsen *et al.*, 1990), System-A amino acid transport was observed only at the abluminal membrane (Sanchez del Pino *et al.*, 1995a,b). This sodium-dependent co-transporter has a higher affinity for small neutral amino acids like alanine (Kilberg, 1986). In addition, another sodium-dependent amino acid transporter was found only at the abluminal membrane, with characteristics of the $B^{o,+}$ system (Sanchez del Pino *et al.*, 1995b). Table 7.1 shows kinetic values for these three carriers (Sanchez del Pino *et al.*, 1995b). As depicted in Fig. 7.4, System L1 provides a

Table 7.1. K_m *or* K_i *values ($\pm$SE) for the different transport systems*

	Transport system			
	L	B$^{o,+}$	A	
Substrate	Phenylalanine	Alanine	Alanine	MeAIB
Inhibitor	*(μM)*	*(mM)*	*(mM)*	*(mM)*
Leucine	17 ±3			
Tryptophan	8 ±1			
Phenylalanine	10 ±2	0.14 ±0.05	10 ±2	8.4 ±1.5
BCH	11 ±2	0.4 ±0.2		151 ±60
Alanine	628 ±117	2.1 ±0.6	0.6 ±0.2	0.6 ±0.1
Glutamine	228 ±51	2.2 ±1.6	0.7 ±0.2	1.2 ±0.2
MeAIB			0.7 ±0.1	0.5 ±0.1

When substrate and inhibitor are the same amino acid, K_m values are given. All others indicate K_i values. MeAIB is *N*-(methylamino)-isobutyric acid. BCH is 2-aminobicyclo(2,2,1)-heptane-2-carboxylic acid. Data reproduced with permission from Sanchez del Pino *et al.*, 1995*b*.

passive mechanism for the delivery of amino acids to the brain, and Systems A and B$^{o,+}$ are positioned to actively remove certain amino acids from the brain.

We recently showed that oxoproline, an intermediate product of the γ-glutamyl cycle (Meister and Anderson, 1983), stimulates the activities of Systems A and B$^{o,+}$ in the blood–brain barrier (Lee *et al.*, 1996). As illustrated in Fig. 7.4, γ-glutamyl cycle activity at the luminal membrane (Orlowski and Green, 1974; Cancilla and DeBault, 1983; Meister and Anderson, 1983; Cotgreave and Schuppe-Koistinen, 1994) would depend upon the concentration of plasma amino acids, which would also correlate with passive transport by the L1-system (Sanchez del Pino *et al.*, 1995*b*; Smith *et al.*, 1987; Weissbach *et al.*, 1982). An increased production of oxoproline during increased blood-to-brain influx of amino acids could serve to regulate their net delivery by stimulating energy-dependent systems that selectively extrude amino acids for which they have affinity.

The isolated membrane vesicle technique has allowed us to observe a sodium-dependent glucose carrier on the abluminal membrane of the blood–brain barrier, as well as facilitative glucose carriers equally distributed between both membrane domains (Lee *et al.*, 1997). The facilitative carriers have an apparent affinity typical of the GLUT-1 transporter (Maher *et al.*, 1994), and their presence on both membranes is consistent with passive movement of glucose between blood and brain. The sodium-dependent glucose carrier is phlorizin inhibitable, and is characterized by a high affinity similar to that of the previously observed sodium–glucose transporter in the rabbit small intestine (Parent *et al.*, 1992). This energy-dependent glucose carrier is positioned to transport glucose from brain extracellular fluid into the endothelial cells of the blood–brain barrier. Its physiological significance remains to be determined.

Concluding remarks

Although the yield of plasma membranes from brain capillary endothelial cells is relatively low, and the technique is clearly laborious, the use of these isolated membranes provides an unusually powerful tool to study the blood–brain barrier. It allows for characterization of the respective luminal and abluminal plasma membrane domains forming the barrier, thus providing a means to quantify the kinetics and distribution of specific transport proteins. Furthermore, regulatory processes at each membrane domain may be studied separately. The use of this technique has led to the discovery of carrier systems not previously known to exist in the blood–brain barrier, including the sodium-dependent $B^{o,+}$ amino acid transporter (Sanchez del Pino *et al.*, 1995*b*), and the sodium–glucose carrier (Lee *et al.*, 1997). With this technique, oxoproline-mediated regulation of amino acid transport was shown to occur only at the abluminal membrane (Lee *et al.*, 1996). These discoveries were made possible by having direct access to the individual plasma membrane domains forming the blood–brain barrier.

Acknowledgment

Supported by NIH grant NS 31017.

References

Betz, A. L. and Goldstein, G. W. (1978). Polarity of the blood–brain barrier: neutral amino acid transport into isolated brain capillaries. *Science*, **202**, 225–6.

Betz, A. L., Firth, J. A. and Goldstein, G. W. (1980). Polarity of the blood–brain barrier: distribution of enzymes between the luminal and antiluminal membranes of brain capillary endothelial cells. *Brain Res.*, **192**, 17–28.

Bradbury, M. W. (1989). Transport across the blood–brain barrier. In *Implications of the Blood–Brain Barrier and its Manipulation*, ed. E. A. Neuwelt, pp. 119–36. New York: Plenum Press.

Brightman, M. W. and Reese, T. W. (1969). Junctions between intimately apposed cell membranes in the vertebrate brain. *J. Cell Biol.*, **40**, 648–77.

Cancilla, P. A. and DeBault, L. E. (1983). Neutral amino acid transport properties of cerebral endothelial cells. *J. Neuropathol.*, **42**, 191–9.

Cotgreave, I. A. and Schuppe-Koistinen, I. (1994). A role for γ-glutamyl transpeptidase in the transport of cystine into human endothelial cells: relationship to intracellular glutathione. *Biochim. Biophys. Acta.*, **1222**, 375–82.

Ennis, S. R., Ren, X.-d. and Betz, A. L. (1996). Mechanisms of sodium transport at the blood–brain barrier studied with in situ perfusion of rat brain. *J. Neurochem.* **66**, 756–63.

Ghandour, M. S., Langley, O. K. and Varga, V. (1980). Immunohistological localization of γ-glutamyltranspeptidase in cerebellum at light and electron microscope levels. *Neurosci. Lett.*, **20**, 125–9.

Hopfer, U. (1989). Tracer studies with isolated membrane vesicles. *Methods Enzymol.*, **172**, 313–21.

Kilberg, M. S. (1986). System A-mediated amino acid transport: metabolic control at the plasma membrane. *Trends Biochem. Sci.*, **11**, 183–6.

Knudsen, G. M., Pettigrew, K. D., Patlak, C. S. *et al.* (1990). Asymmetrical transport of amino acids across the blood–brain barrier in humans. *J. Cereb. Blood Flow Metab.*, **10**, 698–706.

Lee, W.-J., Hawkins, R. A., Peterson, D. R. and Vina, J. (1996). Role of oxoproline in the regulation of neutral amino acid transport across the blood–brain barrier. *J. Biol. Chem.*, **271**, 19129–33.

Lee, W.-J., Peterson, D. R., Sukowksi, E. J. and Hawkins, R. A. (1997). Glucose transport by isolated plasma membranes of the bovine blood–brain barrier. *Am. J. Physiol.*, **272**, C1552–7.

Maher, F., Vannucci, S. J. and Simpson, I. A. (1994). Glucose transporter proteins in the brain. *FASEB J.*, **8**, 1003–11.

Meister, A. and Anderson, M. E. (1983). Glutathione. *Ann. Rev. Biochem.*, **52**, 711–60.

Novogrodsky, A., Tate, S. S. and Meister, A. (1976). γ-Glutamyl transpeptidase, a lymphoid cell-surface marker: relationship to blastogenesis, differentiation, and neoplasia. *Proc. Natl. Acad. Sci. USA*, **73**, 2414–18.

Orlowski, M. and Green, J. P. (1974). Gamma glutamyl transpeptidase in brain capillaries: possible site of blood–brain barrier of amino acids. *Science*, **184**, 66–8.

Pardridge, W. M. (1983). Brain metabolism: a perspective from the blood–brain barrier. *Physiol. Rev.*, **63**, 1481–535.

Parent, L., Supplisson, S., Loo, D. D. F. and Wright, E. (1992). Electrogenic properties of the cloned Na^+/glucose cotransporter: I. Voltage-clamp studies. *J. Membrane Biol.*, **125**, 49–62.

Sanchez del Pino, M. M., Hawkins, R. A. and Peterson, D. R. (1992). Neutral amino acid transport by the blood–brain barrier: membrane vesicle studies. *J. Biol. Chem.*, **267**, 25951–7.

Sanchez del Pino, M. M., Hawkins, R. A. and Peterson, D. R. (1995*a*). Biochemical discrimination between luminal and abluminal enzyme and transport activities of the blood–brain barrier. *J. Biol. Chem.*, **270**, 14907–12.

Sanchez del Pino, M. M., Peterson, D. R. and Hawkins, R. A. (1995*b*). Neutral amino acid transport characterization of isolated luminal and abluminal membranes of the blood–brain barrier. *J. Biol. Chem.*, **270**, 14913–18.

Skopicki, H. A., Fisher, K., Zikos, D. *et al.* (1989). Low-affinity transport of pyroglutamyl-histidine in renal brush-border membrane vesicles. *Am. J. Physiol.*, **257**, C971–C975.

Smith, Q. R., Mommo, S., Aoyagi, M. and Rapoport, S. I. (1987). Kinetics of neutral amino acid transport across the blood–brain barrier. *J. Neurochem.*, **49**, 1651–8.

Tayarani, I., Lefauconnier, J. M., Roux, F. and Bourre, J. M. (1987). Evidence for an alanine, serine, and cysteine system of transport in isolated brain capillaries. *J. Cereb. Blood Flow Metab.*, **7**, 585–91.

Weissbach, L., Handlogten, M. E.,
Christensen, H. N. and Kilberg, M. S.
(1982). Evidence for two Na^+-
independent neutral amino acid
transport systems in primary cultures of
rat hepatocytes. Time-dependent
changes in activity. *J. Biol. Chem.*, **257**,
12006–11.

8 Patch clamp techniques with isolated brain microvessel membranes

HEINZ GÖGELEIN, RÜDIGER POPP and JOACHIM HOYER

- Introduction
- Material and methods
- Results and discussion
- Final remarks

Introduction

Cerebral microvessels possess properties that are typical for peripheral blood vessels, and in addition have properties of epithelial tissues (for review see Joó, 1996). In contrast to the peripheral vasculature, the endothelial cells of brain microvessels are connected by tight junctions and thus provide a permeability barrier between blood and brain interstitial fluid. This so-called blood–brain barrier (BBB) has properties in common with tight epithelia, i.e. an input resistance of $1-2$ k Ω/cm^2, and different transport mechanisms in the luminal and antiluminal (brain-facing) membrane (Betz and Goldstein, 1986). The Na^+/K^+-ATPase is present in the antiluminal membrane and transports Na^+ from inside the cell into the brain interstitial fluid in exchange for K^+ ions (Betz et al., 1980). It has been demonstrated that an amiloride-sensitive Na^+ influx as well as a Na^+/Cl^- co-transport, inhibited by furosemide, is present on the luminal side of the capillaries (Betz, 1983). This enables the transport of salt and water from the luminal to the brain side. However, K^+ transport is mainly directed from the brain to the blood side (Hansen et al., 1977), and it has been concluded that the blood–brain barrier is involved in homeostasis of brain K^+ concentration (Bradbury and Stulcová, 1970; Goldstein, 1979).

The development of the patch-clamp technique by Neher and Sakmann (1976) provided new possibilities to study ion transport across cell membranes. The cell culture technique has primarily been applied to study electrogenic transport systems in endothelial cells. As endothelial cells of the peripheral vascular system are unpolarized, experiments on isolated cells, or cells grown as monolayers, are suitable for investigating ion transport mechanisms in this tissue. For the study of polarized tissue, however, cell cultures are only of limited value. Although cells grow with their basolateral side directed towards the support of the culture plate, and the luminal side faces the medium, one cannot be sure whether all transport mechanisms are distributed in the same manner as in the intact tissue. Culturing of cerebral microvascular cells is possible and has yielded important results about structure and function of these cells (Panula et al., 1978; Goldstein et al., 1984). However, monolayers of cultured BBB cells do not possess the high transendothelial electrical resistance as it is present in intact capillaries (Joó, 1992). Therefore, we looked for possibilities to study ion transport mechanisms in a preparation that is as close as possible to the natural structure of cerebral capillaries. The realization turned out to be rather simple, because intact capillaries are an intermediary product of the process to obtain cultured cells.

After having performed a number of patch-clamp studies with cultured cells, one of the authors (J. Hoyer) directed the patch pipette onto the surface of an isolated capillary, where to his great surprise a seal formed immediately and ion channels could be detected. It now became possible to investigate single ion channels in the blood-facing membrane and to compare the results with those obtained in cultured cells.

Material and methods

Intact cerebral capillaries and cerebral capillary endothelial cells were obtained from porcine or rat brain as has been described (Joó and Karnushina, 1973; Bowman *et al.*, 1981, Mischek *et al.*, 1989; Hoyer *et al.*, 1991). Briefly, the gray matter was minced and incubated with neutral protease dispase II from *Bacillus polymyxa* (Boehringer, Mannheim, FRG). Isolated capillaries were obtained after centrifugation on top of a 15% dextrane solution (Sigma, Munich, FRG, MW 150 000) and stored on ice until use.

Intact isolated capillaries of about 100–200 µm length (Fig. 8.1) were placed in a lucite chamber mounted on the stage of an inverse microscope (Zeiss IM 35), equipped with interference contrast optics. Capillaries were placed into the bath by means of a microliter syringe and were allowed to settle to the glass cover slip. Within about 15 min, the capillaries slightly attached to the glass bottom. As demonstrated in Fig. 8.1, erythrocytes were frequently captured inside the isolated capillaries. When a patch pipette was gently pushed on top of an erythrocyte, it slowly moved away, and thus did not disturb the recording. Gentle superfusion by means of a gravimetrical system and aspiration of the bath fluid with a venturi could be done while a patch pipette had contact to the capillary. The measuring chamber as well as the inflowing solution were electrically heated (electronic device developed by W. Hampel in the workshop of the Max-Planck-Institute for Biophysics, Frankfurt/ Main Germany), so that the temperature in the bath was maintained at 35 ± 1 °C. Experiments were performed with a $\times 40$ objective.

If not otherwise stated the bathing medium consisted of NaCl solution (in mM): 140 NaCl, 4

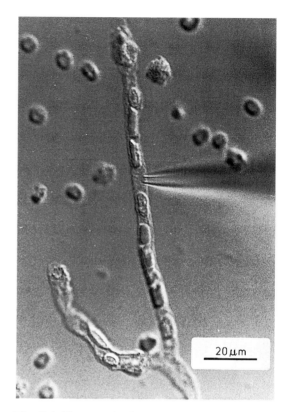

Fig. 8.1. Photograph of an isolated porcine cerebral capillary, with a patch pipette contacting the antiluminal membrane. Erythrocytes are visible inside the capillary. (From Hoyer *et al.* (1991), with permission of the *Journal of Membrane Biology*.

KCl, 1 $MgCl_2$, 1.3 $CaCl_2$, 10 (N-[2-hydroxyethyl]-piperazine-N′-[2-ethanesulfonic acid]) (HEPES), adjusted to pH 7.4 with NaOH. In some experiments all Na^+ in the bathing medium was replaced by K^+. The patch pipette was filled with KCl solution, consisting of (in mM) 145 KCl, 1 $MgCl_2$, 0.73 $CaCl_2$, 1 ethylene glycol-*bis*-(β-aminoethyl ether) $N,N,N′,N′$-tetraacetic acid (EGTA) (free Ca^{2+} concentration 10^{-7} M), 10 HEPES, adjusted to pH 7.4 with KOH.

The capillaries were directly approached by the patch pipette at the antiluminal side (Fig. 8.1), and seal resistance in the order of gigaohms could be easily obtained. Patch-clamp experiments were performed mainly in cell-attached and cell-free (inside-out oriented) configuration (Hamill *et al.*, 1981). In some experiments the slow whole-cell mode was obtained by addition of 200 µg/ml nystatin to the patch pipette filling solution. Patch pipettes (1.5–6 MΩ) were pulled from borosilicate glass capillaries with 0.3 mm wall thickness. Recording and data analysis was as has been described previously (Gögelein and Greger, 1986). Briefly, currents were amplified with a List patch-clamp amplifier EPC-7, A/D converted with a modified Sony PCM 501 and stored on video tape. Data analysis was performed with a LSI 11/23 computer system. Single channel data were low-pass filtered (–3 dB 800 Hz) and sampled with an interval of 0.5 msec. For analysis of single channel recordings, data were displayed (Hewlett-Packard, 1345A) and levels of baseline and channel amplitude were set under optical control. Channel events above half-threshold were considered as open state events and below half-threshold as closed state of a channel. Single channel conductance (g) was determined from linear regression of the current–voltage relationship.

For investigation of stretch-activated ion channels, a negative pressure was applied to the patch pipette by means of a water column. The pressure was monitored by a differential pressure transducer (Hottinger–Baldwin–Messtechnik, Darmstadt, Germany). Single-channel open probability in multichannel patches was calculated as:

$$P_o = (I_{av} - I_o / (I_{max} - I_o)$$

where I_{av} is the average current calculated by the computer, I_o is the baseline level (current where all channels are closed), and I_{max} is the maximal current level occurring at a given clamp potential. I_o and I_{max} were determined visually from the computer display. (The sign of the clamp potential refers to the cytosolic side. The given clamp potentials indicate the voltage between pipette and bath electrode.)

Results and discussion

Inwardly-rectifying potassium channels

Whole-cell current recordings in isolated capillaries were difficult to obtain, but in some experiments current–voltage relationships could be recorded in the slow whole-cell mode. As demonstrated in Fig. 8.2(a), the curve consists of three

distinct parts: a pronounced inward current at negative potentials, little current around zero milli-volt clamp potential, and a nonlinear increase of the outward current at voltages more positive than 30 mV. The cell potential was low (between –10 and –40 mV), which was similar to observations in isolated porcine BBB cells (Hoyer et al., 1991). It is important to note that the current–voltage curve recorded in primary cultured BBB cells was indistinguishable from that obtained in isolated capillaries. The inward-directed current was not studied in isolated capillaries but was investigated in more detail in whole-cell recordings with isolated cells (Hoyer et al., 1991). It has been observed that this current component was due to K^+ ion movement and that it was blocked by 10 mM Ba^{2+}. Addition of 1 μM of angiotensin II or of arginine–vasopressin to the extracellular side caused a time-dependent inhibition of the inwardly rectifying K^+ current. Moreover, application of 100 μM GTP-χ-S to the patch pipette blocked the current, as observed previously in renal juxtaglomerular cells (Kurtz and Penner, 1989). In analogy to other tissues, it can be assumed that the inward-rectifying channels determine the cell's resting potential (Katz, 1949; Sakmann and Trube, 1984). In addition, the influence of the hormones angiotensin II and arginine–vasopressin on the K^+ conductance might indicate an involvement in regulation of salt and water transport across the BBB (Grubb and Raichle, 1981; Raichle and Grubb, 1978).

In cell-attached patches at the antiluminal membrane of isolated capillaries, single K^+ selective channels with a single channel conductance of 30 pS could be recorded. The channel showed distinct inward-rectification, making it a likely candidate to explain the inward-rectifying whole-cell current (Hoyer et al., 1991).

Outwardly-rectifying K^+ channels

The current in the outward direction, activated by positive clamp potentials (Fig. 8.2(a)), was attenuated by 1 mM barium in the bathing solution, indicating that it is carried by K^+ ions. In cell-excised patches, single channels with outward-rectifying properties and g of 8 pS could be observed (Fig. 8.2(b), Popp and Gögelein, 1993). Removing Ca^{2+} ions from the cytosolic side did not affect the

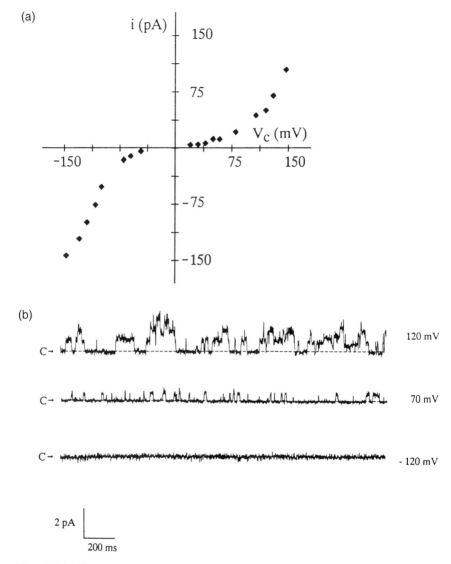

Fig. 8.2. (a) Current–voltage relationship recorded in an isolated porcine cerebral capillary, recorded with the slow whole-cell patch-clamp technique. Voltage pulses of 300 ms duration were applied from the holding potential of 0 mV. The data points were obtained at the end of the voltage pulses. (b) Single outward-rectifying K$^+$ channels recorded in the antiluminal membrane of an isolated porcine cerebral capillary (cell-attached mode). C→ denotes the current where channels are closed (baseline). Both the pipette and the bath contained NaCl solution. The single channel conductance is 8 pS.

current, indicating that these K$^+$ channels were not Ca^{2+} sensitive. The physiological function of these outwardly rectifying K$^+$ channels is unclear. The channel is clearly different from an outward current through ATP-sensitive K$^+$ channels with g of 40 pS, recently described in cultured brain microvascular cells (Janigro *et al.*, 1993).

Stretch-activated nonselective cation channels

In cell-attached patches at the antiluminal side of isolated porcine capillaries, we observed two types of ionic currents that became activated when suction was applied through the patch pipette. The

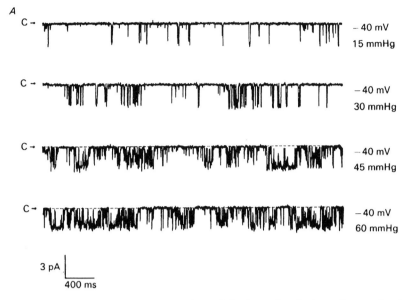

Fig. 8.3. Single stretch-activated ion channels in the antiluminal membrane of an isolated porcine cerebral capillary (cell-attached mode, pipette KCl, bath NaCl solution). The dependence of the channel on various negative pressures is demonstrated. (From: Popp *et al.*, 1992, with permission of the *Journal of Physiology*).

more frequently occurring channel showed slight inward rectification with a single-channel conductance of 37 pS at negative and 24 pS at positive clamp potentials. The mean channel-open probability increased with increasing pressure (Fig. 8.3) and with depolarizing potentials (Popp *et al.*, 1992). The channel was cation selective and permeable to Na^+, K^+, Ba^{2+} and Ca^{2+}. The second type of stretch-activated channels had a single-channel conductance of 87 pS at negative and 35 pS at positive clamp potentials. After excision of the membrane patch, both types of channels rapidly inactivated. In isolated endothelial cells obtained from brain microvessels, cell swelling induced by hypotonic shock evoked the stretch-activated channels in cell-attached experiments. This observation indicates that the stretch-activated channels are probably involved in cell volume regulation. Moreover, it was speculated that these channels could be involved in the K^+ transport from the brain to the blood side. They might be important under cytotoxic brain edema, where increased K^+ concentration and osmolarity in the interstitial fluid could activate the channels in the brain-facing membrane of the capillaries. The lack of specific inhibitors of stretch-activated ion channels makes

it difficult to elucidate their physiological role in *in vivo* models.

Calcium and ATP sensitive nonselective cation channels

After excision of membrane patches from the antiluminal membrane of isolated rat cerebral capillaries, ion channels became active in about 70% of all cases (Popp and Gögelein, 1992). It should be emphasized that these channels could never be observed in cell-attached patches. Ion substitution experiments revealed that the channel was not measurably permeable to Cl^- and the divalent cations Ca^{2+} and Ba^{2+}, but was about equally permeable to Na^+ and K^+ ions. The current–voltage curve was linear in the investigated voltage range (-80 mV to $+80$ mV), and the single-channel conductance was approximately 30 pS (Fig. 8.4). The channel open probability was not dependent on the applied potential. Lowering of Ca^{2+} to 1 µM or below on the cytosolic side inactivated the channel, whereas addition of cytosolic ATP (1 mM) inhibited the channel activity completely and reversibly. The channel was blocked by the inhibitors of nonselective cation channels 3′,5-

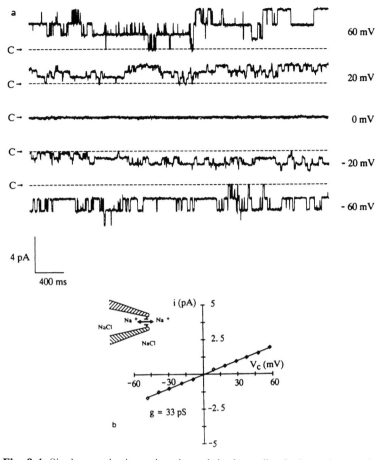

Fig. 8.4. Single nonselective cation channels in the antiluminal membrane of an isolated rat cerebral capillary (cell-excised patch; pipette and bath NaCl solution). At least three channels are present in this patch. The open probability of one channel is approximately 0.65 at all clamp potentials. The lower panel displays the corresponding current–voltage curve for a single channel. The data points were fitted by linear regression, yielding a slope conductance of 33 pS. The symbol in the inset indicates a patch pipette and the ionic conditions. (From: Popp and Gögelein, 1992, with permission of *Biochimica et Biophysica Acta*.)

dichlorodiphenylamine-2-carboxylic acid (DCDPC, 1–10 µM, Gögelein and Pfannmüller, 1989) and by the anti-inflammatory drugs flufenamic acid (10 µM, Gögelein *et al.*, 1990) and tenidap (100 µM), as well by gadolinium (10 µM, Popp and Gögelein, 1992). Application of 100 µM amiloride to the cytosolic side, however, had no effect. Nonselective cation channels with a mean single-channel conductance of 26 pS were also observed in the antiluminal membrane of isolated porcine brain capillaries. It is unlikely that the nonselective cation channels described here are similar to those which were activated by extracellular ATP, as

described by Janigro *et al.* (1996), because the latter ones were also permeable to Ca^{2+} ions.

As in most other tissues, the physiological role of the nonselective cation channels remains unclear. Recent observations in epithelial tissues made it unlikely that the channel is involved in physiological ion transport (Ecke *et al.*, 1996; Slawik *et al.*, 1996). On the other hand, Volk *et al.* (1995), demonstrated recently that nonselective cation channels with similar properties as described in BBB cells were activated under osmotic stress in mouse cortical collecting duct cells, where they might be involved in volume regulatory processes.

Final remarks

Our experiments showed that the patch-clamp technique could be easily applied to the antiluminal membrane of isolated rat or porcine cerebral capillaries. All channels observed in this preparation were also present in isolated cells from primary cultured BBB cells. However, in the latter preparation some additional channels could be observed, such as a K$^+$ channels with $g = 7$ pS (Hoyer *et al.*, 1991), and a stretch-activated channel with $g = 9$ pS, as well as a high conductance Ca^{2+} dependent K$^+$ channel (Popp *et al.*, 1992). It was assumed that these channels are located in the luminal membrane BBB cells.

We made some attempts to obtain recordings from the luminal membrane of isolated cerebral microvessels. We applied the technique of isolated perfused renal tubules (Gögelein and Greger, 1984) to microvessels with diameters of approximately 50 μm to 100 μm. After mechanically rupturing the vessel it was possible to insert a patch pipette into the lumen and to obtain gigaseals in some cases. However, we could not detect single ion channels. We believe that more intense trials with isolated perfused microvessels could lead to successful recordings of ion channels in the luminal membrane.

References

Betz, A. L. (1983). Sodium transport from blood to brain: Inhibition by furosemide and amiloride. *J. Neurochem.*, **41**, 1158–64.

Betz, A. L. and Goldstein, G. W. (1986). Specialized properties and solute transport in brain capillaries. *Ann. Rev. Physiol.*, **48**, 241–50.

Betz, A. L., Firth, J. A. and Goldstein, G. W. (1980). Polarity of the blood–brain barrier: distribution of enzymes between the luminal and antiluminal membranes of brain capillary endothelial cells. *Brain Res.*, **192**, 17–28.

Bowman, P. D., Betz, A. L., Ar, D. *et al.* (1981). Primary culture of capillary endothelium from rat brain. *In Vitro*, **17**, 353–62.

Bradbury, M. W. B. and Stulcová, B. (1970). Efflux mechanism contributing to the stability of the potassium concentration in cerebrospinal fluid. *J. Physiol.*, **280**, 415–30.

Ecke, D., Bleich, M. and Greger, R. (1996). Crypt base cells show forskolin-induced Cl$^-$ secretion but no cation inward conductance. *Pflügers Arch.*, **431**, 427–34.

Gögelein, H. and Greger, R. (1984). Single channel recordings from basolateral and apical membranes of renal proximal tubules. *Pflügers Arch.*, **401**, 424–6.

Gögelein, H. and Greger, R. (1986). A voltage-dependent ionic channel in the basolateral membrane of late proximal tubule of the rat kidney. *Pflügers Arch.*, **407**, S142–S148.

Gögelein, H. and Pfannmüller, B. (1989). The nonselective channel in the basolateral membrane of rat exocrine pancreas. Inhibition by 3′,5-dichlorodiphenylamine-2-carboxylic acid (DCDPC) and activation by stilbene disulfonates. *Pflügers Arch.*, **413**, 287–98.

Gögelein, H., Dahlem, D., Englert, H. C. and Lang, H. J. (1990). Flufenamic acid, mefenamic acid and niflumic acid inhibit single nonselective cation channels in the rat exocrine pancreas. *FEBS Lett.*, **268**, 79–82.

Goldstein, G. W. (1979). Relation of potassium transport to oxidative metabolism in isolated brain capillaries. *J. Physiol.*, **286**, 185–95.

Goldstein, G. W., Betz, A. L. and Bowman, P. D. (1984). Use of isolated brain capillaries and cultured endothelial cells to study the blood–brain barrier. *Federation Proc.*, **43**, 191–5.

Grubb, R. L. and Raichle, M. E. (1981). Intraventricular angiotensin II increases brain vascular permeability. *Brain Res.*, **210**, 426–30.

Hamill, O. P., Marty, A., Neher, E. *et al.* (1981). Improved patch-clamp techniques for high-resolution current recordings from cells and cell-free membrane patches. *Pflügers Arch.*, **391**, 85–100.

Hansen, A. J., Lund-Andersen, H. and Crone, C. (1977). K$^+$ permeability of the blood–brain-barrier, investigated by aid of a K$^+$-sensitive microelectrode. *Acta Physiol. Scand.*, **101**, 438–45.

Hoyer, J., Popp, R., Meyer, J. *et al.* (1991). Angiotensin II, vasopressin and GTP-χ-S inhibit inward-rectifying K$^+$ channels in porcine cerebral capillary endothelial cells. *J. Membr. Biol.*, **123**, 55–62.

Janigro, B., West, G. A., Gordon, E. L. and Winn, H. R. (1993). ATP-sensitive K$^+$ channels in rat aorta and brain microvascular endothelial cells. *Am. J. Physiol.*, **34**, C812–C821.

Janigro, D., Nguyen, T. S., Gordon, E. L. and Winn, H. R. (1996). Physiological properties of ATP-activated cation channels in rat brain microvascular endothelial cells. *Am. J. Physiol.*, **270**, H1423–H1434.

Joó, F. (1992). The cerebral microvessel in culture, an update. *J. Neurochem.*, **58**, 1–17.

Joó, F. (1996). Endothelial cells of the brain and other organ systems: some similarities and differences. *Progr. Neurobiol.*, **48**, 255–73.

Joó, F. and Karnushina, I. (1973). A procedure of the isolation of capillaries from rat brain. *Cytobios.*, **8**, 41–8.

Katz, B. (1949). Les constantes electriques de la membranes du muscle. *Arch. Sci. Physiol.*, **3**, 285–300.

Kurtz, A. and Penner, R. (1989). Angiotensin II induces oscillations of intracellular calcium and blocks anomalous inward-rectifying potassium current in mouse renal juxtaglomerular cells. *Proc. Natl. Acad. Sci. USA*, **86**, 3423–7.

Mischek, U., Meyer, J. and Galla, H.-J. (1989). Characterization of γ-glutamyl transpeptidase activity of cultured endothelial cells from porcine brain capillaries. *Cell Tissue Res.*, **256**, 221–6.

Neher, E. and Sakmann, B. (1976). Single-channel currents recorded from membrane of denervated frog muscle fibres. *Nature*, **260**, 799–802.

Panula, P., Joó, F. and Rechardt, L. (1978). Evidence for the presence of viable endothelial cells in cultures derived from dissociated rat brain. *Experientia*, **34**, 95–7.

Popp, R. and Gögelein, H. (1992). A calcium and ATP sensitive nonselective cation channel in the antiluminal membrane of rat cerebral capillary endothelial cells. *Biochim. Biophys. Acta*, **1108**, 59–66.

Popp, R. and Gögelein, H. (1993). Outward-rectifying potassium channels in endothelial cells from pig cerebral capillaries. *Pflügers Arch.*, **422**, R 120.

Popp, R., Hoyer, J. and Meyer, J. *et al.* (1992). Stretch-activated non-selective cation channels in the antiluminal membrane of porcine cerebral capillaries. *J. Physiol.*, **454**, 435–49.

Raichle, M. E. and Grubb, R. L. (1978). Regulation of brain water permeability by centrally-released vasopressin. *Brain Res.*, **143**, 191–4.

Sakmann, B. and Trube, G. (1984). Conductance properties of single inward-rectifying potassium channels in ventricular cells from guinea-pig heart. *J. Physiol.*, **347**, 641–57.

Slawik, M., Zdebik, A., Hug, M. J. and Greger, R. (1996). The role of non-selective-cation conductance in CCH-induced secretion of rat pancreatic acini. *Pflügers Arch.*, **431**, R 102.

Volk, T., Frömter, E. and Korbmacher, C. (1995). Hypertonicity activates nonselective cation channels in mouse cortical collecting duct cells. *Proc. Natl. Acad. Sci. USA*, **92**, 8478–82.

9 Tissue culture of brain endothelial cells – induction of blood–brain barrier properties by brain factors

CARSTEN T. BEUCKMANN and HANS-JOACHIM GALLA

- Introduction
- Influence of external factors on tight junctions, TEER, and paracellular permeability
- Influence of external factors on expression of BBB-related proteins
- Influence of external factors on three-dimensional structures
- Discussion
- References

Introduction

For several reasons researchers have tried for many years to establish a tissue culture model of the blood–brain barrier (BBB). For ethical reasons the amount of animal experiments should be limited to a reasonable number, and a further consideration is that by simplifying an experimental setting, conditions are much easier to standardize. Because a living animal is of course a complicated organism, many researchers support the idea that isolated brain capillary endothelial cells (BCEC) in culture are a suitable model system, which can be brought to standard conditions more easily, but still give valuable information on how the BBB actually works.

A functioning *in vitro* model of the BBB should display most, if not all, properties of the barrier in living animals. Among these properties are a very high electrical resistance, due to the presence of tight junctions, in other words a very low paracellular permeability for hydrophilic compounds (including ions), expression of BBB-specific marker proteins, and a cellular polar distribution between luminal and abluminal endothelial plasma membranes of these marker proteins, including transporter proteins.

By isolating BCEC and culturing them, these cells keep their endothelial phenotype, still displaying typical properties. They express angiotensin converting enzyme, von Willebrand factor, and internalize acetylated low-density lipoprotein.

Regrettably, BCEC lose BBB-specific features that they possessed *in vivo*. Some examples are a reduced complexity of tight junctions (Tao-Cheng *et al.*, 1987), therefore a low transendothelial electrical resistance (TEER) (Rubin *et al.*, 1991), loss of marker enzymes alkaline phosphatase (ALP) and γ-glutamyl transpeptidase (GGT) (Meyer *et al.*, 1987), or loss of glucose transporter system 1 (GLUT1) (Hemmila and Drewes, 1993).

BBB researchers are focusing their interest on creating culture conditions for BCEC, that mimic the *in vivo* situation the best. But obviously, BCEC *in vitro* lack some brain-derived signals or factors that are necessary for these cells to keep up a differentiated BBB phenotype. Therefore these brain-derived factors have to be identified and tested for their ability to influence BCEC towards an *in vitro* BBB. Because brain capillaries are nearly completely ensheathed by endfeet of astrocytes, these members of the glial family are very likely to be a modulator of BBB-properties in BCEC. Research therefore is mainly focused on astrocytic signals,

79

which might influence cultured BCEC in respect to a differentiated BBB phenotype. Whether these signals are soluble molecules, membrane bound, or a part of the extracellular matrix is still discussed with much controversy.

Influence of external factors on tight junctions, TEER, and paracellular permeability

Tight junctions

BCEC in culture lose the complex network of tight junctions they possess *in vivo*. In the living organism tight junctions of BCEC display a belt-like, continuous appearance with numerous branching points. In culture these structures have not been found; only fragmentary patterns of tight junctions have been documented by Tao-Cheng *et al.* (1987). This group used subcultured bovine BCEC and performed freeze-fracture electron microscopy on these cells. By seeding BCEC onto a confluent bed of rat astrocytes, BCEC regained tight junctions, which were markedly enhanced in length, width, and complexity. These findings could be confirmed by other groups. Tio *et al.* (1990) found an induction of tight junctions in human umbilical cord vein endothelial cells caused by co-culturing these cells together with rat astrocytes in a common compartment without direct cell–cell contacts, where astrocytes continuously conditioned the culture medium. The same effect was achieved with astrocyte-conditioned medium (ACM) without the presence of astrocytes. This is remarkable, because vein endothelial cells do not display tight junctions *in vivo*. Wolburg *et al.* (1994) also confirmed the inductive effect of astrocyte-secreted factors on the complexity of tight junctions of primary cultured bovine BCEC. They found that continuously astrocyte conditioned medium (by culturing BCEC and astrocytes on opposite sides of a filter membrane) or the addition of forskolin to BCEC culture medium could increase tight junction complexity comparable to that of freshly isolated brain capillaries. Therefore cyclic AMP could be one of the second messenger systems involved in the process. On the other hand, phorbol esters, which activate protein kinase C, further decreased tight junction complexity.

TEER and paracellular permeability

TEER and paracellular permeability are an alternative to electron microscopy to look at tight junctions. These two features directly correspond to the 'tightness' of a cell monolayer and can be readily determined.

Several groups report an increase of TEER of bovine BCEC monolayers by astrocytic influence. This was either achieved with subcultured BCEC and rat astrocytes in filter co-cultures (Dehouck *et al.*, 1990), or with cloned BCEC in ACM (Rubin *et al.*, 1991), or with primary cultured BCEC in either filter coculture or in ACM (Wolburg *et al.*, 1994). Raub *et al.*, (1992) did not use astrocytes in their experiments, but used continuous cell lines of astroglial origin in order to produce conditioned media. C_6-glioma and astrocytoma-conditioned media exerted a significant increase of TEER in primary cultured bovine BCEC. Therefore these cell lines still seem to secrete the same factor(s) responsible for junctional tightness in BCEC as primary cultures of astrocytes do. Interestingly, this research group could not find any effects using subcultured BCEC, which seems to be in contrast to other groups, which prefer subcultured cells because of lower contaminations with non-BCEC. Rubin *et al.* (1991) could mimic TEER increase by adding cyclic AMP to BCEC cultures. Cyclic AMP and ACM even showed synergistic effects. This can be explained by later findings that cyclic AMP increases tight junction complexity (Wolburg *et al.*, 1994). Nevertheless, cyclic AMP had no effect on the staining pattern of ZO-1, a tight junction associated protein, which raised the questions of the context of ZO-1 and junction tightness (Rubin *et al.*, 1991).

High TEER corresponds with low paracellular permeability of hydrophilic substances. Several compounds with different molecular weights and therefore sizes have been tested for their ability to traverse a BCEC monolayer on a filter support. ACM decreased the paracellular permeability in BCEC for inulin (Wolburg *et al.*, 1994). C_6-glioma and astrocytoma-conditioned media had similar effects regarding the permeability of sucrose, polyethyleneglycol (molecular weight 4 kDa), and dextran (molecular weight 70 kDa) (Raub *et al.*, 1992).

Influence of external factors on expression of BBB-related proteins

Alkaline phosphatase and γ-glutamyl transpeptidase

Glial influences These two enzymes are well-known as so-called marker enzymes of BBB. Although they are not exclusive markers, having a widespread tissue occurrence, within brain, they show very high specific activity only in capillary endothelial cells. In culture BCEC rapidly lose their ALP and GGT activities due to the cessation of protein *de novo* synthesis (Meyer *et al.*, 1990; Beuckmann et al, 1994).

Several attempts have been made to re-induce these enzyme activities *in vitro*. Bauer *et al.*, (1990) found that C_6-glioma plasma membranes raised GGT-activity in cloned bovine BCEC 10–12-fold. Na–K-ATPase activity could be increased 2-fold. These results were confirmed by Tontsch and Bauer (1991) using cloned porcine BCEC. They described that C_6-glioma plasma membranes or the cells themselves, standing in direct contact to BCEC, reinduced GGT and Na–K-ATPase activities in endothelial cells. Plasma membranes derived from neurons were as efficient as C_6-glioma membranes. This raises the question, if not only astrocytes, but also neurons play a vital role in maintaining the BBB. Interestingly, conditioned media and astrocytes were ineffective. This is in contrast to results of most other researchers involved in this field. These researchers can be divided into two camps. One claims that re-induction of ALP and GGT can be achieved by culturing endothelial cells in glial conditioned media, the other emphasizes the need for direct plasma membrane contacts between the inducing cells and endothelial cells.

By culturing bovine BCEC in the presence of rat astrocytes on different sides of a filter, a GGT-reinduction could be found (Dehouck *et al.*, 1990).

Even human umbilical cord vein endothelial cells have been susceptible to ALP activity induction by culturing them in the presence of astrocytes without direct cell contacts (Tio *et al.*, 1990). Others found that the presence of astrocytes is not necessary in culture. In bovine BCEC C_6-glioma- and astrocytoma-conditioned media could successfully re-induce GGT-activity (Raub *et al.*, 1992). This has also been possible for ALP and GGT activities with cloned immortalized rat BCEC and C_6-glioma conditioned medium. Plasma membranes from C_6-glioma cells and astrocytes were equally effective (Roux *et al.*, 1994).

It has also been possible to induce ALP activity in non-BCEC-like calf pulmonary artery endothelial cells by ACM (Takemoto *et al.*, 1994), although these cells normally possess very low ALP activity in culture. In these experiments, interleukin-6 has been identified as one of the ALP activity inducing factors.

In contrast to results described above, others found that only a direct cell–cell contact between porcine primary cultured BCEC and astrocytes was necessary to reinduce ALP and GGT activities up to levels comparable to freshly isolated cells. The same was found for C_6-glioma cells with respect to ALP activity induction (Meyer *et al.*, 1991; Raub et al, 1992), but not only astrocytes and C_6-glioma cells are able to reinduce ALP activity in BCEC. Neuroblastoma cells and epithelial cells of choroid plexus could also do so; again, direct cell–cell contacts have been necessary to achieve this effect (Beuckmann *et al.*, 1994). The capability to induce ALP activity in BCEC could therefore be a general feature of cells of the neuroectodermal astrocytic family and of neurons.

Non-glial factors By adding cyclic AMP to primary cultured porcine BCEC, ALP activity could be re-induced to the level of freshly isolated cells without the presence of any other inducing cells (Beuckmann *et al.*, 1995). This corresponds to results that cyclic AMP increases TEER in cultured BCEC (Rubin *et al.*, 1991). Although ALP and TEER are two different features of BBB, cyclic AMP seems to be the common second messenger regulating these properties.

Others have shown that the differentiating agent

Table 9.1. *Effects of different 'brain-derived' factors on endothelial cells in vitro*

Species and cell type	Brain derived factor	Property	Reference
Bovine bcec subcultured	A	Tight junctions	Tao-Cheng et al., 1987
Bovine bcec	ACM, cAMP	TEER, $P_{sucrose}$	Rubin et al., 1991
Bovine bcec	Forskolin, phorbol esters, A, ACM	Tight junctions, TEER, P_{inulin}	Wolburg et al., 1994
Bovine bcec 3. passage	A-CCM	TEER, GGT, $P_{sucrose}$, P_{inulin}	Dehouck et al., 1990
Human umbilical vein EC	A-CCM, ACM	ALP, tight junctions	Tio et al., 1990
Bovine bcec	C6-CM, astrocytoma-CM	TEER, $P_{sucrose}$, $P_{dextran}$, P_{peg}, GGT	Raub et al., 1992
Bovine bcec cloned	C6-PM	GGT, NaK-ATPase	Bauer et al., 1990
Porcine bcec cloned	C6, C6-PM, neuron PM	GGT, NaK-ATPase	Tontsch and Bauer, 1991
Porcine bcec primary	A, C6	ALP, GGT	Meyer et al., 1991
Bovine bcec primary	ACM, C6-CM	GLUT-I	Takakura et al., 1991
Human bcec	A	Butyryl-choline esterase	Pakaski and Kara, 1992
Porcine bcec primary	A, C6	ALP, GGT	Rauh et al., 1992
Porcine and murine bcec cloned	Heparin, ECGF	Protein patterns	Amberger et al., 1993
Canine bcec	—	GLUT-I	Hemmila and Drewes, 1993
Bovine bcec cell line	Bovine brain homogenate, TNF-α	GLUT-I, actin	Boado et al., 1994
Bovine bcec cloned	A-CCM	LDL-binding	Dehouck et al., 1994
Porcine bcec primary	A, C6, NB, PE	ALP	Beuckmann et al., 1994
Calf artery EC	ACM, interleukin-6	ALP	Takemoto et al., 1994
Rat bcec immortal	All-*trans*-retinoic acid	GGT, P-glycoprotein	Lechardeur et al., 1995
Porcine bcec primary	cAMP	ALP	Beuckmann et al., 1995
Rat bcec immortal	APM, C6-PM, C6-CM, A-CCM	Capillary-like structures, ALP, GGT	Roux et al., 1994
Mouse bcec	ACM	Glucose uptake	Maxwell et al., 1989
Bovine retinal capillary EC	A, C6	Capillary-like structures	Laterra et al., 1990, 1991
Bovine retinal capillary EC	Steroids, C6	Capillary-like structures	Wolff et al., 1992

Abbreviations: A, astrocyte; ALP, alkaline phosphatase; bcec, brain capillary endothelial cells; C6, C6-glioma; CCM, continuously conditioned medium; CM, conditioned medium; EC, endothelial cells; GF, growth factor; GGT, γ-glutamyl transpeptidase; NB, neuroblastoma; PE, plexus epithelium; peg, polyethyleneglycol; PM, plasma membranes; TEER, transendothelial electrical resistance; TNF, tumor necrosis factor.

all-*trans*-retinoic acid is able to re-induce GGT activity in immortalized rat BCEC (Lechardeur *et al.*, 1995). Another effect was the induction of expression of the endothelial marker P-glycoprotein, which was not expressed in non-treated BCEC. Whether all-*trans*-retinoic acid is also responsible for BBB differentiation *in vivo* has still to be demonstrated.

Glucose transporter system 1

The transport system GLUT1 is expressed in BCEC, but as has already been shown for ALP and GGT, GLUT1 no longer expressed if BCEC are isolated and taken into culture (Hemmila and Drewes, 1993).

Maxwell *et al.*, (1989) showed that constant exposure of BCEC to astrocytic product(s) could significantly increase glucose uptake in endothelial cells. These findings were confirmed by Takakura *et al.* (1991) and explained by the first evidence that ACM and C_6-glioma conditioned medium induced *de novo* synthesis of GLUT1. Another attempt to reinduce GLUT1 expression was made by Boado *et al.* (1994). They also found a loss of GLUT1 in a bovine BCEC line *in vitro* and were able to switch on the transcription of GLUT1-mRNA and actin-mRNA by adding bovine brain homogenate or tumor necrosis factor alpha. In this experimental setting C_6-glioma plasma membranes or conditioned medium were not effective.

Other features

Three other reports need to be mentioned here. Pakaski and Kasa (1992) described an increase in acetylcholinesterase activity in human BCEC by astrocytic factors. ACM can also increase low-density-lipoprotein binding to bovine BCEC (Dehouck *et al.*, 1994). The soluble inducing factor had a molecular weight between 3.5 and 14 kDa. It has to be pointed out, that the described effect of low-density-lipoprotein binding to BCEC could only be exerted by astrocytes that had been co-cultured with BCEC for 12 days. This is one of the few examples where not only an influence of astrocytes on BCEC was seen, but vice versa.

Amberger *et al.* (1993) screened protein patterns of cloned porcine and murine BCEC. In two different cell lines, BBB phenotype was only expressed by the one that had been grown in the presence of heparin and endothelial cell growth factor. These two substances seemed to influence protein pattern and thus cell shape.

Influence of external factors on three-dimensional structures

If bovine retinal capillary cells were seeded onto rat astrocytes or C_6-glioma cells they developed capillary-like structures within several days (Laterra *et al.*, 1990). Direct cell–cell contacts were necessary for this; conditioned media or spatial separation did not cause any effects. If RNA synthesis or protein synthesis was inhibited in culture, capillary formation could be strongly suppressed (Laterra and Goldstein, 1991). However, *in vitro* angiogenesis could be induced without any glial influence by seeding BCEC onto the reconstituted basement membrane protein Matrigel. This suggested two steps in capillary formation: an astroglial-dependent and an independent step. The astroglial influence could be regulated indirectly by steroids, which completely block*ed in vitro* formation of capillaries via C_6-glioma cells (Wolff *et al.*, 1992). Whether the described three-dimensional structures exhibit the necessary polarity of endothelium has yet to be shown.

Discussion

Attempts to examine influences of brain-derived factors on BCEC in tissue culture are numerous and diverse. Therefore it is difficult to classify and to put these different attempts into order. Table 9.1 gives an overview of the different experimental settings mentioned above.

The question of whether glial secreted or plasma membrane bound factors are necessary to induce certain BBB properties in BCEC can still not be resolved. Findings described in the literature are still controversial, sometimes contradictory. But it seems reasonable that more than one inducing factor is responsible for a differentiated BBB phenotype and that not all BBB properties are regulated by a common mechanism.

One of the candidates for an inducing factor is interleukin-6 (Takemoto *et al.*, 1994). This assumption is supported by recent findings, that astrocytes produce interleukin-6 as a response to traumatic injury (Hariri *et al.*, 1994). Thus this cytokine could be part of a repair mechanism of astrocytes in case of emergencies. As far as second messengers are concerned, up to now only cyclic AMP seems to be involved in several regulations of BBB phenotype like high TEER (Rubin *et al.*, 1991) or expression of ALP (Beuckmann *et al.*, 1995), but one has to assume that nature will not rely on one second messenger pathway solely.

Forthcoming research efforts should also focus on the influence of BCEC on astrocytes. This aspect of intercellular communication has been neglected nearly completely so far. So far, tissue culture of BCEC and *in vitro* experimental studies have revealed some aspects of BBB regulation, but certainly maintenance of BBB is a very complex network of interactions between BCEC, astrocytes, and possibly neurons, which still is not understood in full detail.

References

Amberger, A., Lemkin, P. F., Sonderegger, P. and Bauer, H. C. (1993). ECGF and heparin determine differentiation of cloned cerebral endothelial cells in vitro. *Molec. Chem. Neuropathol.*, **20**, 33–43.

Bauer, H. C., Tontsch, U., Amberger, A. and Bauer, H. (1990). Gamma-glutamyl-transpeptidase (GGTP) and Na^+K^+-ATPase activities in different subpopulations of cloned cerebral endothelial cells: responses to glial stimulation. *Biochem. Biophys. Res. Com.*, **168**, 358–63.

Beuckmann, C., Gath, U., Rauh, J. *et al.* (1994). Induction of the blood–brain barrier-related enzyme alkaline phosphatase in cerebral capillary endothelial cells by neuroectodermal cells in vitro. *Mater. Sci. Engin.*, **C2**, 31–5.

Beuckmann, C., Hellwig, S. and Galla, H.-J. (1995). Induction of the blood/brain-barrier-associated enzyme alkaline phosphatase in endothelial cells from cerebral capillaries is mediated via cAMP. *Eur. J. Biochem.*, **229**, 641–4.

Boado, R. J., Wang, L. and Pardridge, W. M. (1994). Enhanced expression of the blood–brain barrier GLUT 1 glucose transporter gene by brain-derived factors. *Molec. Brain Res.*, **22**, 259–67.

Dehouck, B., Dehouck, M.-P., Fruchart, J.-C. and Cecchelli, R. (1994). Upregulation of the low density lipoprotein receptor at the blood–brain barrier: intercommunications between brain capillary endothelial cells and astrocytes. *J. Cell Biol.*, **126**, 465–73.

Dehouck, M.-P., Méresse, S., Delorme, P. *et al.* (1990). An easier, reproducible, and mass-production method to study the blood–brain barrier in vitro. *J. Neurochem.*, **54**, 1798–801.

Hariri, R. J., Chang, V. A., Barie, P. S. *et al.* (1994). Traumatic injury induces interleukin-6 production by human astrocytes. *Brain Res.*, **636**, 139–42.

Hemmila, J. M. and Drewes, L. R. (1993). Glucose transporter (GLUT1) expression by canine brain microvessel endothelial cells in culture: an immunocytochemical study. *Adv. Exp. Med. Biol.*, **331**, 13–18.

Laterra, J. and Goldstein, G. W. (1991). Astroglial-induced in vitro angiogenesis: requirements for RNA and protein synthesis. *J. Neurochem.*, **57**, 1231–9.

Laterra, J., Guerin, C. and Goldstein, G. W. (1990). Astrocytes induce neural microvascular endothelial cells to form capillary-like structures in vitro. *J. Cell. Physiol.*, **144**, 204–15.

Lechardeur, D., Schwartz, B., Paulin, D. and Scherman, D. (1995). Induction of blood–brain barrier differentiation in a rat brain-derived endothelial cell line. *Exp. Cell Res.*, **220**, 161–70.

Maxwell, K., Berliner, J. A. and Cancilla, P. A. (1989). Stimulation of glucose analogue uptake by cerebral microvessel endothelial cells by a product released by astrocytes. *J. Neuropathol. Exp. Neurol.*, **48**, 69–80.

Meyer, J., Mischeck, U., Veyhl, M. *et al.* (1990). Blood–brain barrier characteristic enzymatic properties in cultured brain capillary endothelial cells. *Brain Res.*, **514**, 305–9.

Meyer, J., Rauh, J., and Galla, H.-J. (1991). The susceptibility of cerebral endothelial cells to astroglial induction of blood–brain barrier enzymes depends on their proliferative state. *J. Neurochem.*, **57**, 1971–7.

Pakaski, M. and Kasa, P. (1992). Glial cells in coculture can increase the acetylcholinesterase activity in human brain endothelial cells. *Neurochem. Int.*, **21**, 129–33.

Raub, T. J., Kuentzel, S. L. and Sawada, G. A. (1992). Permeability of bovine brain microvessel endothelial cells in vitro: barrier tightening by a factor released from astroglioma cells. *Exp. Cell Res.*, **199**, 330–40.

Rauh, J., Meyer, J., Beuckmann, C. and Galla, H.-J. (1992). Development of an in vitro cell culture system to mimic the blood–brain barrier. *Prog. Brain Res.*, **91**, 117–21.

Roux, F., Durieu-Trautmann, O., Chaverot, N. *et al.* (1994). Regulation of gamma-glutamyl transpeptidase and alkaline phosphatase activities in immortalized rat brain microvessel endothelial cells. *J. Cell Physiol.*, **159**, 101–13.

Rubin, L. L., Hall, D. E., Porter, S. *et al.* (1991). A cell culture model of the blood–brain barrier. *J. Cell Biol.*, **115**, 1725–35.

Takakura, Y., Trammel, A. M., Kuentzel, S. L. *et al.* (1991). Hexose uptake in primary cultures of bovine brain microvessel endothelial cells. II. Effects of conditioned media from astroglial and glioma cells. *Biochim. Biophys. Acta*, **1070**, 11–19.

Takemoto, H., Kaneda, K., Hosokawa, M. *et al.* (1994). Conditioned media of glial cell lines induce alkaline phosphatase activity in cultured artery endothelial cells. Identification of interleukin-6 as an induction factor. *FEBS Lett.*, **350**, 99–103.

Tao-Cheng, J.-H., Nagy, Z., and Brightman, M. W. (1987). Tight junctions of brain endothelium in vitro are enhanced by astroglia. *J. Neurosci.*, **7**, 3293–9.

Tio, S., Deenen, M. and Marani, E. (1990). Astrocyte-mediated induction of alkaline phosphatase activity in human umbilical cord vein endothelium: an in vitro model. *Eur. J. Morphol.*, **28**, 289–300.

Tontsch, U. and Bauer, H.-C. (1991). Glial cells and neurons induce blood–brain barrier related enzymes in cultured cerebral endothelial cells. *Brain Res.*, **539**, 247–53.

Wolburg, H., Neuhaus, J., Kniesel, U. *et al.* (1994). Modulation of tight junction structure in blood–brain barrier endothelial cells. *J. Cell Sci.*, **107**, 1347–57.

Wolff, J. E. A., Laterra, J. and Goldstein, G. W. (1992). Steroid inhibition of neural microvessel morphogenesis in vitro: receptor mediation and astroglial dependence. *J. Neurochem.*, **58**, 1023–32.

10 Brain microvessel endothelial cell culture systems

KENNETH L. AUDUS, JAYNA M. ROSE, WEN WANG
and RONALD T. BORCHARDT

- Introduction
- Cell culture methods
- Configurations for transport and metabolism studies
- Summary

Introduction

In vitro systems have had an important role in the development of our current understanding of the biochemical properties of the blood–brain barrier (BBB) (Joo, 1985, 1992, 1993). In particular, the development of brain microvessel endothelial cell (BMEC) culture systems, which retain many of the BBB properties *in vitro*, has provided simple, dynamic experimental systems to evaluate and elaborate on the biochemical and molecular basis of the BBB (Laterra and Goldstein, 1993). This chapter focuses on some of the current methodologies for the establishment of primary cultures of BMECs, BMEC and astrocyte co-culture systems, and the configurations available for studying BMEC transport processes.

Cell culture methods

Essentially three types of BMEC cultures are currently used by researchers. These include the primary cultures, co-culture systems, and cell lines. Each has demonstrated and has contributed basic information on cellular, biochemical, and molecular properties of the BBB (Joo, 1985, 1992, 1993; Laterra and Goldstein, 1993). For each system, we have provided a summary of methodologies

involved for establishment and some comments on the advantages and disadvantages of the culture type. For a given researcher, choice of these systems will generally be dictated by the specific BBB application or parameter one wants to investigate.

Primary cultures

BMECs are isolated from bovine brain grey matter by enzymatic digestion as described by Audus and Borchardt (1986, 1987) and Audus *et al.* (1996). Briefly, two fresh bovine brains (~ 30 min after death) are obtained from a local meat processing firm and placed in ice-cold minimum essential medium (MEM) buffered with 50 mM HEPES, pH 7.4, containing 100 μg/ml penicillin G, 100 μg/ml streptomycin, 50 μg/ml polymyxin B, and 2.5 μg/ml amphotericin B. Meninges and large surface vessels are removed from the brains and discarded. The cerebral gray matter is scraped away from the brain, collected, and minced to 1–2 mm cubes with sterile razor blades. The minced gray matter is enzymatically dispersed during a 2.5-h dispase digestion (4 ml dispase solution [12.5%] per 50 g of grey matter) at 37 °C to liberate microvessels from brain tissue. The microvessels are then separated from the tissue debris by dextran (13%) centrifugation. The isolated microvessels are further incubated for 4 h with collagenase/dispase (3 ml of collagenase/dispase [1 mg/ml] per gram of microvessels) to dissociate pericytes and astrocytes from the microvessels. Finally, the microvessels are separated from contaminated cells by Percoll gradient centrifugation. The isolated microvessels are stored at $-70\,°C$ in MEM containing 20% platelet-poor horse serum and 10% DMSO (dimethylsulfoxide). The viability of the isolated microvessel endothelial cells is about 90% as revealed by Trypan Blue exclusion (Audus and Borchardt, 1986). Although this protocol was originally designed for isolating microvessels from bovine brains, it can be applied to the isolation of microvessels from brains of other species (Shi and Audus, 1994).

The isolated brain microvessels can be grown successfully as primary cultures on a substrate-treated solid plastic surface (tissue culture plate), a microporous filter membrane (polycarbonate membrane), or a filter membrane insert (Transwell®). In general, the culture surface is pretreated with rat tail collagen and fibronectin prior to the seeding (Audus and Borchardt, 1986). The BMECs are seeded at $50\,000$ cells/cm^2 in the BMEC medium (45% minimum essential medium, 45% F-12 medium, 10% platelet-poor horse serum, $50\,\mu g/ml$ gentamicin, $125\,\mu g/ml$ heparin). Addition of endothelial cell growth supplements ($25\,\mu g/ml$) to the culture medium is optional. The cells are grown in a 37 °C incubator in 5% CO$_2$ and 95% humidity. The culture medium is changed on the third day after plating and every other day thereafter. The cultured BMECs reach confluence on day 7 or 8 and form a tight monolayer on approximately day 9 or 10. Experiments are typically conducted between days 9 and 12. The cells will begin to undergo noticeable morphological and functional changes after day 16 (Raub *et al.*, 1992).

The primary cultures of BMECs form confluent monolayers that retain many morphological and biochemical properties similar to the BBB *in vivo* (Audus and Borchardt, 1986,1987; Miller *et al.*, 1992) and are functionally polarized (Raub and Audus, 1990; Borges *et al.*, 1994; Wang *et al.*, 1996). The cells grown on solid substrates (e.g. tissue culture plates) are useful for studies of receptor-mediated or transporter-mediated uptake as well as the gene expression of BBB endothelium-specific proteins. BMEC monolayers grown on permeable supports (e.g. microporous polycarbonate membrane or Transwell®) are particularly useful since they allow one to study the transcellular transport of solutes and permit access to both the luminal and abluminal surfaces of the BMEC monolayers (Audus and Borchardt, 1991). This access to both cellular surfaces allows investigation of polarized transporters, receptors, and enzymes as well as other asymmetrically distributed properties that may define the nature of the BBB.

The limitation of primary BMEC cultures has been their higher than desirable paracellular permeability, reflected by the measurement of the electrical resistance across the BMEC monolayer. For instance, the resistance measures 160 Ωcm^2 *in vitro* versus 400–1200 Ωcm^2 *in vivo* (Oleson and Crone, 1986). This apparently results from the development of incomplete tight intercellular junctions in cell culture. It is also noticed that the BMECs undergo some dedifferentiation in cell culture, resulting in down-regulation of the expression of some proteins such as the glucose transporter (Boado and Pardridge, 1990). Since the primary BMEC culture system is free of other environmental inputs (i.e. neuronal and astroglial influence, the cylindrical geometry of the capillary, blood pressure and flow, blood-borne factors, and blood cells), BMEC function and differentiation *in vitro* may not be identical to that of the BBB *in vivo* (Joo, 1992; Reardon and Audus, 1993).

Co-cultures

The influence of astrocytes on BMEC development can be simulated by using astrocyte-conditioned medium or astrocyte co-culture. Astrocyte-conditioned medium is obtained by culturing astrocytes isolated as described by Lillien *et al.* (1988) in MEM containing 10% FCS for two to three days. The astrocyte-conditioned medium is then collected and added to the BMEC culture medium for BMEC culture. The astrocyte co-culture system can be established in two ways, i.e. growing astrocytes with or without direct contact with the BMECs. In a direct contact system, the BMECs are grown directly on the top of the astrocytes layer, or the BMECs are grown on one side of the porous filter membrane and the astrocytes are grown on the other side of the membrane (DeBault, 1981; Tao-Cheng *et al.*, 1987). In an indirect contact system using Transwells®, astrocytes are grown in the bottom chamber of the Transwell® and the BMECs are grown on the insert chamber; where there is no direct contact of the two cell types, but astrocyte-secreted factors can continuously reach the BMECs through the culture medium (Rubin *et al.*, 1991; Raub, *et al.*, 1992).

The advantage of using astrocyte co-culture or conditioned medium is that the incorporation of astrocyte input into the BMEC culture system improves this *in vitro* BBB model so that it more closely mimics the *in vivo* BBB with respect to structural, metabolic, and permeability characteristics (Jantzer and Raff, 1987; Tao-Cheng *et al.*, 1987; Joo, 1992, 1993). However, the more substantial induction effects of astrocytes or conditioned medium on BMECs are observed with the passaged or subcultured cell systems (Raub *et al.*, 1992).

Cell lines

Efforts have been made to establish continuous cell lines representative of BBB endothelium by generating passaged BMECs or transformed BMECs. In general, passaged cells appear to lose the characteristics of BBB endothelial cells during the passages and retain more morphological and biochemical markers for the BBB only when co-cultured with astrocyte, neuron, and/or pericytes or by addition of conditioned medium to the BMEC culture environment (DeBault, 1981; Dehouck *et al.*, 1990; Minikawa *et al.*, 1991; Rubin *et al.*, 1991; Tontsch and Bauer, 1991; Raub *et al.*, 1992).

Several transformed, immortalized BMEC systems that retain some BBB endothelial markers have been established. Rat BMECs transformed by Rous sarcoma virus exhibited anchorage-independent growth and elevated levels of γ-glutamyl transpeptidase (Diglio *et al.*, 1983; Caspers and Diglio, 1984). RBE4 cells, a clone of rat BMECs transfected with a plasmid containing the E1A adenovirus gene, display a nontransformed phenotype, express typical endothelial markers, and remain sensitive to angiogenic and astroglial

factors for the expression of the BBB-related γ-glutamyl transpeptidase activity and alkaline phosphatase activity (Roux *et al.*, 1994). Similar systems developed from mouse and bovine BMECs also demonstrated that transformed BMECs retain certain morphological and biochemical markers of the BBB (Durieu-Trautmann *et al.*, 1991) and have potential in the study of mechanisms related to BMEC growth functions and control (Robinson *et al.*, 1986).

Establishing immortalized BMEC systems would significantly reduce the tedious work required for the isolation of the BMECs; however, these cell systems have not been characterized to the same extent as either the primary or passaged cell culture systems.

Configurations for transport and metabolism studies

While the uptake of substances into the BMECs can be studied with monolayers grown on solid supports, transport studies require culturing the cells onto permeable filters or filter inserts. Metabolism can also be studied on solid supports but many times it is necessary to have a polarized system which is obtained by culturing the cells on permeable filters. The following section outlines three common systems used in metabolism and transport studies of BMECs.

Filter inserts

The most common type of insert used with BMECs is the Costar Transwell® culture-insert system (Costar, Cambridge, MA). Transwell® inserts are available in many sizes but the 24 mm inserts provide the easiest access for transport studies. BMECs are cultured onto Transwell® inserts with a 0.4 μm pore polycarbonate filter. In the Transwell® system, the 3.0 mm pore filters are not recommended since the BMECs can migrate through these pores and form monolayers on both sides of the polycarbonate filter (Raub *et al.*, 1992).

In order to grow BMECs successfully, the endothelial cells must be grown on a substrate-treated surface. Each Transwell® insert is liberally coated with rat-tail collagen (3 mg/ml in 0.1%

acetic acid). All excess collagen is aspirated away with a pipette, leaving a thin wet coating of the surface. The collagen-coated inserts are then exposed to ammonia fumes for 5 min to promote cross-linking of the collagen. The inserts must then be sterilized under UV light for 90 min. After sterilization, bovine fibronectin is added to the surface of the insert for 45 min and the excess is then washed away. The collagen and fibronectin provide a growth surface for the BMECs. The endothelial cells are plated at a density of 50 000–250 000 cells/cm^2 in a volume of 1.5 ml in the insert (donor) chamber with 2.6 ml in the bottom (receiver) chamber (Raub *et al.*, 1992). Confluent monolayers are obtained in 10–14 days under standard culture conditions of 37 °C, 5% CO_2, and 95% humidity. The apical side of the monolayer is defined as the top of the insert and the basolateral side is defined as the side facing the collagen/fibronectin matrix.

Transport and metabolism experiments are performed according to the following procedure: the Transwell® cluster plate is preincubated at 4 °C or 37 °C in pH 7.4 buffer for 15–30 min. The substrate is then added to the apical (insert) side or the basolateral (well) side. Samples (50 µl) can be conveniently taken from the apical or basolateral side at designated time points and replaced with an equivalent volume of buffer. To avoid the effect of an unstirred aqueous layer, the cluster plate can be gently shaken or vortexed. Temperature is maintained by placing the cluster plate in an incubator or water bath (Chikhale *et al.*, 1994; Raub and Newton, 1991; Raub *et al.*, 1992).

The advantages of the Transwell® insert system are its convenience and disposability. The inserts can also be easily removed from the cluster plate and placed into an Endohm apparatus (World Precision Instruments) for transendothelial electrical resistance (TEER) measurements. Disadvantages include the cost, the lack of convenient temperature control, and the inability to sufficiently agitate the solution in the wells to maintain 'well-stirred' conditions. Stirring is partially accomplished by placing the entire cluster plate on an orbital shaker. However, the degree of agitation is greater on the apical side than the basolateral side, which is proportionately more filled with solution and

thus more confined. Also, the design of the Transwell® insert is a vertical diffusion design; therefore, a hydrostatic pressure gradient could also play a role in the transport of substances.

Gas-lift horizontal diffusion chambers

Due to the disadvantages of the Transwell® system, side-by-side diffusion systems are often favored. A new design for one such system, the Costar Snapwell™ and Diffusion Chamber system, is an assembly of Snapwell™ Transwell® inserts (12 mm polycarbonate membrane, 0.4 µm pore) and diffusion chambers placed into a heating block capable of holding six diffusion chambers. The heating block has a 12-channel gas manifold for stirring that can be controlled with individual valves. Electrodes and electrode adapters are also available.

The Snapwells™ are coated using the same procedures as described above for the Transwells®. The cells are plated on the inserts using a volume of 0.5 ml in the insert and a volume of 2.6 ml in the surrounding well. Once confluent monolayers are formed, the bottom section of the Snapwell™ containing the intact cell layer is easily detached for insertion into a diffusion chamber. Figure 10.1 shows a diagram of the Snapwell™ Transwell® system. The diffusion chamber is placed in the heating block and the temperature is maintained with a circulating water bath. The transport buffer is circulated by utilizing gas-lift mixing (usually O_2/CO_2) providing a well-stirred system. Each chamber of the diffusion cell can contain 4.0–6.0 ml of buffer and samples can be easily removed from either side (Karlsson and Artursson, 1992; Hidalgo *et al.* 1991, 1992; Ng *et al.*, 1993).

The horizontal side-by-side orientation of the diffusion system prevents a hydrostatic pressure gradient across the cell layer. The gas-lift system greatly reduces the unstirred aqueous layer adjacent to the cells and the small configuration of the Snapwell™ insert allows for a minimum stagnant layer. A disadvantage of this system is that, although the fluid flow in the chambers is designed to be as laminar as possible to the cell monolayer, some bubbling rates can cause significant mechanical shear to the cells.

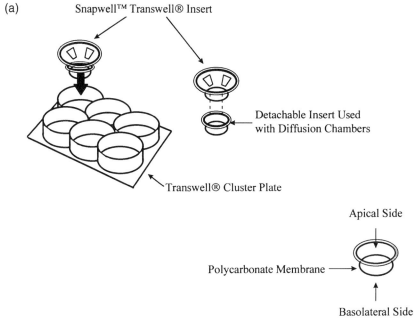

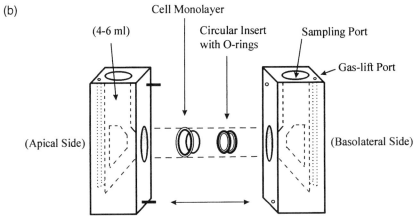

Fig. 10.1 (a). Schematic of the Snapwell™ Transwell® system showing the detachable insert. The insert is shown with the polycarbonate membrane and the apical and basolateral sides defined. (b). Schematic of the diffusion chambers used with the Snapwells™ showing the assembly of the system.

Stirred horizontal diffusion chambers

The third system described here is also a horizontal side-by-side diffusion apparatus. The Side-bi-Side™ diffusion system (Crown Glass, Inc., Somerville, NJ) consists of two glass chambers surrounded by thermal jackets that are maintained at a constant temperature with a circulating water bath (Fig. 10.2). The cells are grown on polycarbonate membranes with a diameter of 13 mm and a pore size of 0.4 μm. The membranes are coated on both sides with rat-tail collagen and placed in a 100 mm culture dish. The dish is UV sterilized for 90 min and then coated with bovine fibronectin. BMECs are plated at a density of 50 000 cells/cm² and confluent monolayers are formed in 10–14 days. The monolayer around the membranes can be examined under a light microscope. Once confluent, each membrane is then placed between the two chambers of the Side-bi-

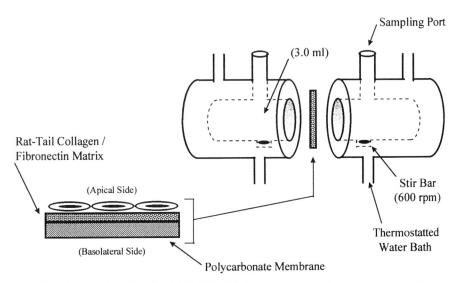

Fig. 10.2. Schematic of the Side-bi-Side™ diffusion apparatus and the placement of the polycarbonate membrane containing confluent monolayers of BMECs.

Side™ diffusion apparatus. The chambers are clamped together and placed onto an external drive console. This console continuously stirs the chambers at 600 r.p.m. using Teflon-coated stir bar magnets. Each chamber contains 3.0 ml buffer, pH 7.4. The apical side of the monolayer is defined as the side facing the solution of the dish and the basolateral side is the side of the monolayer facing the collagen/fibronectin support. Samples are easily removed from either chamber (Guillot and Audus, 1991; Reardon and Audus, 1993; Weber *et al.*, 1993; Borges *et al.*, 1994; Brownson *et al.*, 1994; Dehouck *et al.*, 1995).

The stirring console of the Side-bi-Side™ diffusion apparatus maintains a constant stirring rate of 600 r.p.m. and greatly reduces the unstirred aqueous layer. This stirring has not been found to cause any damage to the cell monolayer. One major disadvantage of this system is the complicated assembly of the diffusion chambers, especially the placement of the membrane. Care must be taken when placing the membrane between the diffusion chambers. The membrane must be removed from the culture dish without disrupting the monolayer and placed between the chambers as quickly as possible. The diffusion chambers must then be clamped together and this does result in crushing of the cells around the circumference of the diffusion cell opening. Generally, an appropriate

passive permeability marker (e.g. sucrose, fluorescein, inulin, dextrans, etc.) is used to normalize permeability data for this source of leakiness.

Summary

The continued importance of the need to direct both conventional drug molecules and the new therapeutic entities developed by the biotechnology industry to the cerebrovasculature or brain for treatment of disease and pathophysiological conditions requires appropriate *in vitro* systems representing the BBB. Provided they are validated for the particular application, the availability of the cell culture methodologies summarized here does permit researchers to investigate some of the fundamental biological properties of the BBB. Moreover, the knowledge of BBB properties generated through investigations employing these cell culture systems is likely to assist researchers in introducing methodological refinements to improve on or develop more appropriate *in vitro* techniques.

Acknowledgment

The authors gratefully acknowledge a Pharmaceutical Research and Manufacturers of America

Foundation, Inc. Predoctoral Fellowship (J.M.R.), an American Foundation for Pharmaceutical Education Predoctoral Fellowship (J.M.R.), a Takeru Higuchi Predoctoral Fellowship (J.M.R.), and research grants from the American Heart Association–Kansas Affiliate, Costar Corporation, and The United States Public Health Service (GM-51633, GM-088359, DA09315).

References

Audus, K. L. and Borchardt, R. T. (1986). Characterization of an *in vitro* blood–brain barrier model system for studying drug transport and metabolism. *Pharmaceut. Res.*, **3**, 81–7.

Audus, K. L. and Borchardt, R. T. (1987). Bovine brain microvessel endothelial cell monolayers as a model system for the blood–brain barrier. *Ann. N.Y. Acad. Sci.*, **507**, 9–18.

Audus, K. L. and Borchardt, R. T. (1991). Transport of macromolecules across the capillary endothelium. *Handbook of Experimental Pharmacology*, **100**, 43–70.

Audus, K. L., Ng, L., Wang, W. and Borchardt, R. T. (1996). Brain microvessel endothelial cell culture systems. In *Model for Assessing Drug Absorption and Metabolism*, ed. R. T. Borchardt, P. L. Smith and G. Wilson, pp. 239–58. New York: Plenum Press.

Boado, R. J. and Pardridge, W. M. (1990). Molecular cloning of the bovine blood–brain barrier glucose transporter cDNA and demonstration of phylogenetic conservation of the 5′-untranslated region. *Molec. Cell. Neurosci.*, **1**, 224–32.

Borges, N., Shi, F., Azevedo, I. and Audus, K. L. (1994). Changes in brain microvessel endothelial cell monolayer permeability induced by adrenergic drugs. *Eur. J. Pharmacol.*, **269**, 243–8.

Brownson, E. A., Abbruscato, T. J., Gillespie, T.J. *et al.* (1994). Effect of peptidases at the blood brain barrier on the permeability of enkephalin. *J. Pharmacol. Exp. Ther.*, **270**, 675–80.

Caspers, M. L. and Diglio, C. A. (1984). Expression of gamma-glutamyl transpeptidase in a transformed rat cerebral endothelial cell line. *Biochim. Biophys. Acta*, **803**, 1–6.

Chikhale, E. G., Ng, K.-Y., Burton, P. S., *et al.* (1994). Hydrogen bonding potential as a determinant of the *in vitro* and *in situ* blood–brain barrier permeability of peptides. *Pharmaceut. Res.*, **11**, 412–9.

DeBault, L. E. (1981). γ-glutamyl transpeptidase induction mediated by glial foot process-to-endothelium contact in co-culture. *Brain Res.*, **220**, 432–5.

Dehouck, M. P., Jolliet-Riant, P., Bree, F. *et al.* (1990). Drug transfer across the blood–brain barrier: Correlation between *in vitro* and *in vivo* models. *J. Neurochem.*, **58**, 1790–7.

Dehouck, M. P., Dehouck, B., Schluep, C. *et al.* (1995). Drug transport to the brain: comparison between *in vitro* and *in vivo* models of the blood–brain barrier. *Eur. J. Pharmaceut. Sci.*, **3**, 357–65.

Diglio, C. A., Wolfe, D. E. and Meyers, P. (1983). Transformation of rat cerebral endothelial cells by Rous sarcoma virus. *J. Cell Biol.*, **97**, 15–21.

Durieu-Trautmann, O., Foignant-Chaverot, N., Perdomo, J. *et al.* (1991). Immortalization of brain capillary endothelial cells with maintenance of structural characteristics of the blood–brain barrier endothelium. *In Vitro Cell. Dev. Biol.*, **27**, 771–8.

Guillot, F. L. and Audus, K. L. (1991). Angiotensin peptide regulation of bovine brain microvessel endothelial cell monolayer permeability. *J. Cardiovasc. Pharmacol.*, **18**, 212–8.

Hidalgo, I. J., Hillgren, K. M., Grass, G. M. *et al.* (1991). Characterization of the unstirred water layer in Caco-2 cell monolayers using a novel diffusion apparatus. *Pharmaceut. Res.*, **8**, 222–7.

Hidalgo, I. J., Grass, G. M., Hillgren, K. M. *et al.* (1992). A new side-by-side diffusion cell for studying transport across epithelial cell monolayers. *In Vitro Cell. Dev. Biol.*, **28A**, 578–80.

Jantzer, R. C. and Raff, M. C. (1987). Astrocytes induce blood–brain barrier properties in endothelial cells. *Nature*, **325**, 253–7.

Joo, F. (1985). The blood–brain barrier *in vitro*: ten years of research on microvessels isolated from the brain. *Neurochem. Int.*, **7**, 1–25.

Joo, F. (1992). The cerebral microvessels in culture, an update. *J. Neurochem.*, **58**, 1–17.

Joo, F. (1993). The blood–brain barrier *in vitro*: The second decade. *Neurochem. Int.*, **23**, 499–521.

Karlsson, J. and Artursson, P. (1992). A new diffusion chamber system for the determination of drug permeability coefficients across the human intestinal epithelium that are independent of the unstirred water layer. *Biochim. Biophys. Acta*, **1111**, 204–10.

Laterra, J. and Goldstein, G. W. (1993). Brain microvessels and microvascular cells *in vitro*. In *The Blood–Brain Barrier: Cellular and Molecular Biology*, ed. W. M. Pardridge, pp. 1–24. New York: Raven Press.

Lillien, L. E., Sendtner, M., Rohrer, H. *et al.* (1988). Type-2 astrocyte development in rat brain cultures is initiated by a CNTF-like protein produced by type-1 astrocytes. *Neuron*, **1**, 485–94.

Miller, D. W., Audus, K. L. and Borchardt, R. T. (1992). Application of cultured endothelial cells of the brain microvasculature in the study of the blood–brain barrier. *J. Tiss. Cult. Meth.*, **14**, 217–24.

Minikawa, T., Bready, J., Berliner, J. *et al.* (1991). *In vitro* interaction of astrocytes and pericytes with capillary-like structure of brain microvessel endothelium. *Lab. Invest.*, **65**, 32–40.

Ng, K. Y., Grass, G. M., Lane, H. *et al.* (1993). Characterization of the unstirred water layer in cultured brain microvessel endothelial cells. *In Vitro Cell. Dev. Biol.*, **29A**, 627–9.

Oleson, S. P. and Crone, C. (1986). Substances that rapidly augment ionic conductance of endothelium in cerebral venules. *Acta Physiol. Scand.*, **127**, 233–41.

Raub, T. J. and Audus, K. L. (1990). Adsorptive endocytosis and membrane recycling by cultured primary bovine brain microvessel endothelial cell monolayers. *J. Cell Sci.*, **97**, 127–38.

Raub, T. J. and Newton, C. R. (1991). Recycling kinetics and transcytosis of transferrin in primary cultures of bovine brain microvessel endothelial cells. *J. Cell Physiol.*, **149**, 141–51.

Raub, T. J., Kuentzel, S. L. and Sawada, G. A. (1992). Permeability of bovine brain microvessel endothelial cells *in vitro*: barrier tightening by a factor released from astroglioma cells. *Exp. Cell Res.*, **199**, 330–40.

Reardon, P. M. and Audus, K. L. (1993). Applications of primary cultures of brain microvessel endothelial cell monolayers in the study of vasoactive peptide interaction with the blood–brain barrier. *s.t.p. Pharma Sciences*, **3**, 63–8.

Robinson, R. A., TenEyck, C. J. and Hart, M. N. (1986). Establishment and preliminary growth characteristics of a transformed mouse cerebral microvessel endothelial cell line. *Lab. Invest.*, **54**, 579–88.

Roux, F., Durieu-Trautmann, O., Chaverot, N. *et al.* (1994). Regulation of gamma-glutamyl transpeptidase and alkaline phosphatase activities in immortalized rat brain microvessel endothelial cells. *J. Cell Physiol.*, **159**, 101–13.

Rubin, L. L., Hall, D. E., Porter, S. *et al.* (1991). A cell culture model of the blood–brain barrier. *J. Cell Biol.*, **115**, 1725–35.

Shi, F. and Audus, K. L. (1994). Biochemical characteristics of primary and passaged cultures of primate brain microvessel endothelial cells. *Neurochem. Res.*, **19**, 427–33.

Tao-Cheng, Nagy, Z. and Brightman, M. W. (1987). Tight junctions of brain endothelium *in vitro* are enhanced by astroglia. *J. Neurosci.*, **7**, 3293–9.

Tontsch, U. and Bauer, H. C. (1991). Glial cells and neurons induce blood/brain barrier related enzymes in cultured cerebral endothelial cells. *Brain Res.*, **539**, 247–53.

Wang, W., Merrill, M. J. and Borchardt, R. T. (1996). Vascular endothelial growth factor affects the permeability of brain microvessel endothelial cells *in vitro. Am. J. Physiol.*, in press.

Weber, S. J., Abbruscato, T. J., Brownson, E. A. *et al.* (1993). Assessment of an *in vitro* blood–brain barrier model using several [Met^5]enkephalin opioid analogs. *J. Pharmacol. Exp. Ther.*, **266,** 1649–55.

11 Intracerebral microdialysis

ELIZABETH C. M. de LANGE, ALBERTUS G. de BOER
and DOUWE D. BREIMER

- Introduction
- Basic principles
- Potentials and limitations
- Technical aspects
- Intracerebral microdialysis and BBB transport studies
- Perspectives and conclusions

Introduction

Transport across the blood–brain barrier (BBB) *in vivo* can be studied by two different experimental strategies. An indirect approach is to measure brain extraction of a compound from blood (or other media) after passage through the brain capillaries, e.g. by the carotid artery single injection technique. A direct means is measuring the concentration of the compound in the brain itself, either after tissue homogenization or by quantitative autoradiography. More sophisticated and noninvasive techniques are PET and NMR. These techniques are however expensive and require specialized equipment and expertise. Another quite appropriate technique is intracerebral microdialysis, which is relatively simple to apply and comparably inexpensive. It allows for the continuous monitoring of levels of compounds within discrete brain regions of a single animal (Ungerstedt, 1984). In recent years the *in vivo* microdialysis technique has been widely used for a variety of applications. It has been used for pharmacological (Jacobson *et al.*, 1985), physiological (Benveniste *et al.*, 1984), and behavioral studies (Gerozissis *et al.*, 1995) to monitor and analyze endogenous compounds such as neurotransmitters, or exogenous compounds. The technique can also be used for the determination of transport of compounds across the BBB (Allen *et al.*, 1992; De Lange *et al.*, 1994, 1995*a–d*). In this chapter the use of intracerebral microdialysis in studying blood–brain barrier (BBB) transport is evaluated. Basic principles, potentials as well as limitations, and technical considerations are presented. Though intracerebral microdialysis is an invasive technique, studies performed on the use of intracerebral microdialysis in BBB transport studies suggest that this method evokes minimal tissue reactions and provides valid information provided that surgical and experimental conditions are carefully optimized and controlled. Pharmacokinetic profiles of compounds in the brain can be obtained in parallel to serial blood sampling. In combination with blood microdialysis, BBB transport can be directly related to actual free concentrations in blood. The technique opens up the possibility for investigations of local BBB functionality under physiological and pathological conditions. Near future technical developments may minimize problems that may sometimes arise in using this technique such as analysis of extreme low concentration/low volume dialysate samples, adsorption of compounds to certain microdialysis membranes, and the quantitation of the dialysis data. However, for already quite a number of cases the technique has demonstrated its practical value and it holds a great promise for automated, continuous sampling of various regions in the brain over prolonged experimental periods.

Basic principles

Intracerebral microdialysis involves the stereotactic implantation of a microdialysis probe in the brain. The probe consists of a semipermeable membrane which can be partly covered by an impermeable coating. Thus, the length and position of the semipermeable part of the probe can be selected to approach the specific area of interest. The probe is perfused continuously with a physiological perfusion solution. Small molecular weight compounds will traverse the semipermeable membrane, either into or out of the perfusate, by diffusion from higher to lower concentrations. The probe can be used in the delivery mode, by adding the compound to the perfusate, or in the sampling mode in which case the perfusate is devoid of the compound of interest (Fig. 11.1). In most applications the probe is used in the sampling mode. The dialysate is collected and can thereafter be analyzed by virtually any technique.

Potentials and limitations

Intracerebral microdialysis offers important advantages over other techniques used for BBB drug transport studies: (1) the concentration of a compound in brain extracellular fluid (ECF) can be measured at multiple time points within an individual animal, which may potentially imply a significant reduction of the number of animals needed to obtain pharmacokinetic profiles; (2) it is possible to use awake and freely moving animals, and thereby possible influences of anesthesia can be reduced or even eliminated; (3) a dialysis membrane with low molecular weight cut off 'purifies' the sample by excluding large molecules; clean-up procedures may therefore be evaded and potential *ex vivo* degradation by enzymes is avoided; (4) the *ex vivo* analysis of the dialysate in principle enables the researcher to select an analysis procedure to determine the levels of the compound of interest in a selective and sensitive way; (5) the dialysate reflects free concentrations of the compound in the ECF of the selected brain area; this is of great value in pharmacological investigations where the free concentrations of the compound are often closely related to the elicited effect; (6) the microdialysis probe can be implanted in virtually any brain region, providing information on the concentration of a compound at the selected site.

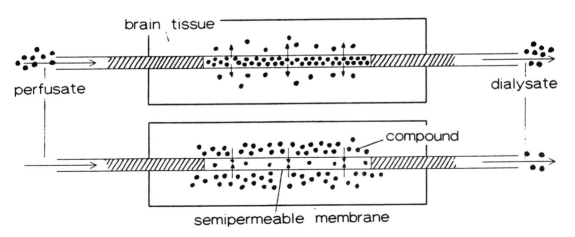

Fig. 11.1. A microdialysis probe is implanted into the brain, with the semipermeable part positioned in the selected area. In the case of concentration differences of a compound between perfusate and periprobe extracellular fluid, diffusion will take place from the higher to the lower concentration. The microdialysis probe can be used in the delivery mode (upper picture) or in the sampling mode (lower picture).

Thus, pharmacokinetic profiles can be obtained in normal brain as well as in affected or diseased brain sites, for example in brain tumors.

However, a number of limitations in the use of this technique should also be considered: (1) it is an invasive technique, and although tissue reactions are minimal, the investigator should be aware of the possible consequences of tissue trauma on the system under investigation; (2) it is a diluting technique that may require very sensitive analytical procedures for quantitative analysis, for example when the compound does not penetrate the brain easily, or when the compound prefers to distribute in compartments other than the extracellular space; (3) if the compound of interest is bound to macromolecules or trapped on or in organelles, some form of tissue analysis might be needed; (4) not only the compound of interest will be removed by the dialysate, also other compounds may traverse the dialysis membrane, and their concentrations may be changed locally ('drainage effect'); (5) the concentrations of the compound in the dialysate reflect their free concentrations in the ECF of the selected brain part, but the relation between these concentrations ('in vivo recovery') not only depends on probe characteristics ('in vitro recovery') but also on periprobe processes like generation, elimination, metabolism, intra/extracellular exchange of the compound. The dialysate concentrations should therefore be considered as semi-quantitative. However, a number of methods exist to estimate 'true' concentrations in the ECF by correcting for in vivo recovery.

Technical aspects

Influence of experimental conditions

Although conceptually simple and straightforward, in vivo microdialysis involves quite a number of factors that may be of influence on the system of investigation. It is of importance to optimize experimental factors so that the data obtained provide valid information.

Probe geometry Microdialysis can be accomplished using a variety of probe geometries. In principle two different designs of intracerebral microdialysis probes can be used: a vertical probe

and a horizontal probe (Fig. 11.2). The choice of probe is generally made on the basis of surgical accessibility of the target tissue. For deep structures a vertical probe, and for superficial structures a horizontal (transversal) probe is usually preferred.

Some in vivo microdialysis experiments are performed with the horizontal probe where the membrane is surgically implanted from one side of the skull to the other, with the aid of a very thin and straight tungsten wire, which is thereafter removed (Imperato and Di Chiara, 1984). These probes are 'home-made' so that the selection of the membrane material and semipermeable part of the membrane can be chosen freely according to the requirements of a particular experiment (Damsma et al., 1988; Di Chiara, 1990; Terasaki et al., 1991; Shimura et al., 1992, Drijfhout et al., 1993, De Lange et al., 1994). For example, the dialyzing part of the horizontal probe can be extended up to about 9 mm for rat cortical brain.

In most laboratories, however, vertical probes are used. These probes are typically made of stainless steel or fused silica tubing, with a short length of semipermeable membrane at the tip (1 to 4 mm). These probes can be used after permanent implantation (fixed) or by (re)insertion via a preimplanted guide (Wellman, 1990). In the latter case the optimal interval between probe insertion and start of the microdialysis experiment can be determined without concomitant effects from anesthesia (Hamilton et al., 1992; Claassen, 1994; Drijfhout et al., 1995), because the animal may have recovered fully from anesthesia at the time of probe insertion. Obviously, probes that can be removed and reimplanted have advantages for chronic studies.

Vertical probes and guides are commercially available (CMA microdialysis AB, Stockholm, Sweden; Europhor, Toulouse, France; Bio Analytical Systems, West Lafayette, IN, USA), but in many cases 'home-made probes' are preferred to suit the specific research needs (Johnson and Justice, 1983; Hernandez et al., 1986; Kapoor and Chalmers, 1987; Kendrick, 1989; Paredes et al., 1989; Nakamura et al., 1990; Wellman, 1990; Frothingham and Basbaum, 1992; Scheyer et al., 1994a; Mason and Romano, 1995).

Membrane materials Dialysis probes are made of semipermeable membranes and a variety of dia-

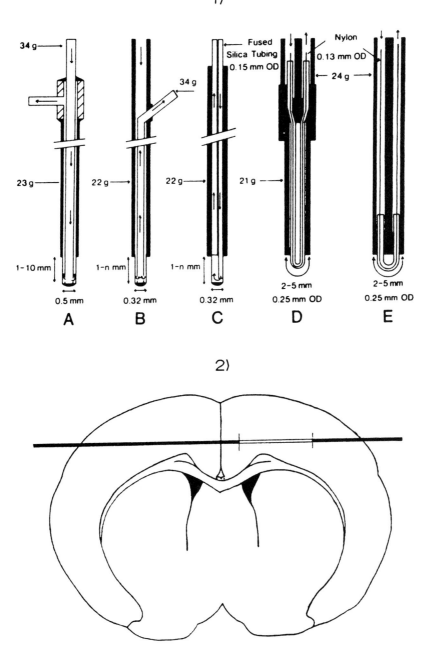

Fig. 11.2. In principle two different designs of intracerebral microdialysis probes can be used: (1) vertical designs A–E: From Kendrick (1989), with kind permission of Academic Press Inc., USA; (2) horizontal (transverse) design.

lyis tubing is commercially available. These differ with respect to outer diameters (150–500 μm) and inner diameters, composition (e.g. celluloses and copolymers like polyacetonitril/sodium methallyl sulfonate and polycarbonate/ether) and molecular mass cut-off (5–50 kDa). The diffusion of a compound over the dialysis membrane will depend on membrane properties and the physico-chemical

Table 11.1 In vitro *extraction (%) with three semi-permeable microdialysis membranes of acid metabolites and acetaminophen (ACET)*

	CMA (*n* = 4)	CUP (*n* = 4)	PAN (*n* = 4)
DOPAC	8.03 ± 1.46	5.99 ± 1.45	13.0 ± 0.88
5-HIAA	9.26 ± 1.33	6.42 ± 1.27	13.4 ± 1.11
HVA	7.17 ± 1.11	5.56 ± 1.26	12.7 ± 1.15
ACET	11.4 ± 1.38	9.80 ± 0.99	16.7 ± 2.23

From: Hsiao *et al.* (1990). With kind permission of Raven Press, New York, USA.

characteristics of the compound (Table 11.1; Hernandez *et al.*, 1986; Benveniste *et al.*, 1989; Levine and Powell, 1989; Maidment *et al.*, 1989; Benveniste and Huttemeier, 1990; Hsiao *et al.*, 1990; Nakamura *et al.*, 1990; Carneheim and Stahle, 1991; Yadid *et al.*, 1993). Specific interactions between compound and membrane material may occur and this may have a profound effect on the relation between the concentration of the compound found in the dialysate and the free periprobe concentrations (Landolt *et al.*, 1991; Tao and Hjorth, 1992).

Perfusion flow rate and recovery The flow rate of the perfusion medium affects the recovery of the compound and the resolution of the time-points. A high flow rate is used to remove or introduce as many molecules as possible per unit of time (absolute recovery) and a low flow is used to obtain a more concentrated dialysate (a higher relative recovery; which is defined as the ratio of the concentration of the compound in the dialysate over that in the periprobe ECF fluid). In general the term recovery refers to the relative recovery. Various *in vitro* experiments have been performed to examine the relationship between flow rate and recovery. Most investigators use a flow rate in the range 1–5 μl/min. The *in vitro* recovery is inversely dependent on the flow rate (Fig. 11.3) and, often linearly, dependent on the concentration in the periprobe fluid (Johnson and Justice, 1983; Jacobson and Hamberger, 1985; Hernandez *et al.*, 1986; Tossman and Ungerstedt, 1986; Levine and Powell, 1989; Lindefors *et al.*, 1989; Nakamura *et al.*, 1990). Then, an increase of the dialysis surface

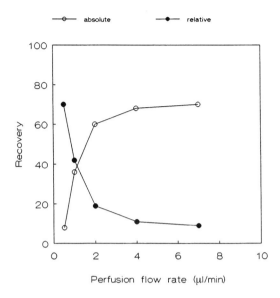

Fig. 11.3. Relationship between perfusion flow rate and relative and absolute recovery.

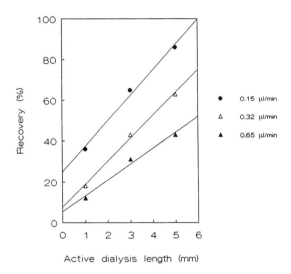

Fig. 11.4. Relationship between active dialysis length and relative recovery at different flow rates. From: Johnson and Justice (1983), with kind permission of Elsevier Science-NL, Sara Burgerhartstraat 25, 1055 KV Amsterdam, The Netherlands.

(length) will increase the recovery (Fig. 11.4; Johnson and Justice, 1983; Lindefors *et al.*, 1989). However, the choice of the length is usually limited by the size of the brain structure to be dialyzed.

A further increase in the flow rate will further

increase the hydrostatic pressure inside the probe, which may result in net transport of fluid across the dialysis membrane. This may counteract the diffusion of the compound into the dialysis fluid. Pressure gradients will be greatly affected by the sequence of dimensions of the perfusate (inlet) tubing and the dialysis (outlet) tubing (Ruggeri *et al.*, 1990). Also the length of the outlet tubing should be considered (Kuipers and Korf, 1994). It is safe to use a sequence of diameters of tubing that slightly increases from the perfusion pump ultimately to the collection side, and to check flow rate with and without the probe interconnected. Another disadvantage of using a high flow rate can be distortion of normal physiology because more substances are removed (Gonzalez-Mora *et al.*, 1991).

While *in vitro* recovery measurements at different flow rates will provide information about permeability of the probe membrane to the compound and a possible interaction between these two, it cannot be used as a reliable measure for recovery *in vivo*, because factors other than membrane properties will affect *in vivo* recovery (see Quantitation of microdialysis data, below).

Composition of the perfusion medium In microdialysis experiments perfusion media are used that vary widely in composition and pH (Benveniste and Huttemeier, 1990; Table 11.2). Ideally the composition, ion strength and pH of the perfusion solution should be as close as possible to those of the ECF of the dialyzed tissue. Extracellular fluids mostly contain only very small concentrations of proteins and can be left out of the perfusion medium, although in some cases proteins have been added to the perfusion medium to prevent peptide sticking to the microdialysis probe and tubings (Kendrick, 1989; Levine and Powell, 1989; Maidment *et al.*, 1989). The composition of the perfusate can be changed in order to study the effects on the system under investigation. It has been shown that deviations in ion composition affect brain dialysate levels of neurotransmitters (Moghaddam and Bunney, 1989; Osborne *et al*, 1990; Timmerman and Westerink, 1991) and drugs (De Lange *et al.*, 1994). The latter investigators have shown that a non-physiological (hypotonic) perfusion medium used in daily repeated

Table 11.2 *Perfusion medium compositions (in mM unless otherwise indicated)*

Distilled water
Saline: 0.9 % NaCl
Saline: 0.9 % NaCl; 1.85% $CaCl_2$ (pH 7.2)
Saline: 0.9 % NaCl; 0.5% bovine serum albumin

Ringers solution
134 NaCl; 5.9 KCl; 1.3 $CaCl_2$; 1.2 $MgCl_2$ (O_2-sat.)
147 NaCl; 2.4 $CaCl_2$; 4 KCl (pH 6.0)
147 NaCl; 3.4 $CaCl_2$; 4 KCl (pH 6.1)
147 NaCl; 1.3 $CaCl_2$; 4 KCl (pH 7.2)
155 NaCl; 2.3 $CaCl_2$; 5.5 KCl
189 NaCl; 3.4 $CaCl_2$; 3.9 KCl

Modified Ringers solution
145 NaCl; 1.2 $CaCl_2$; 2.7 KCl; 1 $MgCl_2$; 0.2 ascorbate (pH 7.4)

Buffered Ringers solution
147 NaCl; 3.4 $CaCl_2$; 2.8 KCl, 1.2 $MgCl_2$; 0.6 K_2HPO_4; 114 µM ascorbate (pH 6.9)

Krebs Ringer solution
147 NaCl; 3.4 $CaCl_2$; 4.0 KCl (pH 6.0)
138 NaCl; 1 $CaCl_2$; 5 KCl; 1 $MgCl_2$; 11 $NaHCO_3$; 1 $NaHPO_4$, 11 glucose (pH 7.5)

Krebs Ringer bicarbonate
122 NaCl; 1.2 $CaCl_2$; 3 KCl, 1.2 $MgSO_4$; 25 $NaHCO_3$; 0.4 KH_2PO_4, (pH 7.4)

Krebs–Henseleit bicarbonate buffer
118 NaCl; 2.5 $CaCl_2$; 4.7 KCl; 0.6 $MgSO_4$; 25 $NaHCO_3$; 1.2 NaH_2PO_4; 11 glucose

Mock-cerebrospinal fluids
120 NaCl; 1.5 $CaCl_2$; 5 KCl; 15 $NaHCO_3$; 1 $MgSO_4$; 6 glucose (pH 7.4)
127 NaCl; 1.1 $CaCl_2$; 2.4 KCl; 0.85 $MgCl_2$; 28 $NaHCO_3$; 0.5 KH_2PO_4; 0.5 Na_2SO_4; 5.9 glucose (pH 7.5)
127 NaCl; 1.3 $CaCl_2$; 2.5 KCl; 0.9 $MgCl_2$; (pH 6.0)
127 NaCl; 1.3 $CaCl_2$; 2.5 KCl; 2
133 NaCl; 3.0 KCl; 24.6 $NaHCO_3$; 6.7 urea; 3.7 glucose

From Benveniste and Huttemeier (1990) with kind permission of Pergamon Press Ltd, Oxford, UK.

experiments resulted in a substantial increase of the dialysate levels of the hydrophilic drug atenolol, presumably reflecting increased BBB permeability.

Temperature of the perfusion medium
While in most *in vitro* studies the effect of temperature is taken into account (Wages *et al.*, 1986), many investigators use perfusion media for *in vivo* experiments at room temperature. This may lead to a temperature gradient between probe and its surroundings, especially at higher flow rates, with potential effects not only on recovery but also on the periprobe tissue. De Lange *et al.* (1994) have investigated the effect of perfusate temperature on drug dialysate levels for a physiological and non-physiological perfusion fluid. In the case of the non-physiological perfusion medium, brain dialysate levels of acetaminophen were significantly affected by perfusate temperature.

Surgical trauma As intracerebral microdialysis is an invasive technique, processes of inflammation and subsequent healing (Coleman *et al*, 1974; Spector *et al.*, 1989) may be evoked following the insertion of a microdialysis probe. These may include neuronal damage, microglial and astroglial reactions, localized hemorrhages, alterations in glucose metabolism, alterations in BBB functionality and local biochemical disturbances (Cavanaugh, 1970; Del Rio Hortega and Penfield, 1972). It was found that following implantation of a microdialysis probe, formation of eicosanoids, local disturbances in cerebral blood flow and glucose metabolism were initially present (Benveniste *et al.*, 1987; Yergey and Heyes, 1990). These changes were more or less normalized one day after surgery. Histological evaluation revealed that glial reactions (gliosis) usually started two or three days after implantation of the probe, being confined mainly to a very small region around the probe (Imperato and Di Chiara, 1984; L'Heureux *et al.*, 1986; Benveniste and Diemer, 1987; Ruggeri *et al.*, 1990; Shuaib *et al.*, 1990; De Lange *et al*, 1995*d*). The perfusion procedure as such also had an effect on the course of tissue reactions (Fig. 11.5; De Lange *et al.*, 1995*d*). It was found that quite different results could be obtained in time, depending on the type and size of the probe (Matlaga *et al.*, 1976; Hamberger *et al.*, 1983; Benveniste and Diemer, 1987; Westerink and De Vries, 1988; Santiago and Westerink, 1990; Fumero *et al.*, 1991), post-surgery interval (Westerink and Tuinte, 1986; De Lange *et al.*, 1994), deviations in the composition

of the perfusate (Moghaddam and Bunney, 1989; Timmerman and Westerink, 1991; De Lange *et al.*, 1994) and the rate of implantation of the probe (Allen *et al.*, 1992).

These results indicate that the optimal period to perform (repeated) intracerebral microdialysis experiments in a particular experimental set-up needs to be determined (O'Connel *et al.*, 1993; De Lange *et al.*, 1994, 1995*d*). In general, the optimal post-surgery interval lies between one and two days after implantation of the probe; after recovery from early tissue reactions, and before the start of long-term reactions.

Quantitation of microdialysis data

A special problem associated with the use of intracerebral microdialysis is the determination of absolute concentrations in the ECF. This is because *in vivo* recovery of the microdialysis probe has to be estimated for each compound in each type of experiment. During the early phases of the microdialysis technique the *in vitro* recovery of a compound from the external medium was used to calculate the concentration in the extracellular space around the probe. However, *in vitro* recovery may deviate importantly from *in vivo* recovery because the latter will be influenced by a number of additional factors such as restricted diffusion through the extracellular space (Benveniste *et al.*, 1989), metabolism, intra/extracellular exchange, microvascular transport and elimination of the compound (Bungay *et al.*, 1990; Morrison *et al.*, 1991; Stahle, 1991). All these factors may vary between experiments. Several methods have been described to determine *in vivo* recovery (Jacobson *et al.*, 1985; Lerma *et al.*, 1986; Lonnroth *et al.*, 1987; Armberg and Lindefors, 1989; Bungay *et al.*, 1990; Larsson, 1991; Morrison *et al.*, 1991; Scheller and Kolb, 1991; Wang *et al.*, 1991, 1993; Ekblom *et al.*, 1992; Yokel *et al.*, 1992; Olson and Justice, 1993; Wong *et al.*, 1993).

Mathematical approach Especially the studies of Bungay *et al.* (1990) and Morrison *et al.* (1991) have provided substantial insight into the processes that govern *in vivo* recovery. Bungay *et al.* (1990) developed a mathematical framework to calculate *in vivo* recovery of compounds at steady-state con-

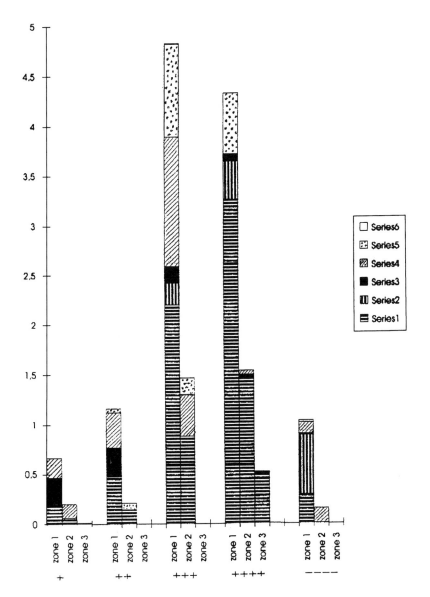

Fig. 11.5. Mean tissue scores of individual parameters for each zone around the probe, for daily repeated perfusion periods of 2.5 hours: (+), perfusion started at 24 hours post surgery; (++), perfusions started at 24 and 48 hours post surgery; (+++), perfusions started at 24, 48 and 72 hours post surgery; (++++), perfusions started at 24, 48, 72 and 96 hours post surgery; (––––) the probe has been present in brain tissue for 96 + 2.5 hours, without perfusion sessions. Series: (1) hypercellularity; (2) pyknosis; (3) hemorrhages; (4) vacuolization; (5) infiltration of granulocytes; (6) exudate.

ditions. They considered the transport of the compound from the ECF into the dialysate being a series of transport steps, each with its own resistance. The transport steps included the transport from the bulk ECF to the probe (R_e), the transport across the semi-permeable membrane (R_m) and the transport into the dialysate (R_d). *In vivo* effectively only R_e needs to be considered, because for the experiments performed up till now this resistance is by far the largest. R_e is the resistance that will depend on diffusion, extracellular-microvascular exchange, metabolism, and intra/extracellular exchange, and it can be deduced that the larger the sum of the rate constants of these factors, the smaller will be R_e, and the larger will be the *in vivo* recovery.

Morrison *et al.* (1991) have extended the steady-state approach to the dynamic situation. Time-dependent expressions for dialysate concentrations and radial concentration profiles were developed. For transient processes dialysis equilibrium is of importance, and it was concluded that the higher the rate of metabolism and/or capillary exchange, the shorter the time needed to obtain equilibrium.

However, to calculate *in vivo* recovery (or C_{ECF}) by these mathematical methods, knowledge of the above-mentioned parameters is needed. These parameters may differ between types of experiments as well as from brain region to brain region. This limits the practical use of these models to calculate *in vivo* recovery.

Practical approach The no-net-flux method (Lonnroth *et al.*, 1987) and the extended no-net-flux method (Olson and Justice, 1993) are practical methods, based on a point of equilibrium at which no assumptions have to be made about periprobe behavior of the compound of interest. For that reason these are of high practical value. The no net flux method requires the presence of steady-state conditions with respect to the concentration of the compound in the ECF (C_{ECF}). In an individual animal the probe is consecutively perfused with different concentrations of the compound (C_{in}), and the resulting dialysate concentrations (C_{out}) are determined. The direction of the diffusion depends on the concentration gradient between the perfusion medium and the periprobe ECF. When C_{in} is larger than C_{ECF}, net diffusion will take place from the perfusion medium into the periprobe tissue (loss). When C_{in} is smaller than C_{ECF}, molecules from the periprobe tissue will diffuse into the perfusion medium (gain). When the difference between C_{out} and C_{in} is plotted as a function of C_{in}, the line will cross the *x*-axis at the value where C_{in} equals C_{ECF} (no net flux conditions). If true steady-state conditions exist, the slope of the line will represent the *in vivo* recovery of the compound (Fig. 11.6).

The extended no-net-flux method is based on the no-net-flux method, but has been adapted so that it is useful under transient conditions. Olson

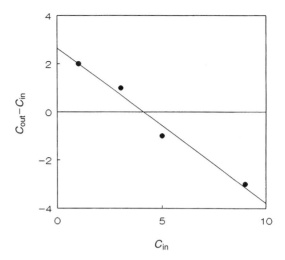

Fig. 11.6. The difference between C_{out} (dialysate concentration) and C_{in} (perfusate concentration) is depicted as a function of C_{in}. The line through the data points will cross the *x*-axis at the value of C_{in} that equals C_{ECF} (the point of no net flux).

and Justice (1993) presented a method by which ECF concentrations and *in vivo* recoveries can be estimated as a function of time. This method is based on the use of a between-group rather than a within-group design. Instead of serial perfusions of the probe with different concentrations of the compound within one animal, a group of animals is perfused with only one selected concentration. Different groups receive different concentrations and the results are combined at each time point. Regression of the mean data points of the different groups at a particular time point will give the actual C_{ECF} at that time. However, for this experimental approach more experimental animals are needed, in part reducing the advantage of minimizing the use of animals by the microdialysis technique.

Using the extended no-net-flux method, Olson and Justice (1993) have shown that *in vivo* recovery may change during the course of an experiment, with or without concomitant changes in ECF concentrations. This is of concern because this has not been taken into account in previous studies.

Components of the microdialysis set-up

Apart from surgical requirements, the basic microdialysis set-up consists of a microdialysis probe, an animal (or human), a perfusion pump, inlet and outlet tubing, and a (refrigerated) microfraction collector. The microdialysis probes can be 'home-made' or purchased commercially. The perfusion pump should be able to provide an exact and pulse-free flow rate in the nl/min and μl/min range, while the microfraction collector should be able to collect volumes exactly according to the pre-set volumes or within a preset time. The perfusate (inlet) tubing and dialysate (outlet) tubing should not interact with the compound of interest. The length and inner diameter of the outlet tubing should be considered to minimize mixing of the dialysate and to prevent hydrostatic pressure build-up across the probe membrane.

The equipment can be extended by a syringe selector, an *in vitro* stand for the probes, swivels for inlet and outlet connection tubing, and an on-line analysis system. A syringe selector accomplishes a change of perfusate syringes without interrupting the flow. An *in vitro* stand is necessary for the safe storage of reusable probes and for testing *in vitro* recovery and may be 'home-made' as well as commercially purchased. The swivels can be used to prevent tangling and twisting of the inlet and out-

let tubing by the freely moving animal. An on-line injector enables direct collection and injection of the microdialysate when the analysis can be performed directly (see below), e.g. by high pressure liquid chromatography (HPLC). An example of an experimental set-up is given in Fig. 11.7.

Analytical considerations

Microdialysis samples are aqueous and their constituents are usually small molecular weight molecules that are moderately to highly soluble in water. The dialysate samples are usually free of endogenous compounds such as lipids and proteins that might interfere with analysis procedures and hence no additional sample preparation is needed.

Perfusion flow rates usually range between 1 and 5 μl/min. Using a 10 min collection interval, sample volumes of 10 to 50 μl are obtained. By on-line analysis sample loss can be minimized, which is important when dealing with very small sample volumes. For on-line sample analysis the analysis time should be shorter than the sample collection time. Sample volumes can be increased by using a higher flow and/or extended collection interval. However, it should be noted that a higher flow reduces recovery. Recovery can be increased by enlargement of the dialysis surface provided that the dialyzed tissue is still homogeneous under those conditions. On the other hand, extension of the collection interval will decrease the time resolution of the measurements. A decrease in the number of time points may be unfavorable for compounds that are subjected to relatively fast changes in their concentrations.

The dialysate collected from the brain by *in vivo* microdialysis can be analyzed by any available analytical procedure. By the use of an appropriate analytical method, parent compound and metabolites can be monitored together (Westerink and Tuinte, 1986; Hurd *et al.*, 1988; Ljungdahl-Stahle *et al.*, 1992; Acworth *et al.*, 1994; Sato *et al.*, 1994; Scheyer *et al.*, 1994*b*; Kurata *et al.*, 1995), while it is also possible to measure a drug together with possibly affected endogenous compounds (Matos *et al.*, 1992; Stain *et al.*, 1995).

In practice, reversed phase HPLC with ultraviolet, fluorescence, or electrochemical detection, or sometimes mass spectroscopy, is mostly used

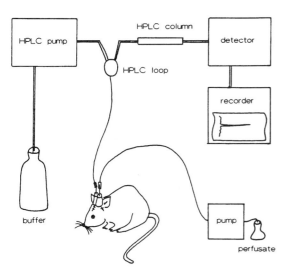

Fig. 11.7. Experimental set-up in the 'on-line' HPLC analysis configuration. By a pump the perfusate is pumped via the inlet tubing through the dialysis probe. Via the outlet tubing the dialysate is collected into an HPLC loop, which is injected onto an HPLC column with pre-set time intervals. The compounds in dialysate samples are separated, detected, and recorded.

because it provides sensitive analysis of small volumes. If compounds are present in the dialysate at very low concentrations, which is often the case, more sensitive analytical techniques are needed. Examples are microbore LC, capillary LC combined with on-column focusing, and capillary electrophoresis (CE) (Tellez et al., 1992; Mock et al., 1993; Lunte and O'Shea, 1994; Robert et al., 1995). These techniques can handle extremely low sample volumes (nanoliters), which means that a lower perfusate flow rate can be used (increasing the recovery) and/or shorter collection intervals can be used (increasing the time resolution). With such low sample volumes evaporation may become a considerable problem and therefore on-line analysis is highly preferred (Deterding et al., 1992; Hogan et al., 1994).

Intracerebral microdialysis and BBB transport studies

Native BBB transport

One of the consequences of the existence of the BBB is the restriction of BBB transport of most relatively hydrophilic compounds as opposed to more lipophilic ones by the presence of tight junctions between the cerebral endothelial cells (Oldendorf, 1974; Levin, 1980; Greenblatt et al., 1983). Also other BBB characteristics such as the presence of the mdrla encoded P-glycoprotein (Cordon-Cardo et al., 1989) may have a major impact on the extent of drug transport into the brain (Schinkel et al., 1994, 1995).

A first question that arises before using intracerebral microdialysis to measure BBB transport is if the BBB is still intact after implantation of a microdialysis probe. Several substances that normally do not pass the BBB have been utilized in microdialysis experiments to verify BBB integrity. The lack of ^{14}C-α-aminoisobutyric acid in brain autoradiograms (except for the sites of the burr holes), and the absense of Na^{99m}TcO$_4$ and ^{14}C-glucose in the dialysate, subsequent to their systemic administration, indicated the absence of important BBB damage (Benveniste et al., 1984; Tossman and Ungerstedt, 1986; Terasaki et al., 1991). In contrast, Major et al. (1990) and Westergren et al.

(1995) found ^{51}Cr-EDTA and ^{3}H-inulin, respectively, present in the dialysate up to 1 day after probe implantation. The latter investigators also detected albumin immunoreactivity at considerable distances from the probe. These results indicate that probe implantation may sometimes injure the BBB. A study of Allen et al. (1992) suggested that BBB injury from probe implantation may result from rapid implantation, stressing the importance of consideration of the implantation procedure.

Studies on drug lipophilicity-dependent BBB transport were performed by Gaykema et al. (1991) and De Lange et al. (1994). The ratio of brain ECF dialysate over total plasma concentrations was determined for a series of alkylamines (C$_2$–C$_8$) (Gaykema et al., 1991). An optimum was found for propylamine. The declining ratio for the more lipophilic alkylamines was attributed to mechanisms that counteract the distribution of the more lipophilic compounds into brain ECF, such as increased plasma protein binding. Levels of acetaminophen (log $P=0.25$) and atenolol (log $P=-1.78$) in brain dialysate and plasma were studied following intravenous bolus administration at 24 hours after probe implantation (De Lange et al., 1994). It was found that the transport of acetaminophen into the brain (18%) was considerably higher than that of atenolol (3.4%), as expected on the basis of their lipophilicity. In previous studies the transport of atenolol into the brain was also restricted (5%) when determined by other experimental approaches (Street et al., 1979; Taylor et al., 1981; Gengo et al., 1989; Agon et al., 1991). BBB transport of acetaminophen was comparable with data obtained by Morrison et al. (1991), who also used microdialysis.

Drug lipophilicity-dependent BBB transport (Fenstermacher et al., 1970, 1974; Sendelbeck and Urquart, 1985) was also demonstrated by the different spatial steady-state distribution profiles of acetaminophen and atenolol in the brain, obtained with microdialysis infusion and sampling probes implanted in parallel at different interprobe distances (De Lange et al., 1995a). Moreover, this study showed that the microdialysis technique measures very locally indeed.

For lipophilic compounds that tend to distribute into compartments other than the ECF, dialysate concentrations may be very low (De

Lange *et al.*, unpublished data) or even not detectable (Carneheim and Stahle, 1991), which makes the microdialysis technique more suitable for studying BBB transport of hydrophilic and lesser lipophilic compounds.

Changes in BBB transport

For compounds that normally do not pass the BBB by restricted paracellular transport, opening of the BBB increases penetration into the brain (Nagy *et al.*, 1981; Neuwelt *et al.*, 1985*a*; Sztriha and Betz, 1991). For evaluation of BBB integrity in microdialysis experiments, opening of the BBB can be used to see if an increase in transport of the compounds is observed also. This would indicate BBB integrity under the control microdialysis conditions. De Lange *et al.* (1995*c*) found a clear increase in atenolol brain dialysate levels selectively at the site of BBB modification by hypertonic mannitol, while Allen *et al.* (1992) could also demonstrate a significant increase in trimethylammonium antipyrine levels in the dialysate after BBB opening by oleic acid infusion. In contrast, the dialysate levels of ^{3}H-inulin could not be increased by using protamine sulphate in the study of Westergren *et al.* (1995). However, as already mentioned, the latter investigators found an extensive albumin immunoreactivity around the probe already under control conditions, indicating BBB injury. These results demonstrate that changes in BBB transport can be investigated provided that BBB integrity in microdialysis experiments is maintained by optimal surgery and experimental conditions (Allen *et al.*, 1992; De Lange *et al.*, 1994).

The technique also offers the possibility to investigate changes in local BBB functionality under pathological conditions. Thus, the penetration of the hydrophilic anticancer drug methotrexate has been measured within normal and tumor-bearing brain (De Lange *et al.*, 1995*b*). It was found that in the presence of the tumor, BBB permeability for methotrexate increased at the ipsilateral side to 250%, while at the contralateral side it was reduced to 65% (Fig. 11.8). Similar data were obtained in studies using other experimental techniques (Shapiro *et al.*, 1985; Neuwelt *et al.*, 1985*b*). Fukuhara *et al.* (1994) studied the 'albumin index' to detect sequential changes in disruption of the

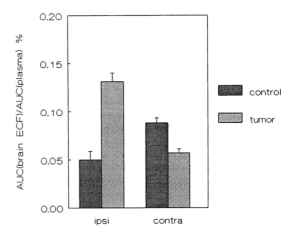

Fig. 11.8. $AUC_{\text{brain ECF}}/AUC_{\text{plasma}}$ (BBB permeability) for the hydrophilic anticancer agent methotrexate in the absence and presence of tumor tissue (left hemisphere), in the ipsi- and contralateral brain of WAG/Rij rats. Methotrexate was administered i.v. (75 mg/kg).

BBB following middle cerebral artery or cold lesion, with only an increase in the albumin index found following the cold lesion.

Increases in the extent of BBB transport of compounds by co-administration of other compounds was demonstrated by microdialysis in studies of Nakashima *et al.* (1992), Dykstra *et al.*, (1993), and Deguchi *et al.* (1995), for the combination of L-DOPA and carbidopa, AZT and probenecid, and baclofen and probenecid respectively (Fig. 11.9). The latter two studies demonstrate that active transport across the BBB can also be studied by intracerebral microdialysis experiments.

Concentrations of drugs in brain may also be influenced by the extent of metabolism as demonstrated by Sato *et al.* (1994). These investigators used intracerebral microdialysis to study the pharmacokinetics of psychotropic agents. Imipramine and its demethylated metabolite desimipramine were measured in brain dialysate after administration of imipramine alone, and following premedication with SKF-525A or concomitant administration of aminopyrine. Aminopyrine, being metabolized by demethylation like imipramine, did not affect the concentration–time profile of imipramine, while desimipramine levels were reduced in a dose-dependent manner probably by competition for demethylation (Fig. 11.10). SKF-

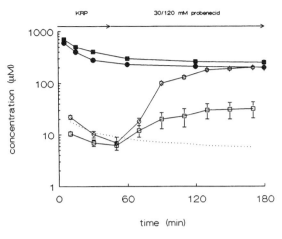

Fig. 11.9. Effects of probenecid on the concentration of baclofen in plasma and hippocampal ECF in rats. The dialysis probe was initially perfused with KRP (pH 7.4) for 60 min after a 50 mg/kg i.v. administration of baclofen. Thereafter, the dialysis solutions were switched from KRP to an isotonic solution containing 30 mM or 120 mM probenecid, and the probe was perfused for another 120 min (as indicated). The dotted line represents the concentration level in control rats. Each data point represents the mean ±SE ($n=3$). (●) plasma and (○) ECF; for 30 mM probenecid. (■) plasma and (□) ECF; for 120 mM probenecid. *$P<0.05$ and **$P<0.001$ versus control in student's test. From Deguchi *et al.* (1995), with kind permission of Plenum Press Corporation, New York, USA.

525A, an inhibitor of cytochrome P450 associated metabolism in the liver, decreased the dialysate levels of desimipramine while increasing those of imipramine. Unfortunately, concomitant plasma levels have not been determined. By that a possible contribution of the inhibitory effects of SKF-525A on brain cytochrome P450 metabolism to the increased brain levels of imipramine could have been determined.

Concentrations in blood

To determine the transport characteristics of compounds across the BBB, their concentrations in blood should also be known. This can be accomplished by serial blood sampling. However, for this purpose, the microdialysis technique may also be suitable. Potentially, free drug concentrations can be determined in parallel to brain ECF concentra-

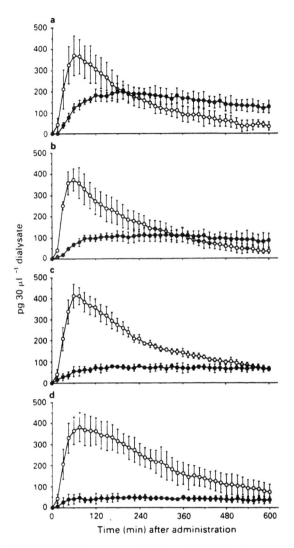

Fig. 11.10. Time-course of imipramine (○) and desimipramine (●) with concomitant administration of aminopyrine (AMP). (a) imipramine only ($n=5$), (b) imipramine + 25 mg/kg AMP ($n=3$), (c) imipramine + 50 mg/kg AMP ($n=4$), (d) imipramine+100 mg/kg AMP ($n=4$). The extracellular concentrations of desimipramine showed significant differences in proportion to the given dosage of AMP (ANOVA, $P<0.0001$), while the concentrations of imipramine were not significantly different with or without administration of AMP. From Sato *et al.* (1994), with kind permission of MacMillan Press, UK.

tions (Wala *et al.*, 1991; Sjoberg *et al.*, 1992; Cheng *et al.*, 1993; Kurata *et al.*, 1995). In cases where drug plasma protein binding is changed by pathological states, drug competition for drug binding,

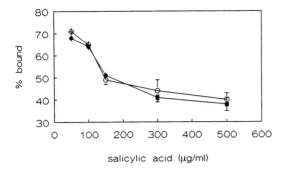

Fig. 11.11. Dependence of binding of salicylate to plasma proteins on the concentration of salicylate (○-○) microdialysis; (●-●) ultrafiltration. From Herrera *et al.* (1990), with kind permission of Plenum Press corporation, New York, USA.

or non-linear protein binding (Fig. 11.11) this will provide additional information which is essential for the appropriate interpretation of transport across the BBB (Dubey *et al.*, 1989; Herrera *et al.*, 1990; Saisho and Umeda, 1991; Ekblom *et al.*, 1992; Telting-Diaz *et al.*, 1992; Chen and Steger, 1993; LeQuellec *et al.*, 1994; Nakashima *et al.*, 1994; Evrard *et al.*, 1996).

Brain concentrations and effects

Intracerebral microdialysis offers the possibility to measure drug levels in the brain of conscious, freely moving animals. Thus, in principle other parameters can be obtained simultaneously during the dialysis experiment. Welty *et al.* (1993) combined intracerebral microdialysis with anticonvulsant action measurements, Stahle *et al.* (1990) with behavioural observations, and Ludvig *et al.* (1992) and Gerozissis *et al.* (1995) with EEG recordings. The study of Gerozissis *et al.* showed that during sleep, prostaglandin E$_2$ (PGE$_2$) first went on dropping and then reincreased towards the values that characterize early periods of wakefulness. In its turn, this reincrease of PGE$_2$ announced the end of sleep and the imminent occurrence of wakefulness.

Perspectives and conclusions

Studies performed on the use of intracerebral microdialysis in BBB transport suggest that this method is of minimal invasiveness and provides valid information if surgical and experimental conditions are carefully checked and controlled. Pharmacokinetic profiles of compounds in the brain can be obtained in parallel to serial blood sampling in individual animals. Especially in combination with blood microdialysis, BBB transport can be directly related to actual free concentrations in blood.

The technique opens up the possibility for investigations of BBB functionality under physiological and pathological conditions. The relationship between local drug concentrations within the brain and their elicited pharmacological effects can be studied, which may be particularly useful for those drugs with late effects or effects that can only be assessed by histological examination, such as those used in cancer chemotherapy.

The efficacy of several strategies designed to increase BBB transport of drugs can be investigated. These include optimizing pharmacokinetics (Shapiro *et al.*, 1975; Kroin and Penn, 1982), osmotic opening of the BBB (Neuwelt and Barnett, 1989), chemical modification of drugs (Greig, 1987), the development of drugs that resemble endogenous compounds for which active transport mechanisms are present on the BBB, incorporation of drugs in liposomes, and the coupling of drugs to antibodies that recognize receptors. Whether these approaches eventually result in increased drug levels within the brain of living animals should be determined *in vivo*, for which intracerebral microdialysis seems to be a suitable technique.

While intracerebral microdialysis is most frequently applied to rats, transgenic or knockout mice can also be used to investigate BBB characteristics. This is of importance because today the concept of the BBB is not limited to specific microanatomical features but expanding to accommodate newly recognized functions. Recently P-glycoprotein expression, which appears to be responsible for multidrug resistance in many tumors, has been found to be present on the BBB (Cordon-Cardo *et al.*, 1989). This may indicate a physiological role for P-glycoprotein (Pgp) in regulating the levels of certain drugs in the brain. Schinkel *et al.* (1994) have recently generated a mouse strain with a homozygous disruption of the *mdr1a* gene. This gene encodes for the only form of Pgp expressed at the BBB and the *mdr1a*(-/-) mice are therefore of special value for BBB transport investigations. It has been shown that *mdr1a*(-/-) disruption results in elevated brain concentrations of many drugs, including vinblastin and digoxin (Schinkel *et al.*, 1994, 1995). De Lange *et al.* (unpublished data) have adapted the microdialysis technique for application in these mice. Currently, experiments are ongoing on the distribution of the Pgp substrate rhodamine-123 in control and *mdr1a*(-/-) mice, and its modulation by co-administration of the Pgp inhibitor SDZ PSC 833.

Although there remain problems in the use of this technique with respect to the measurement of very low concentrations of compounds in the dialysate, possible adsorption of some compounds by certain membranes and quantitation of dialysis data, near future technical developments may minimize such problems. However, for already quite a number of cases the technique has demonstrated its practical value and it holds a great promise for automated, continuous sampling of various regions in the brain over prolonged experimental periods.

References

Acworth, I. N., Yu, J., Ryan, E. *et al.* (1994). Simultaneous measurement of monoamines, amino acids and drug levels, using high pressure liquid chromatography and coulometric array technology: application to *in vivo* microdialysis perfusate analysis. *J. Liq. Chrom.*, **17**, 685–705.

Agon, P., Goethals, P., Van Haver, D. and Kaufman, J.-M. (1991). Permeability of the blood–brain barrier for atenolol studied by positron emission tomography. *J. Pharm. Pharmacol.*, **43**, 597–600.

Allen, D., Crooks, P. A. and Yokel, R. A. (1992). 4-Trimethylantipyrine: a quaternary ammonium nonradionucleide marker for BBB integrity during *in vivo* microdialysis. *J. Pharm. Meth.*, **28**, 129–35.

Armberg, G. and Lindefors, N. (1989). Intracerebral microdialysis: II Mathematical studies of diffusion kinetics. *J. Pharm. Meth.*, **22**, 157–83.

Benveniste, H. and Diemer, N. H. (1987). Cellular reactions to implantation of a microdialysis tube in the rat hippocampus. *Acta Neuropath. (Berl.)*, **74**, 234–8.

Benveniste, H. and Huttemeier, P. C. (1990). Microdialysis – theory and application. *Progress in Neurobiol.*, **35**, 195–215.

Benveniste, H., Drejer, J. Schoesboe, A. and Diemer, N. H. (1984). Elevation of the extracellular concentrations of glutamate and aspartate in rat hippocampus during transient cerebral ischemia monitored by intracerebral microdialysis. *J. Neurochem.*, **43**, 1369–74.

Benveniste, H., Drejer, J. Schoesboe, A. and Diemer, N. H. (1987). Regional cerebral glucose phosphorylation and blood flow after insertion of a microdialyis fiber through the dorsal hippocampus in the rat. *J. Neurochem.*, **49**, 729–34.

Benveniste, H., Hansen, A. J. and Ottosen, N. S. (1989). Determination of brain interstitial concentrations by microdialysis. *J. Neurochem.*, **52**, 1741–50.

Bungay P. M., Morrison P. F. and Dedrick R. L. (1990). Steady-state theory for quantitative microdialysis of solutes and water *in vivo* and *in vitro*. *Life Sci.*, **46**, 105–19.

Carneheim, C. and Stahle, L. (1991). Microdialysis of lipophilic compounds. A methodological study. *Pharmacol. Toxicol.*, **69**, 378–80.

Cavanaugh, J. B. (1970). The proliferation of astrocytes around a needle wound in the rat brain. *J. Anat.*, **106**, 471- 9.

Chen, Z. and Steger, R. W. (1993). Plasma microdialysis: a technique for continuous plasma sampling in freely moving rats. *J. Pharmacol. Toxicol. Methods*, **29**, 111–18.

Cheng, H-Y, Liu, T., Feuerstein, G. and Barone, F. C. (1993). Distribution of spin-trapping compounds in rat blood and brain: *in vivo* microdialysis determination. *Free Rad. Biol. Med.*, **14**, 243–50.

Claassen, V. (1994). Anaesthesia. In *Techniques in the Behavioral and Neural Sciences. Vol. 12: Neglected Factors in Pharmacology and Neuroscience Research*, ed. J. P. Huston. Elsevier Science B. V.

Coleman, D. L., King, R. N. and Anrade, J. D. (1974). The foreign body reaction: a chronic inflammatory response. *J. Biomed. Mater. Res.*, **8**, 199–211.

Cordon-Cardo, C., O'Brien, J. P., Casals, D. *et al.* (1989). Multidrug resistance gene (P-glycoprotein) is expressed by endothelial cells at blood–brain barrier sites. *Proc. Natl. Acad. Sci. USA*, **86**, 695–8.

Damsma, G., Westerink, B. H. C., De Boer, P. *et al.* (1988). Basal acetylcholine release in freely moving rats detected by on-line trans-striatal dialysis: pharmacological aspects. *Life Sci.*, **43**, 1161–8.

Deguchi, Y., Inabe, K., Tomiyasu, K. *et al.* (1995). Study on brain interstitial fluid distribution and blood–brain barrier transport of baclofen in rats by microdialysis. *Pharm. Res.*, **12**, 1838–44.

De Lange, E. C. M., Danhof, M., De Boer, A. G. and Breimer, D. D. (1994). Critical factors of intracerebral microdialysis as a technique to determine the pharmacokinetics of drugs in rat brain. *Brain Res.*, **666**, 1–8.

De Lange, E. C. M., Bouw, M. R., Danhof, M. *et al.* (1995a). Application of intracerebral microdialysis to study regional distribution kinetics of drugs in rat brain. *Br. J. Pharmacol.*, **116**, 2538–44.

De Lange, E. C. M., De Vries, J. D., Zurcher, C. *et al.* (1995b). The use of intracerebral microdialysis for the determination of pharmacokinetic profiles of anticancer drugs in tumor-bearing rat brain. *Pharm. Res.*, **12**, 1924–31.

De Lange, E. C. M., Hesselink, M. B., Danhof, M. *et al.* (1995*c*). The use of intracerebral microdialysis to determine changes in blood–brain barrier transport characteristics. *Pharm. Res.*, **12**, 129–33.

De Lange, E. C. M., Zurcher, C., Danhof, M. *et al.* (1995*d*). Repeated microdialysis perfusions: periprobe tissue reactions and BBB permeability. *Brain Res.*, **702**, 261–5.

Del Rio Hortega, P. and Penfield, W. (1972). Cerebral cicatrix: the reaction of neuroglia and microglia to brain wounds. *Bull. Johns Hopkins Hosp.*, **41**, 278–85.

Deterding, L. J., Dix, K., Burda, L. T. and Tomer, K. B. (1992). On-line coupling of *in vivo* microdialysis with tandem mass spectroscopy. *Anal. Chem.*, **64**, 2636–41.

Di Chiara, G. (1990). In vivo brain dialysis of neurotransmitters. *Trends Pharmacol. Sci.*, **11**, 116–21.

Drijfhout, W. J., Grol, C. J. and Westerink, B. H. C. (1993). Microdialysis of melatonin in the rat pineal gland: methodology and pharmacological applications. *J. Neurochem.*, **61**, 936–42.

Drijfhout, W. J., Kemper, R. H. A., Meerlo, P. *et al.* (1995). Chronic effects of microdialysis probe implantation on the activity pattern and temperature rhythm of the rat. *J. Neurosci. Meth.*, **61**, 191–6.

Dubey R. K., Mcallister, C. B., Inoue, M. and Wilkinson, G. R. (1989). Plasma binding and transport of diazepam across the blood–brain barrier. *J. Clin. Invest.*, **84**, 1155–9.

Dykstra, K. H., Arya, A., Arroila, D. M. *et al.* (1993). Microdialysis study of zidovudine (AZT) transport in rat brain. *J. Pharmacol. Exp. Ther.*, **267**, 1227–36.

Ekblom, M., Hammarlund-Udenaes, M., Lundqvist, T. and Sjoberg, P. (1992). Potential use of microdialysis in pharmacokinetics: a protein binding study. *Pharm. Res.*, **9**, 155–8.

Evrard, P. A., Cumps, J. and Verbeeck, R. K. (1996). Concentration-dependent plasma protein binding of fluriprofen in the rat: an *in vivo* microdialysis study. *Pharm. Res.*, **13**, 18–22.

Fenstermacher, J. D., Rall, D. P., Patlak, C. S. and Levin, V. A. (1970). Ventricular perfusion as a technique for analysis of brain capillary permeability and extracellular transport. In *Capillary Permeability*, ed. C. Crone and N. Lassen, pp. 483–90. Copenhagen: Munkgard.

Fenstermacher, J. D., Patlak, C. S. and Blasberg, R. G. (1974). Transport of material between brain extracellular fluid, brain cells and blood. *Federation Proc.*, **33**, 2070–4.

Frothingham, E. and Basbaum, A. (1992). Construction of a microdialysis probe with attached microinjection catheter. *J. Neurosci. Methods*, **43**, 181–8.

Fukuhara, T., Gotoh, M., Kawauchi, M. *et al.* (1994). Detection of endogenous albumin as an index of blood parenchymal border alterations. *Acta Neurochirurg.*, (S)**60**, 121–3.

Fumero, B., Guadalupe, T., Gonzalez-Mora, J. L. *et al.* (1991). Different dynamics of brain metabolites as assessed by fixed and removable microdialysis probes. In *Monitoring Molecules in Neuroscience. Proceedings 5th International Conference on In Vivo Methods*, ed. H. Rollema, B. Westerink and W. J. Drijfhout, pp. 68–70. The Netherlands: Krips Repro, Meppel.

Gaykema, R. P. A., Koning, H. and Korf, J. (1991). Kinetics of blood brain distribution of drugs in relation to their lipophilicity as monitored with intracerebral dialysis and HPLC. *Monitoring Molecules in Neuroscience. Proceedings 5th International Conference on In Vivo Methods*, ed. H. Rollema, B. Westerink and W. J. Drijfhout, pp. 71–3. The Netherlands: Krips Repro, Meppel.

Gengo, F. M., Fagan, S. C., Hopkins, L. N. *et al.* (1989). Non-linear distribution of atenolol between plasma and cerebrospinal fluid. *Pharm. Res.*, **6**, 248–51.

Gerozissis, K., De Saint Hilaire, Z., Orosco, M. *et al.* (1995). Changes in hypothalamus prostaglandin E_2 may predict the occurrence of sleep or wakefulness as assessed by parallel EEG and microdialysis in the rat. *Brain Res.*, **689**, 239–44.

Gonzalez-Mora, J. L., Guadalupe, T., Fumero, B. and Mas, M. (1991). In *Monitoring Molecules in Neuroscience. Proceedings 5th International Conference on In Vivo Methods*, ed. H. Rollema, B. Westerink and W. J. Drijfhout, pp. 66–7. The Netherlands: Krips Repro, Meppel.

Greenblatt, D. J., Arendt, R. M., Abernethy, D. R. *et al.* (1983). In vitro quantitation of benzodiazepine lipophilicity: relation to *in vivo* distribution. *Br. J. Anaesth.*, **55**, 985–8.

Greig, N. H. (1987). Optimizing drug delivery to brain tumors. *Cancer Treat. Rev.*, **14**, 1–28.

Hamberger, A., Berthold, C. H., Karlsson, B. *et al.* (1983). Extracellular GABA, glutamate and glutamine in vivo. Perfusion-dialysis of the rabbit hippocampus. In *Glutamine, Glutamate and GABA in the Central Nervous System*, ed. L. Hertz, pp. 473–91. New York: Alan R. Liss.

Hamilton, M. E., Mele, A. and Pert, A. (1992). Striatal extracellular dopamine in conscious vs. anesthetized rats: effects of chloral hydrate anesthetic on responses to drugs of different classes. *Brain Res.*, **579**, 1–7.

Hernandez, L., Stanley, B. G. and Hoebel, B. G. (1986). A small removable microdialysis probe. *Life Sci.*, **39**, 2629–37.

Herrera, A. M., Scott, D. O. and Lunte, C. E. (1990). Microdialysis sampling for determination of plasma protein binding of drugs. *Pharm. Res.*, **7**, 1077–81.

Hogan, B. L., Lunte, S. M., Stobaugh, J. F. and Lunte, C. E. (1994). On-line coupling of *in vivo* microdialysis sampling with capillary electrophoresis. *Anal. Chem.*, **66**, 596–602.

Hsiao, J. K., Ball, B. A., Morrison, P. F. *et al.* (1990). Effects of different semipermeable membranes on *in vitro* and *in vivo* performance of microdialysis probes. *J. Neurochem.*, **54**, 1449–52.

Hurd, J. L., Kehr, J. and Ungerstedt, U. (1988). In vivo microdialysis as a technique to monitor drug transport: correlation of extracellular cocaine levels and dopamine overflow in the rat brain. *J. Neurochem.*, **51**, 1314–16.

Imperato, A. and Di Chiara, G. (1984). Trans-striatal dialysis coupled to reverse phase high performance liquid chromatography with electrochemical detection: a new method for the study of *in vivo* release of endogenous dopamine and metabolites. *J. Neurosci.*, **4**, 966–77.

Jacobson, J. and Hamberger, A. (1985). Kanaic acid-induced changes of extracellular amino acid levels, evoked potentials and EEG activity in the rabbit olfactory bulb. *Brain Res.*, **348**, 289–96.

Jacobson, I., Sandberg, M. and Hamberger, A. (1985). Mass transfer in brain dialysis devices – a new method for the estimation of extracellular amino acids concentration. *J. Neurosci. Meth.*, **15**, 263–8.

Johnson, R. D. and Justice, J. B. (1983). Model studies for brain dialysis. *Brain Res. Bull.*, **10**, 567–71.

Kapoor, V. and Chalmers, J. P. (1987). A simple, sensitive method for the determination of extracellular catecholamines in the rat hypothalamus using *in vivo* dialysis. *J. Neurosci. Meth.*, **19**, 173–82.

Kendrick, M. (1989). Use of microdialysis in neuroendocrinology. *Meth. Enzymol.*, **168**, 183–205.

Kroin, J. S. and Penn, R. D. (1982). Intracerebral chemotherapy: chronic microinfusion of cisplatin. *Neurosurg.*, **10**, 349–54.

Kuipers, R. A. and Korf, J. (1994). Flow resistance characteristics of microdialysis probes *in vivo*. *Med. Biol. Eng. Comput.*, **32**, 103–7.

Kurata, N., Inagaki, M., Iwase, M. *et al.* (1995). Pharmacokinetic study of trimethadone and its metabolite in blood, liver and brain by microdialysis in conscious, unrestrained rats. *Res. Commun. Mol. Pathol. Pharmacol.*, **89**, 45–6.

Landolt, H., Langemann, H., Lutz, Th. and Gratzl, O. (1991). Non-linear recovery of cysteine and gluthathione in microdialysis. In *Monitoring Molecules in Neuroscience*, ed. H. Rollema, B. H. C. Westerink and W.-J. Drijfhout, pp. 63–5. The Netherlands: Krips Repro, Meppel.

Larsson, C. I. (1991). The use of an 'internal standard' for control of the recovery in microdialysis. *Life Sci.*, **49**, 1173-8.

LeQuellec, A., Dupin, S., Tufenkji, A. E. *et al.* (1994). Microdialysis: an alternative for *in vitro* and *in vivo* protein binding studies. *Pharm. Res.*, **11**, 835–8.

Lerma, J., Herranz, A. S., Herreras, O. *et al.* (1986). In vivo determination of extracellular concentrations of amino acids in the rat hippocampus. A method based on brain dialysis and computerized analysis. *Brain Res.*, **384**, 145–55.

Levin, V. A. (1980). Relationship of octanol/water partition coefficient and molecular weight to rat brain capillary permeability. *J. Med. Chem.*, **23**, 682–4.

Levine, J. E. and Powell, K. D. (1989). Microdialysis for measurement of neuroendocrine peptides. *Meth. Enzym.*, **168**(K),166–210.

L'Heureux, R., Dennis, T., Curet, O. and Scatton, B. (1986). Measurement of endogenous noradrenaline release in the rat cerebral cortex *in vivo* by transcortical dialysis: effects of drugs affecting noradrenergic transmission. *J. Neurochem.*, **46**, 1794–801.

Lindefors, N., Amberg, G. and Ungerstedt, U. (1989). Intracerebral microdialysis: I. Experimental studies of diffusion kinetics. II. Mathematical studies of diffusion kinetics. *J. Pharmacol. Meth.*, **22**, 141–83.

Ljungdahl-Stahle, E., Guzenda, E., Bottinger, D. *et al.* (1992). Penetration of zidovudine and 3′-fluoro-3′-deoxythymidine into the brain, muscle tissue and veins in cynomolgus monkeys: relation with antiviral action. *Antimicrob. Agents Chemother.*, **36**, 2418–22.

Lonnroth P., Jansson P. A. and Smith U. (1987). A microdialysis method allowing characterization of intercellular water space in humans. *Am. J. Physiol.*, **253**, (Endocrinol. Metab. **16**) E228–E231.

Ludvig, N., Mishra, P. K., Yan, Q. S. *et al.* (1992). The combined EEG-intracerebral microdialysis technique: a new tool for neuropharmacological studies on freely behaving animals. *J. Neurosci. Meth.*, **43**, 129–37.

Lunte, S. M. and O'Shea, T. J. (1994). Pharmaceutical and biomedical application of capillary electrophoresis/ electrochemistry. *Electrophoresis*, **15**, 79–86.

Maidment, N. T., Brumbaugh, D. R., Rudolph, V. D. *et al.* (1989). Microdialysis of extracellular endogenous opioid peptides from rat brain *in vivo*. *Neurosci.*, **33**, 549–57.

Major, O., Shdanova, T., Duffek, L. and Nagy, Z. (1990). Continuous monitoring of blood–brain barrier opening to Cr^{51}-EDTA by microdialysis following probe injury. *Acta Neurochirurg.*, **S51**, 46–8.

Mason, P. A. and Romano, W. F. (1995). Recovery characteristics of a rigid nonmetallic microdialysis probe for use in an electromagnetic field. *Bioelectromagnetics*, **16**, 113–18.

Matlaga, B. F., Yasenchak, L. P. and Salthouse, T. H. (1976). Tissue response to implanted polymers: the significance of sample shape. *J. Biomed. Mater. Res.*, **10**, 391–7.

Matos, F. F., Rollema, H. and Basbaum, A. I. (1992). Simultaneous measurement of extracellular morphine and serotonin in brain tissue and CSF by microdialysis in awake rats. *J. Neurochem.*, **58**, 1773–81.

Mock, K., Hail, M., Mylchreest, I. *et al.* (1993). Rapid high-sensitive mapping by liquid chromatography–mass spectrometry. *J. Chromatogr.*, **646**, 169–74.

Moghaddam, B. and Bunney, B. S (1989). Ionic composition of microdialysis perfusing solution alters the pharmacological responsiveness and basal outflow of striatal dopamine. *J. Neurochem.*, **53**, 652–4.

Morrison P. F., Bungay P. M., Hsiao J. K. *et al.* (1991). Quantitative microdialysis: analysis of transients and application to pharmacokinetics in brain. *J. Neurochem.*, **57**, 103–19.

Nagy, Z., Peters, H. and Huttner, I. (1981). Endothelial surface charge: blood–brain barrier opening to horse radish peroxidase induced by protamine sulphate. *Acta Neuropathol. (Berl.)*, **7**, 7–9.

Nakamura, M., Itano, T., Yamaguchi, F. *et al.* (1990). In vivo analysis of extracellular proteins in rat brains with a newly developed intracerebral microdialysis probe. *Acta Med. Okayama*, **44**, 1–8.

Nakashima, M., Nakano, M., Matsuyama, K. and Ichikawa, M. (1992). An application of the microdialysis system to the pharmacokinetic study on striatal distribution of L-DOPA with or without carbidopa in rats. *Int. J. Pharmaceut.*, **72**, R5–R8.

Nakashima, M., Takeuchi, N., Hamada, M. *et al.* (1994). In vivo microdialysis for pharmacokinetic investigations: a plasma protein binding study of valproate in rabbits. *Biol. Pharm. Bull.*, **17**, 1630–4.

Neuwelt, E. A. and Barnett, P. A. (1989). Blood–brain barrier disruption in the treatment of brain tumors: animal studies. In *Implications of the Blood–Brain Barrier and its Manipulation*, ed, E. A. Neuwelt, Vol. 2, pp. 107–93. New York: Plenum Publishing Corporation.

Neuwelt, E. A., Barnett, P. A., McCormick, C. I. *et al.* (1985*a*). Osmotic blood–brain barrier modification: monoclonal antibody, albumin and methotrexate delivery to cerebrospinal fluid and brain. *Neurosurgery*, **17**, 419–23.

Neuwelt, E. A., Frenkel, E. P. and D'Agostino, A. N. (1985*b*). Growth of human lung tumor in the brain of nude rats as a new model to evaluate antitumor agent delivery across the blood–brain barrier. *Cancer Res.*, **45**, 2827–33.

O'Connel, M. T., Abed, W. T., Alavijeh, M. S. and Patsalos, P. N. (1993). A chronic neuropharmacokinetic study of carbamazepine (CBZ) in rat frontal cortex using microdialysis. *Epilepsia*, **34**(S2), 88–9.

Oldendorf, W. H. (1974). Lipid solubility and drug penetration of the blood–brain barrier. *Proc. Exp. Biol. Med.*, **147**, 813–16.

Olson, R. J. and Justice, J. B. (1993). Quantitative microdialysis under transient conditions. *Anal. Chem.*, **65**, 1017–22.

Osborne, P. G., O'Connor, W. T. and Ungerstedt, U. (1990). Effect of varying the ionic concentration of a microdialysis perfusate on basal striatal dopamine levels in awake rats. *J. Neurochem.*, **56**, 452–6.

Paredes, W., Chen, J. and Gardner, E. (1989). A miniature probe: a new simple construction method for making a chronic, removable and recyclable probe. *Curr. Sep.*, **9**, 94.

Robert, F., Bert, L., Denoroy, L. and Renaud, B. (1995). Capillary zone electrophoreses with laser induced fluorescence detection for the determination of nanomolar concentrations of noradrenaline and dopamine: applications to brain microdialysate analysis. *Anal. Chem.*, **67**, 1838–44.

Ruggeri, M., Zoli, M., Grimaldi, R. *et al.* (1990). Aspects of neural plasticity in the central nervous system – III Methodological studies on the microdialysis technique. *Neurochem. Int.*, **16**, 427–43.

Saisho, Y. and Umeda, T. (1991). Continuous monitoring of unbound floxomef levels in rat blood using microdialysis and its new pharmacokinetic analysis. *Chem. Pharm. Bull.*, **36**, 808–10.

Santiago, M. and Westerink, B. H. C. (1990). Characterization of the *in vivo* release of dopamine as recorded by different types of intracerebral microdialysis probes. *Naunyn-Schmiedberg Arch. Pharmacol.*, **342**, 407–14.

Sato, Y., Shibanoki, S., Sugahara, M. and Ishikawa, K. (1994). Measurement and pharmacokinetics of imipramine and its metabolites by brain microdialysis. *Br. J. Pharmacol.*, **112**, 625–9.

Scheller, D. and Kolb, J. (1991). The internal reference technique in microdialysis: a practical approach to monitoring dialysis efficiency and to calculating tissue concentration from dialysate samples. *J. Neurosci. Meth.*, **40**, 31–8.

Scheyer, R. D., During, M. J., Hochholtzer, J. M. *et al.* (1994*a*). Phenytoin concentrations in the human brain: an *in vivo* microdialysis study. *Epilepsy Res.*, **18**, 227–32.

Scheyer, R. D., During, M. J., Spencer, D. D. *et al.* (1994*b*). Measurement of carbamazepine and carbamazepine epoxide in the human brain using *in vivo* microdialysis. *Neurology*, **44**, 1469–72.

Schinkel, A. H., Smit, J. J. M., Van Tellingen, O. *et al.* (1994). Disruption of the mouse *mdr1a* P-glycoprotein gene leads to a deficiency in the blood–brain barrier and to increased sensitivity to drugs. *Cell*, **77**, 491–502.

Schinkel, A. H., Wagenaar, E., Van Deemter, L. *et al.* (1995). Absence of the mdr1a P-glycoprotein in mice affects tissue distribution and pharmacokinetics of dexamethasone, digoxine and cyclosporin A. *J. Clin. Invest.*, **96**, 1698–705.

Sendelbeck, S. L. and Urquhart, J. (1985). Spatial distribution of dopamine, methotrexate and antipyrine during continuous intracerebral microperfusion. *Brain Res.*, **328**, 251–8.

Shapiro, W. R., Young, D. F. and Metha, B. M. (1975). Methotrexate: distribution into cerebrospinal fluid after intravenous, ventricular and lumbar injections. *N. Engl. J. Med.*, **293**, 161–6.

Shapiro, W. R., Voorhies, R. M., Hiesiger, E. M. *et al.* (1985). Pharmacokinetics of tumor cell exposure to ^{14}C-methotrexate after intracarotid administration without and with hyperosmotic opening of the blood–brain and blood–tumor barriers in rat brain tumors: a quantitative autoradiographic study. *Cancer Res.*, **48**, 694–701.

Shimura, T., Tabata, S., Terasaki, T. *et al.* (1992). In-vivo blood–brain barrier transport of a novel adrenocorticotropic hormone analogue, ebiratide, demonstrated by brain microdialysis and capillary depletion method. *J. Pharm. Pharmacol.*, **44**, 583–8.

Shuaib, A. X., Crain, B., Siren, A.-L. *et al.* (1990). Assessment of damage from implantation of microdialysis probes in the rat hippocampus with silver degeneration staining. *Neurosci. Lett.*, **112**, 149–54.

Sjoberg, P., Olafsson, I. M. and Lundquist, T. (1992). Validation of different microdialysis methods for the determination of unbound steady-state concentrations of theophylline in blood and brain tissue. *Pharm. Res.*, **9**, 1592–8.

Spector, M., Cease, C. and Tong-Li, X. (1989). The local tissue response to biomaterials. *Crit. Rev. Biocompat.*, **5**, 269–95.

Stahle, L. (1991). Drug distribution studies with microdialysis: I. Tissue dependent difference in recovery between caffein and theophylline. *Life Sci.*, **49**, 1835–42.

Stahle, L., Segersvard, S and Ungerstedt, U. (1990). Theophylline concentration in the extracellular space of the rat brain: measurement by microdialysis and relation to behaviour. *Eur. J. Pharmacol.*, **185**, 187–95.

Stain, F., Barjavel, M. J., Sandouk, P. *et al.* (1995). Analgesic response and plasma and brain extracellular fluid pharmacokinetics of morphine and morphine-6-β D-glucuronide in the rat. *J. Pharmacol. Exp. Ther.*, **274**, 852–7.

Street, J. A., Hemsworth, B. A., Roach, A. G. and Day, M. D. (1979). Tissue levels of several labelled ß-adrenoceptor antagonists after intravenous administration in rats. *Arch. Int. Pharmacodyn.*, **237**, 180–90.

Sztriha, L. and Betz, A. L. (1991). Oleic acid reversibly opens the blood–brain barrier. *Brain Res.*, **550**, 257–62.

Tao, R. and Hjorth, S. (1992). Differences in the *in vitro* and *in vivo* 5-hydroxytryptamine extraction performance among three common microdialysis membranes. *J. Neurochem.*, **59**, 1778–85.

Taylor, E. A., Jefferson, D., Carrol, J. D. and Turner, P. (1981). Cerebrospinal fluid concentration of propanolol, pindolol and atenolol in man: evidence for central ß-adrenoceptor antagonists. *Br. J. Clin. Pharmacol.*, **12**, 549–59.

Tellez, S., Forges, N., Roussin, A. and Hernandez, L. (1992). Coupling of microdialysis with capillary electrophoresis: a new approach to the study of drug transfer between two compartments of the body in freely moving rats. *J. Chromatogr.*, **581**, 257–60.

Telting-Diaz, M., Scott, D. O. and Lunte, C. E. (1992). Intravenous microdialysis sampling in awake, freely moving rats. *Anal. Chem.*, **64**, 806–10.

Terasaki, T., Deguchi, Y., Sato, M. *et al.* (1991). In vivo transport of a dynorphine-like analgesic peptide E-2078 through the blood–brain barrier. An application of brain microdialysis. *Pharm. Res.*, **8**, 815–20.

Timmerman, W. and Westerink, B. H. C. (1991). Importance of calcium content infused during microdialysis for effects induced by D2-agonists on the release of dopamine in the striatum of the rat. *Neurosci. Lett.*, **131**, 93–6.

Tossman, U. and Ungerstedt, U. (1986). Microdialysis in the study of extracellular levels of amino acids in the rat brain. *Acta Physiol. Scand.*, **128**, 9–14.

Ungerstedt, U. (1984). Measurement of neurotransmitter release by intracranial dialysis. In *Measurement of Neurotransmitter Release In Vivo*, ed. C. A. Marsden, pp. 210–45. Wiley and Sons Ltd.

Wages, S. A., Church, W. H. and Justice, J. B. Jr. (1986). Sampling considerations for on-line microbore liquid chromatography of brain dialysate. *Anal. Chem.*, **58**, 1649–54.

Wala, E. P., Martin, W. R. and Sloan, J. W. (1991). Distribution of diazepam, nordiazepam and oxazepam between brain extraneuronal space, brain tissue, plasma and cerebrospinal fluid in diazepam and nordiazepam dependent dogs. *Psychopharmacol.*, **105**, 535–40.

Wang, Y., Wong, S. L. and Sawchuck, R. J. (1991). Comparison of *in vitro* and *in vivo* calibration of microdialysis probes using retrodialysis. *Curr. Sep.*, **10**, 87.

Wang, Y., Wong, S. L. and Sawchuck, R. J. (1993). Microdialysis calibration using retrodialysis and zero-net-flux: application to a study of the distribution of zidovudine to rabbit cerebrospinal fluid and thalamus. *Pharm. Res.*, **10**, 1411–19.

Wellman, P. J. (1990). An inexpensive guide cannula and collar for microdialysis experiments. *Brain Res. Bull.*, **25**, 345–6.

Welty, D. F., Schielke, G. P., Vartanian, M. G. and Taylor, C. P. (1993). Gabapentin anticonvulsant action in rats: disequilibrium with peak drug concentrations in plasma and brain dialysate. *Epilepsy Res.*, **16**, 175–81.

Westergren, I., Nystrom, B., Hamberger, A. and Johansson, B. B. (1995). Intracerebral microdialysis and the blood–brain barrier. *J. Neurochem.*, **64**, 229–34.

Westerink, B. H. C. and De Vries, J. B. (1988). Characterization of in vivo dopamine release as determined by brain microdialysis after acute and subchronic implantations: methodological aspects. *J. Neurosci.*, **51**, 683–7.

Westerink, B. H. C. and Tuinte, M. H. J. (1986). Chronic use of intracerebral microdialysis for the in vivo measurements of 3,4,-dihydroxyphenylethylamine and its metabolite 3,4, dihydroxyphenylacetic acid. *J. Neurochem.*, **46**, 181–9.

Wong, S. L., Van Belle, K. and Sawchuck, R. J. (1993). Distributional transport kinetics of zidovudine between plasma and brain extracellular fluid and cerebrospinal fluid blood-barriers in the rabbit: investigation on the inhibitory effect of probenecid utilizing microdialysis. *J. Pharmacol. Exp. Ther.*, **264**, 899–909.

Yadid, G., Pacak, K., Kopin, I. J. and Goldstein, D. S. (1993). Modified microdialysis probe for sampling extracellular fluid and administering drugs *in vivo*. *Am. J. Physiol.*, **265**, R1205–11.

Yergey, J. A. and Heyes, M. P. (1990). Brain eicosanoid formation following acute penetration injury as studied by in vivo microdialysis. *J. Cereb. Blood Flow Metab.*, **10**, 143–6.

Yokel, R. A., Allen, D. D., Burgio, D. E. and McNamara, P. J. (1992). Antipyrine as a dialyzable reference to correct differences in efficiency among and within sampling devices during *in vivo* microdialysis. *J. Pharm. Meth.*, **27**, 135–42.

12 Blood–brain barrier permeability measured with histochemistry

SUKRITI NAG

- Introduction
- Blood–brain barrier permeability to HRP in steady states
- Blood–brain barrier permeability to HRP in pathological states

Introduction

The advent of electron microscopy and the availability of horseradish peroxidase (HRP) as a marker to study vascular permeability to proteins (Graham and Karnovsky, 1966), opened a new era in the study of the blood–brain barrier (BBB). Over the next two decades there was a plethora of studies of BBB permeability to HRP in steady states and in diverse pathological conditions. Horseradish peroxidase, a glycoprotein with a molecular weight of 40 000, can be localized in tissues by both light and electron microscopy. Both the tracer and the HRP reaction product which forms in tissues following a histochemical reaction will be referred to as HRP.

Blood–brain barrier permeability to HRP in steady states

The morphological features unique to cerebral vessels, in contrast to other body vessels, that account for their relative impermeability to plasma proteins and protein tracers such as HRP in steady states, are limited endothelial pinocytosis and the presence of tight junctions along the interendothelial spaces. Other factors affecting BBB permeability to HRP are endothelial surface charge and endothelial cytoskeletal elements.

Pinocytosis

Fluid-phase transcytosis of HRP across endothelium occurs by pinocytotic vesicles, which are membrane-bound spheres, 50–90 nm in diameter. The classic study of Reese and Karnovsky (1967) drew attention to the finding that during steady states, cerebral endothelium contains few pinocytotic vesicles. Vesicles tend to occur in groups irregularly dispersed along the circumference of the endothelial layer. Hence they were quantitated by measuring the entire cross-sectional area of endothelium, and the vesicles in this area were counted to obtain a value for the number of vesicles per μm^2 of endothelium that was found to be five for arteriolar endothelium (Nag et al., 1979, 1980). Another group (Coomber et al., 1988) obtained a quantitative estimate by counting the number of vesicles in selected endothelial segments of individual vessels. These authors obtained a value of 8.8 vesicles per μm^2 of endothelial cytoplasm for microvessels. The number of endothelial pinocytotic vesicles per μm^2 of endothelium did not change significantly in the presence of circulating HRP (Nag et al., 1979).

The observation that there are fewer endothelial pinocytotic vesicles in cerebral vessels as compared with other body vessels was also supported by quantitative studies, which showed one-twelfth fewer vesicles at the capillary luminal plasma membrane in cerebral endothelium (Connell and Mercer, 1974) as compared with myocardial capillaries (Simionescu *et al.*, 1974). However, when all pinocytotic vesicles per μm^2 in endothelial cytoplasm were counted, cerebral endothelium had one fifth the number of vesicles observed in muscle capillaries (Coomber *et al.*, 1988).

Three hypotheses have been proposed to account for transendothelial vesicular passage of non-lipid-soluble macromolecules greater than 10 nm from blood to tissues and in the reverse direction in noncerebral endothelium. The oldest and best known is the 'shuttle hypothesis', according to which single caveolae at the luminal or abluminal surfaces 'bud off' to become free vesicles within the cytoplasm before fusing with the opposite surface (Bruns and Palade, 1968). The second hypothesis is that vesicles fuse to form transendothelial channels for transcytosis of substances from blood to tissues or in the reverse direction (Palade *et al.*, 1979; Predescu and Palade, 1993). The third hypothesis is sometimes referred to as the fusion–fission hypothesis. It suggests that individual vesicles do not move from one surface to the other but merely far enough to fuse and communicate transiently with their immediate neighbors so as to allow intermixing of the vesicular contents, and eventually the contents reach the opposite plasma membrane (Clough and Michel, 1981).

Fusion of vesicles to form transendothelial channels was not observed in normal cerebral endothelium.

Tight junctions

Fusion of the outer leaflets of adjacent plasma membranes at intervals along the interendothelial spaces of neocortical vessels forms 'tight' or 'occluding' junctions (Muir and Peters, 1962). Tracers such as HRP (Reese and Karnovsky, 1967) and microperoxidase (Feder *et al.*, 1969) were not detected in the vascular basement membrane, and this suggested that these junctions extended circumferentially around cerebral endothelial cells, preventing the passage of macromolecules by this route, hence their name zonula occludens. The same kind of junctions between the epithelial cells lining the choroid plexus, and the ependymal cells overlying the median eminence and area postrema,

prevented the entry of HRP into the ventricular cerebrospinal fluid (Brightman *et al.*, 1970). Peroxidase, injected directly into the cerebral ventricles, percolated through the open cerebral interspaces by passing around the discontinuous gap junctions between ependymal cells and glial cells, and even filled the vascular basement membranes. However, the passage of peroxidase into the capillary lumen was prevented by the same endothelial tight junctions that blocked movement from blood into the neuropil (Brightman *et al.*, 1970).

Endothelial surface charge

The normal permeability characteristics of cerebral endothelium are dependent on maintenance of the net negative surface charge, which can be demonstrated by the binding of cationized ferritin (Nag, 1984) or colloidal iron (Nagy *et al.*, 1983) to the endothelial luminal plasma membrane. Peanut agglutinin binding was not demonstrable in normal endothelium, since the ß-D-gal-(1,3)-D-gal *N*-acetyl groups to which peanut agglutinins bind are subterminal to the sialyl groups (Nag, 1986).

Endothelial cytoskeleton

Cerebral endothelial cells, like most eukaryotic cells studied, have a cytoskeleton consisting of microfilaments, intermediate filaments and microtubules. Microfilament bundles have been observed in proximity to cell junctions and tend to be prominent along the abluminal surface of cells or span the cell from the luminal to the abluminal plasma membrane (Nag, 1995). Endothelial microtubules are generally oriented along the long axis of cells and microtubule profiles are seen in cross-section of vessels (Nag, 1995). Some microtubules are oriented from the basal to the apical surface of endothelial cells. The role of the cytoskeleton in BBB permeability alterations will be alluded to later on.

Blood–brain barrier permeability to HRP in pathological states

The routes by which circulating HRP could enter brain in the early phase of BBB breakdown in a pathological state are (1) enhanced pinocytosis and

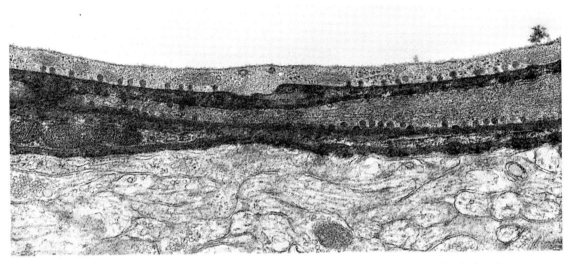

Fig. 12.1. Segment of arteriolar endothelium from a rat with norepinephrine-induced acute hypertension showing increased permeability to HRP resulting in tracer deposition in the endothelial and sarcolemmal basement membranes and in the adventitia. Note the increased numbers of pinocytotic vesicles containing HRP in the endothelial and smooth muscle cells (×21 600).

transendothelial channels; (2) tubulo-canalicular structures; (3) opening of tight junctions. Other factors that increase BBB permeability to HRP in pathological states are reduction of endothelial surface charge and endothelial cytoskeletal alterations.

Enhanced pinocytosis

Numerous studies demonstrated enhanced pinocytosis associated with BBB breakdown to HRP in diverse pathological conditions such as acute (Westergaard *et al.*, 1977; Nag *et al.*, 1977, 1979) and chronic hypertension (Nag, 1984), brain trauma (Povlishock *et al.*, 1978; Lossinsky *et al.*, 1983; Nag, 1996), spinal cord trauma (Beggs and Waggener, 1976), seizures (Hedley-Whyte *et al.*, 1977; Petito and Levy, 1980; Nitsch *et al.*, 1986), excitotoxicity (Nag, 1992) and other pathological states (Brightman *et al.*, 1983; Cervos-Navarro *et al.*, 1983). The type of cerebral vessels showing altered permeability depended on the disease being studied. Increased arteriolar permeability was the dominant finding in seizures (Petito and Levy, 1980) and hypertension (Nag *et al.*, 1977; Westergaard *et al.*, 1977) while in trauma (Beggs and Waggener, 1976; Lossinsky *et al.*, 1983), excitotoxic damage (Nag, 1992) and inflammation it was mainly microvessels that showed BBB breakdown to HRP.

Numerous pinocytotic vesicles (Fig. 12.1) were observed in the cerebral endothelium of arterioles in association with the presence of tracer in the endothelial basement membrane 8 min after the onset of acute hypertension (Nag *et al.*, 1979). However, since pinocytosis is known to be a bi-directional phenomenon, the finding of numerous pinocytotic vesicles containing HRP in cerebral endothelium at one time point gave no indication of the direction of pinocytosis. Studies done at 90 s, an earlier time interval after the onset of acute hypertension, demonstrated numerous endothelial vesicles, many containing HRP, in arterioles that showed no HRP in the basement membrane. In addition, confluent deposits of HRP were observed in pinocytotic vesicles and the adjacent endothelial basement membranes, which did not otherwise contain tracer, suggesting that the vesicles were depositing tracer onto the endothelial basement membranes (Nag *et al.*, 1979) (Fig. 12.2a). This finding observed in all subsequent studies of hypertension (Nag *et al.*, 1980; Nag, 1984, 1986) and other pathological conditions (Beggs and Waggener, 1976; Hedley-Whyte *et al.*, 1977; Raymond *et al.*, 1986; Nag, 1992), allowed no other interpretation than that the tracer crossed the endothelium via the vesicular system.

Quantitative morphometry of cortical arteri-

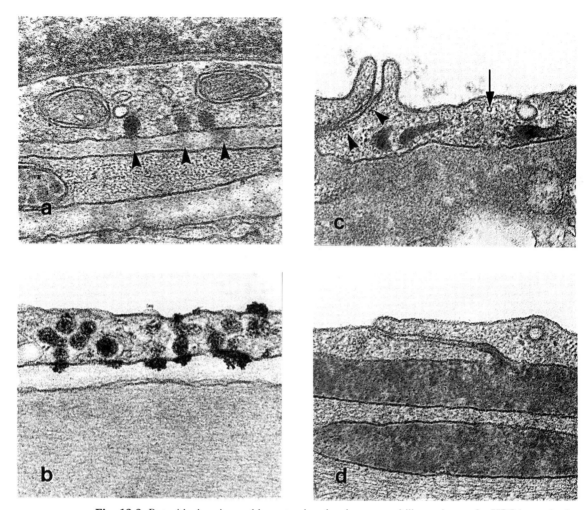

Fig. 12.2. Rat with chronic renal hypertension showing permeability pathways for HRP in cerebral endothelium. (a) Pinocytotic vesicles at the abluminal plasma membrane of endothelium show confluent deposits of HRP in the vesicle and the adjacent basement membrane (arrowheads). (b) Ultracytochemical localization of Ca^{2+}ATPase highlights the increased numbers of endothelial pinocytotic vesicles and the transendothelial channel. (c) Segment of microvessel endothelium showing tubulo-canalicular structures containing HRP. Note the intact tight junction at the luminal end of the interendothelial space. This segment of endothelium contains cross-sectional profiles of all the cytoskeletal elements. Actin filaments (arrowheads) are present along the interendothelial space, the profile of a microtubule is also present (arrow) and cross sectional profiles of intermediate filaments are present at the right-hand side of the electron micrograph. (d) Segment of arteriolar endothelium that is permeable to HRP showing tracer at the abluminal end of an interendothelial space that has intact tight junctions. (a), (b) $\times 66\,000$; (c) $\times 51\,300$; (d) $\times 62\,400$. (Fig. 12.2b is reproduced from Nag, 1993, with permission.)

oles permeable to HRP in experimental hypertension (Table 12.1) consistently demonstrated twice as many endothelial vesicles as compared with the corresponding nonpermeable vascular segments of normotensive control rats (Nag *et al.*, 1979, 1980;

Nag, 1995). In permeable arteriolar segments eight times as many vesicles contained HRP; therefore the overall magnitude of the increase in pinocytosis was 16 times normal. The magnitude of increase in pinocytosis in seizures was observed

Table 12.1 *Quantitative estimate of pinocytosis in cerebral endothelium in pathological conditions*

Experimental conditions	Type of vessel	Mean vesicles/μm^2 of endothelium	
		Control	Test
Counts of total vesicles			
Acute hypertension[a]	arterioles	5.11±1.06	9.85±0.84
Chronic hypertension[b]	arterioles	5.14±0.63	10.28±1.18
Cytochalasin B infusion[c]	arterioles	5.22±1.29	12.12±1.90
Bradykinin infusion[d]	arterioles	4.48±1.80	14.88±5.03
Counts of HRP filled vesicles			
Seizures[e]	capillaries	12.2±5.4	86.7±22.1
	arterioles	6.7±3.0	267.7±46.1
Ischemia[e]	capillaries		52.7±10.6
	arterioles		92.2±33.2
Compression injury[f]	all	3.0	15.0

[a]Nag *et al.*, 1979; [b]Nag *et al.*, 1980; [c]Nag, 1995; [d]Raymond *et al.*, 1986; [e]Petito and Levy, 1980; [f]Beggs and Waggener, 1976.

to be much larger, being 40 times control values (Petito and Levy, 1980). Correlation of vesicle density with arteriolar size showed that arterioles less than 18 μm had a higher density of pinocytotic vesicles as compared with arterioles having diameters greater than 18 μm during bradykinin-induced BBB breakdown (Raymond *et al.*, 1986). Another interesting finding in the latter study was that, when permeability was reduced by drug treatment, fewer arterioles were permeable to HRP, however the magnitude of increase in pinocytosis in those arterioles permeable to HRP was the same as in the non-drug-treated rats.

Fusion of endothelial vesicles to form transendothelial channels extending from the luminal to the abluminal plasma membrane was observed in cerebral endothelium in areas of BBB breakdown in acute (Nag, 1988) and chronic hypertension (Nag, 1990a) (Fig. 12.2b), hyperglycaemia (Shivers and Harris, 1984) and brain trauma (Lossinsky *et al.*, 1989).

The concept of enhanced pinocytosis providing a pathway for passage of HRP across cerebral endothelium in pathological states was not universally accepted. Findings in studies of receptor-mediated transport (Broadwell, 1989)

and studies of frog mesenteric vessels (Frøkjaer-Jensen, 1980), both done in steady states, have been used to discount the role of vesicular transport in increased BBB permeability, with no consideration being given to the heterogeneity existing between endothelia at different locations and that endothelial reactivity may be different in pathological states.

Role of calcium in permeability and pinocytosis Our studies established that in hypertension, early protein transfer into brain occurred by enhanced pinocytosis. What triggered pinocytosis was unclear. Our hypothesis was that permeability and pinocytosis were modulated by intraendothelial influx of ionic Ca^{2+}, which could occur in the following way. Hypertension inhibits the endothelial plasma membrane Na^+,K^+-ATPase resulting in sodium accumulation within the cell. This decreases the efficiency of the Na^+/Ca^{2+} exchanger, leading to intracellular calcium accumulation. Inhibition of the plasma membrane Ca^{2+}-ATPase contributes to further increase of intracellular calcium. Possibly, this increase in intracellular calcium mediates increased endothelial permeability by enhanced pinocytosis.

Ultracytochemical localization of Ca^{2+}-ATPase and Na^+, K^+-ATPase was done using fixed brain slices from acutely hypertensive rats, which were injected with HRP as a marker of BBB permeability alterations (Nag, 1988, 1990*b*). These studies demonstrated reduced localization of both enzymes, indicating reduced activity, only in the arteriolar segments permeable to HRP. Further studies demonstrated that the reduced activity of the endothelial plasma membrane Ca^{2+}-ATPase and Na^+,K^+-ATPase preceded BBB breakdown to endogenous plasma proteins in chronic hypertension (Nag, 1993), thus supporting the hypothesis of the role of Ca^{2+} in increased pinocytosis and permeability. An interesting finding in these studies is the localization of both Ca^{2+}-ATPase and Na^+,K^+-ATPase in the plasma membranes of pinocytotic vesicles. Localization of these enzymes highlighted the increased numbers of endothelial vesicles in arterioles permeable to endogenous serum proteins in chronic hypertension (Fig. 12.2b).

Other agents known to trigger pinocytosis in cerebral endothelium are biogenic amines such as bradykinin (Raymond *et al.*, 1986), histamine (Dux and Joó, 1982), serotonin and cAMP (Westergaard, 1975). Studies of cultured brain endothelium have implicated cAMP, cGMP, PKC and arachidonic acid in the activation of pinocytosis and albumin transport (Joó, 1994).

Tubulo-canalicular structures

Tubulo-canalicular structures are not a common finding in normal endothelium. However, in areas of severe BBB breakdown, such structures containing HRP have been observed in addition to enhanced pinocytosis in the endothelium, of mainly microvessels (Beggs and Waggener, 1976; Nag *et al.*, 1977; Lossinsky *et al.*, 1983; Shivers and Harris, 1984) (Fig. 12.2c). These structures were also seen in microvessels that did not show HRP in the basement membrane, suggesting that this was a pathway by which tracer traversed the endothelium. However, passage of HRP via tubulo-canalicular structures was never observed in the absence of enhanced pinocytosis, and therefore it must be considered as an additional pathway that supplements the vesicular pathway.

Interendothelial junctions

Studies reporting the breakdown of interendothelial junctions in pathological states showed illustrations that demonstrated HRP focally at the luminal or abluminal end of the interendothelial space or in extracellular pools between successive tight junctions that appeared intact (Brightman *et al.*, 1973). There was never convincing demonstration of tracer along the entire length of the junction extending from the luminal to the abluminal end (Fig. 12.2d). This suggests that breakdown of junctions by HRP rarely occurs or else is difficult to demonstrate due to the circumferential nature of these junctions. This applies to the tight junctions between choroidal epithelial cells as well, which, although not as extensive as those of cerebral endothelia, still prevent passage of HRP following intravenous infusion of atrial natriuretic factor (Nag, 1991).

Convincing demonstration of the breakdown of interendothelial junctions was obtained when ionic lanthanum was used as a tracer. This tracer is smaller than HRP, having a molecular weight of 138.9 Da and an ionic radius of 11.5 nm (Harned and Owen, 1958) as compared with a radius of ~ 50 nm for HRP (Karnovsky, 1967). Breakdown of tight junctions by ionic lanthanum was demonstrated in cerebral endothelium following the intracarotid injection of hyperosmotic solutions (Dorovini-Zis *et al.*, 1983) and in choroidal epithelial cells in response to an intravenous infusion of atrial natriuretic peptide (Nag, 1991).

However, it is well-known that prolonged BBB breakdown may be associated with disruption of not only junctions but the entire endothelium. This may explain the finding of diffuse endothelial staining with HRP in areas of BBB breakdown, although the latter appearance has also been attributed to artefact (Brightman *et al.*, 1970; Reese and Karnovsky, 1967).

Endothelial surface charge

Reduction of the net negative charge on the endothelial surface is associated with increased BBB permeability (Nagy *et al.*, 1983; Nag, 1984). In angiotensin-induced acute hypertension, cortical arterioles permeable to HRP at 2.5 min showed enhanced endothelial vesicular activity and marked reduction or loss of cationized ferritin binding to the luminal plasma membrane of endothelium while peanut agglutinin binding occurred (Nag, 1986). Both changes resulted due to loss of the terminal sialic acid groups on the luminal plasma membrane. These changes were rapidly reversible and not demonstrable 10 min after the onset of hypertension, when blood pressures reached resting levels and the BBB was restored. Evidence from the literature indicates that loss of the net negative charge precedes permeability alterations (Nagy *et al.*, 1983).

Endothelial cytoskeleton

Integrity of endothelial actin filaments are important for maintenance of the BBB to protein during steady states since increased permeability to HRP by enhanced pinocytosis occurred in the presence of an actin-disrupting agent, Cytochalasin B (Nag, 1995). The microtubular network, on the other hand, had no demonstrable role during steady states, but disruption of the microtubular network by colchicine had a protective effect and prevented the development of BBB breakdown to HRP in acute hypertension (Nag, 1995). The latter may be due to the postulated role of microtubules in movement of pinocytotic vesicles (Lui *et al.*, 1993);

hence disruption of microtubules hampered the passage of pinocytotic vesicles and prevented BBB breakdown.

In conclusion, tracer studies using HRP have provided insight into the pathways for protein passage from blood into brain and in the reverse direction in steady states and in pathological conditions. Enhanced pinocytosis and tubulo-canalicular channels are pathways for protein passage in the early phase of injury when endothelial cells are still viable and capable of reacting to injury. Prolonged BBB breakdown or severe insults result in breakdown of endothelial junctions and necrosis of endothelium. Immunohistochemical techniques now available for detection of BBB permeability alterations have largely replaced HRP as a marker of BBB permeability alterations, due mainly to the fact that such immunohistochemical studies are less labor intensive, are cheaper and superior for detection of the location and extent of endogenous protein extravasation. Nonetheless, HRP remains a good tracer for detection of the permeability status of cerebral vessels at a particular time point.

Acknowledgment

This work was supported by the Heart and Stroke Foundation of Ontario.

References

Beggs, J. L. and Waggener, J. D. (1976). Transendothelial vesicular transport of protein following compression injury to the spinal cord. *Lab. Invest.*, **34**, 428–39.

Brightman, M. W., Klatzo, I., Olsson, Y. and Reese, T. S. (1970). The blood–brain barrier to proteins under normal and pathological conditions. *J. Neurol. Sci.*, **10**, 215–39.

Brightman, M. W., Hori, M., Rapoport, S. I. *et al.* (1973). Osmotic opening of tight junctions in cerebral endothelium. *J. Comp. Neurol.*, **152**, 317–26

Brightman, M. W., Zis, K. and Anders, J. (1983). Morphology of cerebral endothelium and astrocytes as determinants of the neuronal microenvironment. *Acta Neuropathol.*, Suppl VIII, 21–33.

Broadwell, R. D. (1989). Transcytosis of macromolecules through the blood–brain barrier, a cell biological perspective and critical appraisal. *Acta Neuropathol.*, **79**, 117–28.

Bruns, R. R. and Palade, G. E. (1968). Studies on blood capillaries, Part 2 (Transport of ferritin molecules across the wall of muscle capillaries). *J. Cell Biol.*, **37**, 277–99.

Cervos-Navarro, J., Artigas, J. and Mrsulja, B. J. (1983). Morphofunctional aspects of the normal and pathological blood–brain barrier. *Acta Neuropathol.*, Suppl VIII, 1–19.

Clough, G. and Michel, C. C. (1981). The role of vesicles in the transport of ferritin through frog endothelium. *J. Physiol. (London)*, **315**, 127–42.

Connell, C. J. and Mercer, K. L. (1974). Freeze-fracture appearance of the capillary endothelium in the cerebral cortex of mouse brain. *Am. J. Anat.*, **140**, 595–99.

Coomber, B. L., Stewart, P. A., Hayakawa, K. *et al.* (1988). A quantitative estimate of microvessel ultrastructure in C6 astrocytoma spheroids transplanted to brain and muscle. *J. Neuropath. Exp. Neurol.*, **47**, 299–307

Dorovini-Zis, K., Sato, M., Goping, G. *et al.* (1983). Ionic lanthanum passage across cerebral endothelium exposed to hyperosmotic arabinose. *Acta Neuropathol.*, **60**, 49–60.

Dux, E. and Joó, F. (1982) Effects of histamine on brain capillaries, fine structural and immunohistochemical studies after intracarotid infusion. *Exp. Brain Res.*, **47**, 252–8.

Feder, N., Reese, T. S. and Brightman, M. W. (1969). Microperoxidase, a new tracer of low molecular weight. *J. Cell Bio.*, **43**, 35a-36a.

Frøkjaer-Jensen, J. (1980). Three-dimensional organisation of plasmalemmal vesicles in endothelial cells. An analysis by serial sectioning of frog mesenteric capillaries. *J. Ultrastruct. Res.*, **73**, 9–20.

Graham, R. C. and Karnovsky, M. J. (1966). The early stages of absorption of injected horseradish peroxidase in the proximal tubules of mouse kidney; ultrastructure cytochemistry by a new technique. *J. Histochem. Cytochem.*, **14**, 291–302.

Harned, H. S. and Owen, B. B. (1958). *The Physical Chemistry of Electrolytic Solutions*, 3rd edn, pp. 164, 700, 702. New York: Reinhold.

Hedley-Whyte, E. T., Lorenzo, A. V. and Hsu, D. W. (1977). Protein transport across cerebral vessels during metrazole-induced convulsions. *Am. J. Physiol.*, **233**, C74–C85.

Joó, F. (1994). Insights into the regulation by second messenger molecules of the permeability of the blood–brain barrier. *Microsc. Res. Tech.*, **27**, 507–15.

Karnovsky, M. J. (1967). The ultrastructural basis of capillary permeability studied with peroxidase as a tracer. *J. Cell Biol.*, **35**, 213–36.

Lossinsky, A. S., Vorbrodt, A. W. and Wisniewski, H. M. (1983). Ultracytochemical studies of vesicular and canalicular transport structures in the injured mammalian blood–brain barrier. *Acta Neuropathol.*, **61**, 239–45.

Lossinsky, A. S., Song, M. J., and Wisniewski, H. M. (1989). High voltage electron microscopic studies of endothelial cell tubular structures in the mouse blood–brain barrier following brain trauma. *Acta Neuropathol.*, **77**, 480–8.

Lui, S. M., Magnusson, K.-E. and Sundqvist, T. (1993). Microtubules are involved in transport of macromolecules by vesicles in cultured bovine aortic endothelial cells. *J. Physiol.*, **156**, 311–16.

Muir, A. R. and Peters, A. (1962). Quintuple layered membrane junctions at terminal bars between endothelial cells. *J. Cell Biol.*, **12**, 443–8.

Nag, S. (1984a). Cerebral changes in chronic hypertension, combined permeability and immunohistochemical studies. *Acta Neuropathol.*, **62**, 178–84.

Nag, S. (1984b). Cerebral endothelial surface charge in hypertension. *Acta Neuropathol.*, **63**, 276–81.

Nag, S. (1986). Cerebral endothelial plasma membrane alterations in acute hypertension. *Acta Neuropathol.*, **70**, 38–43.

Nag, S. (1988). Localization of calcium-activated adenosine-triphosphatase (Ca^{2+}-ATPase) in intracerebral arterioles in acute hypertension. *Acta Neuropathol.*, **75**, 547–53.

Nag, S. (1990a). Ultracytochemical localization of Na, K-ATPase in cerebral endothelium in acute hypertension. *Acta Neuropathol.*, **80**, 7–11.

Nag, S. (1990b). Presence of transendothelial channels in cerebral endothelium in chronic hypertension. *Acta Neurochirurg.*, **51**, 335–7.

Nag, S. (1991). Effect of atrial natriuretic factor on permeability of the blood-cerebrospinal fluid barrier. *Acta Neuropathol.*, **82**, 274–9.

Nag, S. (1992). Vascular changes in the spinal cord in *N*-methyl-D-aspartate-induced excitotoxicity, morphological and permeability studies. *Acta Neuropathol.*, **84**, 471–7.

Nag, S. (1993). Cerebral endothelial mechanisms in increased permeability in chronic hypertension. *Ad. Exp. Med. Biol.*, **331**, 263–6.

Nag, S. (1995). Role of the endothelial cytoskeleton in blood–brain barrier permeability to proteins. *Acta Neuropathol.*, **90**, 454–60.

Nag, S. (1996). Cold-injury of the cerebral cortex, immunolocalization of cellular proteins and blood–brain barrier permeability studies. *J. Neuropathol. Exp. Neurol.*, **55**, 880–8.

Nag, S., Robertson, D. M. and Dinsdale, H. B. (1977). Cerebral cortical changes in acute experimental hypertension. An ultrastructural study. *Lab. Invest.*, **33**, 150–71.

Nag, S., Robertson, D. M. and Dinsdale, H. B. (1979). Quantitative estimate of pinocytosis in experimental acute hypertension. *Acta Neuropathol.*, **46**, 107–16.

Nag, S., Robertson, D. M. and Dinsdale, H. B. (1980). Morphological changes in spontaneously hypertensive rats. *Acta Neuropathol.*, **52**, 27–34.

Nagy, Z., Peters, H. and Huttner, I. (1983). Charge-related alterations of the cerebral endothelium. *Lab. Invest.*, **49**, 662–71.

Nitsch, C., Goping, G., Laursen, H. and Klatzo, I. (1986). The blood–brain barrier to horseradish peroxidase at the onset of bicuculline-induced seizures in hypothalamus, pallidum, hippocampus, and other selected regions of the rabbit. *Acta Neuropathol.*, **69**, 1–16.

Palade, G. E., Simionescu, M. and Simionescu, N. (1979). Structural aspects of the permeability of the microvascular endothelium. *Acta Physiol. Scand.*, **463**, 11–32.

Petito, C. K. and Levy, D. E. (1980). The importance of cerebral arterioles in alterations of the blood–brain barrier. *Lab. Invest.*, **43**, 262–8.

Povlishock, J. T., Becker, D. P., Sullivan, H. G. and Miller, J. D. (1978). Vascular permeability alterations to horseradish peroxidase in experimental brain injury. *Brain Res.*, **153**, 223–39.

Predescu, D. and Palade, G. E. (1993). Plasmalemmal vesicles represent the large pore system of continuous microvascular endothelium. *Am. J. Physiol.*, **265**, H725–H733.

Raymond, J. J., Robertson, D. M. and Dinsdale, H. B. (1986). Pharmacological modification of bradykinin induced breakdown of the blood–brain barrier. *Can. J. Neurol. Sci.* **13**, 214–20.

Reese, T. S. and Karnovsky, M. J. (1967). Fine structural localization of a blood–brain barrier to exogenous peroxidase. *J. Cell Biol.*, **34**, 207–17.

Shivers, R. R. and Harris, R. J. (1984). Opening of the blood–brain barrier in *anolis carolinensis*. A high voltage electron microscope protein tracer study. *Neuropathol. Appl. Neurobiol.*, **10**, 343–56.

Simionescu, M., Simionescu, N. and Palade, G. E. (1974). Morphometric data on the endothelium of blood capillaries. *J. Cell Biol.*, **60**, 128–52.

120

Westergaard, E. (1975). The effect of
  serotonin, norepinephrine and cyclic
  AMP on the BBB. *Ultrastructural Res.*, **50**,
  383 .
Westergaard, E., Van Deurs, B. and
  Brondsted, H. E. (1977). Increased
  vesicular transfer of peroxidase across
  cerebral endothelium, evoked by acute
  hypertension. *Acta Neuropathol.*, **37**,
  141–52.

13 Measuring local cerebral capillary permeability–surface area products by quantitative autoradiography

JOSEPH FENSTERMACHER and LING WEI

- Overview of quantitative autoradiography
- Theory of blood–brain barrier permeability measurements
- The quantitative autoradiographic technique

Overview of quantitative autoradiography

Realizing the diversity in neural function, structure, metabolism, and pathology within the central nervous system, Kety, Sokoloff, and coworkers (Landau et al., 1955; Reivich et al., 1969; Sokoloff et al., 1977; and Sakurada et al., 1978) developed quantitative autoradiography (QAR) and used it to demonstrate variations in cerebral blood flow and glucose utilization not only among brain regions but also within them at the level of nuclei, layers, and tracts. In the extreme, QAR can localize and quantitate ^{14}C-radioactivity with reasonable accuracy in a tissue volume of less than $100 \mu m \times 100 \mu m \times 20 \mu m$ when care is taken to minimize intratissue redistribution during and after the experimental period. Because of this ability to localize radioactivity in brain tissue, the measured parameters and functions are often referred to as 'local,' e.g. local cerebral blood flow (LCBF) and local cerebral glucose utilization (LCGU). This localizing capability is the major reason for using quantitative autoradiography in animal studies.

In brief, the technique of quantitative autoradiography involves administering a radiotracer into an experimental animal, usually intravenously, taking a series of blood samples for assessing radioactivity, killing the animal, and rapidly removing and freezing the brain.

Subsequently, the frozen brain is serially sectioned into $20 \mu m$ thick sections (the adult rat brain yields about 1000 such sections), staining some for histologies, placing others inside X-ray cassettes with a sheet of X-ray film for autoradiography, and discarding the remainder (about 75% of the sections). After sufficient exposure, the films (usually two per rat brain) are developed and analyzed for the distribution-quantification of radioactivity by an image analysis system. The resulting data are combined with the blood radioactivity data to calculate a particular function or process.

In addition to spatial localization, the advantages of QAR include the production of histologies of the tissue immediately adjacent to the sections taken for autoradiography and the permanence and completeness of the autoradiographic record, the X-ray film. The histologies can be used to pick out and outline the sites for assaying local radioactivity via the X-ray films and to drive the analysis unbiased by the autoradiographic pictures, which can be beguiling. In turn, the autoradiographic data can be employed to identify areas of interest on the histologies. Most importantly, the structure and state of the tissue in and around the area of interest can also be assessed from the histologies. As for the permanence of the data, the X-ray films last until discarded; they can be read and re-read as long as they are not smudged or scratched (we currently have nearly

20 000 such films, with accompanying histological slides, on file and often go back to reanalyze various sets of them as new questions arise). In the laboratory of Sokoloff and of others including the authors, the entire brain is usually sectioned for autoradiography and matching histologies, and few, if any, brain areas are missed in such a survey. Each film contains an incredible – frankly overwhelming – amount of data.

The drawbacks of the QAR technique mainly involve the immensity of the data analysis. The actual execution of the experiment is only slightly more horrendous in terms of people, time, and space than most other radiotracer experiments; the relatively high doses of radioactivity administered to achieve sufficient 'signal-to-noise' ratios on the X-ray films do, however, add appreciably to the expense of QAR. From this point on, considerable time is consumed. One day is required for careful and complete sectioning of the frozen brain for histologies and autoradiograms by an experienced histological technician. This is followed by exposure periods ranging most commonly from one to three weeks but possibly as short as one to two days and as long as several months. Finally, the analysis of the autoradiograms and the calculation of the various parameters, rates and spaces, consumes a great amount of time. Estimates of the parameter(s) of interest can be made in over 200 brain areas; readings can be made within many structures, e.g. among the six layers of the cortex or the various hypothalamic nuclei. For certain pathological models and physiological alterations, data from ipsilateral (the lesioned or stimulated) and contralateral sides are gathered, analyzed separately, and compared to each other, thus doubling the effort and time. Gradients of radioactivity and related function can be read, for instance, across a lesion such as an area of ischemia or from the third ventricle into the adjacent hypothalamus. After reviewing the initial data, re-reading of some areas and collecting data from new areas of interest is often done. In our recent permeability studies (e.g. Chen *et al.*, 1994*a*, 1994*b*, 1995), two to three days per experiments are spent by one experienced investigator in reading the autoradiograms, calculating the parameters of interest, collating the data, and combining the results from differing groups of experi-

ments to derive other numbers, e.g. calculating the local transfer rate constant (K_1) with the appropriate vascular space correction or the local capillary permeability–surface area (PS) products from LCBF and K_1. Quantitative autoradiography is not for the impatient nor those needing instant gratification; it has, however, been found to be the most appropriate, most sensitive methodology for situations where radiotracer localization in the 100–500 μm range is of importance. With this level of resolution, QAR can be employed in mice, hamsters, and gerbils as well as rats.

Finally, QAR could be said to be the 'mother' of positron emission tomography (PET), magnetic resonance imaging (MRI), and computed tomography (CT) of X-ray contrast agent distribution because many of the markers and approaches used in PET, MRI, and CT were first established by QAR studies of animal models. All three techniques are used in humans to study the state and progression of central nervous system disease and disorders, provide single or multiple slice images of the human brain *in vivo*, and allow repeated image acquisition over time in the same individual. With certain types of measurements, PET and MRI can be used to study brain functions and activities such as learning, motor activity, and addiction. The ultimate payoff of QAR may, thus, be to develop and provide techniques and concepts for studying the human brain.

Theory of blood–brain barrier permeability measurements

The blood–brain barrier is formed by the cerebral capillary wall and greatly limits the blood-to-brain distribution of many solutes. Despite the formidable sound of 'the barrier,' it is not absolute, and both 'impermeable' and 'permeable' materials flux across cerebral capillaries, in some cases facilitated by carriers or transporters. Blood-to-brain influx (defined as the influx rate constant or K_1) depends on the rate of delivery of the exchangeable material to the capillary bed by the blood, the permeability of the capillary wall to the material per unit surface area (P), the surface area of the perfused capillary system (S), and the concentration of the material in plasma water within the capillaries.

Delivery to the capillary bed is a function of both the rate of blood flow (F) and the distribution volume of the exchangeable material within the flowing blood normalized to the plasma water concentration (V_e).

Based on the Krogh single capillary model, Renkin (1959) and Crone (1965) developed a theoretical relationship among these variables; the version of this equation pertinent to QAR measurements of K_i and PS is:

$$K_i = FV_e[1 - \exp(1 - PS/FV_e)] \qquad (13.1)$$

where exp means exponentiation of the following set of terms to the base e. The Renkin–Crone equation in various forms has subsequently been applied in many studies of capillary bed physiology in brain and other tissues. A somewhat jaundiced view of the application of the Renkin–Crone relationship to BBB permeability is, however, called for because capillary beds in brain are not made up of a series of single, unbranching tubes but rather a complex, twisting, and anastomosing array of small microvessels. The Renkin–Crone equation and Krogh model are, at best, only a fair approximation of the real relationship but are currently the only 'show in cerebral capillary town'.

Although seldom stated, measurement of F with a diffusible blood flow marker actually yields an influx rate constant and not a flow rate *per se*. In the case of a 'good' blood flow marker, K_1 is slightly less than the rate of blood flow and is much less than the capillary permeability–surface area product (PS) of the marker (Fenstermacher *et al.*, 1986; Otsuka et al, 1991*a*). To illustrate the size of this error as gauged by the Renkin–Crone equation (Eqn 13.1), the measured K_1 underestimates blood flow by 5% or less when the PS/FV_e ratio > 3.0 and by 10% or less when PS/FV_e > 2.3 (Fenstermacher *et al.*, 1986; Otsuka *et al.*, 1991*a*). Such an error in the estimate of LCBF is tacitly accepted when 'flow-limited' material such as iodoantipyrine (IAP) and butanol are used as markers of cerebral blood flow; this error, however, is generally known to compromise the measurement of F by water, which is often used as a blood flow marker in PET and MRI studies and is less permeable than either IAP or butanol.

All blood-borne materials distribute to some extent in plasma water, and it is their concentration in plasma water that drives the influx across the BBB, thus the normalization given in the definition of V_e above. Exchangeable material may also be carried by plasma proteins and blood cells. Accordingly, V_e is equal to or greater than the plasma water space and can even be greater than the blood volume when the majority of the exchangeable material is plasma protein bound and/or blood cell contained. Red cell carriage of oxygen is an example of the latter case.

The unidirectional extraction (E_i) is another blood–brain transfer number like the influx rate constant and is defined as the amount of solute that influxes across the capillary over a period of time divided by the amount flowing into the capillaries during that period; it is also often referred to as the unidirectional (not net) clearance (Renkin, 1959; Crone, 1965). The unidirectional extraction can either be determined directly as done with the indicator diffusion technique of Crone (1965) and the brain uptake index or BUI technique of Oldendorf (1971) or be calculated by dividing K_1 by FV_e. The extraction fraction version of the Renkin–Crone equation is:

$$E_i = K_1/FV_e = 1 - \exp(1 - PS/FV_e) \qquad (13.2)$$

Incidentally, E_i is less than 1.0 for all materials, since influx cannot exceed delivery.

The influx of a solute that slowly moves across the capillary wall is often referred to as 'permeability-limited'. In this case, K_1 is only weakly dependent on blood flow, is slightly less than PS and much less than FV_e, and approximates PS fairly well. To take two cases, the Renkin–Crone equation suggests that K_1 underestimates PS by less than 10% when $PS/FV_e < 0.2$ and by less than 5% when $PS/FV_e < 0.1$ (Fenstermacher *et al.*, 1986). It is, henceforth, reasonable to say that permeability is limiting when E_i is < 0.2. For the normal BBB, permeability-limited compounds that can be detected by QAR include sucrose, diethylenetriaminepentaacetic acid (DTPA, chelated with an appropriate Auger-electron emitting radioisotope, e.g. [111]In), and α-aminoisobutyric acid (AIB).

The blood-to-brain flux of materials with E_i values = 0.2–0.8 (moderately permeable) depends relatively strongly on both flow and PS product. Over this range of extraction fractions, PS/FV_e varies from 0.22 to 1.60. In various non-QAR studies of the BBB, E_i or K_1 for moderately permeable substances have been measured, and PS products have been calculated, using either measured or assumed values of FV_e. Because of the exponential relationship (Eqns 13.1 and 13.2), a poor estimate of FV_e leads to a sizable error in the calculation of PS, an error that increases as the PS product and PS/FV_e ratio become larger. Antipyrine ($E_i = 0.5$–0.6) is one example of moderately BBB-permeable compounds employable in QAR studies (Chen *et al.*, 1994*a*, 1994*b*, 1995).

The quantitative autoradiographic technique

Introduction to the technique

The preceding theoretical section indicates that both K_i and LCBF need to be measured and used to estimate BBB permeability. For animal studies, this most commonly entails making measurements in two different groups, one for K_i and the other for LCBF. Of importance and great advantage to human studies with *in vivo* 'QAR' techniques such as PET, both influx (either K_i or E_i) and LCBF can be determined sequentially in the same individual.

Two conditions are required for QAR studies of capillary permeability in animals. First, both measurements are to be made by QAR in order to match various experimental parameters such as handling and sectioning the brain and matching tissue areas for analysis. Second, the physiological state of the experimental animals must be carefully monitored and screened. 'Outrider' experiments need to be excluded before calculating PS because the K_i and LCBF groups should be in nearly identical physiological or pathophysiological states as assessed by statistically insignificant differences between the groups. The accurate estimation of PS is impossible with data from physiologically unmatched groups.

One additional variable for measurement, the so-called vascular space correction, must be mentioned. When tissue radioactivity is determined by autoradiography (or tissue dissection and counting,

for that matter), some of the radiolabeled material is in the lumen of the cerebral blood vessels and has not passed into and through the capillary wall, and the remainder has 'fluxed' across the BBB. The latter quantity is the one needed for the calculation of K_i or E_i; accordingly total tissue radioactivity must be corrected for that contained in the vascular space. In QAR this is done by estimating either the plasma space or the whole blood space by autoradiography in 'yet another' group of animals, as will be presented below. Of course, this additional measurement adds to the burden of assessing permeability by QAR.

As might be expected, double-label quantitative autoradiography has been developed and employed by several research groups. Two versions, including one from the author's laboratory (Blasberg *et al.*, 1984), will be briefly reviewed. The procedures to be described below come from nearly twenty years of using quantitative autoradiography; the descriptions reflect the author's interests and applications. Since all anesthetic agents affect brain function and seemingly perturb the processes to be measured, our studies have usually involved awake rats. Also of significant advantage, awake animals regulate their blood gases and blood pressure well, and animal-to-animal variations in physiological state are minimal. Obviously, studies with unanesthetized animals cannot be undertaken without animal care committee approval, which is – of necessity – not readily obtained. If anesthetics are used, then the investigator must be aware that the results may be tainted by this usage. Finally, the extension of the QAR technique to mice, sparked by the existence of transgenic lines, is of utmost importance but has only been taken to a semi-quantitative state.

General animal preparation

Most commonly, young adult rats (weight 250–350 g) are chosen for QAR experiments, and the following presentation applies to such animals. To begin the procedure, the rat is anesthetized with a mixture of 1.5% halothane, 69.0% nitrous oxide, and 29.5% oxygen. While anesthetized, femoral arteries and veins on both sides are catheterized with PE-50 tubing. The incisions are infiltrated with lidocaine hydrochloride and then closed with suture. Subsequently, the rats are immobilized by enclosing the hindquarters and abdomen in a plaster cast. If the experiments are to be done on awake animals, then they are carefully placed in a prone position on a stable base and allowed to recover from anesthesia for two or more hours before administering the radiotracer.

The physiological condition of each rat is determined by measuring blood gases, plasma osmolality, plasma glucose level, and hematocrit; this is done during the recovery period, immediately before beginning the experiment, and during the experimental period, if time and conditions permit. Arterial blood pressure is monitored continuously. Throughout the post-surgical period, behavior such as grooming and exploration, which is common in awake, restrained rats, is observed for signs of abnormality or stress. Rectal temperature is continuously recorded and kept around 37 °C by a heating pad. Radiotracer infusion is begun after sufficient recovery time and, importantly, after achievement of a normal physiological state or the state appropriate for the experimental model.

Local cerebral blood flow

Local cerebral blood flow is best measured by the ^{14}C-iodoantipyrine (IAP) autoradiographic technique of Sakurada *et al.* (1978) as modified by Otsuka *et al.* (1991*a*). Butanol and other alcohols may have high enough BBB permeability to be blood flow markers but cannot be used because of their high volatility and the resulting disappearance from the tissue sections during drying and X-ray film exposure. Two methods of sampling arterial blood have been used. For one, the arterial cannula on one side is shortened as much as possible, and arterial blood is allowed to flow continuously and is serially collected in small tubes or on pieces of filter paper (Sakurada *et al.*, 1978). A correction is applied for time-delay and sample smearing in the cannula. For the other type of 'continuous' blood sampling, an extracorporeal arteriovenous (A-V) shunt is formed by shortening the femoral artery and vein catheters on one side and connecting them with a 1.2 cm length of silicone rubber tubing, which forms a self-sealing

blood sampling chamber (Otsuka *et al.*, 1991*a*). Because flow is brisk through the shunt and only a small portion of the flowing blood is taken, no corrections are needed when sampling by A-V shunt. This approach, which the authors prefer and is described below, has the drawback that shunt blood is delivered to the venous system at 'arterial pressure.' In defense of the shunt, central venous and arterial pressures do not detectably change when used.

To start the experiment, a solution containing 50 µCi of ^{14}C-IAP in 1 ml of saline is intravenously infused over 30 s with an infusion pump according to a schedule that produces a linearly increasing concentration of ^{14}C-IAP in arterial blood over time. During this period, a series of 60–80 µl samples of arterial blood are collected every 5 s by puncturing the silicone tube portion of the A-V loop with a 22-gauge needle attached to a plungerless 1 ml syringe. Blood pressure within the loop gently but quickly drives blood into the syringe with no change in central arterial pressure. The beginning and ending of each sampling period is recorded, most simply by taping the voices of the sampler and a timer. The 'sampling time' is considered to be the midpoint of the sampling intervals.

The rats are decapitated at the completion of the last sampling period, which should come approximately 30 s after starting the IAP infusion to minimize pre-mortem movement of tracer in the tissue and backflux into blood (Patlak *et al.*, 1984; Otsuka *et al.*, 1991*a*). The exact time of decapitation must be carefully measured. Immediately thereafter, the brains are rapidly removed and frozen in 2-methylbutane cooled to −45 °C with dry ice, all of which can and should be done in <45 s. The frozen brains are covered by mounting medium (M-1 Embedding Matrix, Lipshaw, Detroit, MI) and stored at −80 °C in plastic bags until the time of sectioning, which can be as much as 4–5 weeks later when handled in this way. The concentration of radioactivity in blood and/or plasma (c.p.m./ml or c.p.m./µl) from each sample is determined by liquid scintillation counting.

The technique of autoradiograpic assay of tissue radioactivity and the calculation of blood flow is described after the blood space and influx rate experiments.

Local red cell and plasma distribution spaces

The local distribution spaces of red blood cells in brain are best measured with ^{55}Fe-red cells (RBCs), which are obtained from donor rats by the *in vivo* labeling technique of Lin *et al.* (1990). In the past ^{51}Cr-RBCs have been used but are inferior to *in vivo* ^{55}Fe-labeled ones (Lin *et al.*, 1990; Tajima *et al.*, 1992). To begin the RBC experiments, 4 ml of ^{55}Fe- labeled blood (0.3–0.4 mCi/rat) are administered into one femoral vein. The infusion period is about 30 s in length; during this time, 3–4 ml of blood should be simultaneously withdrawn from the femoral artery, thereby maintaining whole body volume constant and mean arterial pressure steady.

For the plasma (albumin) space measurement, 100 µCi of ^{125}I-bovine serum albumin (RISA) in 0.25 ml of saline is infused per animal. The infusion period is around 5 sec. With these dosages and schedules in normal rats, the blood and tissue levels of labeled RBCs and RISA are essentially constant from 45 s onward (Tajima *et al.*, 1992), testifying to the rapidity of mixing within the rat vascular system and justifying the choice of 2–3 min experimental durations for most studies.

For both the RBC and RISA experiments, 50–80 µl samples of blood are obtained at 1 min intervals via a femoral arterial catheter (an A-V shunt is not needed for this since blood levels do not change appreciably after ending the infusion and rapid, repeated sampling is not required). Approximately 3 min after tracer administration, the rat is decapitated by a small animal guillotine, and the brain is quickly removed and prepared for radioassay as described above. Small, accurate volumes of whole blood and plasma are obtained from each blood sample and assayed by liquid scintillation (^{55}Fe) or gamma (^{125}I) counting.

Incidentally, a different method of brain removal and freezing is used for experiments in which microvascular blood volume, not the vascular space correction, is the measurement of interest (Bereczki *et al.*, 1992, 1993*a,b*; Wei *et al.*, 1993). For such studies, the decapitated head is immediately frozen, trapping blood and cerebrospinal fluid in place; subsequently the brain is maintained at −20 °C while being removed from the frozen head, covered with mounting medium, and sectioned. This freezing-brain removal procedure can also be used for studies of the movement of radiolabeled materials such as sucrose, polyethylene glycol (PEG 4000), and peptides through the cerebrospinal fluid (CSF) system and from CSF to brain to blood (Ghersi-Egea *et al.*, 1995).

Local blood-to-brain transfer constants

Local cerebral capillary system transfer constants and *PS* products can be measured by QAR for both slightly permeable compounds such as sucrose and AIB and moderately permeable ones such as antipyrine and 3-*O*-methylglucose (3OMG). The experimental protocols differ for the two classes of compounds and will be described separately; the models or cases in which one or the other group of compounds is selected also varies.

For the moderately permeable compounds, the technique of Otsuka *et al.* (1991*b*), which is virtually identical with the IAP methodology (including the 30 s experimental period), has been used repeatedly by us in normal rats to determine capillary *PS* products under various physiological and pharmacological stresses (Chen *et al.*, 1994*a,b*, 1995). In the main, the protocol is driven by two considerations. First, it should match the IAP technique that provides the LCBF values subsequently used for the calculation of *PS*. The inherent errors and technical problems are, thus, common to both measurements, which is advantageous, in theory, when combining data from two separate sets of experiments. Second, short experimental durations minimize tracer backflux and the need to know the tissue:blood partition coefficient with assurance (Patlak *et al.*, 1984).

Antipyrine and 3OMG have been selected in the past as markers of moderate BBB permeability because their tissue activities can be accurately assessed by QAR (something that is not true for several other moderately permeable ^{14}C-labeled compounds that we have tried) and the processes involved in their distribution differ. Antipyrine crosses the blood–brain barrier by simple diffusion through membrane lipids (lipid-mediated transport), whereas the flux of 3OMG across the BBB is facilitated by the GLUT-1 hexose transporter. The latter process is rather complex, being a function of a number of variables including the concentration of cold glucose in plasma, but is the one desired if glucose transport is of interest.

To initiate these experiments, 50 µCi of ^{14}C-labeled material in 1 ml saline is infused through one femoral vein catheter at a constant rate over 30 s. Everything else in the experimental procedure, from the assessment of the time course of radioactivity in the plasma to the sectioning of the frozen brain for autoradiography, is the same as for the LCBF studies described above and by Otsuka *et al.* (1991*a,b*).

The choice of markers and experimental protocols is a bit more complex for the slightly permeable materials than for moderately permeable ones. Obviously radiolabeled materials in this group cross the normal BBB at slow to very slow rates. To obtain reliable estimates of blood-to-brain transfer constants, the experiments must be run for a relatively long period of time, usually ≥ 10 min, and the vascular space correction must be accurate. The long duration may be sufficient for movement of the marker within the tissue between adjacent areas of dissimilar permeabilities and also from tissue into CSF, processes that obscure local differences in capillary surface area or permeability. Perhaps the safest marker of low BBB permeability for QAR studies is ^{14}C-α-aminoisobutyric acid; AIB crosses the BBB fairly slowly, reaching detectable levels after 10–15 min in brain areas of modest to high capillary density (Blasberg *et al.*, 1983). Of importance, once AIB enters the brain parenchyma it is taken up by neurons and glia and trapped, thereby stopping any further distribution. No further discussion of low permeability materials and the *normal* BBB will follow since interest in such tracers is mainly for investigating abnormal BBB function. To date AIB and RISA are the two most commonly used low-permeability, QAR-detectable markers in studies of BBB abnormality and 'opening.' They clearly have differing virtues and distributional qualities. Other low-permeability markers whose tissue levels can be accurately assayed by QAR include ^{14}C-labeled sucrose and PEG 4000.

These experiments begin by intravenously infusing 0.25 ml of buffered saline, containing either 50 µCi of AIB or 100 µCi of RISA, over 10 s. Small blood samples (50–75 µl) are taken at a set of times that yield an accurate time-course of blood or plasma concentration; the concentration falls over time for AIB but is relatively constant for RISA after the initial 15 s. Typical blood sampling times for AIB are 10, 20, 30, 45, and 60 s plus 2, 5, and 10 min and every 10–15 min thereafter. Less frequent sampling is used for RISA experiments, for example, 15, 30, and 60 s plus 3 and 10 min and every 15–30 min thereafter. The duration of radiotracer circulation is set by the degree of BBB opening, something unknown until the initial set of data are gathered. It is sensible to start with 10 min circulation times for AIB and 30 min for RISA and modify the duration to obtain the best combination of appreciable uptake (> 10 times the vascular correction) and negligible back-flux (estimated interstitial fluid concentration < 1/10 plasma concentration).

After taking a carefully timed final blood sample, the rat is decapitated by a small animal guillotine, and the brain is quickly removed and prepared for sectioning as described above. From each blood sample, known volumes of whole blood and plasma are taken and counted by liquid scintillation or gamma counting. The radioactivity per unit volume is then calculated. Brain radioactivity is determined by QAR.

Quantitative autoradiography

The quantitative autoradiographic procedure has been described many times before (e.g. Otsuka *et al.*, 1991*a,b*; Tajima *et al.*, 1992), and numerous papers can be read for slightly different descriptions, including the classic ones of Sokoloff *et al.* (1977) and Sakurada *et al.* (1978). In all instances 20 µm thick coronal sections are serially cut from the frozen brain in a cryostat set at −17 °C; the sectioning can start at the level of the area postrema and continue through the olfactory bulbs. Customarily, the first and fifth sections are lifted by electrostatic attraction from the knife blade by placing a glass slide immediately above them. They are then virtually instantly dried by putting the slide on a hot plate at 60 °C. These dried sections are stained with, for example, Cresyl Violet, cover slipped, and used to identify the areas of interest and the state of the tissue.

In the same manner, the intervening three

sections are picked up on glass cover slips and dried on the hot plate; they are then glued to Bainbridge board or other poster board of similar thickness, for subsequent QAR analysis. The next 15 sections are then cut and discarded. This sectioning routine is repeated every 400 μm, which produces nearly 50 sets of sections (two histologic and three autoradiographic images per set) for the entire rat brain. The redundancy in this procedure is necessary because the sections often have flaws such as small tears, wrinkles, and bubbles. With sufficient practice, this repetitious slicing and saving of sections provides at least one good autoradiographic measure for virtually every area and structure in the brain from each experiment.

The boards with the dried sections for autoradiography are placed in X-ray cassettes along with a sheet of X-ray film and a set of radioactive standards. For ^{14}C-experiments, sets of calibrated ^{14}C-methylmethacrylate standards covering a range of radioactivity can be purchased from any of several radiochemical suppliers. For both ^{125}I- and ^{55}Fe-experiments, the sets of standards are made for each batch of radiotracer received and employed. This is done by adding decreasing amounts of radioactivity to a series of calf brain homogenates in small plastic centrifuge tubes, freezing the mixtures within the tubes, mounting the frozen 'tubes of homogenate' upright on planchets, and sectioning them as described above for the frozen brain (Lin *et al.*, 1990).

After sealing the cassettes and exposing the films for sufficient time (usually 7–21 days), the latter are developed. Local tissue radioactivity is assessed from the autoradiograms by an image analysis system such as those sold by Imaging Research Inc. (St. Catharines, Ontario, Canada). For each autoradiogram, the image processor generates a mathematical relationship between optical density and radioactivity from the standard data by a spline-fit routine and, based on this curve, converts the optical density reading from a specific tissue site to radioactivity. The sites to be read can be outlined either by hand or by a cursor-controlled rectangular or circular reading frame. When possible, readings should be made for each area of interest on 3–6 sections and averaged to produce a mean value. For the rat brain, areas of interest can be identified with a stereotaxic atlas

(e.g. Paxinos and Watson, 1982) and the adjacent histological sections.

Calculations

Local cerebral blood flow is calculated from the iodoantipyrine data from blood (plasma can also be used because the concentrations of IAP are virtually identical in the two fluids) and tissue and the equation of Sakurada *et al.* (1978):

$$A(T) = F \int_0^T C(t) \{ \exp[-F(T-t)/\lambda] \} \, dt \quad (13.3)$$

where $A(T)$ is the amount of radiolabeled IAP per unit weight tissue at the end of the experimental period, T, as determined by QAR; F is LCBF; λ is the tissue:blood partition coefficient of IAP; and $C(t)$ is the concentration of IAP in plasma or whole blood at time after starting the experiment, t. The IAP partition coefficient is set at 0.8 ml/g for both white and gray matter in accordance with the measurements of Sakurada *et al.*

The distribution spaces of RISA and RBC are calculated by the standard equations (Tajima *et al.*, 1992; Bereczki *et al.* 1993a) and are employed for the vascular space correction of the tissue radioactivity of the 'BBB permeable' material. For the RISA space (V_{RISA}):

$$V_{RISA} = A(T)/C(T) \quad (13.4)$$

where $A(T)$ is the amount of RISA activity per unit weight tissue at the end of the experimental period, T, as assayed by QAR, and $C(T)$ is the concentration of RISA in plasma. For the RBC space (V_{RBC}):

$$V_{RBC} = A(T)/C(T) \quad (13.5)$$

where $A(T)$ is the amount of RBC activity per unit weight tissue at the end of the experimental period, T, as assayed by QAR, and $C(T)$ is RBC radioactivity in the final blood sample. The whole blood space, V_{bld}, equals the sum of V_{RISA} and V_{RBC}.

The influx constant, K_1, is estimated from the blood or plasma and tissue data for the 'BBB permeability' marker and the following equation (Namba *et al.*, 1987; Otsuka *et al.* 1991b):

$$A(T) = K_1 \exp(-TK_1/\lambda) \int_0^T C(t) \, [\exp(tK_1/\lambda)] \, dt \quad (13.6)$$

129

where $A(T)$ is the amount of radiolabeled material (e.g. antipyrine or 3OMG) in brain parenchyma (namely, outside of the lumens and walls of the blood vessels in the tissue section) at the end of the experimental period, T; λ is the tissue:blood partition coefficient of the substance; and $C(t)$ is the concentration of the substance in plasma or whole blood at time after starting the experiment, t. To obtain $A(T)$, the total tissue radioactivity assayed by QAR is 'corrected' by subtracting the amount of radioactivity contained in the blood vessels within the tissue (vascular radioactivity).

The correction factor depends on the intravascular partitioning of the marker of interest, whole blood, plasma only, or blood cells (with negligible amount in plasma) and the concentration of that material in its blood compartment at the end of the experiment, $C(T)$. To illustrate this with 3OMG (or glucose), the plasma space is multiplied by the plasma concentration for rat brain because rat RBCs do not carry appreciable glucose, whereas for human studies the blood volume is multiplied by the blood concentration because human red cells carry exchangeable glucose. For other examples, RISA and AIB distribute in only plasma, whereas antipyrine is contained in all blood compartments.

The tissue:blood partition coefficient also varies among molecular species and conditions. In normal rat brain, λ equals 0.9 for antipyrine (Sakurada et al., 1978), 0.55 for 3OMG (Namba et al., 1987), 0.15 (the extracellular space) for RISA (Nakagawa et al., 1987), and >3.0 for AIB (Blasberg et al., 1983). These values undoubtedly change under various – perhaps most – pathological conditions. If the experiments can be designed to minimize backflux (done by shortening the experimental time), then an exact value of λ is not key to the estimation of K_1 (Eqn 5), a point previously emphasized by Chen and coworkers (1994a,b, 1995).

To calculate PS products from K_1 data, another form of the Renkin–Crone equation is used:

$$PS = -FV_e \ln(1 - K_1/FV_e) \qquad (13.7)$$

where FV_e is the volume flow through the capillaries of all the compartments of the blood that contain exchangeable material normalized to radiotracer concentration in plasma, as previously discussed. The plasma concentration is the driving force for influx and consequently sets the influx rate (Fenstermacher et al., 1986). As stated above, this 'normalized flow', FV_e, is never less than plasma water flow but can be greater than blood flow if a large portion of the exchangeable material is reversibly bound to plasma proteins and/or red cell constituents. For the curious, Chen et al. (1994a,b, 1995) have presented a slightly different treatment of measuring and applying the normalized flow.

Statistical analysis

A single 'permeability' experiment does not simply and directly produce a transfer constant and a PS product. Rather, the data from each experiment are combined with mean values from other groups of animals (in particular, first, the mean plasma or red cell or blood spaces to make the vascular space correction and calculate K_1 and, second, the mean LCBF rate to estimate PS). In turn, the estimations of the means and standard errors of K_1 and PS for each brain area should take into account the variations embedded in the mean spaces and mean flow rates. This is done with formulae for approximating the standard errors of sums and ratios that can be found in treatises on statistics such as Kendall and Stuart's (1958); the assistance of a good statistician is generally required, however, to do this with any assurance and efficacy. The significance of the differences in K_1 and PS between groups (control versus experimental) and among brain areas are tested by analysis of variance with repeated measures. Again the investigator will need the assistance of a competent statistician in this testing.

Double-label quantitative autoradiography

There are two versions of double-label QAR that merit some discussion. Using two different exposure periods, Blasberg et al. (1984) concurrently measured LCBF (with ^{131}I-IAP) and ^{14}C-AIB transfer across the capillaries of the avian sarcoma virus-induced (ASV) rat brain tumor model. For the initial exposure, a thin sheet of plastic (Mylar, 3 mm thick, 16 mg/cm^2) was inserted between the tissue sections and X-ray film. The ^{14}C-emissions were absorbed or blocked by the plastic sheet and the resulting autoradiogram represented the distribution of ^{131}I-IAP from which LCBF was estimated. After waiting four months for the disappearance of the ^{131}I (approximately 16 half-lives), the tissue sections were placed in the cassette without the thin plastic sheet and an autoradiogram of ^{14}C-distribution was produced. The two sets of autoradiographic data were co-imaged and maps of K_1 and *PS* products of AIB were generated. There were 19 brain tumors among the seven rats in this study; their histologies, LCBFs, K_1s, and *PS* products varied greatly, which clearly justified the double-label approach despite its complications and shortcomings.

Ginsberg *et al.* (1986) have developed a different double-label technique and used it to simultaneously determine LCBF and LCGU with ^{14}C-IAP and ^{14}C-2-deoxyglucose (2DG), respectively. This approach was based on two exposures and washing the sections between exposures with chloroform to remove IAP and unphosphorylated 2DG from the tissue. The authors meticulously varied solvents, exposure times, and dosages of IAP and 2DG. The recommended and subsequently employed combination was 20 µCi of 2DG and 50 µCi of IAP, four days of initial exposure and ten days of final exposure, and a five-day washing period with continuous gentle agitation in technical grade chloroform between the exposures. Although not perfect, this double-label approach yielded LCBFs and LCGUs comparable to the ones measured by single-label QAR. With the choice of a BBB permeability marker that is not eluted from the tissue by the solvent (RISA?), it is conceivable that the Ginsberg *et al.* version of double-label QAR might work for simultaneous measurements of LCBF and K_1 values and the subsequent calculation of *PS* products.

References

Bereczki, D., Wei, L., Acuff, V., *et al.* (1992). Technique-dependent variations in cerebral microvessel blood volumes and hematocrits in the rat. *J. Appl. Physiol.*, **73**, 918–24.

Bereczki, D., Wei, L., Otsuka, T. *et al.* (1993*a*). Hypoxia increases velocity of blood flow through parenchymal microvascular systems in rat brain. *J. Cereb. Blood Flow Metab.*, **13**, 475–86.

Bereczki, D., Wei, L., Otsuka, T. *et al.* (1993*b*). Hypercapnia slightly raises blood volume and sizably elevates flow velocity in brain microvessels. *Am. J. Physiol.*, **264**, H1360–H1369.

Blasberg, R., Fenstermacher, J. and Patlak, C. (1983). Transport of α-aminoisobutyric acid across brain capillary and cellular membranes. *J. Cereb. Blood Flow Metab.*, **3**, 8–32.

Blasberg, R., Molnar, P., Groothuis, D. *et al.* (1984). Concurrent measurements of blood flow and transcapillary transport in avian sarcoma virus-induced experimental brain tumors: implications for chemotherapy. *J. Pharmacol. Exp. Ther.*, **231**, 724–35.

Chen, J.-L., Acuff, V., Bereczki, D. *et al.* (1994*a*). Slightly altered permeability-surface area products imply some cerebral capillary recruitment during hypercapnia. *Microvasc. Res.*, **48**, 190–211.

Chen, J.-L., Wei, L., Bereczki, D. *et al.* (1994*b*). Virtually unaltered permeability-surface area products imply little capillary recruitment in brain with hypoxia. *Microcirculation*, **1**, 35–47.

Chen, J.-L., Wei, L., Bereczki, D. *et al.* (1995). Nicotine raises the influx of permeable solutes across the rat blood–brain barrier with little or no capillary recruitment. *J. Cereb. Blood Flow Metab.*, **15**, 687–98.

Crone, C. (1965). The permeability of brain capillaries to non-electrolytes. *Acta Physiol. Scand.*, **64**, 407–17.

Fenstermacher, J., Blasberg, R. and Patlak, C. (1986). Methods for quantifying the transport of drugs across brain barrier systems. In *Membrane Transport of Antineoplastic Agents: The International Encyclopedia of Pharmacology and Therapeutics*, ed I. D. Goldman, pp. 113–46. Oxford: Pergamon.

Ghersi-Egea, J.-F., Gorevic, P., Ghiso, J. *et al.* (1995). Fate of cerebrospinal fluid-borne amyloid β-peptide: rapid clearance into blood and appreciable accumulation by cerebral arteries. *J. Neurochem.*, **67**, 880–3.

Ginsberg, M., Smith, D., Wachtel, M. *et al.* (1986). Simultaneous determination of local cerebral glucose utilization and blood flow by carbon-14 double-label autoradiography: method of procedure and validation studied in the rat. *J. Cereb. Blood Flow Metab.*, **6**, 273-85.

Kendall, M. and Stuart, A. (1958). *The Advanced Theory of Statistics*, Vol. 1. New York: Hafner.

Landau, W., Freygang, W., Rowland, L. *et al.* (1955). The local circulation of the living brain: values in the unanesthetized and anesthetized cat. *Trans. Am. Neurol. Assoc.*, **80**, 125–9.

Lin, S.-Z., Nakata, H., Tajima, A. *et al.* (1990). Quantitative autoradiographic assessment of ^{55}Fe-RBC distribution in rat brain. *J. Appl. Physiol.*, **69**, 1637–43.

Nakagawa, H., Groothuis, D., Owens, E. *et al.* (1987). Dexamethasone effects on [^{125}I] albumin distribution in experimental RG-2 gliomas and adjacent brain. *J. Cereb. Blood Flow Metab.*, **7**, 687–701.

Namba, H., Lucignani, G., Nehlig, C. *et al.* (1987). Effects of insulin on hexose transport across the blood–brain barrier in normoglycemia. *Am. J. Physiol.*, **252**, E299–E303.

Oldendorf, W. (1971). Brain uptake of radiolabeled amino acids, amines, and hexoses after arterial injection. *Am. J. Physiol.*, **221**, 1629–39.

Otsuka, T., Wei, L., Acuff, V. *et al.* (1991*a*). Variation in local cerebral blood flow response to high-dose pentobarbital sodium in the rat. *Am. J. Physiol.*, **261**, H110–H120.

Otsuka, T., Wei, L., Bereczki, D. *et al.* (1991*b*). Pentobarbital produces dissimilar changes in glucose influx and utilization in the brain. *Am. J. Physiol.*, **261**, R265–R275.

Patlak, C., Blasberg, R. and Fenstermacher, J (1984). An evaluation of errors in the determination of blood flow by the indicator fractionation and tissue equilibration (Kety). methods. *J. Cereb. Blood Flow Metab.*, **4**, 47–60.

Paxinos, G. and Watson, C. (1982). *The Rat Brain in Stereotaxic Coordinates*. New York: Academic Press.

Reivich, M., Jehle, J., Sokoloff, L. and Kety, S. (1969). Measurement of regional cerebral blood flow with antipyrine-^{14}C in awake cats. *J. Appl. Physiol.*, **27**, 296–300.

Renkin, E. M. (1959). Transport of potassium-42 from blood to tissue in isolated mammalian skeletal muscles. *Am. J. Physiol.*, **197**, 1205–10.

Sakurada, O., Kennedy, C., Jehle, J. *et al.* (1978). Measurement of local cerebral blood flow with iodo[^{14}C]antipyrine. *Am. J. Physiol.*, **234**, H59–H66.

Sokoloff, L., Reivich, M., Kennedy, C. *et al.* (1977). The [^{14}C]deoxyglucose method for the measurement of local cerebral glucose utilization: theory, procedure, and normal values in the conscious and anesthetized albino rat. *J. Neurochem.*, **28**, 897–916.

Tajima, A., Nakata, H., Lin, S.-Z. *et al.* (1992). Differences and similarities in albumin and red cell flows through cerebral microvessels. *Am. J. Physiol.*, **262**, H1515–H1524.

Wei, L., Otsuka, T., Acuff, V. *et al.* (1993). The velocities of red cell and plasma flows through parenchymal microvessels of rat brain are decreased by pentobarbital. *J. Cereb. Blood Flow Metab.*, **13**, 487–97.

14 Measurement of blood–brain barrier in humans using indicator diffusion

GITTE M. KNUDSEN and OLAF B. PAULSON

- Introduction
- Intravenous bolus injection
- Comparison to other methods
- Future applications of the indicator diffusion technique

Introduction

The terms indicator diffusion, double-indicator, single injection or indicator dilution have been used interchangeably for this technique, the principles of which were outlined by Chinard *et al.* (1955) and first applied in the brain by Crone, who also provided the first quantitative measurements of capillary permeability and demonstrated a carrier-mediated transport of D-glucose across the blood–brain barrier (BBB) (Crone, 1965). In 1971, the method was applied in humans by Lassen and co-authors, and later used in several clinical studies (Bolwig *et al.*, 1977; Paulson *et al.*, 1977; Hertz and Paulson, 1980, 1982; Knudsen *et al.*, 1990*a*,*b*, 1991, 1995; Hasselbalch *et al.*, 1995, 1996). In 1994, the intravenous indicator diffusion method was developed (Knudsen *et al.*). A more detailed description of its application in humans has been given previously (Knudsen, 1994*b*).

The indicator diffusion technique for BBB permeability measurements has classically been applied as follows (Fig. 14.1): An intracarotid bolus injection of isotopically labeled test and BBB impermeable reference substance is given, immediately followed by a rapid series of blood sampling from the internal jugular vein in humans or from the sagittal sinus in rats. If closely matching tracer substances have been chosen and the ven-

ous concentration of each tracer is normalized with the injectate concentration then the time course of the brain outflow curves of the test and reference substances are known. During the initial phase of tracer uptake the extraction, $E([C_{ref} - C_{test}]/C_{ref})$, has been assumed to be unidirectional. Hence, the permeability surface area product, PS, for the test substance is determined by

$$PS = -\phi \cdot CBF \cdot \ln(1-E) \qquad (14.1)$$

where CBF is the cerebral blood flow and ϕ is the apparent distribution volume for the substance in whole blood. The influence of the different factors in Eqn (14.1) will be discussed below.

Value of ϕ

The value of ϕ must be known since it may have major impacts for PS in the case of protein binding, red blood cell carriage, or ionized compounds.

Many substances of importance for the central nervous system, such as hormones, fatty acids, and drugs are protein bound. If the drug–protein dissociation rate is very slow as compared to the capillary transit time, then the bound concentration can be regarded as constant and *in vitro* measurements of the degree of protein binding may be directly incorporated in the calculations (Pardridge and Landaw, 1984). Conversely, if the drug is

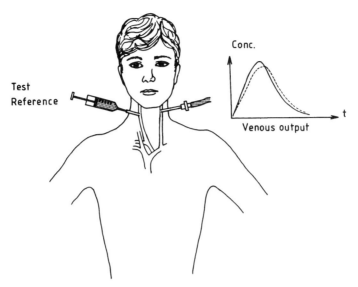

Fig. 14.1. Diagram of the classical indicator diffusion technique with intracarotid injection. Modified from Knudsen *et al.* (1994*b*), with permission.

extremely rapidly released as compared to the capillary transit time then the protein-bound fraction constitutes an extra source of the compound and hence ϕ is 1/(free fraction).

If the equilibration across the cell membrane, in particular of the red blood cell, is slow as compared to the capillary transit time, the erythrocyte compartment must be considered in the assessment of the brain input function; this applies especially for high- and medium-permeable substances.

Since a major part of the BBB consists of lipid membranes, lipophilic substances readily cross it. The unionized fraction of the total amount of an acid, C_u/C_t, is determined by the equation (Knudsen *et al.*, 1991)

$$C_u/C_t = 1/(1 + 10^{(pH-pK_a)}) \qquad (14.2)$$

Variations in pH may therefore have an important impact upon the barrier permeability.

Cerebral blood flow

For the determination of transfer variables, knowledge of CBF is required. The most exact method currently available for quantitation of global CBF in humans is probably the Kety–Schmidt technique with correction for incomplete tracer equilibrium (Madsen *et al.*, 1993). In animal studies, repeated CBF measurements may be carried out by intraarterial xenon injection, followed by external detection of isotope washout.

Extraction

The different factors influencing extraction are discussed below.

Representativeness of internal jugular blood After intracarotid injection the venous outflow curves presumably represent the extractive properties of brain tissues supplied from that carotid artery. In rats, it is of particular importance to ensure ligation of arterial branches supplying extracranial tissue and to avoid suction from the sagittal sinus since this may lead to backflux from neck veins and thereby extracerebral contamination. With the intravenous indicator diffusion method, correct placement of the catheter in the bulb of the internal jugular vein is important since placement just a few centimeters below this point may lead to extracerebral blood contamination (Jakobsen and Enevoldsen, 1989).

A different problem arises from the BBB-free areas in the brain, for example the choroid plexus. In spite of the relatively high resistance of cerebral endothelium to the transport of small ions, an extraction of small ions of up to 2% may be observed. That is, although the BBB-free areas quantitatively constitute a minute fraction of the brain weight they contribute measurably to the outflow curves, presumably because of the high perfusion of these regions. In reality, the BBB-free areas set the lower limit for the measurement of low-permeable substances that must have a minimum extraction of about 5% in order to be reliably determined.

Matching test and reference substance One of the basic assumptions for utilization of the indicator diffusion technique is that within the capillary, the test and reference substances behave identically. The two intravascular separation phenomena, interlaminar diffusion due to differences in molecular size and erythrocyte carriage, may be accounted for by applying several references of which the curves are weighted, to minimize the potential influence of intravascular separation of test and reference substance. Corrections for the intravascular separation phenomena by using several simultaneous reference substances have been described in detail (Hertz and Paulson, 1980). For most test substances the corrections are, however, small and without major impact for the results (Knudsen *et al.*, 1994*b*).

Radiochemical purity and metabolism The radiochemical purity of the test substance must remain high during the passage of the cerebral capillary and no significant metabolism must take place before reaching the brain capillary. This is particularly critical while employing the intravenous injection approach.

Recirculation It has usually been assumed that recirculation does not contribute significantly before it becomes visible in the outflow curves (Zierler, 1963) and the problem has conventionally been solved by semi-logarithmic extrapolations of the venous outflow curves, although this approach may be of doubtful validity.

Capillary heterogeneity and tracer backflux Two more factors further complicate the validation of the tracer extraction. As a function of time the extraction is not constant but increases until

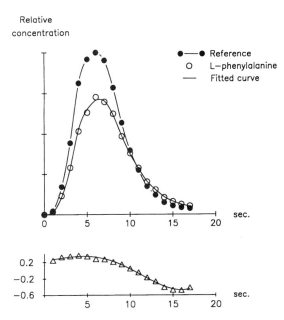

Fig. 14.2. Intracarotid indicator diffusion experiment: relative concentrations of L-phenylalanine and the averaged reference curve. Below is the corresponding extraction curve for L-phenylalanine.

backflux dominates (Fig. 14.2). Such a heterogeneity of transit times was first emphasized in the heart (Rose and Goresky, 1976) and later recognized in the human brain by Hertz and Paulson (1980). This heterogeneity could be caused by heterogeneous pathway lengths through the brain or by regional differences in the linear capillary plasma flow or in the permeability. We will not deal with the latter complicated possibility. Regional variations in the linear capillary plasma flow are probably insignificant since the regional number of perfused capillaries correlates well with regional CBF (Klein *et al.*, 1986). Equation (1) is based on a single capillary and it is implicitly assumed that the equation is valid for a sum of capillaries with identical extractive properties per unit volume. If so, heterogeneity of extraction at the organ level would be fully characterized by the distribution of transit times of the reference substance.

Backflux is reflected in the tail of the venous outflow curves by a decreasing extraction of the test substance (Fig. 14.2). The backflux phenomenon is especially pronounced for substances with a much higher permeability out of than into the brain (Knudsen *et al.*, 1990*b*). Generally, as permeability increases, it becomes increasingly difficult to assess unidirectional influx since the equilibration across the BBB takes place more rapidly.

In order to accommodate capillary heterogeneity as well as tracer backflux, the extraction at the peak of the curve has traditionally been considered to be the best estimate for unidirectional flux. However, the more meaningful measure of extraction, the average extraction, is not always well approximated by the peak extraction due to the capillary heterogeneity and tracer backflux.

In order to account for backflux, the E_o method was suggested by Martín and Yudilevich in 1964. With this approach, the extraction at the first venous appearance of the tracers is used for the estimation of PS_1, and the later part of the curve is only used to improve the estimate by backward extrapolation. Using only the initial increasing part of the curve, however, does not provide an improved estimate of the unidirectional flux due to the existence of capillary heterogeneity. Realizing this heterogeneity, Bass and Robinson in 1982 suggested another strategy for the calculation of PS_1 where different kinds of heterogeneity were taken into account. By this approach the backflux problem was, however, not fully addressed and estimates of PS_1 were limited to lower bound estimates.

A more complex mathematical solution, which incorporated the influence of heterogeneous capillary and large-vessel transit times as well as backflux, was introduced in 1989 by Sawada and coworkers to be applied in experimental BBB studies of highly permeable substances. According to this model, the transit time heterogeneity, the distribution volume and transfer variables for transport across the BBB determine the time course of the outflow curves. At the same time this approach was extended and used in double indicator studies in humans after intracarotid or intravenous tracer injection (Knudsen *et al.*, 1990*b*). Two models were developed, the non-mixed and the mixed models (Fig. 14.3). In the non-mixed model, the BBB is considered as a double membrane barrier consisting of the luminal and the abluminal endothelial cell membranes, and consequently different permeabilities in and out of the endothelial cell may be present. The well-mixed model represents the

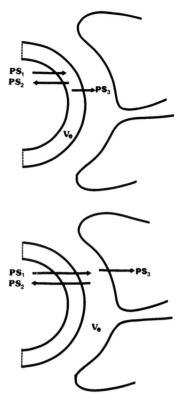

Fig. 14.3. Diagram of the transfer constants in the non-mixed model (upper) and the well-mixed model (lower). PS_1 is the transport from blood to the endothelial cell (or interstitial fluid); PS_2 is the transport from the endothelial cell (or interstitial fluid) back to the blood; PS_3 is the transport from the endothelial cell into the interstitial fluid (or from the interstitial fluid into the cells); V_e is the distribution volume of the tracer within the measurement period.

classical concept that the BBB, though anatomically consisting of two separate membranes, is considered as a single membrane that separates the blood from the brain interstitial fluid (Fig. 14.3). The estimates of the parameters that result in the best fit to the measured test curve and the standard errors of the estimates are obtained by means of a weighted least squares procedure: weighted differences between the theoretical curve evaluated at the estimates and the measured test outflow curve are minimized by means of the simplex method. The two models were evaluated for D-glucose (Knudsen *et al.*, 1990*a*) and for large neutral amino acids (Knudsen *et al.*, 1990*b*). As for the fitting, both models yielded similar sum of squares values. Moreover, both models also gave similar results for the four fitted parameters, signifying that in spite of the different assumptions, similar parameter estimates are obtained by both methods.

Intravenous bolus injection

The inherent limitations of the intracarotid injection method in humans led to the development of an intravenous approach (Knudsen *et al.*, 1994*b*).

The principles of the intravenous indicator diffusion technique are illustrated in Fig. 14.4. After intravenous tracer injection, blood from a peripheral artery is sampled to determine the cerebral input curves, and blood from the internal jugular vein is sampled to obtain the cerebral outflow curves. The differences in the arterial input between the test and reference substances are corrected by the calculation of a Dirac impulse response for passage through the cerebrovascular bed, which is obtained in terms of a five-parameter model, the lagged normal density curve (Bassingthwaighte *et al.*, 1966) where an additional parameter is included in order to obtain better curve fitting (Knudsen *et al.*, 1994*b*). The response is used in conjunction with a brain model to yield a theoretical time course for the venous output of the test substance from the brain for a Dirac impulse arterial input of the test substance. The resulting theoretical output can then be mathematically convoluted with the actual arterial input of the test substance to yield a theoretical venous outflow time course of the test material. This can be iteratively compared to the actual output of the test substance in order to determine the parameters of the system model.

The intravenous approach was validated by comparison of the results obtained in the same individual with intravenous and intracarotid injections, respectively (Knudsen *et al.*, 1994*b*). Similar results with the two injections regimes were found for D-glucose and for L-phenylalanine, in the latter provided that the erythrocyte compartment was taken into account. Data obtained following intravenous injection of leucine and water yielded similar results when compared to previous intracarotid data. Although the calculated standard errors for the individual estimates are comparable for the intravenous and the intracarotid injection techniques, it is our impression that the scatter of the estimates of the model parameters is larger with the intravenous injection. This may be caused by differences in curve dispersion between the cerebral arteries and the arterial measurement site.

Generally, PS_1 is well determined and shows good reproducibility in repeated experiments (Knudsen *et al.*, 1994*b*). PS_2 is well determined for

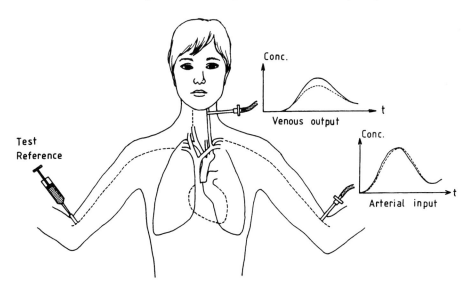

Fig. 14.4. Diagram of the indicator diffusion technique with intravenous injection. Modified from Knudsen *et al.* (1994*b*), with permission.

a group (Knudsen *et al.*, 1993) whereas a significant correlation between repeated measurements of PS_2 can generally not be established.

Comparison to other methods

The average unidirectional extraction for glucose obtained with the indicator diffusion method is about 17%, which is in agreement with a simultaneously published study applying $[1–^{11}C]$D-glucose in dynamic PET scannning (Blomqvist *et al.*, 1990). The indicator diffusion technique was in our laboratory validated against dynamic PET measurements by a series of simultaneous measurements of transfer rates for the glucose analog fluoro-deoxyglucose (FDG). A statistically significant correlation was found between K_1 values obtained with PET as compared to the indicator diffusion method but dynamic PET yielded significantly different K_1 values that on average were 15% lower than with the intravenous indicator diffusion method (unpublished results). The difference is probably due to the longer experimental time in dynamic PET studies, which leads to an underestimation of backflux and, consequently, a lower rate constant for the transport from blood to brain.

High time resolution experiments are required for determination of BBB transport of the large neutral amino acids and for that purpose the indicator diffusion method is especially well suited. For a number of methods, the backflux of large neutral amino acids impedes a valid estimation of the unidirectional transport across the BBB; until now this has actually been ignored in most studies dealing with large neutral amino acid transport where studies using a circulation time of 2–4 min have been assumed to yield estimates for the unidirectional transport. Estimates for the amino acid carriers V_{max} and the apparent K_m may be provided by varying the plasma concentrations (Knudsen *et al.*, 1995).

For substances with a rapid metabolism in blood it is necessary to correct the tracer input and output curves for the metabolism that takes place during the indicator diffusion experiment. The magnitude of these time constants heavily influ-

ences the calculation of the actual brain extraction of a given flow tracer. Based upon estimates of the time constant for drug conversion in blood and the input time delay, an algorithm that allows for such a correction has been derived (Knudsen *et al.*, 1994*a*).

Future applications of the indicator diffusion technique

With the increasing complexity of new techniques and models it is of major importance to confirm models and estimates of parameters. Assumptions are almost always made and especially under pathological circumstances these assumptions are prone to violations. The intravenous indicator diffusion technique offers the possibility for testing some of these assumptions. The ethical aspects of the method have been thoroughly considered previously (Knudsen, 1994).

The indicator diffusion technique does not provide information about the regional distribution of the BBB permeability as in PET or MR studies but it enables rapid and repeated determinations of BBB permeability in human subjects prone to different physiological situations. Since the permeability is determined from a single passage through the brain, the indicator diffusion method has limited sensitivity for substances with a unidirectional extraction below about 5%, and methods with longer circulation times are more appropriate for determination of brain extractions below this limit. For the investigation of very lipophilic substances, however, the technique has proven to give both sensible and reproducible results for highly permeable substances.

In conclusion, the intravenous indicator diffusion technique is a valid method for estimation of BBB transport and it offers a high temporal resolution. It is rapid and allows for comparison of several test substances in the same experiment as well as repeated examinations within a few minutes. The method has the potential for usage of non-radioactive tracers, does not require advanced instruments, is relatively inexpensive, and allows for bed-side investigations.

References

Bass, L. and Robinson, P. J. (1982). Capillary permeability of heterogenous organs: a parsimonious interpretation of indicator diffusion data. *Clin. Exp. Pharmacol. Physiol.*, **9**, 363–88.

Bassingthwaighte, J. B., Ackerman, F. H. and Wood, E. H. (1966). Applications of the lagged normal density curve as a model for arterial dilution curves. *Circ. Res.*, **18**, 398–415.

Blomqvist, G., Stone-Elander, S., Halldin, C. *et al.* (1990). Positron emission tomographic of glucose utilization using [1-^{11}C]D-glucose. *J. Cereb. Blood Flow Metabol.*, **10**, 467–83.

Bolwig, T. G., Hertz, M. M., Paulson, O. B. *et al.* (1977). The permeability of the blood–brain barrier during electrically induced seizures in man. *Eur. J. Clin. Invest.*, **7**, 87–93.

Chinard, F. P., Vosburgh, G. J. and Enns, T. (1955). Transcapillary exchange of water and of other substances in certain organs of the dog. *Am. J. Physiol.*, **183**, 221–34.

Crone, C. (1965). Facilitated transfer of glucose from blood into brain tissue. *J. Physiol. Lond.*, **181**, 103–13.

Hasselbalch, S., Knudsen, G. M., Jakobsen, J. *et al.*(1995). Blood–brain barrier permeability of glucose and ketone bodies during short-term starvation in humans. *Am. J. Physiol.*, **268**, E1161–E1166.

Hasselbalch, S., Knudsen, G. M., Holm, S. *et al.* (1996). Transport of D-glucose and 2-fluorodeoxyglucose across the blood–brain barrier in humans. *J. Cereb. Blood Flow Metabol.*, **16**, 659–66.

Hertz, M. M. and Paulson, O. B. (1980). Heterogeneity of cerebral capillary flow in man and its consequences for estimation of blood–brain barrier permeability. *J. Clin. Invest.*, **65**, 1145–51.

Hertz, M. M. and Paulson, O. B. (1982). Transfer across the human blood–brain barrier, evidence for capillary recruitment and for a paradox glucose permeability increase in hypocapnia. *Microvasc. Res.*, **24**, 364–76.

Jakobsen, M. and Enevoldsen, E. (1989). Retrograde catheterization of the right internal jugular vein for serial measurements of cerebral venous oxygen content. *J. Cereb. Blood Flow Metab.*, **9**, 717–20.

Klein, B., Kuschinsky, W., Schröck, H. and Vetterlein, F. (1986). Interdependency of local capillary density, blood flow, and metabolism in rat brains. *Am. J. Physiol.*, **251**, H1333–H1340.

Knudsen, G. M. (1994). Application of the double-indicator technique for measurement of blood–brain barrier permeability in humans. *Cerebrovasc. Brain Metab. Rev.*, **6**, 1–30.

Knudsen, G. M., Pettigrew, K., Paulson, O. B *et al.* (1990*a*). Kinetic analysis of blood–brain barrier transport of D-glucose in man, Quantitative evaluation in the presence of tracer backflux and capillary heterogeneity. *Microvasc. Res.*, **39**, 28–49.

Knudsen, G. M., Pettigrew, K., Patlak, C. S. *et al.* (1990*b*). Asymmetrical transport of amino acids across the blood–brain barrier in man. *J. Cereb. Blood Flow Metabol.*, **10**, 698–706.

Knudsen, G. M., Paulson, O. B., Hertz, M. M. (1991). Kinetic analysis of the human blood–brain barrier transport of lactate and its influence by hypercapnia. *J. Cereb. Blood Flow Metabol.*, **11**, 581–6.

Knudsen, G. M., Schmidt, J. F., Almdal, T. *et al.* (1993). The passage of amino acids and glucose across the blood–brain barrier in patients with hepatic encephalopathy. *Hepatology*, **6**, 987–92.

Knudsen, G. M., Andersen, A. R., Somnier, F. E. *et al.* (1994*a*). Brain extraction and distribution of ^{99m}Tc-bicisate in humans and in rats. *J. Cereb. Blood Flow Metabol.*, **14**(Suppl), S12–S18.

Knudsen, G. M., Pettigrew, K., Patlak, C. S. and Paulson, O. B. (1994*b*). Blood–brain barrier permeability measurements by double-indicator method using intravenous injection. *Am. J. Physiol.*, 266, H987–H999.

Knudsen, G. M., Hasselbalch, S., Toft, P. *et al.* (1995). Blood–brain barrier transport of amino acids in healthy controls and in patients with phenylketonuria. *J. Inher. Metab. Dis.*, **18**, 653–64.

Lassen, N.A., Trap-Jensen, J., Alexander, S. C. *et al.* (1971). Blood–brain barrier studies in man using the double-indicator method. *Am. J. Physiol.*, **220**, 1627–33.

Madsen, P. L., Holm, S., Herning, M. and Lassen, N. A. (1993). Average blood flow and oxygen uptake in the human brain during resting wakefulness, a critical appraisal of the Kety-Schmidt technique. *J. Cereb. Blood Flow Metab.*, **13**, 646–55.

Martín, P. andYudilevich, D. L. (1964). A theory for the quantification of transcapillary exchange by tracer-dilution curves. *Am. J. Physiol.*, **207**, 162–8.

Pardridge, W. M. and Landaw, E. M. (1984) Tracer kinetic model of blood–brain barrier transport of plasma protein-bound ligands. *J. Clin. Invest.*, **74**, 745–52

Paulson, O. B., Patlak, C. S. and Hertz, M. M. (1977). Filtration and diffusion of water across the blood–brain barrier in man. *Microvasc. Res.*, **13**, 113–24.

Rose, C. P., and Goresky, D. A. (1976). Vasomotor control of capillary transit time heterogeneity in the canine coronary circulation. *Circ. Res.*, **39**, 541–54.

Sawada, Y., Patlak, C. S. and Blasberg, R. G. (1989). Kinetic analysis of cerebrovascular transport based on indicator diffusion technique. *Am. J. Physiol.*, **256**, 794–812.

Smith, Q. R., Momma, S., Aoyagi, M. and Rapoport, S. I. (1987). Kinetics of neutral amino acid transport across the blood–brain barrier. *J. Neurochem.*, **49**, 1651–8.

Zierler, K. L. (1963). Theory of use of indicators to measure blood flow and extracellular volume and calculation of transcapillary movement of tracers. *Circ. Res.*, **12**, 464–71.

15 Measurement of blood–brain permeability in humans with positron emission tomography

SUNG-CHENG HUANG, CARL HOH, JORGE R. BARRIO
and MICHAEL E. PHELPS

- Introduction
- Basic principles
- PET tracers for BBB measurements
- Study procedures and data analysis methods
- Additional considerations
- Summary

Introduction

The importance of blood–brain barrier (BBB) integrity has long been recognized and BBB permeability has been measured using invasive tracer techniques in experimental animals. Since the development of positron emission tomography (PET), non-invasive measurement of BBB permeability in humans has become feasible. Although the integrity of the BBB in man has also been examined using contrast CT, MRI, and radioscintigraphy, the results are mostly qualitative, i.e. they do not provide the permeability–surface area product (referred to simply as permeability in this chapter) in terms of ml/min/g. Without a quantitative measure, BBB changes due to disease progression, treatment, and pharmacological interventions cannot be easily assessed. PET has been successfully employed to examine BBB permeability in man in various diseases and pharmacological interventions (Brooks et al., 1984; Hawkins et al., 1984; Lockwood et al., 1984; Iannotti et al., 1987; Schlageter et al., 1987; Pozzilli et al., 1988; Ott et al., 1991; Black et al., 1997). In the following, the basic principles used in these techniques are introduced and the procedure, requirements, and typical results are reviewed.

Basic principles

For a systemically administered tracer to get to the extra-vascular space of the brain tissue, the tracer needs to be delivered first to the capillaries in the brain tissue by cerebral blood flow (or perfusion) (CBF) and then transported across the BBB. However, if the BBB transport is much slower than the CBF perfusion, the influx of the tracer from blood/plasma to tissue is primarily determined by the blood/plasma concentration of the tracer and the permeability across the BBB. This can be shown easily by the following analysis. According to the Renkin–Crone equation (Renkin, 1959; Crone, 1963) that describes the relationship of tracer extraction and blood flow in a capillary model, the flux of a tracer extracted into tissue as a function of blood flow and capillary permeability is

$$R = F(1 - \exp(-PS/F))C_a \qquad (15.1)$$

where F is CBF in ml/min/g, P is permeability in cm/min, and S is the surface area of the capillary wall in units of cm^2/g, and C_a is the concentration of tracer in blood/plasma. PS (in ml/min/g) is commonly called the permeability–surface area product for the tracer. For $PS \ll F$, the flux of tracer extracted into the extravascular space is approximately equal to PSC_a. It should be noted that the permeability discussed here is a combined measure that includes the effects of the tracer's crossing of blood cell membranes, dissociation from specific/non-specific bindings in blood, and the crossing of the capillary wall.

If C_a is not a constant, but a function of time, then the flux would also be time dependent. In such a case, the total amount of tracer taken up by tissue from blood/plasma (assume no back flux or clearance of tracer from tissue) is equal to PS times the integral of $C_a(t)$ from time zero of tracer injection to the measurement time T, i.e.,

$$M = PS \int_0^T C_a(t)\mathrm{d}t \quad (15.2)$$

or

$$PS = M/(\int_0^T C_a(t)\mathrm{d}t) \quad (15.3)$$

Since $C_a(t)$ can be measured from blood samples and M, the amount of tracer accumulated in tissue, can be measured by PET or, in the case of experimental animals, by autoradiography, the value of PS can be easily calculated. In either case, M is the amount of tracer in the extravascular tissue space. If the vascular space contains a significant amount of tracer as compared with what is taken up in the extravascular space, the vascular component needs to be subtracted from the total tissue tracer concentration measured by PET to give the quantity M in Eqn (15.3). This vascular component is usually estimated as the product of the vascular volume times the concentration of the tracer in the blood at the measurement time T. In the case of the tracer not taken up by blood cells, it is also equal to the product of the plasma volume times the plasma concentration of the tracer.

The derivation of the above equation assumes that the tracer is trapped irreversibly. However, in reality, few tracers satisfy the assumption rigorously. To remove this restriction, compartmental modeling (Huang and Phelps, 1985) is usually used. With this approach, the uptake and clearance of the tracer in tissue is described as shown in Fig. 15.1. The rate of tracer clearance from tissue at time t is assumed to be proportional to the tracer concentration in tissue at that time. k_2 is the proportionality constant and is commonly called the rate con-

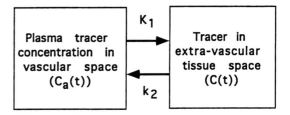

Fig. 15.1. A compartmental model commonly used to describe the tracer kinetics in tissue for quantitative measurement of BBB permeability.

stant of tracer clearance from tissue. K_1 is equal to PS of Eqns (15.1)–(15.3). According to this model, the amount of tracer in tissue, $C(T)$ as measured by PET, is a function of time and is equal to

$$C(T) = C_e(T) + \mathrm{CPV}\,C_a(T)$$
$$= K_1 \int_0^T C_a(t)\mathrm{d}t - k_2 \int_0^T C_e(t)\mathrm{d}t + \mathrm{CPV}\,C_a(T) \quad (15.4)$$

where CPV is the plasma volume in tissue (assuming tracer is not taken up by blood cells), C_a is plasma concentration of the tracer, and C_e ($= C - \mathrm{CPV}\,C_a$) is the tracer concentration in the extravascular space. The first term on the right hand side represents the total amount of tracer crossing the BBB from plasma to the extravascular space from time zero to T; the second term represents the total amount of tracer cleared from the extravascular space back to plasma; the third term represents the amount of tracer in the vascular space at time T. $C_e(T)$ in the above equation can be solved in terms of $C_a(T)$, and $C(T)$ becomes

$$C(T) = K_1 \int_0^T C_a(t)\exp(-k_2(T-t))\mathrm{d}t + \mathrm{CPV}\,C_a(T) \quad (15.5)$$

Since PET measurements are taken over a finite scan time, the quantity corresponding to PET measurements is the the average value $(C_{\mathrm{pet}}(T))$ over that duration, as

$$C_{\mathrm{pet}}(T) = \frac{1}{\mathrm{DT}} \int_{T'}^{T''} C(s)\mathrm{d}s$$
$$= \frac{K_1}{\mathrm{DT}} \int_{T'}^{T''} (\int_0^s C_a(t)\exp(-k_2(s-t))\mathrm{d}t)\mathrm{d}s$$
$$+ \frac{\mathrm{CPV}}{\mathrm{DT}} \int_{T'}^{T''} C_a(s)\mathrm{d}s \quad (15.6)$$

where $T' = T - \mathrm{DT}/2$ and $T'' = T + \mathrm{DT}/2$ are, respectively, the beginning and ending times of the scan, and DT = $(T'' - T')$ is the scan duration. Therefore, when the total tissue tracer concentration is measured with multiple scans at different time points, the values of K_1, k_2 and CPV can be estimated simultaneously according to the above equation, using least-squares data fitting available in most data processing computer software packages today.

PET tracers for BBB measurements

For BBB permeability measurement with PET, there are two commonly used tracers: Ga-68 EDTA and Rb-82. These two tracers have different physical and chemical properties and their use depends on the application desired. Ga-68 has a physical half-life of 68 min, and is produced from the decay of Ge-68 in a generator. The first-pass extraction fraction of Ga-68 EDTA across normal BBB is very low, in the order of 0.04% . Rb-82, on the other hand, is considered as a potassium analog (Love et al., 1954; Kilpatrick et al., 1956), with a larger first-pass extraction fraction through the brain tissue (~2% (Brooks et al., 1984)). Rb-82 is available from Sr-82/Rb-82 generators and has an extremely short half life (75 seconds).

The permeability values measured with these two tracers are not the same, because of their large differences in chemical properties and in molecular size. Rb-82's short half-life allows the measurement to be repeated quickly (within minutes), but the measurement time that is generally short yields high measurement noise. Rb-82 generator needs to be replaced monthly and is expensive. Ga-68 EDTA measures the passive physical permeability of the BBB for molecules of its comparable size. Although its extraction fraction in normal brain tissue is low (yielding low measurement counts), its extraction into tissue with BBB disruption can be relatively high (>10 times higher) and can give images with a high contrast between abnormal tissue and normal tissue regions. Also, because of its longer half-life, tissue distribution can be imaged over a long period (e.g. >60 minutes) to provide a good-quality measurement of the tracer kinetics in tissue regions of interest. Ga-68 generator has a half-life of about 275 days, thus is more economical than Rb-82 generator (half-life 25 days).

Tracers used for measurement of BBB permeability are not restricted to the above two (e.g. C-11 atenolol was used by Agon et al. (1991); N-13 ammonia by Phelps et al. (1981) and Lockwood et al. (1984)). The only necessary requirement for a tracer to be suitable for such measurement is that its uptake and delivery into brain tissue is not flow-limited. For tracers that are not inert and participate in tissue biochemical processes, the problem of measuring BBB permeability can be greatly simplified if the tissue trapping of the tracer (after crossing the BBB) is rapid (like Rb-82). With this property, the early part of the tracer kinetics in tissue would be primarily related to BBB permeability. However, many tracers cross the BBB by carrier-mediated facilitated transport; the BBB permeability obtained with these tracers (e.g. K_1 of F-18 fluoro-L-DOPA (Huang et al., 1991)) is not the permeability by passive diffusion as provided by Ga-68 EDTA.

Study procedures and data analysis methods

Depending on the tracer used along with other practical considerations, different PET study procedures have been used at different institutions. Many data analysis methods to calculate PS have thus been devised. Since Ga-68 EDTA is most commonly used, we will focus our discussion to procedures and methods that use this tracer. For methods using Rb-82, the readers are referred to the papers by Yen et al. (1982), Brooks et al. (1984), Lammertsma et al. (1984), and Zunkeler et al. (1996).

For Ga-68 EDTA studies, dynamic scanning is usually used. The PET scanning of multiple frames (gradually increased from 1 to 5 minutes with a total scanning time of about 60 min) is started at the time of Ga-68 injection (5–7 mCi, administered intravenously as a bolus). Plasma tracer concentration as a function of time ($C_a(t)$) over the same period is measured from arterial blood samples using a well counter. Sometimes, because of its convenience, venous blood sampling may be used to avoid arterial puncture. After the dynamic images of all scan frames are reconstructed, regions-of-interest (ROI) are defined and are projected to images of all scan frames to give the tracer kinetics in the ROI ($C_{\text{pet}}(t)$).

Once properly calibrated, the measured ROI curve can be fitted by the model equation of Eqn (15.6) to give the values of K_1, k_2 and CPV of the model that are most consistent with the data. The K_1 value so obtained represents the *PS* value of the tracer in the brain region defined by the ROI. This approach was first used by Hawkins *et al.* (1984) to measure the BBB permeability of brain tumors. Typical *PS* values obtained were 0.0029 ml/min/g. In a recent study at UCLA that used the same approach, a *PS* value of 0.0002 ml/min/g was obtained for normal brain tissue and the values for whole tumor regions ranged from 0.0007 to 0.0068 ml/min/g (Black *et al.*, 1996; Zhou *et al.*, 1996).

The reason that CPV can be estimated simultaneously with the other parameters is because the plasma curve has a drastically different dynamics (or shape) from the component due to the extravascular activity (the first term on the right-hand side of Eqn (15.6). However, this requires the PET measured tissue activity to have sufficiently fine sampling (≤ 1 min frame rate at the beginning). Otherwise, reliable CPV value cannot be obtained from Ga-68 determinations. If this is the case, CPV should be measured or estimated separately and then fixed to the independently estimated value in the curve-fitting step. Similar problem and solution apply to the estimation of k_2. The total scan time of the dynamic scanning needs to be fairly long (~ 60 min) to give enough information for estimation of k_2.

In studies where the value of k_2 is small (i.e. not much tracer clearance from tissue during the study interval), a graphical approach using Patlak analysis (Patlak *et al.*, 1983) can be used to estimate K_1 ($= PS$). Patlak analysis uses linear regression to estimate the slope of a transformed tissue time activity curve. With this type of analysis, the value of k_2 is assumed to be zero and the value of CPV only affects the intercept of the regression and does not need to be estimated (either simultaneously or separately). This approach has been used by Iannotti *et al.* (1987) and Pozzilli *et al.* (1988). In both studies, a *PS* value of about 0.0003 ml/min/g was obtained for normal brain tissue. In the study by Pozzilli *et al.* (1988), a *PS* value of 0.0012 ml/min/g

was also obtained for focal lesion regions of multiple sclerosis. Iannotti *et al.* (1987) had also compared the use of ROI curve in the superior sagittal sinus against the use of plasma curve from arterial blood sampling, and found the superior sagittal sinus curve plus a venous blood sample in late times gave comparable results as those from arterial blood curves. Schlageter *et al.* (1987) used the Patlak approach to study Alzheimer patients and estimated a *PS* value of 0.00012 ml/min/g that is not significantly different from the value they measured in normal tissue. With a normal surface area of 100 cm^2/g (Raichle *et al.*, 1976), this corresponds to a permeability of about 2×10^{-8} cm/s.

In the analysis of tumor tissue regions, the k_2 is not negligible, but an adjustment method originally proposed by Patlak to account for non-zero k_2 is generally used (Patlak *et al.*, 1983). With this adjustment, Iannotti *et al.* (1987) obtained *PS* values of up to 0.012 ml/min/g in brain tumors.

Because of its robustness, the Patlak graphical approach can be applied to Ga-68 images on a pixel-by-pixel basis to give parametric images of BBB permeability (i.e. image of the *PS*). In normal tissue regions, the *PS* value can also be calculated from PET measurements by adopting the autoradiographic method (Eqn 15.3) (Zhou *et al.*, 1996). However, for regions that have significantly increased permeability, the tracer clearance from tissue is not negligible and the method would give *PS* estimates that are highly dependent on the exact time of measurement.

Additional considerations

Reliability of the measured permeability from PET is much related to (a) the physical characteristics of the PET scanner used; (b) how the study procedure was performed; and (c) the various image processing procedures involved. Many physical factors, such as scattered radiation, random coincidence, deadtime, and partial volume effect (Hoffman *et al.*, 1979), can affect the accuracy of PET determinations (Phelps *et al.*, 1985). In general, PET scanners with high detection efficiency, high spatial resolution (both in-plane and axially) and high temporal sampling capability are preferable. Careful control of the patient movement

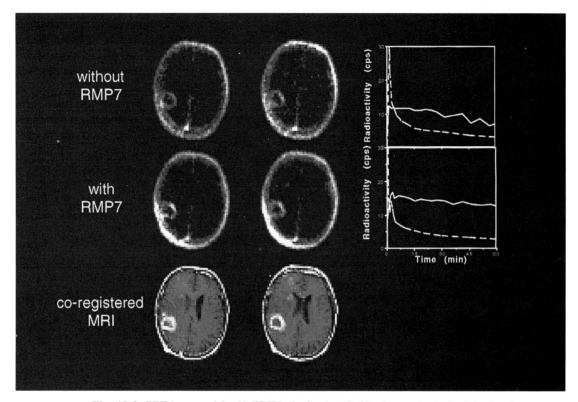

Fig. 15.2. PET images of Ga-68 EDTA distribution (0–60 min post i.v. bolus injection) in two transaxial cross-sections (3.125 mm apart) of the head of a tumor patient. Images on the top row were obtained under baseline. Images in the middle row were obtained with intra-arterial injection of RMP7. The top and the middle images were three-dimensionally co-registered to the MR images shown in the bottom. The graphs in the right column are the tissue curves obtained from a MR-based ROI that encompassed the entire tumor. The plasma time activity curves (dashed lines) of the study are also shown.

during the study to minimize the amount of movement between the transmission scanning (for measuring attenuation correction factors) and the emission scan, as well as during the course of the dynamic scan is critical to give reliable tissue kinetics (Huang *et al.*, 1979; Yu *et al.*, 1994).

In order to define the ROIs more objectively and consistently, co-registration of PET and MR images can be used (Lin *et al.*, 1994). Figure 15.2 shows the results of a study to evaluate the BBB permeability changes in brain tumors due to intra-arterial injection of an experimental drug, RMP7 (an analog of bradykinin). The patient was studied twice in two separate days with Ga-68 PET, one as a baseline study and one with intra-arterial RMP7 injection. PET images of both studies were co-registered to the MR image of the same subject

and ROI was defined based on the MR images, which had a more defined anatomical delineation of the tumor. The graphs in Fig. 15.2 are the tissue curves obtained from a MR-based ROI that encompassed the entire tumor visible on the MR images. After model fitting analysis, BBB permeability of the tumor was shown to be increased by 88% due to intra-arterial RMP7 administration in this particular case. Without careful attention to many aspects of the study, it would not have been easy to assess this pharmacological effect of the drug.

Due to the relatively low spatial resolution and the tissue heterogeneity in the region of interest, the tissue curve obtained from the PET measurement may represent the combination of different kinetics from heterogeneous tissues. Therefore, a multiple-compartment model may be more appropriate to use to describe the PET measured tissue curves (Zhou *et al.*, 1996). Also, partial volume effects may need to be corrected, e.g. with MRI-based correction methods (Muller-Gartner *et al.*, 1992; Yang *et al.*, 1996), especially if comparison across tissue regions of difference sizes, e.g. different size tumors, is desired.

Summary

Quantitative measurement of BBB permeability with PET commonly uses Ga-68 EDTA as the tracer and requires a dynamic PET scanning to give the tracer kinetics in tissue. A plasma tracer curve is usually obtained from sequential blood samples. A model-based curve fitting or some simplified graphical method is used to calculate BBB permeability. Careful attention needs to be paid to every step in the study procedure to ensure reliability of the results. Since Ga-68 is produced with commercial generators of long usable life (>275 days), the study can be performed conveniently without the need of an on-site cyclotron.

Extensive efforts on instrumentation and reconstruction algorithms are being devoted in Nuclear Medicine to making measurements from single photon emission tomography (SPECT) quantitative. When it becomes truly so, SPECT could also be used to measure BBB permeability *in vivo* in man, using analogous methodology to that discussed above for PET. Recent work on the use of MR imaging with Gadolinium-DTPA as a tracer has revealed that BBB permeability in tumors may also be quantitated using dynamic MR imaging (Kenney *et al.*, 1992). However, the same principles discussed in this chapter are used in these study methods, and the same care should be exercised in every step of the procedure. It is premature to speculate whether these methods can yet provide results as reliable as those obtained by PET. In the near future, however, PET will remain the primary methodology for quantitative *in vivo* measurement of BBB permeability in man. Results obtained with PET will also serve as the gold standard for development and validation of newer methods.

Acknowledgment

The authors would like to thank Mr. Y. Zhou for preparing Fig. 15.2 and for doing the image processing shown in the figure. They also want to acknowledge the support from DOE (contract DE-FC03–87-ER60615) that has facilitated the continued advancement of the PET methodology. The authors are also partially supported by NIH grants (NS33356, CA01669, CA56655). The pharmacological evaluation data illustrated in Fig. 15.2 was taken from a project directed by Dr. Keith Black of the neurosurgery department at UCLA School of Medicine and partially supported by Alkermes Inc., Mass.

References

Agon, P., Goethals, P., Van Haver, D. and Kaufman, J.-M. (1991). Permeability of the blood–brain barrier for atenolol studied by positron emission tomography. *J. Pharm. Pharmacol.*, **43**, 597–600.

Black, K., Cloughsey, T., Huang, S. C. *et al.* (1996). Intracarotid infusion of RMP-7, a bradykinin analog, increases transport of gallium-68 EDTA into human gliomas. *J. Neurosurg.*, **86**, 603–9.

Brooks, D. J., Beaney, R. P., Lammertsma, A. A. *et al.* (1984). Quantitative measurement of blood–brain barrier permeability using Rb-82 and positron emission tomography. *J. Cereb. Blood Flow Metabol.*, **4**, 535–45.

Crone, C. (1963). The permeability of brain capillaries to non-electrolytes. *Acta Physiol. Scand.*, **64**, 407–17.

Hawkins, R. A., Phelps, M. E., Huang, S. C. *et al.* (1984). A kinetic evaluation of blood brain permeability in human brain tumors with Ga-68 EDTA and positron computed tomography. *J. Cereb. Blood Flow Metabol.*, **4**, 507–15.

Hoffman, E. J., Huang, S. C. and Phelps, M. E. (1979). Quantitation in positron emission computed tomography. 1. Effect of object size. *J. Comput. Assist. Tomogr.*, **3**, 299–308.

Huang, S. C. and Phelps, M. E. (1985). Principles of tracer kinetic modeling in positron emision tomography and autoradiography. In *Positron Emission Tomography and Autoradiography*, ed. M. E. Phelps, J. Mazziotta, H. R. Schelbert, pp. 287–346. Raven Press.

Huang, S. C., Hoffman, E. J., Phelps, M. E. and Kuhl, D. E. (1979). Quantitation in positron emission computed tomography. 2. effects of inaccurate attenuation correction. *J. Comput. Assist. Tomogr.*, **3**, 804–14.

Huang, S. C., Yu, D. C., Barrio, J. R, et al. (1991). Kinetics and modeling of 6-[F-18]fluoro-L-DOPA in human positron emission tomographic studies, *J. Cereb. Blood Flow Metab.*, **11**, 898–913.

Iannotti, F., Fieschi, C., Alfano, B. et al. (1987). Simplified, noninvasive PET measurement of blood–brain barrier permeability, *J. Comput. Assist. Tomog.*, **11**, 390–7.

Kenney, J., Schmiedl, U., Maravilla, K. et al. (1992). Measurement of blood–brain barrier permeability in a tumor model using magnetic resonance imaging with Gadolinium-DTPA. *Magnet. Reson.Med.*, **27**, 68–75.

Kilpatrick, R., Renschler, H. E., Munro, D. S. and Wilson, G. M. (1956). A comparison of the distribution of K-42 and Rb-86 in rabbit and man. *J. Physiol.*, **133**, 194–201,.

Lammertsma, A. A., Brooks, D. J., Frackowiak, R. S. J. et al. (1984). A method to quantitate the fractional extraction of Rb-82 across the blood–brain barrier using positron emission tomography. *J. Cereb. Blood Flow Metabol.*, **4**, 523–34.

Lin, K. P., Huang, S. C., Baxter, L. and Phelps, M. E. (1994). A general technique for inter-study registration of multi-function and multimodality images. *IEEE Trans. Nucl. Sci.*, **41**, 2850–5.

Lockwood, A. H., Bolomey, L. and Napoleon, F. (1984). Blood-brain barrier to ammonia in humans. *J. Cereb. Blood Flow Metabol.*, **4**, 516–22.

Love, W. D., Romney, R. B. and Burch, G. E. (1954). A comparison of the distribution of potassium and exchange-able Rubidium in the organs of the dog, using Rubidium-86. *Circ. Res.*, **2**, 112–22.

Muller-Gartner, H. W., Links, J. M., Prince, J. L. et al. (1992). Measurement of radiotracer concentration in brain gray matter using positron emission tomography: MRI-based correction for partial volume effects. *J. Cereb Blood Flow Metab.*, **12**, 571–83.

Ott, R. J., Brada, M., Flower, M. A. et al. (1991). Measurements of blood–brain barrier permeability in patients undergoing radiotherapy and chemotherapy for primary cerebral lymphoma. *Eur. J. Cancer*, **27**, 1356–61.

Patlak, C. S. and Blasberg, R. G. (1985). Graphical evaluation of blood-to-brain barrier transfer constants from multiple time uptake data. Generalizations. *J. Cereb Blod Flow Metab.*, **5**, 584–90.

Patlak, C. S., Blasberg, R. G. and Fenstermacher, J. D. (1983). Graphical evaluation of blood-to-brain transfer constants from multiple-time uptake data. *J. Cereb Blood Flow Metab.*, **3**, 1–7.

Phelps, M. E., Huang, S. C., Kuhl, D. E. et al. (1981). Cerebral extraction of N-13 ammonia, its dependence on cerebral blood flow and capillary permeability. *Stroke*, **12**, 607–19.

Phelps, M. E., Mazziotta, J. and Schelbert, H. R. (1985). *Positron Emission Tomography and Autoradiography*. Raven Press.

Pozzilli, C., Bernardi, S., Mansi, L. et al. (1988). Quantitative assessment of blood–brain barrier permeability in multiple sclerosis using 68-Ga-EDTA and positron emission tomography. *J. Neurol. Neurosurg. Psychiat.*, **51**, 1058–62.

Raichle, M. E., Eicking, J. O., Straatman, M. G. et al. (1976). Blood–brain barrier permeability of C-11 labelled alcohols and O-15 labelled water. *Am. J. Physiol.*, **230**, 543–52.

Renkin, E. M. (1959). Transport of potassium-42 from blood to tissue in isolated mammalian skeletal muscles. *Am J. Physiol.*, **197**, 1205–10.

Schlageter, N. L., Carson, R. E. and Rapoport, S. I. (1987). Examination of blood–brain barrier permeability in dementia of the Alzheimer type with [Ga-68]EDTA and positron emission tomography. *J. Cereb. Blood Flow Metab.*, **7**, 1–8.

Yang, J., Huang, S. C., Mega, M. et al. (1996). Investigation of partial volume correction methods for brain FDG-PET studies. *IEEE Trans. Nucl. Sci.*, **43**, 3322–7,

Yen, C.-K., Yano, Y., Budinger, T. F. et al. (1982). Brain tumor evaluation using Rb-82 and positron emission tomography. *J. Nucl. Med.*, **23**, 532–7.

Yu, D. C., Huang, S. C., Lin, K. P. et al. (1994). Movement correction of FDOPA PET dynamic studies using frame-to-frame registration, *Biomed. Engin. – Applic. Basis Comm.*, **6**, 660–71.

Zhou, Y., Huang, S. C., Hoh, C. K. et al. (1996). Gallium-68 EDTA PET study of brain tumor BBB permeability changes induced by intra-arterial RMP7. *J. Nucl. Medi.*, **37**, 146.

Zunkeler, B., Carson, R. E., Olson, J. et al. (1996). Hyperosmolar blood–brain barrier disruption in baboons: an in vivo study using positron emission tomography and rubidium-82. *J Neurosurg.*, **84**, 494–502.

16 Magnetic resonance imaging of blood–brain barrier permeability

CLIVE P. HAWKINS

- Introduction
- Quantitative measurement of blood–brain barrier breakdown in the multiple sclerosis lesion
- Modification and evaluation of the standard quantitative method

Introduction

Magnetic resonance imaging is a sensitive method to detect disease in the central nervous system and monitor its progress. The magnetic resonance technique particularly reflects the amount of tissue water predominantly in the extracellular compartment. Experimental studies have shown its ability to monitor inflammation in the tissue (Hawkins *et al.*, 1990) and also to discriminate extracellular from intracellular edema, and gliosis (Barnes *et al.*, 1987, 1988).

With the introduction of the contrast agent gadolinium-DTPA, it is possible to detect blood–brain barrier breakdown *in vivo* (Weinmann *et al.*, 1984; Hawkins *et al.*, 1990, 1992). For example, in multiple sclerosis gadolinium enhancement has been shown to be a frequent, early and important feature of the evolving multiple sclerosis plaque and has been used in recent treatment trials as a marker of inflammatory disease activity (Grossman *et al.*, 1986; Gonzalez-Scarano *et al.*, 1987; Kappos *et al.*, 1988; Miller *et al.*, 1988; Kermode *et al.*, 1990) – see Fig. 16.1.

In early studies gadolinium enhanced MRI was used to assess the degree and distribution of blood–brain barrier breakdown in experimental allergic encephalomyelitis, an animal model similar to multiple sclerosis. The pattern of barrier breakdown in the acute phase of the condition was compared to that of chronic relapsing disease (Hawkins *et al.*, 1991).

In multiple sclerosis it has been possible to develop a theoretical model of the blood–brain barrier and its breakdown in relation to signal intensities seen on magnetic resonance imaging and change in signal following a bolus administration of gadolinium-DTPA (Tofts and Kermode, 1991). In essence the enhancement curve following administration of the contrast agent was fitted to a theoretical model with triexponential decay based on compartmental analysis.

Quantitative measurement of blood–brain barrier breakdown in the multiple sclerosis lesion

The transfer constant, defined as permeability surface area per unit volume of tissue (k), and leakage space per unit volume of tissue (v_1) are measured. Results for the transfer constant are in general agreement with values obtained by other methods ($k = 0.050$ per minute and 0.013 per minute; v_1, 21% and 49%). The theoretical compartmental model is based on DTPA kinetics following bolus injection and involves a plasma volume connected to a large extracellular space distributed throughout

(a)

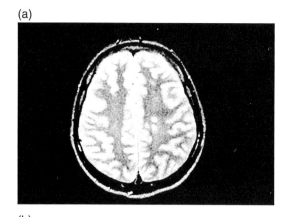

(b)

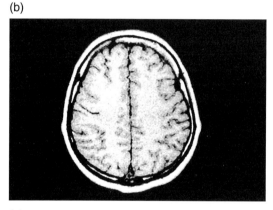

(c)

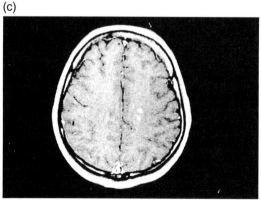

Fig. 16.1. Axial brain MRI of a patient with early relapsing remitting MS. (a) T_2 weighted image revealing two high signal areas in the left periventricular white matter (SE 2468/80). (b) Corresponding T_1 weighted image from the same patient (SE 550/10) before gadolinium–DTPA injection. (c) T_1 weighted image after gadolinium–DTPA injection (0.1 mmol/kg) showing two areas of enhancement indicating blood–brain barrier breakdown. (Kind permission of Dr Brendan Davies, Research Fellow, Department of Neurology, Royal Infirmary, Stoke on Trent.)

much of the body except the brain. The kidney is considered to drain tracer from the plasma and hence from the extracellular space. A fourth component is added, the multiple sclerosis plaque, in continuity with the plasma through a breached blood–brain barrier. However, this fourth component is small enough not to influence the overall plasma concentration. It is assumed there would be fast mixing of the bolus injection of tracer within the plasma. An assumption is made that capillary flow in the lesion is high enough to prevent plasma concentration from depletion by leakage of tracer through the blood–brain barrier, i.e. all tracer within the compartment is well mixed.

The final equation from which k and v_1 can be estimated follows –

$$C_t(t) = D\{b_1\exp(-m_1 t) + b_2\exp(-m_2 t) + b_3\exp(-m_3 t)\}$$

where C_t is the concentration of the tracer in tissue and D is the DTPA dose (mmol/kg body weight) where

$$m_3 = k/v_1$$
$$b_1 = ka_1/(m_3 - m_1)$$
$$b_2 = ka_2/(m_3 - m_2)$$
$$b_3 = -(b_1 + b_2)$$

and a_1, a_2, m_1, m_2 have been determined empirically from the plasma curve.

The initial slope of the curve is given by

$$dC_t(0_t)/dt = kD(a_1 + a_2)$$

With different values of k and v_1, differing $C_t(t)$ curves are obtained. Increased permeability leads to an increase in the initial slope of the concentration curve as expected from the equation shown, and for a fixed permeability, increasing the leakage space has no effect on the initial slope but does alter the maximum concentration reached and delays the time to maximum enhancement (see Fig. 16.2).

In the aforementioned method, Tofts and Kermode (1991) used mean values measured in ten normal subjects to obtain values for the plasma concentration following bolus injection, whilst Larsson *et al.* (1990), using a similar theoretical model, measured this directly using arterial catheterization and concentrations were measured using neutron activation. There were other

BBB PERMEABILITY USING DYNAMIC MRI

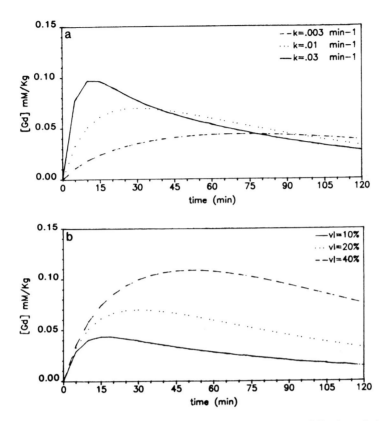

Fig. 16.2. Model triexponential lesion concentration curves, following a bolus injection of 0.1 mmol/kg of gadolinium–DTPA. (a) Fixed leakage space $v_1 = 20\%$, varying permeability k. (b) Fixed permeability $k = 0.01$ per min, varying leakage space v_1. (From Tofts and Kermode, 1991, with kind permission of Dr Paul S. Tofts and *Magnetic Resonance in Medicine*.)

differences relating to assumptions made about the magnetic resonance techniques employed (Larsson and Tofts, 1992).

Modification and evaluation of the standard quantitative method

Tofts and Berkowitz (1993) described modifications in the analysis of the standard compartmental model previously described in measurement of blood–brain barrier permeability but also blood–retinal barrier lesions. The initial slope method involved a linear approximation to the known equation with errors estimated at between 17% and 26%. The second was an early enhancement method taking into account all non linearities and

iterative computation is required, its accuracy limited without knowledge of size of the leakage space. The third was a simplified early enhancement method appropriate for retinal lesions taking into account only the plasma decay curve on the basis that this is likely to represent the major source of curvature using short magnetic resonance echo time, because the leakage space is large in the form of the vitreous humour. The latter has been used to measure blood retinal barrier breakdown *in vivo* with permeability values comparable to those measured by other techniques (Berkowitz *et al.*, 1992).

The alternatives of bolus injection or constant infusion methods were compared to measure capillary permeability from the gadolinium enhancement curve. Using the simplified early enhancement

149

method applicable to retinal lesions it was shown by computer simulation that a constant infusion is unable to establish a constant plasma concentration in an acceptable time period *in vivo* although a hybrid injection of bolus and infusion can achieve this.

In addition, it was demonstrated that the bolus injection achieves a higher tissue concentration and hence signal enhancement on scan than does the same dose given as infusion, and the bolus injection allows a given tissue concentration in a shorter time than the same dose as infusion (Tofts and Berkowitz, 1994).

It should be possible to apply the described methods to the individual requirements of study. Conditions other than multiple sclerosis associated with blood–brain barrier breakdown, for example stroke, intracranial tumours and vasculitis disorders, may be similarly studied. It would be possible to measure blood–brain barrier permeability using these techniques in treatment trials to assess the efficacy of putative drugs at different time points, and compare with other measures of disease activity in multiple sclerosis, stroke and intracranial malignancy.

References

Barnes, D., McDonald, W. I., Johnson, G. *et al.* (1987). Quantitative nuclear magnetic resonance imaging; characterisation of experimental cerebral oedema. *J. Neurol., Neurosurg. Psych.*, **50**, 125–33.

Barnes, D., McDonald, W. I., Landon, D. N. and Johnson, G. (1988). The characterisation of experimental gliosis by quantitative nuclear magnetic resonance imaging. *Brain*, **101**, 83–94.

Berkowitz, B. A., Tofts, P. S., Sen, H. A. *et al.* (1992). Accurate and precise measurement of blood–retinal barrier breakdown using dynamic Gd-DTPA MRI. *Invest. Ophthalmol. Vis. Sci.*, **33**, 3500–6.

Gonzalez-Scarano, F., Grossman, R. I., Galletta, S. *et al.* (1987). Multiple sclerosis disease activity correlates with gadolinium enhanced magnetic resonance imaging. *Ann. Neurol.*, **21**, 300–6.

Grossman, R. I., Gonzalez-Scarano, F., Atlas, S. W. *et al.* (1986). Multiple sclerosis: gadolinium enhancement in MR imaging. *Radiology*, **161**, 71–5.

Hawkins, C. P., Munro, P. M. G., Mackenzie, F. *et al.* (1990). Duration and selectivity of blood–brain barrier breakdown in chronic relapsing experimental allergic encephalomyelitis studied by gadolinium – DTPA and protein markers. *Brain*, **113**, 365–78.

Hawkins, C. P., Mackenzie, F., Tofts, P. S. *et al.* (1991). Patterns of blood–brain barrier breakdown in inflammatory demyelination. *Brain*, **114**, 801–10.

Hawkins, C. P., Munro, P. M. G., Landon, D. N. and McDonald, W. I. (1992). Metabolically dependent blood–brain barrier breakdown in chronic relapsing experimental allergic encephalomyelitis. *Acta Neuropathol.*, **83**, 630–5.

Kappos, L., Stadt, D., Rohrbach, E. and Keil, W. (1988). Gadolinium – DTPA-enhanced magnetic resonance imaging in the evaluation of different disease courses and disease activity in MS. *Neurology, Cleveland*, **38** (supplement 1), 255.

Kermode, A. G., Thompson, A. J., Tofts, P. S. *et al.* (1990). Breakdown of the blood–brain barrier precedes other MRI signs of new lesions in multiple sclerosis: pathogenetic and clinical implications. *Brain*, **113**, 1477–89.

Larsson, H. B. W., Stubgaard, N., Frederiksen, J. L. *et al.* (1990). Quantitation of blood–brain barrier defect by magnetic resonance imaging and gadolinium DTPA in patients with multiple sclerosis and brain tumours. *Magnet. Reson. Med.* **16**, 117–131.

Larsson, H. B. W. and Tofts, P. S. (1992). Measurement of blood–brain barrier permeability using dynamic gadolinium DTPA scanning – a comparison of methods. *Magnet. Reson. Med.*, **24**, 174–6.

Miller, D. H., Rudge, P., Johnson, G. *et al.* (1988). Serial gadolinium enhanced magnetic resonance imaging in multiple sclerosis. *Brain*, **111**, 927–39.

Tofts, P. S. and Kermode, A. G. (1991). Measurement of the blood–brain barrier permeability and leakage space using dynamic MR imaging. 1. Fundamental concepts. *Magnet. Reson. Med.*, **17**, 357–67.

Tofts, P. S. and Berkowitz, B. A. (1993). Rapid measurement of capillary permeability using the early part of the dynamic gadolinium–DTPA MRI enhancement curve. *J. Magnet. Reson., Series B*, **102**, 129–36.

Tofts, P. S. and Berkowitz, B. A. (1994). Measurement of capillary permeability from the gadolinium enhancement curve: a comparison of bolus and constant infusion injection methods. *Magnet. Reson. Imag.*, **12**, 81–91.

Weinmann, H. J., Laniado, M. and Mutzel, W. (1984). Pharmacokinetics of Gd–DTPA/dimeglumine after intravenous injection into healthy volunteers. *Phys. Chem. Phys. Med. NMR*, **16**, 167.

17 Molecular biology of brain capillaries

RUBEN J. BOADO

- Introduction
- BBB-specific genes
- Analysis of BBB-gene transcripts
- Isolation of BBB–RNA transcripts
- Isolation of RNA from capillary-depleted total brain
- Northern blot analysis of BBB-transcripts
- Quantitative polymerase chain reaction of BBB-transcripts
- Analysis of BBB-gene products (proteins)
- Molecular cloning of BBB-specific genes
- BBB-reporter genes
- Summary

Introduction

The brain microvascular endothelium represents the blood–brain barrier (BBB) *in vivo* (Brightman, 1977), and the expression of BBB-specific genes provides the anatomical and biochemical properties of this barrier (i.e. tight junctions, nutrient transporters, etc.). Because only lipophilic molecules of less than 600 Da diffuse through the BBB (Pardridge, 1995), the brain is protected against peripheral neurotransmitters (i.e. noradrenaline), cytotoxins, and microorganisms. From the pharmacological point of view, the protective properties of the BBB represent a disadvantage for brain drug delivery of hydrophilic therapeutics (for example, AZT, antisense oligodeoxynucleotides, nerve growth factor) for the treatment of cerebral HIV–AIDS, brain tumors, Alzheimer's disease and other brain disorders (Boado, 1995a; Pardridge, 1995). On the contrary, polar nutrients, as in the case of glucose and amino acids, and peptides like insulin, gain access to the brain through specific transporters

located on both lumenal and ablumenal membranes of the BBB (see Chapter 6). Although the mechanism of gene expression of BBB-specific proteins appears to be directed by factors released by brain cells (i.e. astrocytes) and sequestered by the endothelium (Stewart and Wiley, 1981), little is known in regards to either the identification or isolation of these putative brain trophic factors. This intellectually stimulating field has captivated the attention of several groups of investigators over the last couple of decades, and the progress has been limited to the development of reproducible cell culture models and to the initial characterization of brain-derived complex fractions possessing trophic properties. The activity of γ-glutamyl transpeptidase (γ-GTP) in brain endothelial cultured cells has been reported to be augmented by condition medium or plasma membrane fractions obtained from cultures of either astrocytes or glioma cells (Arthur *et al.*, 1987; DeBault and Cancilla, 1980; Janzer and Raff, 1987; Tontsch and Bauer, 1991), and the expression of the BBB-GLUT1 (glucose transporter

151

type I) gene in brain endothelial cultured cells has been either increased or stabilized by brain derived factors (Boado et al., 1994a; Boado, 1995b).

In vivo, the expression of BBB-specific genes has been correlated with barrier properties; for example, GLUT1 protein parallels the expression of tight junctions during development (Dermietzel et al., 1992; Bauer et al. 1995; Bolz et al., 1996), and the levels of either immunoreactive GLUT1 or γ-GTP activity and barrier properties in brain microvessels are inversely correlated with the grade of malignancy of human gliomas and damage following brain injury (Guerrin et al., 1990; Rosenstein and More, 1994). Interestingly, when brain capillary endothelial cells are grown in tissue culture, the expression of BBB-specific genes (i.e. tight junctions, GLUT1, γ-GTP) are markedly down-regulated or absent (DeBault and Cancilla, 1980; Arthur et al., 1987; Janzer and Raff, 1987; Boado and Pardridge, 1990a, 1994a; Tontsch and Bauer, 1991; Nagashima et al., 1994). This has led to the hypothesis that the lack of correlation between *in vivo* and culture cell models to study the expression of BBB-specific genes and the transport of molecules through the BBB is related to the absence of brain-derived trophic factors in tissue cultures, that maintain the levels of expression of BBB-specific genes, and consequently barrier functions.

It is clear that the isolation of brain trophic factors represents a complex and difficult task; however, it may result from a careful investigation and understanding of the molecular mechanisms involved in the expression of BBB-specific genes (i.e. GLUT1, γ-GTP). In addition, these factors may also provide potential treatments for restoration of barrier properties *in vivo* following stroke or brain injury, as well as providing *in vitro* models to be used as animal alternatives for testing and development of new therapeutics and drug delivery systems for brain. Overall, the aim of this chapter is to provide a comprehensive overview of molecular biology strategies available for analysis of the expression and cloning of BBB-specific genes.

BBB-specific genes

The expression of BBB markers, for example GLUT1 and γ-GTP, as models of BBB-specific

genes have been investigated by different laboratories (Arthur et al., 1987; Boado et al., 1994a; Boado, 1995b; DeBault and Cancilla, 1980; Janzer and Raff, 1987; Tontsch and Bauer, 1991). The criteria for selecting these genes as BBB-specific is based on the fact that even though they are expressed in other tissues, within the brain, they are principally, if not exclusively, expressed at the BBB (Boado and Pardridge, 1990b; DeBault and Cancilla, 1980; Pardridge et al., 1990). The enzymatic activity of BBB-γ-GTP has been extensively used to investigate the effect of putative brain trophic factors in brain microvascular endothelial cultured cells (Arthur et al., 1987; DeBault and Cancilla, 1980; Janzer and Raff, 1987; Tontsch and Bauer, 1991). However, changes in the activity of this enzyme may not parallel changes in the abundance of γ-GTP protein or gene expression (Taniguchi et al., 1985).

Molecular mechanisms related to the expression of BBB–GLUT1 as a model of a BBB-specific gene have been investigated. Although expression of the GLUT1 gene has been described in choroid plexus and scattered astrocytes (Bondy et al., 1992; Pardridge and Boado, 1993), it has been demonstrated that the GLUT1 transcript is absent in RNA samples obtained from capillary-depleted brain cortex from bovine, rabbit, and rat (Boado and Pardridge, 1990b; Pardridge and Boado, 1993; Kumagai et al., 1995), suggesting that the GLUT1 gene is principally expressed at the BBB within the brain. In addition, quantitative Western blot analysis in comparison with cytochalasin B binding assay have shown that GLUT1 is the principal glucose transporter expressed at the BBB, and that this transporter is responsible for more than 90% of the transportation of glucose to the brain (Pardridge et al., 1990; Pardridge and Boado, 1993). Because the BBB only represents a small fraction of the total brain surface area (~ 10 μl/g brain), the BBB–GLUT1 is the limiting step in the transportation of glucose to brain (Pardridge and Boado, 1993). Based on cytochalasin B binding studies (Pardridge et al., 1990), the number of binding sites for glucose per gram of tissue, independent of the GLUT isoform, can be calculated in both capillary-depleted total brain and BBB membranes, respectively. These numbers are: 500 and 10 pmol/g for brain cells and BBB, respectively, which represents a 50-fold increase in the number of binding sites for glucose in non-microvascular cells, confirming that indeed the BBB–GLUT1 is the limiting step in the transport of glucose from blood to brain. The expression of the BBB GLUT1 gene has been found to be altered in different pathophysiological conditions including hypoglycemia, diabetes mellitus, brain tumors, and development (Harik and Roessmann, 1991; Nagamatsu *et al.*, 1993; Boado and Pardridge, 1993; Pardridge and Boado, 1993 Boado *et al.*, 1994*b*). The regulatory mechanism of BBB–GLUT1 gene expression has been found to be exerted at either the gene transcriptional level or post-transcriptional stabilization of GLUT1 mRNA (Boado and Pardridge, 1993; Boado *et al.*, 1994*a*). However, post-transcriptional modification of this gene appears to be the the principal site of regulation in the majority of the investigated conditions (Boado and Pardridge, 1993; Sandouk *et al.*, 1993; Boado *et al.*, 1994*b*, Boado, 1995*b*).

Analysis of BBB-gene transcripts

As discussed above, the volume of brain capillaries only represents a small fraction of total brain. Consequently, the levels of BBB-specific gene transcript in a total brain RNA preparation may be under the limit of detection of particular assays. For example, the brain microvascular 1.7 kb smooth muscle α-actin transcript is undetected by Northern blotting in a Poly(A)$^+$ mRNA preparation of total brain, whereas in contrast, this transcript is evident using a brain capillary mRNA isolate (Fig. 17.1C) (Boado and Pardridge, 1994*b*). Therefore, a careful analysis of BBB-specific gene transcripts requires isolation of brain capillaries prior to analysis of gene products (Figs. 17.1, 17.2). Methods for isolation of brain microvessels under RNase-free conditions have been extensively published (Boado and Pardridge, 1990*b*, 1991), and they are similar to the ones described in detail in Chapter 6. Modifications include: (a) RNase free solutions and buffers preincubated at 4 °C for > 15 hours, (b) sterile and disposable plasticware, (c) glassware and surgical material baked for 20 hours at 230 °C, and (d) the procedure is generally performed in a cold-room with the aid of a Waring

blender as in the case of bovine brain (Boado and Pardridge, 1990*b*).

Isolation of BBB–RNA transcripts

Molecular cloning and analysis of the expression of BBB-specific transcripts may begin with the isolation of BBB–RNA (Fig. 17.1, IV and VI), and methods for isolation of BBB–Poly(A)$^+$ mRNA in either one or multiple steps have been successfully used. Typically, in a conventional two-step method, total RNA is isolated from brain capillaries by homogenization in guanidine thiocyanate (GIT) (Boado and Pardridge, 1990*b*) followed by purification of RNA from contaminant DNA and proteins through a CsCl ultracentrifugation (Chirgwin *et al.*, 1979) or phenol:chloroform extraction/alcohol precipitation (Chomczynski and Sacchi, 1987) (Fig. 17.1, VI). In the second step, the Poly(A)$^+$ mRNA is isolated from total RNA using an oligo-d(T) column (Fig. 17.1, IV). The yield of total RNA obtained using the GIT/CsCl method is relatively low, and approximately 100 μg of total RNA have been isolated per one bovine cortical shell (approximately 180 g), which resulted in the production of 1–2 μg Poly(A)$^+$ mRNA following oligo-d(T) selection in the second step (Boado and Pardridge, 1990*a*). Therefore, 13 bovine brains have been processed in order to obtain enough Poly(A)$^+$ mRNA for the synthesis of a BBB-λgt11 expression library (see below). The total yield of RNA using the GIT/acid phenol/alcohol precipitation method has been reported to be slightly better than the procedure based on GIT/CsCl centrifugation, and approximately 200–500 μg total RNA are usually obtained from one bovine cortical shell (Boado and Pardridge, 1994*a*). However, this material may contain significant DNA contamination, and the treatment of the sample with RNase-free DNaseI is required if the material is used for RT Q-PCR (reverse transcriptase quatitative polymerase chain reaction) (Boado and Pardridge, 1994*a*, Boado, 1995*b*). The yield of Poly(A)$^+$ mRNA isolated from bovine brain capillaries was markedly improved by the introduction of the one-step procedure for isolation of Poly(A)$^+$ transcript (Boado and Pardridge, 1991). This method utilizes a combination of SDS (sodium

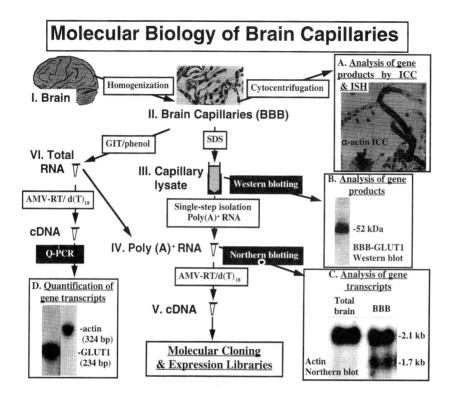

Fig. 17.1. Molecular biology of brain capillaries. Since the volume of brain capillaries only represents a small fraction of total brain, the molecular cloning and analysis of the expression of BBB-specific genes begins with isolation of brain microvessels by homogenization of brain (I) followed by centrifugation of brain capillaries (II). Brain capillary Poly(A)$^+$ mRNA (IV) may be isolated by the conventional two-step procedure wherein total RNA (VI) is obtained following disruption of cells with either GIT/phenol and alcohol precipitation or GIT/CsCl ultracentrifugation, and Poly(A)$^+$ mRNA (IV) is then selected using an oligo-d(T) column. Alternatively, Poly(A)$^+$ mRNA may be obtained in a single-step procedure using a combination of SDS (III), proteinase K , and oligo-d(T) cellulose. This method allows for determination of both proteins and transcripts by Northern (C) and Western blotting (B), respectively, if an aliquot of the sample is obtained prior to addition of proteinase K to the capillary lysate (III). Poly(A)$^+$ mRNA may be used for either measurement of the abundance of a transcript of interest by Northern blot analysis, or synthesis of cDNA (V) using AMV-RT and oligo d(T)$_{18}$ primer. cDNA may be employed for molecular cloning and construction of expression libraries. In addition, cDNA may be used for quantification of BBB-specific mRNAs by RT Q-PCR as in the case of GLUT1 and actin transcripts (D). Isolated brain capillaries may also be subjected to cytocentrifugation followed by an immunocytochemistry (A) technique that combines determination of the abundance of a particular gene product with its cellular localization. A. Immunocytochemical detection of smooth muscle α-actin in cytospun isolated brain capillaries. This protein is expressed at the pre-capillary arterioles, whereas both endothelial and pericytes (arrows) were negative. B. Western blot analysis of BBB–GLUT1 shows the characteristic 52 kDa protein corresponding to the glycosylated form of brain capillary GLUT1 protein. C. Northern blot analysis of Poly(A)$^+$ mRNA isolated from total brain and brain capillaries with an actin cDNA probe. Both samples contain a 2.1 kb band corresponding to cytoplasmic β/γ-actin transcript; however, because BBB-specific transcripts are diluted in the total brain mRNA pool, the 1.7 kb microvascular smooth muscle α-actin is solely detected in the BBB-Poly(A)$^+$ mRNA preparation.
D. Quantification of GLUT1 and actin transcripts by RT Q-PCR. Autoradiogram shows single PCR products of 234 and 324 bp corresponding to BBB–GLUT1 and γ-actin, respectively. For more details see text. From Boado and Pardridge, 1994*a*, 1994*b*; Pardridge *et al.* 1990, with permission of Lippincott-Raven Publishers; Wiley-Liss Inc.; and the American Society for Biochemistry & Molecular Biology.

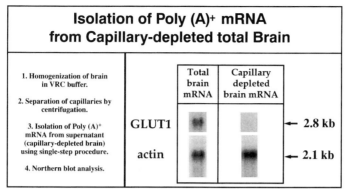

Fig. 17.2. Isolation of RNA from capillary-depleted total brain. In order to determine that transcripts measured in a total brain RNA pool arc indeed from BBB origin, RNA may be obtained from a capillary-depleted total brain sample (Boado and Pardridge, 1990*b*) as summarized on the left-hand side of the figure. Northern blot analysis of rat total brain and capillary-depleted brain demonstrates that the BBB–GLUT1 transcript is absent in capillary-depleted brain (right-hand side of figure), and that this is not due to poor quality of the RNA preparation since re-probing of membranes with an actin probe showed intact 2.1 kb transcript corresponding to cytoplasmic β/γ-actin isoform. From Kumagai *et al.*, 1995, with permission.

dodecyl sulfate) and proteinase K for lysis and digestion of cellular proteins. SDS, as well as urea, at concentrations of 1–2%, markedly stimulates the proteinase K activity and inhibits the activity of cellular RNases (Hilz *et al.*, 1975). This method also allows for quantification of both protein and RNA, if an aliquot of material is obtained after the homogenization with SDS buffer and prior to addition of proteinase K (Fig. 17.1, II and III). After digestion of proteins is completed (typically 45 minutes at 45 °C), the ionic concentration of the solution is adjusted to 0.5 M sodium chloride, which represents the optimal ionic concentration for binding of Poly(A)$^+$ mRNA to oligo-d(T) cellulose (Boado and Pardridge, 1991). The selection of Poly(A)$^+$ mRNA is performed in the same tube by addition of oligo-d(T) cellulose. Following washing of Poly(A)$^-$ RNA (i.e. ribosomal and transfer RNAs) with 0.5 and 0.1 M sodium chloride buffers, Poly(A)$^+$ transcripts are obtained with the aid of a Spin-X filter unit (Boado and Pardridge, 1991). The yield of Poly(A)$^+$ mRNA ranged from 14–17 µg of mRNA per batch of capillaries isolated from a single bovine cortical shell, which represents > 10-fold increase compared to the conventional 2-step method (see above). In addition, this method has also been used for isolation of Poly(A)$^+$ mRNA from bovine choroid plexus, human, rat and bovine brain, with a yield of 15–19 µg/g weight (Boado and Pardridge, 1991, 1994*b*; Boado *et al.*, 1992, 1994*b*; Boado, 1995*b*; Kumagai *et al.*, 1995; Kannan *et al.*, 1996). The yield for brain endothelial cultured cells and other cell lines was in the range of 6–12 µg/10^7 cells (Boado and Pardridge, 1991; Boado *et al.*, 1992).

Isolation of RNA from capillary-depleted total brain

If the limit of detection allows, it is possible to determine the abundance of BBB-specific transcripts in a total brain RNA preparation, assuming that those transcripts are solely expressed at the BBB. It is, however, possible to demonstrate that transcripts measured in a total brain RNA pool are indeed from BBB origin. For example, Northern blot analysis of RNA isolated from total brain or capillary-depleted total brain from bovine, rabbit, or rat (Fig. 17.2) demonstrated the absence of detectable GLUT1 transcript in the capillary-depleted sample (Boado and Pardridge, 1990*b*; Pardridge and Boado, 1993; Kumagai *et al.*, 1995). The failure to detect GLUT1 mRNA in these samples was not due to poor quality of the RNA preparation since re-probing of membranes with an actin probe showed intact 2 to 2.1 kb transcript corresponding to cytoplasmic β/γ-actin isoforms in the capillary-depleted sample. The single step method for isolation of Poly(A)$^+$ mRNA has been successfully adapted for isolation of Poly(A)$^+$ transcripts from capillary-depleted brain preparations (Fig. 17.2) (Kumagai *et al.*, 1995). However, it has to be emphasized that the initial homogenization in the capillary depletion step produces a massive release of cellular RNases; therefore, this procedure must be carefully performed at 4 °C in the presence of the RNase inhibitor, vanadyl ribonucleoside complex (VRC) (Fig. 17.2) (Boado and Pardridge, 1990*b*).

Northern blot analysis of BBB-transcripts

The single step method for isolation of Poly(A)$^+$ mRNA (Fig. 17.1, IV) has been extensively used for quantification of BBB transcript by Northern blotting (Fig. 17.1, C). Northern blot analysis performed at high stringency conditions (0.3 M Na$^+$) has allowed for determination of GLUT1, actin, and tubulin transcripts during development, in diabetes mellitus, in chronic hypoglycemia (Pardridge and Boado, 1993); and for demonstration of post-transcriptional stabilization of GLUT1 transcript in hypoglycemia and by brain-derived factors (Boado, 1995*b*; Boado and Pardridge, 1993). In addition, this method has been used to demonstrate a positive correlation between the expression of GLUT3 and GLUT1 and the malignancy of human gliomas (Boado *et al.*, 1994*b*). Along the same line, the expression of 5-lipoxygenase was also correlated with the grade of astrocytoma, and evidence for the expression of a 5-lipoxygenase multi-transcript family has also been demonstrated (Boado *et al.*, 1992). Transcript measured following isolation of Poly(A)$^+$ mRNA by the single-step method was in the range 1–10 kb (Boado *et al.*, 1992; Palos *et al.*, 1996), suggesting that this method is useful for isolation and quantification of mRNAs comprised of a variety of sizes in the absence of partially degraded transcripts.

Quantitative polymerase chain reaction of BBB-transcripts

The study of the expression of BBB-specific genes (i.e. GLUT1, γ-GTP) in brain capillary endothelial cells in tissue culture is made difficult owing to the significant downregulation of transcripts compared to that in brain capillaries *in vivo*. For example, detection of GLUT1 mRNA by Northern blot analysis requires isolation of Poly(A)$^+$ mRNA from confluent 150 mm diameter dishes, as approximately 7 μg Poly(A)$^+$ mRNA are obtained from these cells (Boado and Pardridge, 1991, 1993). This limitation makes difficult the analysis of GLUT1 mRNA or other BBB-specific transcripts in brain endothelial culture cells, particularly when multiple sample experiments are to be analyzed. A potential solution to this problem is offered by reverse transcriptase quantitative polymerase chain reaction. A method for quantification of the concentration of bovine GLUT1 and cytoplasmic γ-actin mRNA has been established using RT Q-PCR assay (Fig. 17.1, D) (Boado and Pardridge, 1994*a*). In this method, total RNA is isolated from endothelial cultured cells incubated in either 10 or 25 mm dishes by the method of GIT/phenol/alcohol precipitation followed by synthesis of cDNA using AMV-RT and oligo-d(T) primer (Fig. 17.1, VI). The sense and antisense primers for PCR amplification were comprised of 20-mer oligodeoxynucleotides corresponding to nucleotides 277–296 and 491–510 or the bovine GLUT1 mRNA, respectively. The set for actin primers correspond to nucleotides 22–41 and 344–363 of the bovine γ-actin cDNA sequence. Therefore, PCR results in amplification of DNA fragments of 234 and 342 nucleotides for GLUT1 and actin, respectively (Fig. 17.1, D). Quantification of actin transcript was used as a standard control in lieu of synthetic artificial mRNA (Heuvel *et al.*, 1993). Even though artificial mRNA may be useful in determination of sample to sample variation, quantification of the housekeeping gene, actin, provides the following advantages: (a) information in regards to the quality of isolated RNA; on the other hand, competitive PCR of artificial RNA with degraded target RNA is interpreted as undetectable transcript; and (b) when results are expressed as GLUT1/actin mRNA ratio, the quantification of GLUT1 transcript is independent of any variation in the optical densitometry grading performed for the initial determination of the RNA concentration. This is of particular importance considering that the photometric reproducibility of spectro-

Table 17.1. *Molecular cloning of BBB transcripts using viral and plasmid cDNA libraries.*

Reference	Origin of cDNA	Vector	Isolated clone(s)
Boado and Pardridge (1990)	Bovine brain capillaries	λgt11	Full length GLUT1
Dechert *et al.* (1994)	Porcine brain capillaries	λ-ZAP	Partial protein kinase
Papandrikopoulou *et al.* (1989)	Porcine brain capillaries	λgt10	Full length γ-GTP
Weiler-Gütter *et al.* (1989)	Porcine brain capillaries	λgt10	Partial GLUT1
Weiler-Gütter *et al.* (1990) [& Zinke *et al.* (1992)]	Porcine brain capillaries subtracted with lung	pUC19	Partial Apo A-1 [GLUT1 & glial markers]

photometers approximates 0.5 % of absorbance (260 nm) values of >0.100 or 4 µg RNA. Therefore, if the target/housekeeping gene PCR product ratio is not obtained, following a standard PCR protocol of 30 cycles in which each original molecule of single-stranded cDNA produces $2^{(cycle-2)}$ $-(cycle-2)$ or 2.68×10^8 molecules, the initial variation in A_{260} readings is translated into significant variation among samples. RT Q-PCR has been used to provide further evidence that GLUT1 transcript is markedly downregulated in endothelial cultured cells compared to fresh isolated brain capillaries, and the GLUT1/actin mRNA ratio in brain capillaries was found to be 20-fold higher than cultured cells (Boado and Pardridge, 1994*a*). This method has also been used for investigating the effect of brain-derived factors and TNFα on the expression of BBB GLUT1 in brain endothelial cultured cells (Boado and Pardridge, 1994*a*; Boado, 1995*b*).

Analysis of BBB-gene products (proteins)

As depicted in Fig. 17.1 (II and III), a single-step method for isolation of Poly(A)$^+$ mRNA allows for co-determination of transcripts and proteins by Northern and Western blotting, respectively, if an aliquot of the sample is obtained following homogenization with SDS and prior to addition of proteinase K (Fig. 17.1, B). Quantitative Western blot analysis, using antibodies directed to either the 13 amino acid carboxyl terminal of GLUT1 or to the human GLUT1 protein, has been used for quantification of the GLUT1 gene product in isolated brain capillaries from bovine brain, from rabbit

brain during development, and from diabetic and hypoglycemic rat brain (Pardridge and Boado, 1993; Kumagai *et al.*, 1995).

The quantification of products of BBB-specific genes has been performed in isolated brain capillaries subjected to cytocentrifugation followed by immunocytochemistry (Fig. 17.1, A). This powerful technique combines the determination of the abundance of a particular gene product with its cellular localization within the brain microvasculature (i.e. endothelial, pericyte or smooth muscle cells). Using this approach, it has been demonstrated that the smooth muscle α-actin protein is expressed at pre-capillary arterioles of isolated brain microvessels (Fig. 17.1, A), whereas no immunostaining was observed in either capillary endothelial cells or in pericytes (arrows in Fig. 17.1, A,) of normal brain capillaries (Boado and Pardridge, 1994*b*). Whether these cell types express smooth muscle α-actin under pathological conditions is at present unknown. Since capillaries are isolated under RNase-free conditions, this preparation may be suitable for conventional or fluorescence *in situ* hybridization, or *in situ* PCR.

Molecular cloning of BBB-specific genes

Isolation of Poly(A)$^+$ mRNA by either the two-step method or the single-step method allows for the synthesis of complementary DNA using AMV-RT (AMV is avian myeloblastosis virus) and oligo-d(T) primer (Fig. 17.1, IV and V), and this material has been employed for the preparation of BBB-cDNA libraries (Table 17.1). Using 10 µg Poly(A)$^+$ mRNA isolated using the conventional two-step method, a BBB-λgt11 cDNA expression library has been prepared, and the bovine GLUT1 cDNA was isolated (Boado and Pardridge, 1990a). This BBB-λgt11 cDNA library was comprised of 1.32×10^6 independent clones and 88% recombinants. The insert size has been described to be from 0.6 to >4 kb with an average insert size of 1.7 kb. A clone containing an insert size of approximately 2.2 kb corresponding to bovine GLUT1 has been isolated with a rat cDNA probe and it corresponded to the 3′ end of the 2619 nucleotide long GLUT1 mRNA. The 5′ end of the bovine GLUT1 transcript has been isolated in a secondary screening of the same library to complete the full-length bovine GLUT1 mRNA (Boado and Pardridge, 1990a). The position of the start site of the transcript of the bovine BBB–GLUT1 has been determined by primer extension analysis, and found to correspond to the beginning of the cDNA clone isolated from this λgt11 cDNA library (Boado and Pardridge, 1990a). Other authors have used similar techniques for the preparation of λgt10 cDNA libraries, and the isolation of clones corresponding to porcine GLUT1 and porcine γ-GTP have been reported (Table 17.1). Preparation of cDNA libraries in the vector λgt11 or λ-ZAP allows for both cloning with DNA probes and expression cloning with antibodies, whereas λgt10 libraries are designed for screening with DNA probes only. A strategy for preparation of cDNA libraries enriched in a particular transcript, for example, low abundant transcripts or tissue-specific transcripts, is named subtraction cloning. In this approach, Poly(A)⁺ RNA is isolated from tissue or cell line of interest (i.e. brain capillaries) and is used as a template to synthesize cDNA. This cDNA is then annealed to Poly(A)⁺ RNA extracted from a second cell line or tissue in which the gene of interest is not expressed. The cDNAs that do not form hybrids during hybridization (specific genes) are then purified and used for the construction of cDNA libraries. This approach was used for the cloning of BBB-specific genes using lung Poly(A)⁺ mRNA in this subtraction procedure (Weiler-Gütter et al., 1990). Nineteen randomly selected clones were isolated from a library of 20 000 independent recombinants. DNA sequence analysis showed that two of these clones were GLUT1, one was Apo (i.e. apolipoprotein)

A-1, and other clones were related to glial-specific mRNA species, which the authors have speculated to correspond to a minor glial content in the brain capillary preparation (Weiler-Gütter et al., 1990; Zinke et al. 1992). Although no new specific BBB clones have been reported using this approach, this technique may be of potential benefit for isolation of BBB-specific genes.

BBB-Poly(A)⁺ RNA may be used for direct injection into *Xenopus laevis* oocytes for identification and cloning of BBB-specific genes. Kannan et al. (1996) have recently reported the existence of the sodium-dependent glutathione transporter using bovine brain capillary mRNA, which is different from γ-glutamyl transpeptidase and the facilitative glutathione transporter.

The PCR technique has also been used for either cloning or generation of specific regions of BBB transcripts as in the case of GLUT1 5′-UTR and cloning of BBB-protein kinase (Boado et al., 1996; Dechert et al., 1994).

BBB-reporter genes

The availability of BBB-specific cDNAs by either cloning of novel BBB transcript or identification of known BBB-specific genes as in the case of GLUT1, γ-GTP, and Apo A-1, provides the opportunity for construction of BBB-reporter genes. Vectors containing regulatory sequences of BBB-transcripts may be employed for either the investigation of their function at the molecular level or for the identification of brain trophic factors involved in their regulation. For example, it has been demonstrated that the expression of the BBB–GLUT1 gene is exerted at the post-transcriptional level in different pathophysiological conditions. Thus, glucose deprivation increased the abundance of GLUT1 transcript through a mechanism mediated by mRNA stabilization without changes in the transcriptional rate of this gene (Boado and Pardridge, 1993). In addition, dissociation between the levels of GLUT1 mRNA and protein has been described during development, in brain tumors and in diabetes mellitus (Pardridge and Boado, 1993; Boado et al., 1994b, Nagamatsu et al., 1993). Moreover, deletion of 171 nucleotides of the 5′-UTR of human GLUT1 mRNA, which is comprised of 179 nucleotides, produced a marked decrease in the translation efficiency of this transcript, suggesting that this region of the BBB–GLUT1 contains control elements involved in the translational regulation of the GLUT1 expression (Boado *et al.*, 1996). In order to functionally characterize *cis*-acting elements involved in the translational control of the GLUT1 transcript, a series of vectors containing different fragments of human GLUT1 5′-UTR have been prepared with the aid of PCR. Fragments of GLUT1 5′-UTR ranging from 18 to 171 nucleotides have been generated containing *Hin*dIII restriction endonuclease sequence at both ends for direct subcloning into the single *Hin*dIII site of the luciferase expression vector pGL2 promoter (Boado *et al.*, 1996). The firefly luciferase is preferred to the bacterial chloramphenicol acetyltransferase as reporter gene because it is two orders of magnitude more sensitive, rapid and the determination of its enzymatic activity does not require the use of radioactive substrates.

Different BBB–GLUT1 reporter gene constructs have been used for transfection of brain endothelial cultured cells and these vectors yielded the transcripts shown in Fig. 17.3, A. Transfection with the luciferase construct containing nucleotides 1–171 of the human GLUT1 5′-UTR resulted in more than 3-fold increase in luciferase expression (Fig. 17.3, B). The stimulatory effect has been further localized at nucleotides 1–96 and 123–153 of human GLUT1 5′-UTR. On the contrary, disruption of the luciferase leading sequence with an unrelated 171 nucleotide fragment has decreased expression of this protein, suggesting that the stimulatory effect of 5′-UTR of human GLUT1 has been exerted in a sequence-specific manner, probably through a *cis-/trans*-acting interaction (Boado *et al.*, 1996). In addition, this luciferase expression construct containing the human GLUT1 translational control elements may be used for characterization of brain-derived factors involved in the molecular expression of this gene. For example, increased stability of BBB GLUT1 mRNA by brain-derived factors in a neurotropic preparation (Cerebrolysin, EBEWE, Austria) possessing neurotrophic factor-like action (Akai *et al.*, 1992; Ruther *et al.*, 1994) has been recently associated with augmented gene expression using a

BBB–GLUT1 reporter gene in brain capillary endothelial cultured cells (Boado, 1995*b*, 1996).

Furthermore, RNA/cytosolic protein complexes of 88–120 kDa have recently been identified in human and rat brain tumors that bind to a specific sequence in the 3′-UTR of both bovine and human GLUT1 transcripts (Dwyer *et al.*, 1996; Tsukamoto *et al.*, 1996). This region has been located at nucleotides 2180–2197 of bovine GLUT1 mRNA, which is 100% conserved among species. Since the malignancy of human brain gliomas has been correlated with expression of GLUT1 and GLUT3 transcripts in the tumor parenchyma, and since these tumors did not produce GLUT1 protein, it is possible that understanding of the function of the 88–120 kDa GLUT1 RNA/cytosolic protein complex may provide insights into the post-transcriptional regulation of GLUT1 gene. In order to test this hypothesis, the 200 base pairs encompassing this *cis*-acting element have been introduced in the unique PflMI site within the 3′-UTR of the luciferase pGL2 promoter vector. Transfection of C6 rat glioma cells has resulted in a 6-fold increase in luciferase expression compared to the parental pGL2 construct without bovine GLUT1 insert or with a construct containing the bovine GLUT1 inserted in reverse orientation. This data provides evidence suggesting that indeed the post-transcriptional regulation of GLUT1 gene expression may be mediated by interaction of cytosolic-specific proteins within the GLUT1 mRNA 3′-UTR. Whether this cytoplasmic *trans*-acting factor is present in normal brain capillaries or decreased in brain microvessels surrounding brain tumors is at present unknown.

Summary

The BBB evolved to protect the brain against peripheral neurotransmitter cytotoxins and microorganisms, and the highly differentiated properties of this barrier arise from the expression of BBB-specific genes. Downregulation of these genes (i.e. GLUT1, γ-GTP), has been associated with lack of barrier functions, as in the case of brain tumors, injury, or brain microvascular endothelial cultured cells. Identification of brain trophic factors involved

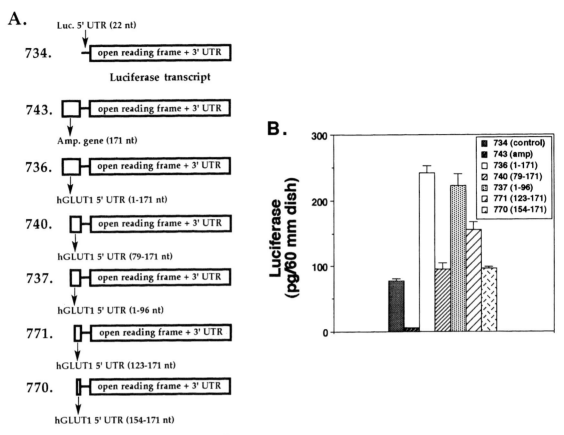

Fig. 17.3. Effect of GLUT1 5′-UTR on the expression of luciferase in brain endothelial cultured cells. A series of cDNA fragments corresponding to the human GLUT1 5′-UTR were generated by PCR and subcloned into the single *Hin*dIII site of the luciferase expression vector pGL2. In addition, 171 nucleotides of the ampicillin resistant gene (negative control) were also generated by PCR and subcloned in pGL2. Bovine endothelial cultured cells were plated in 60 mm dishes and transfected with 5 μg plasmid and 25 μg transfectam reagent. Transfection of cells with the various luciferase expression vectors yielded the transcript depicted in (A); numbers on the left-hand side represent number of clones assigned in this laboratory. Luciferase activity was determined 48 hours after transfection and expressed as pg/dish in (B). Bars represent mean ±S.E. (*n* = 3). Insertion of the hGLUT1 5′-UTR (736) produced a marked increase in the luciferase expression compared to the control without inserted cDNA (734). Disruption of the luciferase leader RNA with the 171 nucleotides corresponding to the ampicillin resistant gene decreased luciferase expression (743). Most of the hGLUT1 5′-UTR stimulatory effect was retained by clones 737 and 771. From Boado *et al.*, 1996, with permission of Lippincott-Raven Publishers.

in the expression of BBB-specific genes may be of importance for both augmentation of gene expression of BBB-specific genes and restoration of barrier properties. The understanding of the expression of these tissue-specific genes may result from the investigation of the molecular biology of brain capillaries. The expression of BBB-specific genes may be studied at both the protein and transcript levels following a simple one-step procedure for isolation of BBB proteins and Poly(A)$^+$ mRNA. BBB-transcripts may be quantified by Northern blotting or RT Q-PCR, or used for molecular cloning and construction of expression libraries. Preparation of BBB-reporter gene may markedly increase the sensitivity of detection reducing the number of cells required, and may be used for investigating gene function or screening of brain trophic factors involved in their regulation. In addition, cytocentrifugation followed by immuno-cytochemistry allows for determination of the cellular localization of gene products.

Acknowledgments

Emily Yu typed the manuscript. The author is indebted to Dr W. Pardridge for many valuable discussions. This research was supported by NIH grant P01-NS25554, American Heart Association (Los Angeles Affiliate) grant 1025-GI, and EBEWE Pharmaceuticals.

References

Akai, F., Himura, S., Sato, T. *et al.* (1992). Neurotrophic factor-like effect of FPF1070 on septal cholinergic neurons after transections of fimbria-fornix in the rat. *Histol. Histopathol.*, **7**, 213–21.

Arthur, F. E., Shivers, R. R. and Bowman, P. D. (1987). Astrocyte-mediated induction of tight junctions in brain capillary endothelium: an efficient in vitro model. *Dev. Brain Res.*, **36**, 155–9.

Bauer, H., Sonnleitner, U., Lametschwnatner, A. *et al.* (1995). Ontogenic expression of the erythroid-type glucose transporter (Glut 1) in the telencephalon of the mouse: correlation to the tightening of the blood–brain barrier. *Dev. Brain Res.*, **86**, 317–25.

Boado, R. J. (1995a). Antisense drug delivery through the blood–brain barrier. *Adv. Drug Deliv. Rev.*, **15**, 73–107.

Boado, R. J. (1995b). Brain-derived peptides regulate the steady state levels and increase stability of the blood–brain barrier GLUT1 glucose transporter mRNA. *Neurosci. Let.*, **197**, 179–82.

Boado, R. J. (1996). Brain-derived peptides increase the expression of a blood–brain barrier (BBB) GLUT1 glucose transporter reporter gene. *Neurosci. Lett.*, **220**, 53–6.

Boado, R. J., and Pardridge, W. M. (1990a). Molecular cloning of the bovine blood–brain barrier glucose transporter cDNA and demonstration of phyloge-netic conservation of the 5′-untranslated region. *Molec. Cell. Neurosci.*, **1**, 224–32.

Boado, R. J., and Pardridge, W. M. (1990b). The brain-type glucose transporter mRNA is specifically expressed at the blood–brain barrier. *Biochem. Biophys. Res. Comm.*, **166**, 174–9.

Boado, R. J. and Pardridge, W. M. (1991). A one-step procedure for isolation of (A)⁺ mRNA from isolated brain capillaries and endothelial cells in culture. *J. Neurochem.*, **57**, 2136–9.

Boado, R. J., and Pardridge, W. M. (1993). Glucose deprivation causes post-transcriptional enhancement of brain capillary endothelial glucose transporter gene expression via GLUT1 mRNA stabilization. *J. Neurochem.*, **60**, 2290–6.

Boado, R. J., and Pardridge, W. M. (1994a). Measurement of blood–brain barrier GLUT1 glucose transporter and actin mRNA by a quantitative polymerase chain reaction assay. *J. Neurochem.*, **62**, 2085–90.

Boado, R. J. and Pardridge, W. M. (1994b). Differential expression of α-actin mRNA and immunoreactive protein in brain microvascular pericytes and smooth muscle cells. *J. Neurosci. Res.*, **39**, 430–5.

Boado, R. J., Pardridge, W. M., Vinters, H. V. and Black, K. L. (1992). Differential expression of arachidonate 5-lipoxygenase transcripts in human brain tumors: evidence for the expression of a multitranscript family. *Proc. Natl. Acad. Sci. USA*, **89**, 9044–8.

Boado, R. J., Wang, L. and Pardridge, W. M. (1994a). Enhanced expression of the blood–brain barrier GLUT1 glucose transporter gene by brain-derived factors. *Molec. Brain Res.*, **22**, 259–67.

Boado, R. J., Black, K. L. and Pardridge, W. M. (1994b). Gene expression of GLUT3 and GLUT1 glucose transporters in human brain tumors. *Molec. Brain Res.*, **27**, 51–7.

Boado, R. J., Tsukamoto, H. and Pardridge, W. M. (1996). Evidence for transcriptional control elements in 5′-untranslated region of GLUT1 glucose transporter mRNA. *J. Neurochem.*, **67**, 1335–43.

Bolz, S., Farrell, C. L., Dietz, K. and Wolburg, H. (1996). Subcellular distribution of glucose transporter (GLUT-1) during development of the blood–brain barrier in rats. *Cell Tiss. Res.*, **284**, 355–65.

Bondy, C. A., Lee, W.-H. and Zhou, J. (1992). Ontogeny and cellular distribution of brain glucose transporter gene expression. *Molec. Cell. Neurosci.*, **3**, 305–14.

Brightman, M. W. (1977). Morphology of blood–brain interfaces. *Exp. Eye Res.*, **25**, 1–25.

Chirgwin, J. M., Przybyla, A. E., MacDonald, R. J. and Rutter, W. J. (1979). Isolation of biologically active ribonucleic acid from sources enriched in ribonuclease. *Biochemistry*, **18**, 5294–9.

Chomczynski, P. and Sacchi, N. (1987). Single step method of RNA isolation by acid guanidinium thiocyanate-phenol-chloroform extraction. *Anal. Biochem.*, **162**, 156–9.

DeBault, L. E. and Cancilla, P. A. (1980). Gamma glutamyl transpeptidase in isolated brain endothelial cells: induction by glial cells in vitro. *Science*, **207**, 653–5.

Dechert, U., Weber, P., König, B. *et al.* (1994). A protein kinase isolated from porcine brain microvessels is similar to a class of heat-shock proteins. *Eur. J. Biochem.*, **225**, 405–9.

Dermietzel, R., Krause, D., Kremer, M. *et al.* (1992). Pattern of glucose transporter (Glut 1) expression in embryonic brains is related to maturation of blood–brain barrier. *Dev. Dyn.*, **193**, 152–63.

Dwyer, K. J., Boado, R. J. and Pardridge, W. M. (1996). Cis-element/cytoplasmic protein interaction within the 3'-untranslated region of the GLUT1 glucose transporter mRNA. *J. Neurochem.*, **66**, 449–58.

Guerrin, C., Laterra, J., Hruban, R. H. *et al.* (1990). The glucose transporter and blood–brain barrier of human brain tumors. *Ann. Neurol.*, **28**, 758–65.

Harik, S. I. and Roessmann, U. (1991). The erythrocyte-type glucose transporter in blood vessels of primary and metastatic brain tumors. *Ann. Neurol.*, **29**, 487–91.

Heuvel, J. P. V., Tyson, F. L. and Bell, D. A. (1993). Construction of recombinant RNA templates for use as internal standards in quantitative RT-PCR. *Biotechniques*, **14**, 395–8.

Hilz, H., Weigers, U. and Adamietz, P. (1975). Stimulation of proteinase K action by denaturing agents: application to the isolation of nucleic acids and the degradation of masked proteins. *Eur. J. Biochem.*, **56**, 103–8.

Janzer, R. C. and Raff, M. C. (1987). Astrocytes induce blood–brain barrier properties in endothelial cells. *Nature*, **325**, 253–7.

Kannan, R., Yi, J. R., Tang, D. *et al.* (1996). Evidence for the existence of a sodium-dependent glutathione (GSH) transporter. Expression of bovine brain capillary mRNA and size fractions in *Xenopus laevis* oocytes and dissociation from γ-glutamyltranspeptidase and facilitative GSH transporters. *J. Biol. Chem.*, **271**, 9754–8.

Kumagai, A. K., Kang, Y-S, Boado, R. J. and Pardridge, W. M. (1995). Upregulation of blood–brain barrier GLUT1 glucose transporter protein and mRNA in experimental chronic hypoglycemia. *Diabetes*, **44**, 1390–404.

Nagamatsu, S., Sawa, H., Wakizaka, A. and Hoshino, T. (1993). Expression of facilitated glucose transporter isoforms in human brain tumors. *J. Neurochem.*, **61**, 2048–53.

Nagashima, T., Shigin, W., Mizoguchi, A. *et al.* (1994). The effect of leukotriene C4 on the permeability of brain capillary endothelial cell monolayer. *Acta Neurochirurg.* [Suppl.] **60**, 55–7.

Palos, T. P., Ramachandran, B., Boado, R. and Howard, B. D. (1996). Rat C6 and human astrocytic tumor cells express a neuronal type of glutamate transporter. *Molec. Brain Res.*, **37**, 297–303.

Papandrikopoulou, A., Frey, A. and Gassen, H. G. (1989). Cloning and expression of γ-glutamyl transpeptidase from isolated porcine brain capillaries. *Eur. J. Biochem.*, **183**, 693–8.

Pardridge, W. M. (1995). Transport of small molecules through the blood–brain barrier: biology and methodology. *Adv. Drug Del. Rev.*, **15**, 5–36.

Pardridge, W. M. and Boado, R. J. (1993). Molecular cloning and regulation of gene expression of blood–brain barrier glucose transporter, in *The Blood–Brain Barrier: Cellular and Molecular Biology*, pp. 395–440. New York: Raven Press.

Pardridge, W. M., Boado, R. J. and Farrell, C. R. (1990). Brain-type glucose transporter (GLUT-1) is selectively localized to the blood–brain barrier. Studies with quantitative western blotting and in situ hybridization. *J. Biol. Chem.*, **265**, 18035–40.

Rosenstein, J. M. and More, N. S. (1994). Immunocytochemical expression of the blood–brain barrier glucose transporter (GLUT-1) in neural transplants and brain wounds. *J. Comp. Neurol.*, **350**, 229–40.

Ruther, E., Ritter, R., Apecechea, M. *et al.* (1994). Efficacy of the peptidergic nootropic drug Cerebrolysin in patients with senile dementia of the Alzheimer type (SDAT). *Pharmacopsychiatry*, **27**, 32–40.

Sandouk, T., Reda, D. and Hofmann, C. (1993). The antidiabetic agent pioglitazone increases expression of glucose transporters in 3T3-F442A cells by increasing messenger ribonucleic acid transcript stability. *Endocrinology*, **133**, 352–9.

Stewart, P. A. and Wiley, M. J. (1981). Developing nervous tissue induces formation of blood–brain barrier characteristics in invading endothelial cells: a study using quail-chick transplantation chimera. *Dev. Biol.*, **84**, 183–92.

Taniguchi, N., Lizuka, S., Zhe, Z. N. *et al.* (1985). Measurement of human serum immunoreactive γ-glutamyl transpeptidase in patients with malignant tumors using enzyme-linked immunosorbent assay. *Cancer Res.*, **45**, 5835–9.

Tontsch, U. and Bauer, H. C. (1991). Glial cells and neurons induce blood–brain barrier related enzymes in cultured cerebral endothelial cells. *Brain Res.*, **539**, 247–53.

Tsukamoto, H., Boado, R. J. and Pardridge, W. M. (1996). Differential expression in glioblastoma multiforme and cerebral hemangioblastoma of cytoplasmic proteins that bind two different domains within the 3'-untranslated region of the human glucose transporter 1 messenger RNA. *J. Clin. Invest.*, **97**, 2823–32.

Weiler-Gütter, H., Zinke, H., Möckel, B. *et al.* (1989). cDNA cloning and sequence analysis of the glucose transporter from porcine blood–brain barrier. *Biol. Chem. Hoppe-Seyler*, **370**, 467–73.

Weiler-Gütter, H., Sommerfeldt, M., Papandrikopoulou, A. *et al.* (1990). Synthesis of apolipoprotein A-1 in pig brain microvascular endothelial cells. *J. Neurochem.*, **54**, 444–50.

Zinke, H., Möckel, B., Frey, A. *et al.* (1992). Blood–brain barrier: a molecular approach to its structural and functional characterization. In *Progress in Brain Res.*, ed. A. Ermisch, R. Landgraf and H.-J. Rühle, Vol. 91, pp. 103–15.

PART II

Transport biology

18 Biology of the blood–brain glucose transporter

LESTER R. DREWES

- Introduction
- Structure
- How GLUT1 works
- GLUT1 expression
- Regulatory mechanisms
- Summary

Introduction

During the past decade there has been remarkable advancement in our knowledge about the molecular components involved in the fundamental biological function of membrane transport, the movement of a molecule (or two different molecules as in co-transport) from one side of an impermeable biological membrane to the other side. Despite these advancements, scientists only now are poised to discover the answers to key questions regarding the actual mechanism of transport of simple hydrophilic molecules, the regulation of intrinsic transporter activity, the pathways of intracellular trafficking of transporters and their targeting to specific plasma locations, and the factors that signal transporter expression in a cell-specific and a temporal-specific manner.

The system of glucose transport in the brain ranks with high importance in neuroscience because of two fundamental observations made previously. First, the brain exhibits a nearly exclusive appetite for blood-borne glucose to sustain a high rate of aerobic metabolism. Secondly, the brain vasculature is lined with a layer of endothelial cells that form tight junctional contacts and thus prevent any gaps or spaces between cells that would allow

for the free movement of blood-borne glucose (or other hydrophilic substances) into the brain extracellular space. The existence of this so called blood–brain barrier led to the suggestion that this substrate enters the brain by transcellular transport systems, a hypothesis that was proposed, tested and reported in the now classic pioneering studies of Professor Christian Crone of the University of Copenhagen (Crone, 1965).

Structure

Blood–brain transport of D-glucose occurs by transcellular transport through the endothelial cells that line the brain vasculature. It is carried out by an integral membrane protein embedded in the endothelial cell plasma membrane located on both the luminal (blood–endothelial cell interface) and abluminal (endothelial cell–extracellular matrix interface) sides of the cell. The glucose transporter protein, known as GLUT1, is the product of a single gene consisting of 10 (or 11 depending on the species) exons spanning about 30 kb of chromosomal DNA. In humans the gene is assigned to a chromosomal location at chromosome 1p33. In most species studied, the brain vascular GLUT1

Table 18.1. *Sequence similarities of the blood–brain glucose transporter (GLUT1) in mammalian species*

Species	Sequence similarity to human cDNA (%)	Sequence similarity to human amino acid (%)	Genbank accession number
Human	100	100	K03195
Rabbit	93	96	M21747
Cow	92	96	M60448
Mouse	89	96	M22998
Rat	89	97	M13979
Pig	85	89	X17058
Chicken	78	88	L07300

mRNA is a single transcribed product of 2.7–2.9 kb in length with a sequence encoding a protein that contains 492 amino acids. Of the seven species for which the GLUT1 sequence has been reported, the mRNA sequence is greatly conserved and ranges from 93% to 78% identical when compared to the human sequence (Table 18.1). The GLUT1 protein is similarly conserved with most species having amino acid sequences identical by 96% or greater. Pig and chicken sequences are slightly less than 90% in identity to the human protein sequence.

The fundamental importance of glucose as a substrate and energy resource for higher organisms has led to the evolutionary development of multiple membrane proteins that transport D-glucose and are closely related to GLUT1. This family of transporters add significant redundancy to this basic process, allow very specific spatial and temporal expression patterns, and incorporate unique regulatory mechanisms. In addition to GLUT1, there are five other members of the glucose transporter family that, on the basis of their sequences and resulting biochemical characteristics, are related. The expression of GLUT2 in adult tissues is primarily in liver and pancreatic β cells and has the highest K_m (lowest affinity) while GLUT3 is nearly exclusively in neuronal cells of the nervous system and has a relatively low K_m. Under basal conditions GLUT4 is the major transporter present in adipose and muscle cells, but it is not functionally active in the plasma membrane until it is recruited in response to insulin stimulation. The intestine is the location for significant expression of GLUT5, a transporter that shares affinity with the ketohexose, D-fructose, and is probably responsible for dietary absorption of this sugar. GLUT6 is a misnomer because it contains stop codons and frame shifts within its coding sequence and is, therefore, classified a pseudogene. However, GLUT7 is a novel transporter because it is the only transporter not targeted for the plasma membrane, but rather the membrane of the endoplasmic reticulum where it is believed to function in association with glucose 6-phosphatase in the process of gluconeogenesis and glycogenolysis to transport glucose from inside the cellular organelle to the cytoplasm. A short amino acid sequence on the carboxyl terminal end is believed to be the signal for directing this protein to the endoplasmic reticular membrane. Several excellent reviews that compare and contrast the six members of the GLUT family have appeared in recent years (Bell *et al.*, 1993; Gould and Holman, 1993; Olson and Pessin, 1996).

Additional details of GLUT structures have been revealed from studies using peptide specific antibodies, glycohydrolases, affinity probes, and deduction from sequence analysis (Holman, 1989). As an integral membrane protein, GLUT1 contains multiple membrane spanning segments with the carboxyl- and amino-terminal ends extending from the cytoplasmic side. The estimates for the number of transmembrane segments varies between 12 and 16 depending on the extent of α-helical or β-sheet conformation attributed to the spanning segments (Fig. 18.1). Standard hydropathy profiles suggest the smaller number, but structural analogies to the bacterial porins, for which X-ray crystallographic analyses are complete suggests up to 16 hydrophobic segments arranged in a circular array with a glucose binding site in the channel-like core (Fischbarg *et al.*, 1993). A single *N*-glycosylation site is located at asparagine 45 between transmembrane segments 1 and 2 on the exofacial side of the membrane. The nature of the attached carbohydrate may vary in quality and quantity and results in distinct molecular species that can be distinguished as separate GLUT1 forms by electrophoresis on SDS gels. The GLUT1 located in the brain endothelium resembles the human erythrocyte form in having an average apparent

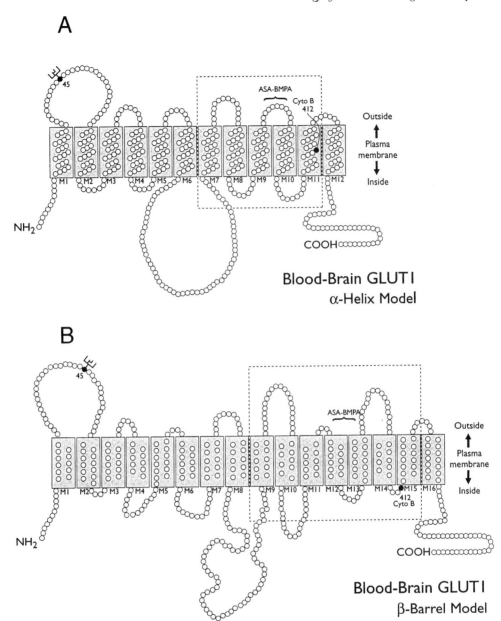

Fig. 18.1. Models of membrane embedded GLUT1 structures. Two alternative structures have been proposed. (A) The α-helix model is based primarily on a hydropathy profile of the GLUT1 amino acid sequence and consists of 12 transmembrane α-helixes of about 21 amino acids each. The locations of the transport inhibitors cytochalasin b (Cyto B, amino acid 412) and the bis-mannitol compound (ASA-BMPA) are shown. The rectangle with dashed line border is believed to enclose the transmembrane segments most directly involved in sugar binding and translocation. (B) The antiparallel β-barrel model is based primarily on antibody binding studies and secondary structure similarity to bacterial porins that have been subjected to X-ray crystallographic analysis. Inhibitor binding sites and rectangle are as in (A).

weight of 55 000 daltons. In contrast, the GLUT1 of the choroid plexus (blood–CSF barrier) has a much lower apparent weight of 46 000 daltons, a size similar to that of the GLUT1 form that is primarily associated with brain astrocytes (Dick *et al.*, 1984; Kumagai *et al.*, 1994; Maher *et al.*, 1994; Vannucci *et al.*, 1994).

A relatively long hydrophilic loop about midway in the GLUT1 sequence also has a cytoplasmic orientation. This central loop contains potential phosphorylation sites and hydrophilic amino acids that may be important for GLUT1 interactions with enzymes of carbohydrate metabolism such as the hexokinases or with cytoskeletal elements and other cytoplasmic proteins. Based on substrate and inhibitor binding data it is believed that substrate binding and translocation occurs with the carboxyl terminal half of the transporter.

Eukaryotic expression systems such as the yeast system and the baculovirus-infected insect cell system are now available that yield large quantities of homogeneous GLUT1. For a definitive picture of the three-dimensional organization of the GLUT1 polypeptide and its associated membrane environment, subsequent development of crystallization techniques for membrane proteins such as GLUT1 are needed.

How GLUT1 works

GLUT1, located in the luminal and abluminal membranes of the brain endothelial cells, serves as a facilitative carrier with a K_m of 2–5 mM for glucose and variable affinity for other sugars and inhibitors (Table 18.2).

Glucose travels transcellularly down its concentration gradient from about 5 mM in blood to about 0.5–3.5 mM in the brain extracellular fluid. Extensive kinetic analysis combined with detailed chemical and proteolytic studies of GLUT1 indicate that the functional protein exists in the membrane as a tetrameric homo-oligomer with one catalytically active binding site per subunit (Coderre *et al.*, 1995). However, at any instant two binding sites are presented on the extracellular side and two on the cytoplasmic side. It is hypothesized that when sugar binds to one subunit and is transported, there is a simultaneous generation of a new binding site on the opposite side of the membrane

Table 18.2. *Kinetic parameters of the blood–brain facilitative glucose transporter (GLUT1)*

Substrate	K_m (mM)	IC$_{50}$ (mM)
D-Glucose	2–5	5
2-Deoxyglucose	7	—
3-O-Methylglucose	26	—
D-Galactose	17	—
D-Fructose	N.T.	—
Cytochalasin B	N.D.	0.0001

From *in vitro* studies of *Xenopus* oocytes expressing GLUT1 and *in vivo* measurements (Gould and Holman 1993).
N.T. = Not transported.
N.D. = Not determined.

by an adjoining subunit. This cooperative property is specific to the tetrameric GLUT1 forms because dimeric forms lack cooperativity. Thus, transport requires the cooperative interaction of tetrameric subunits and the coupling of subunit binding sites. The use of substrate analogs in kinetics experiments indicates that the D-pyranose ring structure is the preferred substrate of GLUT1 and that glucose carbon positions C-1, C-3, and C-6 are critically important in binding (Silverman, 1991). Interaction of sugar with the GLUT1 binding site likely involves the breaking of hydrogen bonds between the glucose hydroxyls and water and the formation of new hydrogen bonds between the sugar and polar amino acid side chains lining the transporter passageway. The activation energy for substrate binding (~ 11 kcal/mol) and the network of polar amino acids located in several transmembrane segments of GLUT1 are consistent with a substrate-induced conformational change that results in a transmembrane sugar translocation. Availability in the future of a three-dimensional structure of GLUT1 will make an understanding of the chemical mechanism much less speculative.

GLUT1 expression

Endothelial cell location and subcellular distribution

There is considerable overlap in the tissue distribution and expression of the various GLUT family

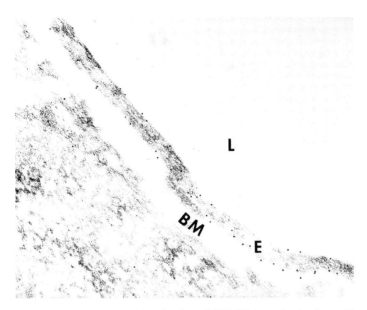

Fig. 18.2. Ultrastructural localization of GLUT1 in canine brain capillary. Canine cerebellum was subjected to post-embedding immunogold labeling (anti-GLUT1 antibody) as described previously for dog cerebral cortex (Gerhart *et al.*, 1989). Gold particles are localized primarily on the luminal and abluminal membranes with some distributed over cytoplasmic regions. L, capillary lumen; E, endothelial cell; BM, basement membrane.

members. However, GLUT1 is expressed at high levels in probably all fetal tissues. In adult human tissues GLUT1 expression decreases, but is detectable in adipose, muscle and liver tissues. GLUT1 remains elevated in endothelial cells of the brain and in the erythrocytes, cells in which only one isoform of glucose transporter is present. It has been estimated that the amount of GLUT1 relative to the total erythrocyte membrane protein may be as high as 5%, a figure that is comparable to the amount of GLUT1 in brain endothelial cell membranes as well (Dick *et al.*, 1984). Immuno-electron microscopy of brain endothelial cells reveals that most GLUT1 is located in the luminal and abluminal membranes and in some species is asymmetrically distributed (Gerhart *et al.*, 1989) (Fig. 18.2). In rat brain, for example, the ratio of abluminal to luminal GLUT1 is nearly 4 to 1 (Farrell and Pardridge, 1991). A significant amount (18–45%) of the total GLUT1 is also detected in cytoplasmic regions of the endothelial cell. The significance of this has not yet been clarified, although it has been suggested that this represents a storage site for GLUT1 transporter available for recruitment to the plasma membrane or an intermediate form of GLUT1 in transit between the two asymmetric cell membranes. Such a system would be analogous to the insulin-sensitive GLUT4 system of adipocytes and muscle in which GLUT4 transporters in the basal state exist in tubular vesicular structures below the cell surface and are rapidly fused into the plasma membrane as functional transporters in response to insulin receptor activation. It would follow from the brain GLUT1 hypothesis that redistribution of GLUT1 molecules in the endothelial cell would increase the blood–brain glucose transport capacity of the cell in response to an external chemical signal. Such a signaling mechanism would increase local blood–brain glucose transport during periods when local glucose consumption increases several-fold as a result of neuronal activation. Altern-atively, the cytoplasmic immunoreactive elements may represent biosynthetic precursors of GLUT1 or proteolytic products of GLUT1 degradation. Further studies are needed to explore these alter-native hypotheses.

Development

Brain endothelial GLUT1 has been examined in rats at stages of development from late embryonic

L. R. DREWES

Table 18.3. *Changes in vascular GLUT1 expression in brain in response to various stimuli or stress conditions*

Stimulus/Stress	Response in blood–brain GLUT1 expression
Development, CNS maturation	Increase
Glioma	Decrease
Hypoxia	Increase
Ischemia	Increase
Hyperglycemia–spontaneous	Decrease
Hyperglycemia–diabetic	Variable
Hypoglycemia	Increase
Seizures (epilepsy)	Increase
Endothelial cell transplant to CNS	Increase

periods through adulthood (Devaskar *et al.*, 1991; Dermietzel *et al.*, 1992; Vannucci *et al.*, 1994). GLUT1 protein and mRNA levels gradually increase from about 40% of their adult levels at birth and reach near adult levels by 21 days of age soon after weaning. Thus, the expression closely follows the changes in cerebral glucose utilization rate rather than anatomical or other developmental changes (Vannucci *et al.*, 1994). Not only does the microvascular GLUT1 increase rapidly between ages 7 and 21 days, but the functional activity of the protein also increases in a parallel manner as determined by *in vivo* transport measurements using radioactively labeled 2-deoxyglucose. In contrast to other brain structures, the microvessels of the circumventricular organs do not contain a tight endothelium and lack the barrier properties associated with the brain microvasculature (Zeller *et al.*, 1996). Accordingly, GLUT1 is absent from the capillary endothelium of the circumventricular organs and the choroid plexus of the adult rat. The absence of GLUT1 exists during all stages of postnatal development, although in the area postrema and subfornical organ, GLUT1, present at birth, is rapidly lost.

Brain tumors

Brain tumors, either spontaneous or experimentally induced from immortalized cells lines, are classified into several categories primarily based on their rate of cell division and growth. Tumor cell metabolism is dependent on a sufficient nutrient supply and vascular delivery system that expands by neovascularization of the enlarging tumor mass. The vascular endothelium of brain tumors loses its tight junctions and associated barrier properties as well as the expression of the blood–brain glucose transporter GLUT1. In human brain tumors classified according to their growth rate it was found that the expression of vascular GLUT1 was inversely proportional to the rate of tumor growth with the most aggressive glioblastoma multiforme having the least immunoreactive transporter (Guerin *et al.*, 1990; Harik and Roessmann, 1991). A similar observation was made in a series of experimentally induced rat brain gliomas (Guerin *et al.*, 1992). Thus, it appears that blood–brain glucose transport is unnecessary for tumor nutrient supply when the endothelium lacks barrier properties. However, an exception in humans may be the relatively rare hemangioblastoma in which the endothelium is leaky, but the GLUT1 expression in the endothelium remains high (Cornford *et al.*, 1995*a*).

Hypoxia/ischemia

Cerebral energy metabolism is highly dependent on the aerobic metabolism of glucose. Therefore, under conditions of limited oxygen supply, a shift toward anaerobic glycolytic metabolism and increased glucose consumption will occur. Under conditions of prolonged hypoxia created by reducing the atmospheric pressure to one-half normal, significant adaptations were observed in rat brain after one week including an estimated 25% increase in microvessel GLUT1 (Harik *et al.*, 1994). Expression of vascular GLUT1 has also been examined following acute forms of oxygen deprivation, namely ischemia induced by transient or permanent vascular occlusion. Under transient conditions no significant alteration of vascular GLUT1 is observed (Gerhart *et al.*, 1994). However, a stronger ischemic insult such as occurs following middle cerebral artery occlusion in rat results in significantly increased GLUT1 mRNA after 24 hours (McCall *et al.*, 1996; Urabe *et al.*, 1996). The modest increases in GLUT1 mRNA, however, may correlate to substantial changes in the expression of GLUT1 protein, which is also increased after 24 hours and remains elevated for 4 days. Similar findings of increased vascular GLUT1 have been observed within 4 hr after ischemic insult with a maximum response after 24 hours in 7-day-old rat pups (Vannucci *et al.*, 1996).

Hypo- and hyperglycemia

The relationship between plasma glucose levels and expression of blood–brain glucose transporter is scientifically interesting and also potentially relevant to understanding the underlying mechanisms in the diabetic subject. Studies based primarily on difficult or complex *in vivo* transport measurements have led to some controversies regarding changes in blood–brain glucose transport under conditions of altered glucose and insulin levels (for review see Pelligrino *et al.*, 1992). Several initial studies of blood–brain glucose transport have concluded that in chronic hyperglycemia transport capacity is diminished. Subsequent, also carefully executed, studies have found no evidence for this decline and have even suggested a possible increase in transport capacity. Although yet unresolved, recent studies have provided additional information regarding the expression of the GLUT1 protein in cerebral microvessels and the corresponding mRNA. It now appears likely that some forms of hyperglycemia (spontaneous) lead to a quantitative decrease in glucose transport capacity and a significant down regulation of the expression of blood–brain glucose transporters (Cornford *et al.*, 1995). However, chemically induced diabetes may involve additional factors other than elevated glucose levels such as the chemical toxicity of the inducing agent, the biological action of the *db* gene product leptin, or other unknown factors. It may turn out that the pathological response to diabetes (chronic hyperglycemia) may be heterogeneous as has been observed for vascular GLUT1 expression in the blood–retinal barrier of human diabetics where a subpopulation of endothelial cells express normal amounts of GLUT1 and others exhibit hyperexpression by more than 18 times normal (Kumagai *et al.*, 1996). It is clear that additional experimental work in this area is needed to clarify the pathophysiological processes at work.

In contrast, chronic hypoglycemia is a condition that has not been as extensively studied. Hypoglycemia sustained in rats for up to one week by slow insulin infusion results in a significant increase in *in vivo* blood–brain glucose transport (Pelligrino *et al.*, 1990; Kumagai *et al.*, 1995). Furthermore, analysis of microvessel GLUT1 protein and mRNA content revealed an estimated 50% decrease when compared to matched controls. Thus, upregulation of GLUT1 occurs during chronic hypoglycemia.

Seizures

Another condition in which there is hypermetabolism of glucose is epileptic-like seizures. Intense neuronal and synaptic excitation is coupled to major energy-consuming processes involving increased glucose metabolism. Maintenance of brain ATP levels under such conditions requires a ready supply of glucose made available via the blood–brain transport system. Under conditions of repeated seizures it might be hypothesized that blood–brain GLUT1 is increased to match the glucose demand. Recent studies in which mild seizures were induced in rats demonstrated that blood–brain GLUT1 expression as well as brain GLUT3 expression are significantly increased following seizure induction (Gronlund *et al.*, 1996). These experimental findings are supported by observations of clinical material from a patient with intractable seizure activity (Cornford *et al.*, 1994). Immunoelectron microscopy of a brain biopsy from this patient indicated a many-fold increase in the density of GLUT1 in brain endothelial cell luminal and abluminal membranes.

Human genetic GLUT1 disorder

Because glucose is such an essential fuel for brain energy metabolism it was believed that any defect in the GLUT1 gene would be fatal and incompatible with life. However, in a landmark paper (DeVivo *et al.*, 1991) two unrelated pediatric patients were described with persistent hypoglycorrhachia, seizures, and delayed brain development. Based on cytochalasin B binding, erythrocyte glucose uptake, immunoblot analysis, and response to a ketogenic diet it was proposed that a partially defective GLUT1 was expressed and resulted in poor transport of glucose into the brain. This may represent a forerunner of additional diseases related to blood–brain transporter defects.

Regulatory mechanisms

Blood–brain GLUT1 and its characteristic high level of expression in the brain endothelium is the result of multiple regulatory mechanisms operating at several levels.

Transcriptional regulation

At the transcriptional level it is believed that brain-derived trophic factors exert their effect on endothelial cells by inducing the expression of blood–brain barrier specific genes. These factors are brain-specific and may consist of soluble and insoluble components that work in concert. Based on the close contact between endothelial cells and astrocytic endfeet, it has been suggested that the factors inducing brain endothelial cell GLUT1 may be astrocytic in origin. This hypothesis has been supported with experimental evidence, although the *in vitro* effects have not been robust and specific effector molecules have not yet been identified.

Based on gene activation mechanisms in other systems, trophic factors operate through membrane receptors and activate signaling pathways involving intracellular kinases and signaling intermediates. Activated transcription factors then associate with DNA response element sequences located upstream of the target gene to initiate transcription. Several known response elements have been identified in the upstream region of the GLUT1 gene and presumably are involved in upregulation of GLUT1 transcription. Several growth factors and a brain-derived extract have been shown to exhibit some enhanced expression of GLUT1 in a cultured brain endothelial cell model (Boado *et al.*, 1994; Boado, 1995).

Translational regulation

The transcription of any gene results in an mRNA molecule consisting of a coding sequence flanked by a 5′- and 3′-untranslated terminal region (UTR). The UTRs are believed to be involved in translational events such as ribosomal binding, polymerase initiation, etc. Alignment of the 5′- and 3′-UTRs for the GLUT1 molecules from various species indicates a striking conservation of sequence and suggests that these sequences may also function in post-transcriptional events. The importance of several specific sequences in the 5′- and 3′-UTRs is beginning to be recognized. For example, all GLUT1 species contain in their 3′-UTR an AUUUA motif in the context of an AU-rich region. This motif, or *cis*-regulatory sequence, is a binding site for a cytoplasmic protein (know as adenosine-uridine-binding factor, AUBF) that makes this mRNA less susceptible to degradation. AUBF, a *trans*-acting factor, may be present in endothelial cell cytoplasm or in neural cell extracts. Recently, a group of cytosolic proteins derived from extracts of cells of neural origin have been identified that associate with multiple sites on the 5′- and 3′-UTRs of GLUT1 (Boado and Pardridge, 1993). In addition, evidence has been presented that a 3′-UTR cis-regulatory sequence is functionally important in promoting translation (Dwyer *et al.*, 1996; Tsukamoto *et al.*, 1996). Thus, it appears that the mRNA–cytosolic protein interactions may prove to be critically important in the stability of mRNA and subsequently the level of expression of the GLUT1 protein by brain endothelial cells.

Intrinsic activity

The transport activity of GLUT1 molecules embedded in the plasma membrane does not appear to be altered acutely except in small degrees. To date no significant effect has been seen by endogenous inhibitors, phosphorylation, or other covalent modification, or association with other proteins or low molecular weight molecules. However, the asymmetric kinetic properties of GLUT1 may be worth examining in terms of the location and direction of net transport. It has been proposed that because influx kinetics are different than efflux kinetics the location of GLUT1 in either the luminal or abluminal membrane of the endothelial cell may make an important difference in the capacity for net transcellular glucose flux.

Thus, the potential intracellular trafficking and redistribution of the blood–brain glucose transporter (GLUT1) as discussed above may have significant consequences.

Summary

The primary transport system for blood–brain glucose transport is GLUT1 located in both the luminal and abluminal sides of the vascular endothelial cell. Expression of GLUT1 increases or decreases depending on the pathophysiological state and a defect in its synthesis may be responsible for a genetically-related neurological disease of infants and young children. Although major advances have been made in our understanding of blood–brain GLUT1, several additional questions remain. These include, what is the molecular mechanism for glucose binding and translocation? What is the endothelial cell glucose concentration and how does glucose avoid phosphorylation during transcellular transport? What is the molecular signal for targeting delivery of newly synthesized transporter specifically to either the luminal membrane or abluminal membrane? What are the trophic factors that induce GLUT1 gene transcription? What are the cytoplasmic components that stabilize or destabilize GLUT1 mRNA? What are the developmental cues that cause tissue-specific and temporal-specific expression of GLUT1? What is the mechanism of intracellular trafficking and recycling of GLUT1 protein? What effect would overexpression of blood–brain GLUT1 have on cerebral metabolism in normal animals or in neurodegenerative states? These and other questions will be answered with the continued pace of advancement in cerebral vascular biology.

Acknowledgments

The author gratefully acknowledges the important contributions of Dr. David Z. Gerhart in the studies described here and in the preparation of this manuscript. Apologies are extended to those authors who because of space constraints were unable to be cited for their important works. Also appreciated is the funding support of the National Institutes of Health with grants NS-27229, NS-32754 and NS-33824.

References

Bell, G. I., Burant, C. F., Takeda, J. and Gould, G. W. (1993). Structure and function of mammalian facilitative sugar transporters. *J. Biol. Chem.*, **268**, 19161–4.

Boado, R. J. (1995). Brain-derived peptides regulate the steady state levels and increase stability of the blood–brain barrier GLUT1 glucose transporter mRNA. *Neurosci. Lett.*, **197**, 179–82.

Boado, R. J. and Pardridge, W. M. (1993). Glucose deprivation causes posttranscriptional enhancement of brain capillary endothelial glucose transporter gene expression via GLUT1 mRNA stabilization. *J. Neurochem.*, **60**, 2290–6.

Boado, R. J., Wang, L. and Pardridge, W. M. (1994). Enhanced expression of the blood–brain barrier GLUT1 glucose transporter gene by brain-derived factors. *Mol. Brain Res.*, **22**, 259–67.

Boado, R. J., Tsukamoto, H. and Pardridge, W. M. (1996). Evidence for translational control elements within the 5′-untranslated region of GLUT1 glucose transporter mRNA. *J. Neurochem.*, **67**, 1335–43.

Coderre, P. E., Cloherty, E. K., Zottola, R. J. and Carruthers, A. (1995). Rapid substrate translocation by the multisubunit, erythroid glucose transporter requires subunit associations but not cooperative ligand binding. *Biochemistry*, **34**, 9762–73.

Cornford, E. M., Hyman, S. and Swartz, B. E. (1994). The human brain GLUT1 glucose transporter: Ultrastructural localization of the blood–brain barrier endothelia. *J. Cereb. Blood Flow Metab.*, **14**, 106–12.

Cornford, E. M., Hyman, S., Black, K. L. *et al.* (1995a). High expression of the Glut1 glucose transporter in human brain hemangioblastoma endothelium. *J. Neuropathol. Exp. Neurol.*, **54**, 842–51.

Cornford, E. M., Hyman, S., Cornford, M. E. and Clare-Salzler, M. (1995b). Down-regulation of blood–brain glucose transport in the hyperglycemic nonobese diabetic mouse. *Neurochem. Res.*, **20**, 869–73.

Crone, C. (1965). Facilitated transfer of glucose from blood into brain tissue. *J. Physiol. (Lond.)*, **181**, 103–13.

Dermietzel, R., Krause, D., Kremer, M. *et al.* (1992). Pattern of glucose transporter (Glut 1) expression in embryonic brains is related to maturation of blood–brain barrier tightness. *Dev. Biol.*, **193**, 152–63.

Devaskar, S., Zahm, D. S., Holtzclaw, L. *et al.* (1991). Developmental regulation of the distribution of rat brain insulin-insensitive (Glut 1) glucose transporter. *Endocrinology*, **129**, 1530–40.

DeVivo, D. C., Trifiletti, R. R., Jacobson, R. I. *et al.* (1991). Defective glucose transport across the blood–brain barrier as a cause of persistent hypoglycorrhachia, seizures, and developmental delay. *N. Engl. J. Med.*, **325**, 703–9.

Dick, A. P. K., Harik, S. I., Klip, A. and Walker, D. M. (1984). Identification and characterization of the glucose transporter of the blood–brain barrier by cytochalasin B binding and immunological reactivity. *Proc. Natl. Acad. Sci. USA*, **81**, 7233–7.

Dwyer, K. J., Boado, R. J. and Pardridge, W. M. (1996). *Cis*-Element/cytoplasmic protein interaction within the 3′-untranslated region of the GLUT1 glucose transporter mRNA. *J. Neurochem.*, **66**, 449–58.

Farrell, C. L. and Pardridge, W. M. (1991). Blood–brain barrier glucose transporter is asymmetrically distributed on brain capillary endothelial luminal and abluminal membranes: an electron microscopic immunogold study. *Proc. Natl. Acad. Sci. USA*, **88**, 579–83.

Fischbarg, J., Cheung, M., Czegledy, F. *et al.* (1993). Evidence that facilitative glucose transporters may fold as β-barrels. *Proc. Natl. Acad. Sci. USA*, **90**, 11658–62.

Gerhart, D. Z., LeVasseur, R. J., Broderius, M. A. and Drewes, L. R. (1989). Glucose transporter localization in brain using light and electron immunocytochemistry. *J. Neurosci. Res.*, **22**, 464–72.

Gerhart, D. Z., Leino, R. L., Taylor, W. E. *et al.* (1994). GLUT1 and GLUT3 gene expression in gerbil brain following brief ischemia: An in situ hybridization study. *Mol. Brain Res.*, **25**, 313–22.

Gould, G. W. and Holman, G. D. (1993). The glucose transporter family: structure, function and tissue-specific expression. *Biochem. J.*, **295**, 329–41.

Gronlund, K. M., Gerhart, D. Z., Leino, R. L. *et al.* (1996). Chronic seizures increase glucose transporter abundance in rat brain. *J. Neuropathol. Exp. Neurol.*, **55**, 832–40.

Guerin, C., Laterra, J., Drewes, L. R. *et al.* (1992). Vascular expression of glucose transporter in experimental brain neoplasms. *Am. J. Path.*, **140**, 417–25.

Guerin, C., Laterra, J., Hruban, R. H. *et al.* (1990). The glucose transporter and blood–brain barrier of human brain tumors. *Ann. Neurol.*, **28**, 758–65.

Harik, S. I. and Roessmann, U. (1991). The erythrocyte-type glucose transporter in blood vessels of primary and metastatic brain tumors. *Ann. Neurol.*, **29**, 487–91.

Harik, S. I., Behmand, R. A. and LaManna, J. C. (1994). Hypoxia increases glucose transport at blood–brain barrier in rats. *J. Appl. Physiol.*, **77**, 896–901.

Holman, G. D (1989). Side-specific photolabelling of the hexose transporter. *Biochem. Soc. Trans.*, **17**, 438–40.

Kumagai, A. K., Dwyer, K. J. and Pardridge, W. M. (1994). Differential glycosylation of the GLUT1 glucose transporter in brain capillaries and choroid plexus. *Biochim. Biophys. Acta*, **1193**, 24–30.

Kumagai, A. K., Kang, Y.-S., Boado, R. J. and Pardridge, W. M. (1995). Upregulation of blood–brain barrier GLUT1 glucose transporter protein and mRNA in experimental chronic hypoglycemia. *Diabetes*, **44**, 1399–404.

Kumagai, A. K., Vinores, S. A. and Pardridge, W. M. (1996). Pathological upregulation of inner blood-retinal barrier Glut1 glucose transporter expression in diabetes mellitus. *Brain Res.*, **706**, 313–17.

Maher, F., Vannucci, S. J. and Simpson, I. A. (1994). Glucose transport proteins in brain. *FASEB J.*, **8**, 1003–11.

McCall, A. L., Van Bueren, A. M., Nipper, V. *et al.* (1996). Forebrain ischemia increases Glut1 protein in brain microvessels and parenchyma. *J. Cereb. Blood Flow Metab.*, **16**, 69–76.

Olson, A. L. and Pessin, J. E. (1996). Structure, function, and regulation of the mammalian facilitative glucose transporter gene family. *Annu. Rev. Nutr.*, **16**, 235–56.

Pelligrino, D. A., Segil, L. J. and Albrecht, R. F. (1990). Brain glucose utilization and transport and cortical function in chronic vs. acute hypoglycemia. *Am. J. Physiol.*, **259**, E729–E735.

Pelligrino, D. A., LaManna, J. C., Duckrow, R. B. *et al.* (1992). Hyperglycemia and blood–brain barrier glucose transport. *J. Cereb. Blood Flow Metab.*, **12**, 887–99.

Silverman, M. (1991). Structure and function of hexose transporters. *Annu. Rev. Biochem.*, **60**, 757–94.

Tsukamoto, H., Boado, R. J. and Pardridge, W. M. (1996). Differential expression of glioblastoma multiforme and cerebral hemangioblastoma of cytoplasmic proteins that bind two different domains within the 3′-untranslated region of the human glucose transporter 1 (GLUT1) messenger RNA. *J. Clin. Invest.*, **97**, 2823–32.

Urabe, T., Hattori, N., Nagamatsu, S., Sawa, H. and Mizuno, Y. (1996). Expression of glucose transporters in rat brain following transient focal ischemic injury. *J. Neurochem.*, **67**, 265–71.

Vannucci, S. J., Seaman, L. B., Brucklacher, R. M. and Vannucci, R. C. (1994). Glucose transport in developing rat brain: Glucose transporter proteins, rate constants and cerebral glucose utilization. *Mol. Cell. Biochem.*, **140**, 177–84.

Vannucci, S. J., Seaman, L. B. and Vannucci, R. C. (1996). Effects of hypoxia-ischemia on GLUT1 and GLUT3 glucose transporters in immature rat brain. *J. Cereb. Blood Flow Metab.*, **16**, 77–81.

Zeller, K., Vogel, J. and Kuschinsky, W. (1996). Postnatal distribution of Glut1 glucose transporter and relative capillary density of blood–brain barrier structures and circumventricular organs during development. *Dev. Brain Res.*, **91**, 200–8.

19 Glucose transporters in mammalian brain development

HANNELORE BAUER

- Introduction
- Glucose transporters in the brain
- Developmental regulation of glucose transporters
- Conclusion and outlook

Introduction

The uptake of glucose into mammalian cells is a necessity, and, regardless of the cell type, occurs either by facilitative diffusion along a natural glucose concentration gradient or by an active sodium-coupled transport system against the glucose concentration gradient. During the past decade, the molecular structure, function and location of glucose transporters (GTs) has been extensively studied, leading to a rather detailed knowledge of the mechanisms underlying sugar transport in biological tissues (for review see Bell *et al.*, 1990; Kasanicki and Pilch 1990; Thorens *et al.*, 1990; Bell *et al.*, 1993; Partridge and Boado, 1993).

Collectively, the sodium-independent 'facilitative' glucose transporters form a small multigene family of structurally and functionally related integral transmembrane proteins. Despite their close relationship, facilitative GTs exhibit distinct kinetic properties and show a pronounced tissue-specific expression pattern. To date, seven members of the facilitative GT family have been described and their cDNAs have been cloned and sequenced. These sequences, including one non-functional pseudosequence (Glut 6) (Kayano *et al.*, 1990), were termed Glut 1 to Glut 7, referring to the order in which they were identified.

This chapter focuses on the developmental expression of the major facilitative glucose transporters in the mammalian brain. Facilitative GTs of tissues other than the brain are not discussed further.

Glucose transporters in the brain

In the brain, blood-borne glucose provides nearly the entire energy source needed to guarantee proper neuronal and glial function. Numerous immunological and biochemical studies have suggested that various GTs are active in the brain, obviously reflecting heterogeneity in glucose utilization and oxidative metabolism among different regions of the CNS (Sokoloff *et al.*, 1977; Huang *et al.*, 1980). So far, three major types of facilitative GTs (Glut 1, Glut 3 and Glut 5) and two types of GTs that are only transiently expressed or expressed to a minor extent (Glut 2 and Glut 4) have been found in the brain (Maher *et al.*, 1993) (Fig. 19.1).

Glut 1

Glut 1 was the first member of facilitative glucose transporters to be cloned and sequenced (Mueckler *et al.*, 1985), and was shown to be expressed in all cell types, with an exceptionally high abundance in tissue with barrier function, such as brain

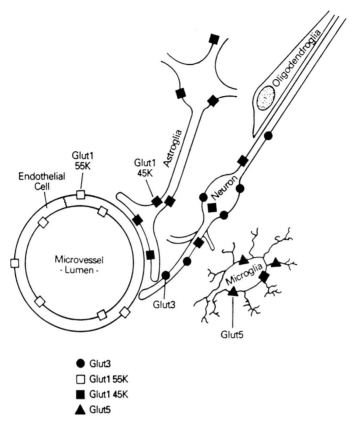

Fig. 19.1. Schematic representation of the cellular localization of glucose transporter isoforms in the brain. Reprinted from Maher *et al.* (1993).

microvessels and retinal capillaries (Harik *et al.*, 1990*a,b*; Farrell *et al.*, 1992). Actually, Glut 1 was isolated from a cDNA library of transformed liver cells (HepG2) using an antiserum to the purified human erythrocyte glucose transporter (Lienhard *et al.*, 1982). Its sequence was shown to be 98% homologous to a cDNA isolated from rat brain (Birnbaum *et al.*, 1986). Thus, Glut 1 is alternatively referred to as the 'erythroid-type', 'HepG2-type' or 'rat brain-type' isoform.

Glut 1 was shown to be modulated by insulin or insulin-like growth in rat adipocytes (Oka *et al.*, 1988) and fetal lung and muscle (Simmons *et al.*, 1993) as well as in primary cultures of neuronal and glial cells (Werner *et al.*, 1989; Masters *et al.*, 1991). Also, when expressed in Chinese hamster ovary cells, Glut 1 was found to be responsive to insulin (Asano *et al.*, 1989). However, the transport of glucose across the endothelial plasma membrane *in vivo* is apparently not under hormonal

regulation (Brooks *et al.*, 1986; McCall *et al.*, 1986; Gerhart *et al.*, 1989).

SDS-PAGE of whole brain tissue revealed that in the brain, Glut 1 occurs as two molecular mass forms, a 55 kDa and a 45 kDa form, which differ in their distribution pattern. The 55 kD form is expressed in the microvascular endothelium of the CNS, commonly related to the blood–brain barrier (Harik *et al.*, 1990*a*; Pardridge *et al.*, 1990; Pardridge and Boado, 1993), with a 4-fold greater abundance on the abluminal membrane as compared to the luminal membrane (Farrell and Pardridge, 1991).

In contrast to the 55 kDa form, the 45 kDa Glut 1 form is not found in brain microvasculature but constitutes by far the greatest proportion of total Glut 1 protein present in the adult brain. Expression of the 45 kDa Glut 1 (neuronal/glial Glut 1) has been demonstrated in vascular-free membrane fractions from CNS tissue, choroid plexus and synaptosomes (for review see Maher *et al.*, 1993), as well as in cultured neurons and glial cells (Walker *et al.*, 1988; Mudd *et al.*, 1990; Maher *et al.*, 1991).

Glut 3

Glut 3 (human fetal skeletal muscle type glucose transporter) shares a 64.4% amino acid sequence homology with the HepG2 type but is distinct from the adult skeletal muscle Glut protein since it is not insulin responsive. Glut 3 was originally cloned from a human fetal skeletal muscle cell line (Kayano *et al.*, 1988). To date, several homologs have been identified, isolated from mouse, rat and chicken brain (White *et al.*, 1991; Nagamatsu *et al.*, 1992; Krishnan and Haddad, 1995). Several studies have demonstrated that Glut 3 appears specific to neurons, suggesting a role in neuronal maturation, which includes the metabolic supply for dendritic and axonal traffic (Maher *et al.*, 1991, 1992; Bondy *et al.*, 1992; Nagamatsu *et al.*, 1992). Only minor Glut 3 immunoreactivity was found in astrocytes, oligodendrocytes and microglia (Maher *et al.*, 1991, 1992), however inducibility of Glut 3 expression was demonstrated in malignant glial cells (Yamamoto *et al.*, 1990; Nishioka *et al.*, 1992; Boado *et al.*, 1994).

There are several lines of evidence indicating that Glut 3 is also expressed in brain microvasculature (Gerhart *et al.*, 1992; Mantych *et al.*, 1992). Interestingly, this expression appeared to be species specific, since Glut 3 was found in many canine cerebral endothelial cells in cerebellum and brain stem but was absent from gerbil and rat brain microvasculature (Gerhart *et al.*, 1995).

There are still difficulties concerning the confinement of Glut 3 expression in the brain due to discrepancies between data obtained from *in vivo* and *in vitro* studies. This was attributed to a different epitope accessibility for Glut 3 antibodies *in situ* compared to *in vitro* systems. (For further discussion see Maher *et al.*, 1993).

Glut 5

The jejunal/kidney glucose transporter isoform Glut 5 has actually been described as a fructose transporter, originally cloned from human small intes-

tine cells (Kayano *et al.*, 1990) and has since been shown to be expressed at high levels on apical membranes of the absorptive epithelial cells of the small intestine, kidney, testis and sperm (Burant *et al.*, 1992; Rand *et al.*, 1993), but also in differentiated human macrophages (Maher *et al.*, 1993). However, besides its ability to mediate high affinity fructose transport, Glut 5 was also found to transport glucose, though at very low levels (Kayano *et al.*, 1990; Rand *et al.*, 1993). Unexpectedly, Glut 5 expression was also demonstrated in brain tissue (Rand *et al.*, 1993; Mantych *et al.*, 1993; Payne *et al.*, 1993). By use of immunofluoroescence studies, Glut 5 was found in brain cerebral microvascular endothelial cells, similar to the blood–brain barrier-related Glut 1. However, only some of the Glut 1 positive microvascular endothelial cells simultaneously stained positive for Glut 5, suggesting different distribution patterns for these two facilitative glucose transporters.

Other glucose transporters expressed in the brain

Immunocytochemical studies have demonstrated that Glut 2 (the liver-type glucose transporter), actually known to mediate glucose transport in hepatocytes and insulin-producing β cells (Fukumoto *et al.*, 1988; Thorens *et al.*, 1988; Orci *et al.*, 1989; Thorens *et al.*, 1990; Unger, 1991), appears to be expressed in various brain regions though at apparently low levels (Brant *et al.*, 1993; Leloup *et al.*, 1994). Highest Glut 2 expression was detected in the pituitary and optic chiasma of isolated rat brain tissue suggesting a β-cell-like glucose sensing mechanism in certain cell populations in the brain (Brant *et al.*, 1993).

The insulin-regulatable glucose transporter (IRGT) Glut 4 (muscle/fat facilitative glucose transporter) was actually described in both brown and white adipose tissues as well as cardiac, skeletal and smooth muscle (Birnbaum, 1989; Charron *et al.*, 1989; Fukumoto *et al.*, 1989; James *et al.*, 1989; Kaestner *et al.*, 1989) but not in endothelial cells (Slot *et al.*, 1990). Moreover, Glut 4 has been suggested to be absent from both the liver and the brain (Liu *et al.*, 1992). In contrast, data reported by Brant *et al.* (1993) showed that Glut 4 is expressed in the pituitary, the hypothalamus and the medulla, regions that are outside the blood–brain barrier. A hypothalamic Glut 4 expression was also demonstrated by Livingstone *et al.* (1995). However, whether or not glucose transport in these brain regions is partly responsive to insulin has remained unclear.

Developmental regulation of glucose transporters

Glucose transporters in preimplantation embryos

Preimplantation mouse embryos preferably utilize pyruvate and lactate as energy sources until the stage of compaction (eight-cell stage) and there are lines of evidence indicating that glucose may act even as an inhibitor on early cleavage embryos (Chatot *et al.*, 1989; Seshagiri and Bavister, 1989). Low levels of glucose were already detected in preimplantation embryos from the one-cell stage on (Gardner and Leese, 1988). Following compaction, embryos switch to a glucose-based metabolism (Gardner and Leese, 1986, 1988) and from the late morula stage onwards embryonic development becomes more and more dependent on glucose as a main energy source (Biggers and Borland, 1976; Wordinger and Brinster, 1976).

Glut 1 was found to be the earliest appearing glucose transporter in the mouse embryo and was detected from the egg throughout preimplantation development (Hogan *et al.*, 1991; Aghayan *et al.*, 1992). Its upregulation was quantitated by Morita *et al.* (1994), showing an 11-fold increase in Glut 1 mRNA in blastocysts compared to two-cell embryos. At the eight-cell stage, expression of Glut 2 appears, apparently as a reaction to the increased amount of glucose needed (Hogan *et al.*, 1991). At the blastocyst stage, Glut 1 and Glut 2 already display different cellular localization. While Glut 1 exhibits a widespread distribution in both the trophectoderm and the inner cell mass, Glut 2 is restricted on trophectoderm membranes, suggesting a different functional significance for these transporters (Aghayan *et al.*, 1992).

Although the expression of the insulin receptor gene has been detected in preimplantation embryos (Rosenblum *et al.*, 1986; Mattson *et al.*,

1988; Heyner *et al.*, 1989a,b), Glut 4 was not detectable during preimplantation or early postimplantation development (Hogan *et al.*, 1991; Aghayan *et al.*, 1992). Expression of Glut 1 and Glut 2 in the preimplantation mouse embryo was also demonstrated by Rao *et al.* (1990) using Western blot analysis and immunocytochemistry. As known from human studies and from experiments in a rat model, lack of sufficient glucose supply caused by uteroplacental insufficiency results in an asymmetric growth retardation of the embryo, leaving the brain unaffected (Ogata *et al.*, 1986). This suggests a different regulation of glucose transporter expression in the nervous tissue.

Glucose transporters in the developing mammalian brain

Expression of glucose transporters during brain ontogenesis has been studied in several animal models, including mouse, rat and rabbit (Sivitz *et al.*, 1989; Sadiq *et al.*, 1990; Devaskar *et al.*, 1991; Dermietzel *et al.*, 1992; Dwyer and Pardridge, 1993; Harik *et al.*, 1993; Nagamatsu *et al.*, 1994; Trocino *et al.*, 1994; Vannucci, 1994; Bauer *et al.*, 1995; Bolz *et al.*, 1996) and there is evidence that alterations in the cellular localization of GTs occur, obviously in concert with the changing glucose metabolic needs of the brain.

Glut 1 in postimplantation embryos

Particular attention has been paid to the developmental regulation of Glut 1, not only because glucose transport across cerebral microvessels is a rate limiting step in sugar movement from the blood to the brain and virtually all cerebral functions are affected and/or rate limited by this blood–brain barrier (BBB) establishment and BBB function in brain microvascular endothelial cells.

A recent biochemical and histochemical study on the tissue-specific expression and localization of Glut 1 protein in the rat embryo has revealed that from embryonic day 9.5 to day 11.5, i.e. the main periods of neurulation, Glut 1 immunoreactivity was observed predominantly in the neuroepithelial cells (Trocino *et al.*, 1994). During advanced embryonic development, Glut 1 expression was localized mainly to intraneural microvessels with a persisting Glut 1 staining in neuroepithelial cells. This specific confinement of Glut 1 to cerebral microvessels, and the concomitant reduction of Glut 1 immunoreactivity in neuroepithelial cells between E12 and E16 was reported to be characteristic for the developing rodent brain (Dermietzel *et al.*, 1992; Harik *et al.*, 1993; Bauer *et al.*, 1995).

Interestingly, there are lines of evidence indicating that the redistribution of Glut 1 from neuroepithelial cells to the cerebral microvasculature takes place in regions of the neural tube that mature first. Ventral regions, for instance, whose neurons become postmitotic earlier, lose Glut 1 expression before dorsal regions. This was histochemically demonstrated by Harik *et al.* (1993), showing that at E12 to E14 a stronger Glut 1 immunoreaction was detectable in the dorsal telencephalon, compared to the ventral telencephalon.

The early localization of BBB Glut 1 to cerebral microvessels in the developing rat brain was once more confirmed by a recently performed electron microscopic study. From E13 on, Glut 1 immunoreactivity was demonstrated to be restricted to the capillary endothelial cells and was shown to occur at both the luminal and abluminal plasma membranes. In the course of embryonic development, vessels decreased in size, and the BBB Glut 1 was found to be upregulated at different rates on the luminal and abluminal membranes, pointing towards the establishment of a vectorial glucose transport system across the endothelial cells. In fact, the occurrence of Glut 1 shifted to the abluminal vessel wall, resulting in a 3- to 4-fold increase in density on the abluminal membrane compared to the luminal membrane. This is consistent with earlier studies, showing an asymmetric distribution of Glut 1 in rat capillaries, with 12% of the immunoreactive Glut 1 on the luminal endothelial membrane, 48% on the abluminal membrane, and 40% in the cytoplasm (Farrell and Pardridge, 1991; Cornford *et al.*, 1993).

Upregulation of Glut 1 has been suggested to occur in two phases. Initially, during early intrauterine development, there is a 4-fold increase in the density of the Glut 1 transporter in brain vessel profiles, and later, from E19 to adult life, there is a further 2-fold increase. This increase in density was suggested to be due to an increase in absolute amounts of Glut 1 protein and to a concomitant reduction in vessel size, which in consequence, also appears as 'upregulation' (Bolz *et al.*, 1996).

Glut 1 expression from neonatal to adult stage

Immunohistochemical staining revealed that, compared to the fetus and adult, a relative decrease in the *in situ* expression of Glut 1 is evident in the brain of the neonatal rat and rabbit (Sivitz *et al.*, 1989; Sadiq *et al.*, 1990; Devaskar *et al.*, 1991; Devaskar *et al.*, 1992). Immediately after birth, the total amount of immunoreactive Glut 1 protein in a rat brain membrane fraction was decreased approximately 5-fold, primarily due to a loss of the higher 55 kDa (BBB Glut 1) component with a relatively smaller decrease in the 43 kDa band (Sivitz *et al.*, 1989). This was also confirmed by studies with neuronal and glial cells, derived from developing rabbit brains (Sadiq *et al.*, 1990); the peak abundance of brain-type Glut 1 protein was found in the adult, followed next by the fetus. An apparent nadir in Glut 1 expression in the newborn rabbit was clearly demonstrated by Dwyer and Pardridge (1993) using quantitative Western blotting of microvessels from rabbit brains on postnatal day 1, 14, 28 and 70. Between birth and day 14, a significant decrease in Glut 1 expression followed by a subsequent upregulation between 14 and 70 days was detectable.

Additional evidence to suggest a constant increase in cerebral Glut 1 expression throughout development has come from immunogold electron microscopy studies with fetal and newborn rabbits (Cornfold *et al.*, 1993). The authors have shown that immunolocalizable Glut 1 expression increased throughout development (gestational day 14 to adulthood) and positively correlated with the developmental status of the capillaries. This was further exemplified by the age-correlated increases in immunogold-localized Glut 1 per square micron of cytoplasm, per micron of abluminal membrane, and per micron of luminal membrane (Cornford *et al.*, 1993).

Discrepancies concerning the developmental alteration of BBB Glut 1 expression in the newborn rat brain were reported by Devaskar *et al.*

(1991). The authors have studied Glut 1 protein levels within whole brain homogenate, crude brain membranes and microvasculature-enriched fractions from developing rat brains, beginning at gestational day 18. While the relative amount of microvascular Glut 1 protein in crude brain membranes was found to decline at the neonatal stage compared to the adult and fetus, quantitation of Glut 1 abundance in whole brain homogenate (45 kDa form) or in microvessels (55 kDa form) revealed a gradual developmental upregulation of both Glut 1 types.

In the developing rat brain, the relative amount of the 2.8 kb glucose transporter mRNA (corresponding to the 55 kDa Glut type) was found to be decreased approximately 4-fold by day 4 after birth compared to that on gestational day 19, and was restored to fetal levels within 60 days post delivery, suggesting a transcriptional regulation of Glut 1 expression during development (Sivitz et al., 1989). These findings directly contrast with other reports, demonstrating that the concentration of Glut 1 mRNA in the rabbit brain remained virtually unchanged between day 14 and 70, though the amount of Glut 1 protein increased during this period (Dwyer and Pardridge, 1993). Obviously, the regulation of Glut 1 expression is mediated at both transcriptional and non-transcriptional levels (reviewed by Pardridge and Boado, 1993).

Controversial results have also been obtained from cytochalasin-B binding studies, reflecting the total amount of all of the different glucose transporters present in the brain (Dick et al., 1984). Data reported by Sivitz et al. (1989) have indicated that cytochalasin-B binding to brain membranes was not significantly different among fetal, neonatal and adult rat brain, suggesting that various glucose transporters may be active in the neonatal brain, compensating for the observed Glut 1 depression during the early postnatal stage. On the other hand, there are other reports demonstrating that the assessment of Glut levels by cytochalasin B binding revealed higher ligand binding sites in the brain of adult rats than in neonates (Morin et al., 1988).

No significant regional variation in total (vascular and non-vascular) Glut 1 content was found in the cortex, hippocampus, thalamus, and hypothalamus during fetal and postnatal development.

Total Glut 1 content in the forebrain was demonstrated to increase from 15% of the adult levels at postnatal day 1 to 20% at day 14, attaining adult levels at day 30. As for the 55 kDa Glut 1, similar expression levels were observed: BBB Glut 1 protein in isolated brain microvessels at E19 was 13% of adult value but increased to 30% at postnatal day 1. This level remained unchanged throughout the first postnatal week, before increasing again to adult levels by 21–30 days (Vanucchi, 1994).

Detection of low levels of vascular Glut 1 in the newborn animal is in keeping with the comparably low capacity of glucose uptake from the blood to the brain at this stage (Daniel et al., 1978; Spatz et al., 1978; Fuglsang et al., 1986; Dyve and Gjedde, 1991). In fact, substrate requirements for the generation of metabolic energy change during brain development. While the adult brain is entirely dependent on glucose as metabolic substrate, the neonatal rat brain preferentially uses ketones as its primary source (Hawkins et al., 1971; Sokoloff, 1973; Patel and Owen, 1976). Concomitantly, the activity of several glycolytic enzymes is low in newborn rat brains but progressively increases throughout the first days to weeks after birth (Leong and Clark, 1984).

Similar to the vascular Glut 1, the 45 kDa Glut 1 type increases with development (Sivitz et al., 1989; Bondy et al., 1992; Vannucci, 1994). However, the increase of 45 kDa Glut 1 is more gradual and has been suggested to reflect overall brain growth. Non-vascular Glut 1, which is obviously a glial glucose transporter (Bondy et al., 1992) is substantially expressed throughout the brain parenchyma, and no regional variation in the levels of non-vascular Glut 1 protein was observed in the forebrain during development (Vannucci, 1994).

Glut 1 in the choroid plexus

In contrast to the blood–brain barrier, the blood–CSF barrier is fully developed in the fetus (Sturrock, 1979). As evidenced by Northern blotting, all of the Glut 1 found in the choroid plexus was suggested to be the 45 kDa Glut 1 form, which is located exclusively in the tight junction-forming choroid epithelium (Vannucci, 1994). This is in line with earlier results from immunohistochemical studies, revealing a distinct staining of

Glut 1 in the basal membranes of the choroidal epithelial cells of adult rats (Harik *et al.*, 1990*a*; Farrell *et al.*, 1992; Harik *et al.*, 1993). No Glut 1 staining has been observed in the choroid microvessels, which are known to be devoid of any barrier properties.

It has been demonstrated that Glut 1 expression in the choroid plexus is also developmentally regulated (Dwyer and Pardridge, 1993; Vannucci, 1994). In the developing rat brain, Glut 1 levels in the choroid epithelium were shown to be highest during gestation followed by a 50% decline by day 1 and a further depression throughout the first postnatal week, which obviously reflects similar decreases in the cerebral glycogen content of the developing rat brain (Kohle and Vannucci, 1977). Adult Glut 1 levels are attained by day 21 (Vannucci, 1994). The high levels of Glut protein present at the late gestational stages in the embryonic rat were suggested to be related to a high glycogen store found in the fetal brain (Kohle and Vannucci, 1977).

Glut 3 in postimplantation, neonatal and adult stage

In the early mouse embryo, no Glut 3 expression has been detected so far (Smith and Gridley, 1992), and some studies have even failed to detect Glut 3 mRNA or protein during advanced embryonic development of the rat CNS (Nagamatsu *et al.*, 1994). On the other hand, there is experimental evidence indicating that Glut 3 is expressed in differentiating neurons of the developing rat brain after blood–brain barrier formation (i.e. around gestational day 16) (Bondy *et al.*, 1992). Within the rabbit CNS, Glut 3 mRNA was found to be most abundant in the 10-day-old neonate and adult, followed next by the early neonate, with little in the fetus (Sadiq *et al.*, 1990). The extent of Glut 3 expression obviously coincides with neuronal maturation (Mantych *et al.*, 1992; Nagamatsu *et al.*, 1994; Vanucci, 1994).

In contrast to BBB Glut 1, a steady, almost linear increase in Glut 3 expression from the first postnatal days to adulthood was observed (Vanucci, 1994). Variable levels of Glut 3 expression were detected in different neuronal populations in the mammalian brain (Bondy *et al.*, 1992) but no Glut 3 staining was found in regions that lack neuronal elements, such as white matter, adenohypophysis, pineal gland, and cerebral microvessels (Maher *et al.*, 1992; Brant *et al.*, 1993). As evidenced by immunoblotting techniques, highest Glut 3 levels were present in isolated membranes from the thalamus and hypothalamus during the first 3 prenatal weeks, a fact that has been suggested to be due to an early functional maturation.

To further elaborate these findings, Glut 3 levels were quantified in the brainstem and the cerebellum, two regions of the rat brain known to mature differentially. In the brainstem, which is relatively mature at birth, Glut 3 levels were about 30% of the adult value at pd 7, and adult levels were attained at pd 14. In contrast, in the cerebellum, which is characterized by later neuronal migration and differentiation, Glut 3 was barely detectable at pd 7, and its level was still lower than 60% of the adult value by pd 21 (Vanucci, 1994).

Glut 1 in the developing blood–brain barrier

It was shown previously that expression of Glut 1 is high in tissue with barrier function and strongly correlates with the occurrence of occluding interendothelial or epithelial tight junctions (Harik *et al.*, 1990*a*,*b*). Thus, it is intriguing to speculate that the embryonic CNS endothelium acquires a high density of Glut 1 at the time that the BBB is established. Since the question concerning the timing and the onset of BBB function in the mammalian CNS has not been settled yet, any correlation of Glut 1 expression to BBB function in the mammalian embryo appears difficult. However, there are several clues to suggest a rather 'mature' embryonic BBB, that is created very early during embryonic development (Dziegielewska *et al.*, 1979; Mollgard *et al.*, 1988; Bauer *et al.*, 1995).

Using intravascularly injected HRP and labeled dextran, Dermietzel and his group (1992) showed that redistribution of Glut 1 from the parenchymal cells to microvascular endothelium appeared first in the hindbrain and the parieto-temporal regions of the hemispheres, regions that are known to be vascularized early on. Interestingly, these regions were shown previously to be equipped first with a

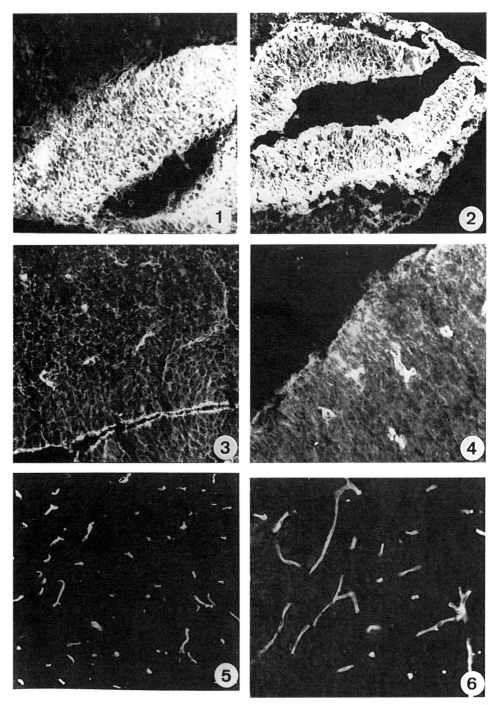

Fig. 19.2. Glut 1 immunoreactivity in the telencephalon of the embryonic mouse: (1) Intraneural and perineural domain of a 9-day-old mouse embryo. (2) Intraneural and perineural domain of a 10-day-old mouse embryo. A uniform distribution of Glut 1 immunoreactivity is found in the intraneural domain, with only minor staining in the perineural area. (3) Enlargement of an area from the intraneural domain at embryonic day 11, showing that Glut 1 is specifically localized to endothelial cells. (4) Enlargement of an area from the intraneural domain at embryonic day 12, (5) embryonic day 16, and (6) adult.

functioning BBB (Wakai and Hirokawa, 1978; Risau *et al.*, 1986). From tracer experiments it has become clear that the observed loss of Glut 1 in the neuroectoderm is paralleled by a tightening of the BBB endothelium. At E14.5 only those neuroepithelial domains in the developing rat brain were found to possess a high level of BBB Glut 1 immunoreactivity where intracerebral blood vessels were still permeable to HRP (Dermietzel *et al.*, 1992). However, whether or not there is a direct causal relationship between Glut 1 redistribution and BBB maturation has remained debatable. Moreover, it has since been observed that the 'leaky' nonparenchymal vessels of the perineural plexus also show intense Glut 1 immunoreactivity (Dermietzel *et al.*, 1992; Harik *et al.*, 1993).

A correlation of Glut 1 expression pattern to the maturation of BBB function in the developing mouse brain was done by Bauer *et al.* (1995). Similar to the rat, strong Glut 1 immunoreactivity was detected in the telencephalon from the ninth intrauterine day on. However, only minor if any staining was observed in the perineural domain, which is in contrast to data reported previously (Harik *et al.*, 1993). At E11, shortly after intraneural neovascularization, Glut 1 expression disappeared from neuroepithelial cells and was found to be restricted to intraneural capillaries (Fig. 19.2). Accordingly, permeability studies have demonstrated that tracer substances are already largely excluded from the mouse CNS at gestational day 12, suggesting that BBB establishment occurs shortly after, or probably during intraneural neovascularization. This notion agrees well with previous findings, demonstrating that capillaries that invaded the neuroectoderm at E10 in the embryonic mouse were already devoid of fenestrations (Bauer *et al.*, 1993). Accordingly, it has been suggested that the restriction of Glut 1 expression to cerebral capillaries indicates a specialization of the endothelial plasma membrane and most likely reflects the onset of BBB function in the embryonic CNS.

Conclusion and outlook

Except in the neonate, the developing mammalian brain is entirely dependent on glucose as a metabolic substrate, and from early developmental stages onwards is well equipped with a variety of facilitative glucose transporters. To date, the developmental regulation of glucose transporters in both neuronal and non-neuronal cell populations of the brain has well been established, and there is accumulating evidence that regionalization of distinct glucose transporter types in the CNS reflects maturational changes and concomitant alterations in glucose metabolism of various brain cells.

Future research on glucose transporter expression in the developing brain will probably have to focus on several areas, such as (i) the identification and characterization of so far unknown or poorly described glucose transporter types; (ii) the better understanding of glucose transporter diversity in different brain cell populations; (iii) the elucidation of the functional significance of insulin-regulatable glucose transporter expression in the mammalian CNS; and (iv) the identification of regulatory glucose-sensing mechanisms at the blood–brain interface, maintaining sugar homeostasis in the brain under non-pathological conditions. Thus, glucose transporters will remain an interesting class of membrane proteins in the years to come.

Acknowledgments

This work was supported by the Austrian Ministry of Sciences and Art and by the Austrian Programme for Advanced Research and Technology (APART) of the Austrian Academy of Sciences.

References

Aghayan, M., Rao, L. V., Smith, R. M. *et al.* (1992) Developmental expression and cellular localization of glucose transporter molecules during mouse preimplantation development. *Development*, **115**, 305–12.

Asano, T., Shibasaki, Y., Ohno, S. *et al.* (1989). Rabbit brain glucose transporter responds to insulin when expressed in insulin-sensitive Chinese hamster ovary cells. *J. Biol. Chem.*, **264**, 3416.

Bauer, H. C., Bauer, H., Lametschwandtner, A. *et al.* (1993). Neovascularization and the appearance of morphological characteristics of the blood–brain barrier in the embryonic mouse central nervous system. *Dev. Brain. Res.*, **75**, 269–78.

Bauer, H., Sonnleitner, U., Lametschwandtner, A. *et al.* (1995). Ontogenic expression of the erythroid-type glucose transporter (Glut 1) in the telencephalon of the mouse: correlation to the tightening of the blood–brain barrier. *Dev. Brain. Res.*, **86**, 317–25.

Bell, G. I., Kayano, T., Buse, J. B. *et al.* (1990). Molecular biology of mammalian glucose transporters. *Diabetes Care*, **13**, 198–208.

Bell, G. I., Burant, Ch. F., Takeda, J. and Gould, G. W. (1993). Structure and function of mammalian facilitative sugar transporters. *J. Biol. Chem.*, **268**, 19161–4.

Biggers, J. D. and Borland, R. M. (1976). Physiological aspects of growth and development of the preimplantation embryo. *Ann. Rev. Physiol.*, **38**, 95–119.

Birnbaum, M. J. (1989). Identification of a novel gene encoding an insulin-responsive glucose transporter protein. *Cell*, **57**, 305–15.

Birnbaum, M. J., Haspel, H. C. and Rosen, O. M. (1986). Cloning and characterization of a cDNA encoding the rat brain glucose-transporter protein. *Proc. Natl. Acad. Sci. USA.*, **83**, 5784–8.

Boado, R. J., Black, K. L. and Pardridge, W. M. (1994). Gene expression of GLUT 3 and GLUT 1 glucose transporters in human brain tumors. *Brain Res. Mol. Brain Res.*, **27**, 51–7.

Bolz, S., Farrell, C. L., Dietz, K. and Wolburg, H. (1996). Subcellular distribution of glucose transporter (GLUT-1) during development of the blood–brain barrier in rats. *Cell Tissue Res.*, **284**, 355–65.

Bondy, C. A., Lee, W. H. and Zhou, J. (1992). Ontogeny and cellular distribution of brain glucose transporter gene expression. *Mol. Cell. Neurosci.*, **3**, 305–14.

Brant, A. M., Jess, Th. J., Milligan, G. *et al.* (1993). Immunological analysis of glucose transporters expressed in different regions of the rat brain and central nervous system. *Biochem. Biophys. Res. Commun.*, **192**, 1297–302.

Brooks, D. J., Gibbs, J. S., Sharp, P. *et al.* (1986). Regional cerebral glucose transport in insulin dependent diabetic patients studied using 13-C-3-O-methyl-D-glucose and positron emission tomography. *J. Cereb. Blood Flow Metab.*, **6**, 240–4.

Burant, Ch. F., Takeda, J., Brot-Laroche, E. *et al.* (1992). Fructose transporter in human spermatozoa and small intestine in Glut 5. *J. Biol. Chem.*, **267**, 14523–26.

Charron, M. J., Brosius, F. C., Alper, S. L. and Lodish, H. F. (1989). A glucose transport protein expressed predominantly in insulin-responsive tissues. *Proc. Natl. Acad. Sci. USA*, **86**, 2535–9.

Chatot, C. L., Ziomek, C. A., Bavister, B. D. *et al.* (1989). An improved culture medium supports development of random-bred 1-cell mouse embryos in vitro. *J. Reprod. Fert.*, **86**, 679–88.

Clarke, D. W., Boyd Jr, F. T., Kappy, M. S. and Raizada, M. K. (1984). Insulin binds to specific receptors and stimulates 2-deoxy-D-glucose uptake in cultured glial cells from rat brain. *J. Biol. Chem.*, **259**, 11672.

Cornford, E., Hyman, S. and Pardridge, W. M. (1993). An electron microscopic immunogold analysis of developmental up-regulation of the blood–brain barrier GLUT 1 glucose transporter. *J. Cereb. Blood Flow Metab.*, **13**, 841–54.

Daniel, P. M., Love, E. R. and Pratt, O. E. (1978). The effect of age upon the influx of glucose into the brain. *J. Physiol. (Lond.)*, **274**, 141–8.

Dermietzel, R., Krause, D., Kremer, M. *et al.* (1992). Pattern of glucose transporter (Glut 1) expression in embryonic brains is related to maturation of blood–brain barrier tightness. *Dev. Dynam.*, **193**, 152–63.

Devaskar, S., Zahm, D. S., Hortzclaw, L. *et al.* (1991). Developmental regulation of the distribution of rat brain insulin-insensitive (Glut 1) glucose transporter. *Endocrinology*, **129**, 1530–40.

Devaskar, S., Chundu, K., Zahm, D. S. *et al.* (1992). The neonatal rabbit brain glucose transporter. *Dev. Brain Res.*, **67**, 95–103.

Dick, A. P., Harik, S. I., Klip, A. and Walker, D. M. (1984). Identification and characterization of the glucose transporter of the blood–brain barrier by cytochalasin B binding and immunologic reactivity. *Proc. Natl. Acad. Sci. USA*, **81**, 7233–7.

Dwyer, K. J. and Pardridge, W. M. (1993). Developmental modulation of blood–brain barrier and choroid plexus GLUT 1 glucose transporter messenger ribonucleic acid and immunoreactive protein in rabbits. *Endocrinology*, **132**, 558–65.

Dyve, S. and Gjedde, A. (1991). Glucose metabolism of fetal rat brain in utero, measured with labeled deoxyglucose. *Acta Neurol. Scand.*, **83**, 14–19.

Dziegielewska, K. M., Evans, C. A. N., Malinowska, D. H. *et al.* (1979). Studies on the development of brain barrier systems to lipid insoluble molecules in fetal sheep. *Nature*, **292**, 207–31.

Farrell, C. L. and Pardridge, W. M. (1991). Blood–brain barrier glucose transporter is asymmetrically distributed on brain capillary endothelial lumenal and ablumenal membranes: an electron microscopic study. *Proc. Natl. Acad. Sci. USA*, **88**, 5779–83.

Farrell, C. L., Yang, J. and Pardridge, W. M. (1992). Glut-1 glucose transporter is present within apical and basolateral membranes of brain epithelial interfaces and in microvascular endothelia within tight junctions. *J. Histochem. Cytochem.*, **40**, 193–9.

Fuglsang, A., Lomholt, M. and Gjedde, A. (1986). Blood–brain transfer of glucose analogs in newborn rats. *J. Neurochem.*, **46**, 1417–28.

Fukumoto, H., Seino, S., Imura, H. *et al.* (1988). Sequence, tissue distribution, and chromosomal localization of mRNA encoding a human glucose transporter-like protein. *Proc. Natl. Acad. Sci. USA*, **85**, 5434–8.

Fukumoto, H., Seino, S., Imura, H. *et al.* (1988). Characterization and expression of human HepG2/erythrocyte glucose-transporter gene. *Diabetes*, **37**, 657–61.

Fukumoto, H., Kayano, T., Buse, J. B. *et al.* (1989). Cloning and characterization of the major insulin-responsive glucose transporter expressed in human skeletal muscle and other insulin-responsive tissues. *J. Biol. Chem.*, **264**, 7776–9.

Gardner, D. K. and Leese, H. J. (1986). Non-invasive measurement of nutrient uptake by single cultured preimplantation mouse embryos. *Hum. Reprod.*, **1**, 25–7.

Gardner, D. K. and Leese, H. J. (1988). The role of glucose and pyruvate transport in regulating nutrient utilization by preimplantation embryos. *Development*, **104**, 423–9.

Gerhart, D. Z., LeVasseur, R. J., Broderius, M. A. and Drewes, L. R. (1989). Glucose transporter localization in brain using light and electron immunocytochemistry. *J. Neurosci. Res.*, **22**, 464–72.

Gerhart, D. Z., Broderius, M. A., Borson, N. D. and Drewes, L. R. (1992). Neurons and microvessels express the brain glucose transporter protein GLUT 3. *Proc. Natl. Acad. Sci. USA*, **89**, 733–7.

Gerhart, D. Z., Leino, R. L., Borson, N. D. *et al.* (1995). Localization of glucose transporter Glut 3 in brain: comparison of rodent and dog using species-specific carboxyl-terminal antisera. *Neurosci.*, **66**, 237–46.

Gould, G. W. and Holman, G. D. (1993). The glucose transporter family: structure, function and tissue-specific expression. *Biochem. J.*, **295**, 329–41.

Harik, S. I., Kalaria, R. N., Andersson, L. *et al.* (1990a). Immunocytochemical localization of the erythroid glucose transporter: abundance in tissues with barrier functions. *J. Neurosci.*, **10**, 3862–72.

Harik, S. I., Kalaria, R. N., Whitney, P. M. *et al.* (1990b). Glucose transporters are abundant in cells with 'occluding' junctions at the blood–eye barriers. *Proc. Natl. Acad. Sci. USA*, **87**, 4261–4.

Harik, S. I., Hall, A. K., Richey, P. *et al.* (1993). Ontogeny of the erythroid/HepG2-type glucose transporter (Glut-1) in the rat nervous system. *Dev. Brain. Res.*, **72**, 41–9.

Hawkins, R. A., Williamson, D. H. and Krebs, H. A. (1971). Ketone-body utilization by adult and suckling rat brain in vivo. *Biochem. J.*, **133**, 13–18.

Heyner, S., Rao, L. V., Jarret, L. and Smith, R. M. (1989a). Preimplantation mouse embryos internalize maternal insulin via receptor-mediated endocytosis: pattern of uptake and functional correlation. *Dev. Biol.*, **134**, 48–58.

Heyner, S., Smith, R. M. and Schultz, G. A. (1989b). Temporally regulated expression of insulin and insulin-like growth factors and their receptors in early mammalian development. *BioEssays*, **11**, 171–8.

Hogan, A., Heyner, S., Charron, M. J. *et al.* (1991). Glucose transporter gene expression in early mouse embryos. *Development*, **113**, 363–72.

Huang, S. C., Phelps, M. E., Hoffman, E. J. *et al.* (1980). Non-invasive determination of local cerebral metabolic rate of glucose in man. *Am. J. Physiol.*, **238**, E69–E82.

James, D. E., Strube, M. and Mueckler, M. (1989). Molecular cloning and characterization of an insulin-regulatable glucose transporter. *Nature*, **338**, 83–7.

Kaestner, K. G. H., Christy, R. J., McLenithan, J. C. *et al.* (1989). Sequence, tissue distribution, and differential expression of mRNA for a putative insulin-responsive glucose transporter in mouse 3T3-L1 adipocytes. *Proc. Natl. Acad. Sci. USA*, **86**, 3150–4.

Kalaria, R. N., Gravina, J. W., Schmidley, J. W. *et al.* (1988). The glucose transporter of the human brain and the blood–brain barrier. *Ann. Neurol.*, **24**, 756–64.

Kasanicki, M. A. and Pilch, P. F. (1990). Regulation of glucose-transporter function. *Diabetes Care*, **13**, 219–27.

Kayano, T., Fukumoto, H., Eddy, R. L. *et al.* (1988). Evidence for a family of human glucose transporter-like proteins. *J. Biol. Chem.*, **263**, 15245–8.

Kayano, T., Burant, Ch. F., Fukumoto, H. *et al.* (1990). Human facilitative glucose transporters. *J. Biol. Chem.*, **265**, 13276–82.

Kohle (Vannucci), S. J. and Vannucci, R. C. (1977). Glycogen metabolism in fetal and postnatal rat brain: influence of birth. *J. Neurochem.*, **28**, 441–3.

Krishnan, S. N. and Haddad, G. G. (1995). Cloning of glucose transporter-3 (Glut3) cDNA from rat brain. *Life Sci.*, **56**, 1193–7.

Leloup, C., Arluison, M., Lepetit, N. *et al.* (1994). Glucose transporter (Glut 2) expression in specific brain nuclei. *Brain Res.*, **638**, 221–6.

Leong, S. F. and Clark, J. B. (1984). Regional enzyme development in rat brain: enzymes of energy metabolism. *Biochem. J.*, **218**, 139–45.

Lienhard, G. E., Kim, H. H., Ransome, K. J. and Gorga, J. C. (1982). Immunological identification of an insulin-responsive glucose transporter. *Biochem. Biophys. Res. Commun.*, **105**, 1150–6.

Liu, M. L., Olson, A. L., Moye-Rowley, W. S. *et al.* (1992). Expression and regulation of the human GLUT/4 muscle-fat facilitative glucose transporter gene in transgenic mice. *J. Biol. Chem.*, **267**, 11673–6.

Livingstone, C., Lyall, H. and Gould, G. W. (1995). Hypothalamic GLUT 4 expression: a glucose- and insulin-sensing mechanism. *Mol. Cell. Endocrinol.*, **107**, 67–70.

Maher, F., Davies-Hill, T. M., Lysko, P. G. *et al.* (1991). Expression of two glucose transporters, Glut 1 and Glut 3, in cultured cerebellar neurons: evidence for neuron-specific expression of Glut1. *Mol. Cell Neurosci.*, **2**, 351–60.

Maher, F., Vannucci, S., Takeda, J. and Simpson, I. A. (1992). Expression of mouse Glut 3 and human Glut 3 glucose transporter proteins in brain. *Biochem. Biophys. Res. Commun.*, **182**, 703–11.

Maher, F., Vannucci, S. J. and Simpson, I. A. (1993). Glucose transporter proteins in brain. *FASEB J.*, **8**, 1003–11.

Mantych, G. J., James, D. E., Chung, H. D. and Devaskar, S. U. (1992). Cellular localization and characterization of Glut 3 glucose transporter isoform in human brain. *Endocrinology*, **131**, 1270–8.

Mantych, G. J., James, D. E. and Devaskar, S. U. (1993). Jejunal/kidney transporter isoform (Glut 5) is expressed in the human blood–brain barrier. *Endocrinology*, **132**, 35–40.

Masters, B. A., Werner, H., Roberts, Ch. T. Jr (1991). Developmental regulation of insulin-like growth factor-1-stimulated glucose transporter in rat brain astrocytes. *Endocrinology*, **128**, 2548–57.

Mattson, B. A., Rosenblum, I. Y., Smith, R. M. and Heyner, S. (1988). Autoradiographic evidence for insulin and insulin-like growth factor binding to early mouse embryos. *Diabetes*, **37**, 585–9.

McCall, A. L., Fixman, L. B., Fleming, N. *et al.* (1986). Chronic hypoglycemia increases brain glucose transport. *Am. J. Physiol.*, **251**, E442–E447.

Mollgard, K., Dziegielewska, K. M., Saunders, N. R., Zakut, H. and Soreq, H. (1988). Synthesis and localization of plasma proteins in the developing human brain. *Dev. Biol.* **128**, 207–21.

Morin, A. M., Dwyer, B. E., Fujikawa, D. G. and Wasterlain, C. G. (1988). Low (^{3}H) cytochalasin B binding in the cerebral cortex of newborn rats. *J. Neurochem.*, **51**, 206–11.

Morita, Y., Tsutsumi, O., Oka, Y. and Taketani, Y. (1994). Glucose transporter GLUT 1 mRNA expression in the ontogeny of glucose incorporation in mouse preimplantation embryos. *Biochem. Biophys. Res. Commun.*, **199**, 1525–31.

Mudd, L. M., Werner, H., Shen-Orr, Z. *et al.* (1990). Regulation of rat Brain/HepG2 glucose transporter gene expression by phorbol esters in primary cultures of neuronal and astrocytic glial cells. *Endocrinology*, **126**, 545–9.

Mueckler, M., Caruso, C., Baldwin, S. A. *et al.* (1985). Sequence and structure of a human glucose transporter. *Science*, **229**, 941–5.

Nagamatsu, S., Kornhauser, J. M., Burant, Ch. B. *et al.* (1992). Glucose transporter expression in brain. *J. Biol. Chem.*, **267**, 467–72.

Nagamatsu, S., Sawa, H., Nakamichi, Y. *et al.* (1994). Developmental expression of GLUT 3 glucose transporter in the rat brain. *FEBS Lett.*, **346**, 161–4.

Nishioka, T., Oda, Y., Seino, Y. *et al.* (1992). Distribution of the glucose transporters in human brain tumors. *Cancer Res.*, **52**, 3972–9.

Ogata, E. S., Bussey, M. and Finlay, S. (1986). Altered gas exchange, limited glucose, branched chain amino acids, and hypoinsulinism retard fetal growth in the rat. *Metabolism*, **35**, 950–77.

Oka, Y., Asano, T., Shibasaki, Y. *et al.* (1988). Studies with antipeptide antibody suggest the presence of at least two types of glucose transporter in rat brain and adipocyte. *J. Biol. Chem.*, **263**, 13432–9.

Orci, L., Thorens, B., Ravazzola, M. and Lodish, H. F. (1989). Localization of the pancreatic β cell glucose transporter to specific plasma membrane domains. *Science*, **245**, 259–97.

Pardridge, W. M. and Boado, R. J. (1993). Molecular cloning and regulation of gene expression of blood–brain barrier glucose transporter. In *The Blood Brain Barrier*, ed. W. M. Pardridge, pp. 395–440. New York: Raven Press Ltd.

Pardridge, W. M., Boado, R. J. and Farrell, Ch. R. (1990). Blood-type glucose transporter (Glut-1) is selectively localized to the blood–brain barrier. *J. Biol. Chem.*, **265**, 18035–40.

Patel, M. S. and Owen, O. E. (1976). Lipogenesis from ketone bodies in rat brain. Evidence for conversion of acetoacetate into acetylcoenzyme A in the cytosol. *Biochem. J.*, **156**, 603–7.

Payne, J., Mattiaci, L. A., Maher, F. *et al.* (1993). Expression of Glut 5 on microglia in normal and AD brain. *Soc. Neurosci. Abstr.*, **19**, 1042.

Rand, E. B., Depaoli, A. M., Davidson, N. O. *et al.* (1993). Sequence, tissue distribution, and functional characterization of the rat fructose transporter GLUT 5. *Am. J. Physiol.*, **264**, G1169–76.

Rao, L. V., Smith, R. M., Charron, M. J. and Lodish, H. F. (1990). Expression of glucose transporter isoforms during mouse preimplantation development. (Abstr.). *J. Cell. Biol.*, **111**, 359a.

Risau, W., Hallmann, R. and Albrecht, U. (1986). Differentiation dependent expression of proteins in brain endothelium during development of the blood–brain barrier. *Dev. Biol.*, **117**, 537–45.

Rosenblum, I. Y., Mattson, B. A. and Heyner, S. (1986). Stage-specific insulin binding in preimplantation embryos. *Dev. Biol.*, **116**, 261–3.

Sadiq, F., Holzclaw, L., Chundu, K. *et al.* (1990). The ontogeny of the rabbit brain glucose transporter. *Endocrinology*, **126**, 2417–24.

Seshagiri, P. B. and Bavister, B. D. (1989). Glucose inhibits development of hamster 8-cell embryos in vitro. *Biol. Reprod.*, **40**, 599–606.

Simmons, R. A., Flozak, A. S. and Ogata, E. S. (1993). The effect of insulin and insulin-like growth factor 1 on glucose transport in normal and small for gestational age fetal rats. *Endocrinology*, **133**, 1361–8.

Sivitz, W., DeSautel, S., Walker, P. S. and Pessin, J. E. (1989). Regulation of the glucose transporter in developing rat brain. *Endocrinology*, **124**, 1875–80.

Slot, J. W., Moxley, R., Geuze, H. J. and James, D. E. (1990). No evidence for expression of the insulin-regulatable glucose transporter in endothelial cells. *Nature*, **346**, 369–71.

Smith, D. E. and Gridley, Th. (1992). Differential screening of a PCR-generated mouse embryo cDNA library: glucose transporters are differentially expressed in early postimplantation mouse embryos. *Development*, **116**, 555–61.

Sokoloff, L. (1973). Metabolism of ketone bodies by the brain. *Ann. Rev. Med.*, **24**, 271–80.

Sokoloff, L., Reivich, M., Kennedy, C. *et al.* (1977). The ^{14}C-deoxyglucose method for the measurement of local glucose utilization: theory, procedure, and normal values in the conscious and anaesthetized albino rat. *J. Neurochem.*, **28**, 897–916.

Spatz, M., Micic, D., Mrsulja, B. B. *et al.* (1978). Changes in the capillary lactate and 2-deoxy-glucose uptake in developing brain. *Brain Res.*, **151**, 619–22.

Sturrock, R. R. (1979). A morphological study of the development of the mouse choroid plexus. *J. Anat.*, **129**, 777–93.

Thorens, B., Sarkar, H. K., Kaback, H. R. and Lodish, H. F. (1988). Cloning and functional expression in bacteria of a novel glucose transporter present in liver, intestine, kidney, and β-pancreatic islet cells. *Cell*, **55**, 281–90.

Thorens, B., Charron, M. J. and Lodish, H. F. (1990). Molecular physiology of glucose transporters. *Diabetes Care*, **13**, 209–18.

Trocino, R. A., Akazawa, S., Takino, H. *et al.* (1994). Cellular-tissue localization and regulation of the GLUT-1 protein in both the embryo and the visceral yolk sac from normal and experimental diabetic rats during the early post-implantation period. *Endocrinology*, **134**, 869–78.

Unger, R. H. (1991). Diabetic hyper-glycemia: link to impaired glucose transport in pancreatic β cells. *Science*, **251**, 1202–5.

Vannucci, S. J. (1994). Developmental expression of Glut 1 and Glut 3 glucose transporters in brain. *J. Neurochem.*, **62**, 240–6.

Wakai, S. and Hirokawa, N. (1978). Development of the blood–brain barrier to horseradish peroxidase in the chick embryo. *Cell Tissue Tes.*, **195**, 195–203.

Walker, P. S., Donavan, J. A., Van Ness, B. G. *et al.* (1988). Glucose dependent regulation of glucose transport activity, protein and mRNA in primary cultures of rat brain glial cells. *J. Biol. Chem.*, **263**, 15594–601.

Werner, H., Raizada, M. K., Mudd, L. M. and Foyt, H. L. (1989). Regulation of rat brain/HepG2 glucose transporter gene expression by insulin and insulin-like growth factor 1 in primary cultures of neuronal and glial cells. *Endocrinology*, **125**, 314–20.

White, M. K., Rall, T. B. and Weber, M. J. (1991). Differential regulation of glucose transporter isoforms by the src oncogene in chicken embryo fibroblasts. *Mol. Cell. Biol.*, **11**, 4448–54.

Wordinger, R. J. and Brinster, R. L. (1976). Influence of reduced glucose levels on the in vitro hatching, attachment and trophoblast outgrowth of the mouse blastocyst. *Dev. Biol.*, **53**, 294–6.

Yamamoto, T., Seino, Y., Fukumoto, H., Koh, G. *et al.* (1990). Overexpression of facilitative glucose transporter genes in human cancer. *Biochem. Biophys. Res. Commun.*, **170**, 223–30.

20 Blood–brain barrier amino acid transport

QUENTIN R. SMITH and JAMES STOLL

- Introduction
- Blood–brain barrier transport systems
- Sodium-independent systems
- Sodium-dependent systems
- Low activity systems
- Conclusions

Introduction

Amino acids serve critical roles in brain and are required for normal brain development and function. However, marked differences exist among amino acids, in the roles they serve and metabolic handling within the nervous system.

For example, glutamate, aspartate, glycine, and GABA operate as neurotransmitters in brain and may, in fact, be the predominant neurotransmitters at over 90% of central nervous system synapses (Smith and Cooper, 1992). As a result, they are synthesized locally in neurons and their release and re-uptake are regulated closely to maintain synaptic efficiency. In contrast, most large neutral and basic amino acids, including arginine, lysine, tryptophan, leucine, isoleucine, valine, methionine and phenylalanine, cannot be synthesized in brain, yet are required for brain protein synthesis and as precursors for serotonin (tryptophan), nitric oxide (arginine) and the catecholamines (tyrosine). These 'essential' amino acids must be delivered to the brain from the circulation to ensure normal cerebral growth and metabolism.

The handling of amino acids at the blood–brain barrier reflects this dichotomy. Most dietary 'nonessential' small neutral and anionic (acidic) amino acids have very slow rates of uptake into brain, and, in fact, may be shuttled out of brain by active transport (Oldendorf, 1971; Pardridge, 1983; Al-Sarraf et al., 1995). Due to their low blood–brain barrier 'permeability,' acute changes in plasma levels of nonessential amino acids are generally not reflected in parallel changes in brain concentrations, except in 'nonbarrier' regions. In contrast, most large neutral and basic amino acids show rapid rates of brain uptake (Oldendorf, 1971; Smith et al., 1987; Stoll et al., 1993), with half-times for plasma-to-brain equilibration of 1–10 min. These dietary 'essential' amino acids are shuttled quickly into brain by facilitated exchange systems to ensure adequate substrate availability to neurons and glia under most normal in vivo conditions.

Blood–brain barrier transport systems

The differences that exist among amino acids in delivery to brain arise from the special distribution and activity of amino acid transport systems at the membranes of the blood–brain barrier, especially the brain capillary endothelium (Pardridge, 1983; Smith and Cooper, 1992). The brain capillary

AMINO ACID TRANSPORT SYSTEMS

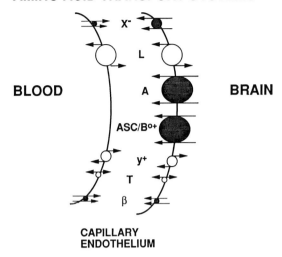

Fig. 20.1. Diagram of amino acid transport systems at the brain capillary endothelium and their localization to the capillary luminal (plasma-facing) or abluminal (brain-facing) membranes. Shaded systems are sodium dependent, whereas unshaded systems are sodium independent.

endothelium represents the primary exchange interface for solute movement from plasma to brain extracellular fluid. In the past 25 years, over eight separate amino acid transport systems have been identified at brain capillaries (see Fig. 20.1).

In vivo studies have shown that most 'essential' large neutral and basic α-amino acids are taken up into brain from plasma by the 'large neutral amino acid' (System L1) or 'cationic (basic) amino acid' (System y⁺) carriers (Oldendorf, 1971; Oldendorf and Szabo, 1976; Pardridge, 1983; Smith *et al.*, 1987; Stoll *et al.*, 1993). These carriers are sodium-independent facilitative exchange systems that are located at both the capillary luminal and abluminal membranes (Sánchez del Pino *et al.*, 1992, 1995) (Fig. 20.1). *In vitro* studies using isolated brain capillaries and capillary membrane vesicles have also provided evidence for the presence of three sodium-dependent, active transport systems for neutral amino acids, including System A, System B⁰⁺, and System ASC (Betz and Goldstein, 1978; Tayarani *et al.*, 1987; Sánchez del Pino *et al.*, 1995). Systems A, ASC, and B⁰⁺ are thought to be located primarily at the capillary abluminal membrane (Fig. 20.1) and to contribute to amino acid efflux

from brain. Systems A and ASC show preference for small neutral amino acids, whereas System B⁰⁺ expresses affinity for both neutral and basic amino acids (Guidotti and Gazzola, 1992). Finally, thyroid hormones, β-amino acids (e.g., β-alanine and taurine), and anionic amino acids (e.g., glutamate and aspartate) are shuttled into brain capillaries by three separate carriers of low capacity, Systems T, β, and X⁻, respectively (Hutchinson *et al.*, 1985; Tayarani *et al.*, 1989; Hokari *et al.*, 1995; Tamai *et al.*, 1995).

Sodium-independent systems

System L1

Most of the natural plasma neutral amino acids are taken up into brain by the sodium-independent, System L exchange transporter. This carrier was characterized initially in Ehrlich cells by Oxender and Christensen (1963) and later shown by Oldendorf and colleagues to mediate the brain uptake of 14 of the 16 primary neutral amino acids (Oldendorf, 1971; Oldendorf and Szabo, 1976; Pardridge, 1983).

Transport via the L carrier is saturable, stereospecific (preferring L to D), bi-directional and sodium/energy independent (Fig. 20.2) (Momma *et al.*, 1987; Greenwood *et al.*, 1989). The carrier operates principally via substrate-coupled antiport, though it can mediate net influx (Guidotti and Gazzola, 1992). System L at the blood–brain barrier shares many of the characteristics of the L System transporter in other tissues, including preference for α-neutral amino acids with large, bulky side chains, trans-stimulation, and inhibition by 2-aminobicyclo[2.2.1]heptane-2-carboxylic acid (BCH) (Smith *et al.*, 1987; Aoyagi *et al.*, 1988; Hargreaves and Pardridge, 1988). The two carriers differ, however, in apparent transport affinity ($1/K_m$) for most substrates. For example, the K_m for L-phenylalanine uptake into brain (~ 10 μM; Momma *et al.*, 1987; Sánchez del Pino *et al.*, 1995; Shulkin *et al.*, 1995) is 100–1000 times less than that in other tissues. Based on this difference, it has been proposed that the blood–brain barrier L System represents a separate isoform – designated System L1. A comparable high affinity system has been identified at the choroid plexus (Segal *et al.*, 1990).

BRAIN PERFUSION METHOD

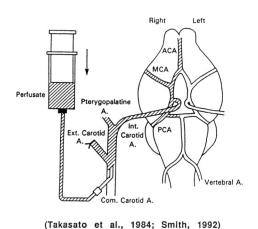

(Takasato et al., 1984; Smith, 1992)

SATURABLE TRANSPORT

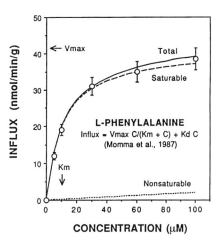

CONCENTRATION (µM)

Fig. 20.2. Left: Schematic of brain perfusion method (Smith *et al.*, 1987) and Right: concentration-dependence of saturable L-phenylalanine uptake into brain (Momma *et al.*, 1987). Most blood–brain barrier amino acid transporters follow Michaelis Menten kinetics, where: Influx $= V_{max}C/(K_m + C)$ and C=perfusate amino acid concentration. In addition, there often is a small component of 'nonsaturable' or 'low affinity' uptake, designated as: Influx$= K_D C$ (Pardridge, 1983; Momma *et al.*, 1987)

Michaelis–Menten constants (V_{max} and K_m) have been reported for the brain neutral amino acid uptake into brain. Table 20.1 lists values obtained using the *in situ* rat brain perfusion technique (Smith *et al.*, 1987; Aoyagi *et al.*, 1988; Takada *et al.*, 1992). V_{max} differs among amino acids by ~2 fold and averages ~50 nmol/min/g wet brain. K_m, on the other hand, varies to a far greater extent (>1000-fold) with some values as low as ~5 µM and other values >1 mM. Transport 'affinity' (estimated as $1/K_m$) for the L1 carrier is strongly influenced by amino acid side chain hydrophobicity and conformation. Hydrophobic 'meta' analogs of phenylalanine (e.g., D,L-NAM) are especially preferred (Smith, 1995).

Uptake via this blood–brain barrier L1 System carrier is quite sensitive to competition because nine or more amino acids share the system and because the transporter is heavily saturated (>95%) with amino acids as a group at normal plasma concentrations ($\Sigma(C/K_m)>20$) (Table 20.1). As a consequence, any condition that produces a selective increase in plasma concentration of one or more large neutral amino acids will reduce influx rates for all those competitors for which plasma concentrations do not change. A classic example of this is phenylketonuria, in which elevated

plasma phenylalanine markedly depresses brain delivery of other neutral amino acids and contributes to the development of mental retardation in infants. Imbalances also occur in liver failure, diabetes and uremia (Smith and Cooper, 1992). However, competition does not produce marked imbalances in brain amino acid uptake or concentrations when plasma amino acid concentrations all change in the same direction as a group, such as after ingestion of a protein balanced meal (Peters and Harper, 1987; Smith *et al.*, 1987).

The L1 System transport protein has not been isolated and the gene that encodes for the carrier has not been identified or cloned. Tate *et al.* in 1992 reported a rat kidney cDNA clone (initially termed NAA-Tr and later named rBAT), which when expressed in *Xenopus* oocytes enhanced uptake of neutral amino acids. However, subsequent work identified this as a related mechanism, possibly System b^{o+} – a sodium-independent variant of System B^{o+} that mediates both neutral and basic amino acid transport (Guidotti and Gazzola, 1992), or a regulatory subunit/accessory protein that modulates both neutral and basic amino acid transport (Wells and Hediger, 1992; Bertran *et al.*, 1993; Palacín, 1994). Mutations in the corresponding human gene have been linked to the

Table 20.1. *Blood–brain barrier transport constants for brain uptake of neutral amino acids, basic amino acids and thyroid hormones, as measured by the* in situ *rat brain perfusion technique*

Amino acid	Plasma concentration (μM)	K_m (μM)	V_{max} (nmol/ min/g)	K_m (app) (μM)	Influx (nmol/ min/g)
Neutral amino acids (System L1)					
Phe	81	11	41	170	13.2
Trp	82	15	55	330	8.2[a]
Leu	175	29	59	500	14.5
Met	64	40	25	860	1.7
Ile	87	56	60	1210	4.0
Tyr	63	64	96	1420	4.1
His	95	100	61	2220	2.5
Val	181	210	49	4690	1.8
Thr	237	220	17	4860	0.8
Gln	485	880	43	19900	1.0
Basic amino acids (System y$^+$)					
Arg	117	56	24	302	6.7
Lys	245	70	22	279	10.3
Orn	98	109	26	718	3.1
Thyroid hormones (System T)					
T3		0.26	0.16		

Values are taken from Smith *et al.* (1987), Stoll *et al.* (1993) and Hokari and Smith (1996). [a]Estimated assuming ~ 70% of albumin-bound Trp contributes to brain uptake. V_{max} is the maximal saturable transport capacity, K_m is the half-saturation concentration in the absence of competitors, K_m(app) is the 'apparent' K_m under normal physiological conditions (i.e. in the presence of normal concentrations of plasma amino acids: K_m (app) $= K_m(1 + \Sigma(C_i/K_m i))$, and influx is the unidirectional amino acid flux rate from plasma to brain. Apparent K_ms *in vivo* are much greater than true K_ms because of transport saturation and competition (Pardridge, 1983).

cause of human cystinuria (Calonge *et al.*, 1994). Further, a cell surface protein (4F2hc), which appears to enhance System L and System y$^+$ activity, has been identified (Bertran *et al.*, 1992; Bröer *et al.*, 1995), though its exact function has not been determined (Palacín, 1994).

The L System carrier is known to be modulated by amino acid availability, hormones and second messengers (Ramamoorthy *et al.*, 1992). Transport activity is down-regulated in some *in vitro* brain endothelial monolayers (Pardridge *et al.*, 1990), but up-regulated *in vivo* in liver failure and development (Smith and Cooper, 1992).

System y$^+$

Next to the cerebrovascular L1 carrier, the System y$^+$ exhibits the greatest transport capacity for amino acid uptake into brain. System y$^+$ mediates the brain uptake of three cationic amino acids (arginine, lysine, and ornithine) with a V_{max} of ~ 24 nmol/min/g and K_m of 56–110 μM (Stoll *et al.*, 1993). The V_{max} is approximately half that obtained for System L1, whereas the K_m values are on the same order of magnitude (Table 20.1).

System y$^+$ transport is stereospecific (preferring L to D), sodium/energy independent, bi-directional and subjects to trans-stimulation (Fig. 20.3). The System apparently can mediate accumulation against a concentration gradient because of a sensitivity to membrane potential (Kavanaugh, 1993). Affinity is primarily for amino acids with cationic side chains, though some short chain neutral amino acids interact weakly with the transporter in the presence of sodium. 4-Amino-1-guanyl-piperi-dine-4-carboxylic acid (GPA) has been proposed as a System y$^+$ model substrate.

System y$^+$ transport has been demonstrated in brain capillaries both *in vivo* and *in vitro*, and it is thought that the carrier is located at both the capillary luminal and abluminal membranes. A similar transport carrier was subsequently identified at the basolateral membrane of the choroid plexus epithelium and may mediate cationic amino acid uptake into CSF (Segal *et al.*, 1990; Preston and Segal, 1992).

The cDNA for the System y$^+$ transporter was cloned serendipitously by Albritton *et al.* (1989) and shown to encode a murine retrovirus receptor (Fig. 20.4). Based on a predicted structural homology with yeast histidine and arginine permeases, Kim *et al* (1991) and Wang *et al* (1991) injected the cRNA for the receptor into frog oocytes and demonstrated that it led to enhanced cationic amino acid transport activity with characteristics

BRAIN L-[^{14}C]LYSINE UPTAKE

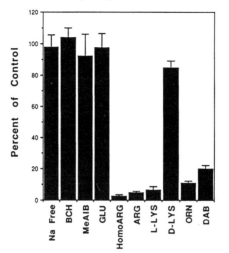

COMPARISON OF K_m VALUES

Amino Acid	Rat Blood-Brain Barrier	Murine Ecotropic Retrovirus Receptor (*Xenopus* Oocyte)
	(µM)	(µM)
HomoArginine	33 ± 2	----
Arginine	52 ± 5	77 ± 2
L-Lysine	70 ± 4	73 ± 8
Ornithine	114 ± 8	105 ± 2
D-Lysine	>5000	21,100

Values are mean ± SEM for n=6-25. Data for murine ecotropic retrovirus receptor are from Wang et al. (1992). Data for the rat blood-brain barrier are from Stoll et al. (1993).

Fig. 20.3. Left: Sodium-dependence and inhibitor selectivity of L-lysine uptake into rat brain as measured using *in situ* perfusion (Stoll *et al.*, 1993), and right: comparison of K_m values obtained for *in vivo* uptake into rat brain with values reported for expression of CAT-1, the ecotropic retrovirus receptor, in *Xenopus* oocytes (Wang *et al.*, 1992; Stoll *et al.*, 1993). DAB, diamino butyric acid.

virtually identical to that reported for System y$^+$. Subsequently, the corresponding human and rat genes (CAT-1 for cationic amino acid transporter) have been cloned and shown to share >88% sequence identity with the murine sequence (Yoshimoto *et al.*, 1992; Stoll *et al.*, 1993; Puppi and Henning, 1995). The human gene maps to chromosome 13q12-q14 and consists of 10 introns and 11 exons coding for a mRNA of approximately 9 kb (Albritton *et al.*, 1992). The human cDNA sequence predicts a 629 amino acid protein with 12–14 transmembrane spanning regions. The corresponding mouse sequence predicts a protein of 622 amino acids (Fig. 20.4).

Messenger RNA studies have shown that CAT-1 is not ubiquitously expressed in tissues, but varies tremendously with highest values in bone marrow, intestine, kidney, testes, and brain and with essentially no expression in liver (Kim *et al.*, 1991; Kakuda *et al.*, 1993; Stoll *et al.*, 1993; Puppi and Henning, 1995). In brain, expression is ~40-fold enriched in cerebral microvessels, consistent with the critical role of the blood–brain barrier in the delivery of essential cationic amino acids to brain. A Northern blot of rat capillary CAT-1 expression is shown in Fig. 20.5.

BASIC AMINO ACID TRANSPORTER (CAT-1)
System y$_1$+

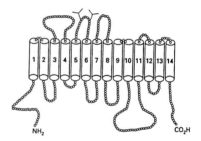

622 Amino Acids   Mr = 67,087 daltons

Murine Ecotropic Retrovirus Receptor (EcoR) (Albritton et al., 1989)

System y$_1$+ Basic Amino Acid Transporter (Kim et al., 1991; Wang et al., 1991)

Fig. 20.4. Model of proposed structure of murine CAT-1 in the plasma membrane. The transporter is proposed to have 14 transmembrane spanning regions (Kim *et al.*, 1991).

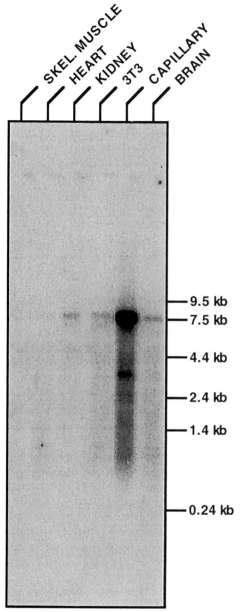

.**Fig. 20.5.** Northern blot of CAT-1 mRNA in rat skeletal muscle, heart, kidney, NIH 3T3 cells, brain capillaries (isolated microvessels) and whole brain.

Subsequent work has identified a second gene for a cationic amino acid transporter (CAT-2), which encodes for two transporter proteins of low and high affinity based on alternative splicing (Closs *et al.*, 1993*a,b*; Kakuda *et al.*, 1993). CAT-2 is differentially expressed in tissues, including brain, but does not appear to be enriched at the blood–brain barrier. Messenger RNA levels for CAT-2 in cerebral microvessels are fairly low and

comparable to that of whole brain. This suggests that CAT-1 may be the primary basic amino acid transporter of the blood–brain barrier.

CAT-1 transporter mRNA and System y^+ activity are increased in proliferating cells and during development of the blood–brain barrier, consistent with the enhanced need of the developing brain of amino acids for growth and protein synthesis. System y^+ activity and message levels are also influenced by phorbol esters, calcium ionopores, and protein kinase C inhibitors (Yoshimoto *et al.*, 1992) and thus are actively regulated by second messengers.

Sodium-dependent systems

System A

For many years, System L was thought to be the only transporter for neutral amino acids at the blood–brain barrier. However, with the advent of methods using isolated brain microvessels, it became apparent that brain capillaries are also loaded with sodium-dependent transport systems that have affinity for neutral amino acids.

System A was the first sodium-dependent amino acid transport system described at the blood–brain barrier (Betz and Goldstein, 1978; Tayarani *et al.*, 1987; Hargreaves and Pardridge, 1988; Sanchez del Pino *et al.*, 1995). Like many amino acid carriers, it does not show absolute substrate selectivity, but prefers neutral amino acids with small, polar side chains (e.g. proline, alanine, glycine, methionine and glutamine) (Guidotti and Gazzola, 1992). The transporter is unique in that it accepts N-methylated substrates, and thus the nonmetabolizable analog, N-methylisobutyric acid (MeAIB) has become the defining substrate for this system. Transport is generally low affinity ($K_m \sim 1$ mM) by $1:1$ sodium-coupled symport. In many cells, uptake by the A System is sensitive to membrane potential, and is greatly inhibited by reduced pH or substrates in the 'trans' compartment (i.e. transinhibition) (Guidotti and Gazzola, 1992).

Based on the fact that most *in vivo* studies showed little evidence of appreciable A System transport into brain (Oldendorf and Szabo, 1976), Betz and Goldstein (1978) proposed that the brain capillary A System was confined to the capillary abluminal membrane (Fig. 20.1). This was confirmed recently by Sánchez del Pino *et al.* (1995) using isolated brain capillary luminal and abluminal membranes. In that preparation, sodium-dependent, MeAIB-sensitive alanine transport was found only at the capillary abluminal membrane

Ennis *et al.* (1994) in a careful brain perfusion study confirmed the absence of a System A component of *in vivo* aminoisobutyric acid (AIB) uptake into rat brain. Removal of sodium from the perfusate or addition of 2 mM MeAIB did not affect brain AIB uptake, whereas influx was markedly reduced by addition of 2 mM phenylalanine, consistent with L system transport.

Because the A System is located at the capillary abluminal membrane and mediates active intracellular accumulation, it may have an important role in removal of amino acids from the brain extracellular fluid. Furthermore, a number of amino acids exhibit substantial affinity for both the L and the A Systems (e.g. methionine), and it is possible that such substrates may serve to link the transport function of both mechanisms.

In many tissues the A System is known to be very sensitive to hormones and amino acid availability. The A System at the blood–brain barrier may also be modulated by enzymes of the γ-glutamyl cycle, as oxyproline, an intermediate in the cycle, markedly stimulates System A transport (Lee *et al.*, 1996).

System ASC or B^{o+}

Isolated brain microvessels also have been noted to express a component of neutral amino acid uptake that is sodium dependent but not inhibitable by MeAIB. Tayarani *et al.* (1987) first noted this component *in vitro* using isolated rat cerebral microvessels and attributed it to System ASC, due to its preference for small neutral amino acids, including alanine, serine and cysteine. Hargreaves and Pardridge (1988) described a similar component of leucine uptake using isolated human brain microvessels and attributed it also to System ASC. The mechanism was presumed to be at the capillary abluminal membrane, as System ASC transport activity has not been observed in most studies of *in vivo* brain uptake (Wade and Brady, 1981; Tovar *et al.*, 1988; Cornford *et al.*, 1992).

However, recently, Sánchez del Pino *et al.* (1995) have challenged this position using isolated bovine brain capillary membranes. In their system, Sánchez del Pino *et al.* found no evidence for System ASC uptake, but instead observed a sodium-dependent, BCH-sensitive component of alanine uptake which they attributed to System B^{o+} and which was confined exclusively to the capillary abluminal membrane. This discrepancy may reflect species differences or an incomplete analysis of transport selectivity. If the sodium-dependent component observed by Sánchez del Pino *et al.* was mediated by System B^{o+}, it should be inhibitable by cationic amino acids (Guidotti and Gazzola, 1992). Importantly, both Tayarani *et al.* (1987) and Hargreaves and Pardridge (1988) reported no effect of cationic amino acids on neutral amino acid uptake in their preparations.

A gene (ASCT1) that may encode the human System ASC System transporter was recently cloned and traced to chromosome 2p13-p15 (Arriza *et al.*, 1993; Hofmann *et al.*, 1994). The cDNA codes for a 532 amino acid sequence with a predicted size of ~56 kDa. The brain was shown to contain mRNA for the protein by Northern blot analysis. The presence of either System ASC or B^{o+} at the abluminal membrane of the blood–brain barrier would not be surprising as they are expressed in many tissues and may have a role in amino acid transport out of the central nervous system. The transporters may serve to accumulate amino acids in the endothelium or to transport amino acids out of brain extracellular fluid.

Low activity systems

System T

Thyroid hormones (T3 and T4) are taken up into brain by a saturable mechanism distinct from System L1 as their influx is blocked by 10 μM TRIAC (triiodothyroacetic acid) but not by 1 mM BCH (Hokari and Smith, 1994). The transport capacity of the thyroid hormone transporter is some 40 times less than that of System L1 (Table 20.1). While T3 is not taken up into brain by the L1 transporter, it expresses significant affinity for the System L1 transporter, with a 50% inhibition concentration (K_i) of 1.0 ± 0.1 µM (Hokari and Smith, 1996). The System T transporter may therefore be necessary to allow thyroid hormones into brain, where they exert significant activity, especially in developing animals.

System β

Taurine is also taken up slowly into brain capillaries by a high-affinity, low-capacity transporter which has been localized to brain capillaries (Tayarani *et al.*, 1989; Tamai *et al.*, 1995). This transporter is both sodium- and chloride-dependent and mediates active transport (Tamai *et al.*, 1995) of β-amino acids. A cDNA for a sodium- and chloride-dependent taurine transporter has been cloned and the transporter has been shown to be highly expressed in brain (Uchida *et al.*, 1992).

System X⁻

Finally, anionic amino acids (i.e., glutamate and aspartate) are taken up into brain and brain microvessels at slow rates by a sodium-dependent, high-affinity system, tentatively identified as System X⁻ ($K_m = 1.9$ µM for L-glutamate) (Oldendorf and Szabo, 1976; Hutchinson *et al.*, 1985; Al-Sarraf *et al.*, 1995). As these amino acids are neuroexcitatory and toxic at high concentrations,

System X⁻ may function to pump anionic amino acids out of brain, as originally proposed by Pardridge (1979). A family of anionic amino acid transporters have been cloned and identified in brain (Kanai *et al.*, 1994).

Conclusions

Over the past 25 years, significant progress has been made in the identification and characterization of blood–brain barrier amino acid transport systems, using primarily physiological methods. However, with the advent of the cloning and identification of the first blood–brain barrier amino acid transport protein and gene (System y⁺) in 1993, a new era has been ushered in to the investigation of barrier amino acid transport systems. It is hoped that these new approaches will provide novel, more selective tools and probes to study the transport systems and evaluate their regulation. With these new molecular biological approaches, it may be possible ultimately to modify blood–brain barrier amino acid transport expression to treat human disease.

Acknowledgments

This work was supported by the NIA Intramural Program.

References

Albritton, L. M., Tseng, L., Scadden, D. and Cunningham, J. M. (1989). A putative murine ecotropic retrovirus receptor gene encodes a multiple membrane-spanning protein and confers susceptibility to virus infection. *Cell*, **57**, 659–66.

Albritton, L. M., Bowcock, A. M., Eddy, R. L. *et al.* (1992). The human cationic amino acid transporter (ATRC1): Physical and genetic mapping to 13q12-q14. *Genomics*, **12**, 430–4.

Al-Sarraf, H., Preston, J. E. and Segal, M. B. (1995). The entry of acidic amino acids into brain and CSF during development using in situ brain perfusion in the rat. *Dev. Brain Res.*, **90**, 151–8.

Aoyagi, M., Agranoff, B. W., Washburn, L. C. and Smith, Q. R. (1988). Blood–brain barrier transport of 1-aminocyclohexanecarboxylic acid, a nonmetabolizable amino acid for in vivo studies of brain transport. *J. Neurochem.*, **50**, 1220–6.

Arriza, J. L., Kavanaugh, M. P., Fairman, W. A. *et al.* (1993). Cloning and expression of a human neutral amino acid transporter with structural similarity to the glutamate transporter gene family. *J. Biol. Chem.*, **268**, 15329–32.

Bertran, J., Magagnin, S., Werner, A. *et al.* (1992). Stimulation of system y⁺-like amino acid transport by the heavy chain of human 4F2 surface antigen in *Xenopus laevis* oocytes. *Proc. Natl. Acad. Sci., USA*, **89**, 5606–10.

Bertran, J., Werner, A., Chillarón, J. *et al.* (1993). Expression cloning of a human renal cDNA that induces high affinity transport of L-cystine shared with dibasic amino acids in *Xenopus* oocytes. *J. Biol. Chem.*, **268**, 14842–9.

Betz, A. L. and Goldstein, G. W. (1978). Polarity of the blood–brain barrier: neutral amino acid transport into isolated brain capillaries. *Science*, **202**, 225–7.

Bröer, S., Bröer, A. and Hamprecht, B. (1995). The 4F2hc surface antigen is necessary for expression of system L-like neutral amino acid transport activity in C6-BU-1 rat glioma cells: Evidence from expression studies in *Xenopus laevis* oocytes. *Biochem. J.*, **312**, 863–70.

Calonge, M. J., Gasparini, P., Chillon, M., *et al.* (1994). Cystinuria caused by mutations in rBAT, a gene involved in the transport of cystine. *Nature Genet.*, **6**, 420–5.

Closs, E. I., Albritton, L. M., Kim, J. W. and Cunningham, J. M. (1993*a*). Identification of a low affinity, high capacity transporter of cationic amino acids in mouse liver. *J. Biol. Chem.*, **268**, 7538–44.

Closs, E. I., Lyons, C. R., Kelly, C. and Cunningham, J. M. (1993*b*). Characterization of a third member of the MCAT family of cationic amino acid transporters. *J. Biol. Chem.*, **268**, 20796–800.

Cornford, E. M., Young, D., Paxton, J. W. *et al.* (1992). Melphalan penetration of the blood–brain barrier via the neutral amino acid transporter in tumor-bearing brain. *Cancer Res.*, **52**, 138–43.

Ennis, S. R., Ren, X. and Betz, A. L. (1994). Transport of α-aminoisobutyric acid across the blood–brain barrier studied with in situ perfusion of rat brain. *Brain Res.*, **643**, 100–7.

Greenwood, J., Hazell, A. S. and Pratt, O. E. (1989). The transport of leucine and aminocyclopentanecarboxylate across the intact, energy-depleted rat blood–brain barrier. *J. Cereb. Blood Flow Metab.*, **9**, 226–33.

Guidotti, G. G. and Gazzola, G. C. (1992). Amino acid transporters: systematic approach and principles of control. In *Mammalian Amino Acid Transport*, ed. M. S. Kilberg & D. Haussinger, pp. 3–30. New York: Plenum Press.

Hargreaves, K. M. and Pardridge, W. M. (1988). Neutral amino acid transport at the human blood–brain barrier. *J. Biol. Chem.*, **263**, 19392–7.

Hofmann, K., Düker, M., Fink, T. *et al.* (1994). Human neutral amino acid transporter ASCT1: Structure of the gene (SLC1A4) and localization to chromosome 2p13-p15. *Genomics*, **24**, 20–6.

Hokari, M. and Smith, Q. R. (1994). Thyroid hormones express high affinity for both the thyroid hormone and large neutral amino acid transporters of the blood–brain barrier. *Soc. Neurosci. Abstr.*, **20**, 1335.

Hutchison, H. T., Eisenberg, H. M. and Haber, B. (1985). High affinity transport of glutamate in rat brain microvessels. *Exper. Neurol.*, **87**, 260–9 .

Kakuda, D. K., Finley, K. D., Dionne, V. E. and Macleod, C. L. (1993). Two distinct gene products mediate y+ type cationic amino acid transport in Xenopus oocytes and show different tissue expression patterns. *Transgene*, **1**, 91–101.

Kanai, Y., Smith, C. P. and Hediger, M. A. (1994). A new family of neurotransmitter transporters: the high affinity glutamate transporters. *FASEB J.*, **8**, 1450–9.

Kavanaugh, M. P. (1993). Voltage dependence of facilitated arginine flux mediated by the System y+ basic amino acid transporter. *Biochemistry*, **32**, 5781–5.

Kim, J. W., Closs, E. I., Albritton, L. M. and Cunningham, J. M. (1991). Transport of cationic amino acids by the mouse ecotropic retrovirus receptor. *Nature (Lond.).* **35**, 725–8.

Lee, W. J., Hawkins, R. A., Peterson, D. R. and Viña, J. R. (1996). Role of oxyproline in the regulation of neutral amino acid transport across the blood–brain barrier. *J. Biol. Chem.*, **271**, 19129–33.

Momma, S., Aoyagi, M., Rapoport, S. I. and Smith, Q. R. (1987). Phenylalanine transport across the blood–brain barrier as studied with the in situ brain perfusion technique, *J. Neurochem.*, **48**, 1291–300.

Oldendorf, W. H. (1971). Brain uptake of radiolabeled amino acids, amines and hexoses after arterial injection. *Am. J. Physiol.*, **221**, 1629–39.

Oldendorf, W. H. and Szabo, J. (1976). Amino acid assignment to one of three blood–brain barrier amino acid carriers. *Am. J. Physiol.*, **230**, 94–8.

Oxender, D. L. and Christensen, H. N. (1963). Distinct mediating systems for the transport of neutral amino acids by the Ehrlich cell. *J. Biol. Chem.*, **238**, 3686–99.

Palacín, M. (1994). A new family of proteins (rBAT and 4F2hc) involved in cationic and zwitterionic amino acid transport: A tale of two proteins in search of a transport function. *J. Exp. Biol.*, **196**, 123–37.

Pardridge, W. M. (1979). Regulation of amino acid availability to brain: selective control mechanisms for glutamate. In *Glutamic Acid: Advances in Biochemistry and Physiology*, ed. L. J. Filer, Jr, pp. 125–37. New York: Raven Press.

Pardridge, W. M. (1983). Brain metabolism: a perspective from the blood–brain barrier. *Physiol. Rev.*, 63, 1481–535.

Pardridge, W. M., Triguero, D. and Cancilla, P. A. (1990). Comparison of *in vitro* and *in vivo* models of drug transcytosis through the blood–brain barrier. *J. Pharmacol. Exp. Ther.*, **253**, 884–91.

Peters, J. C. and Harper, A. E. (1987). Acute effects of dietary protein on food intake, tissue amino acids and brain serotonin. *Am. J. Physiol.*, **252**, R902–R914.

Preston, J. E. and Segal, M. B. (1992). The uptake of anionic and cationic amino acids by the isolated perfused sheep choroid plexus. *Brain Res.*, **581**, 351–5.

Puppi, M. and Henning, S. J. (1995). Cloning of the rat ecotropic retroviral receptor and studies of its expression in intestinal tissues. *Proc. Soc. Exp. Biol. Med.*, **209**, 38–45.

Ramamoorthy, S., Leibach, F. H., Madresh, V. B. and Ganapathy, V. (1992). Modulation of activity of amino acid transport system L by phorbol esters and calmodulin antagonists in a human placental choriocarcinoma cell line. *Biochim. Biophys. Acta*, **1136**, 181–8.

Sánchez del Pino, M. M., Hawkins, R. A. and Peterson, D. R. (1992). Neutral amino acid transport by the blood–brain barrier. *J. Biol. Chem.*, **267**, 25951–7.

Sánchez del Pino, M. M., Hawkins, R. A. and Peterson, D. R. (1995). Neutral amino acid transport characterization of isolated luminal and abluminal membranes of the blood–brain barrier. *J. Biol. Chem.*, **270**, 14913–18.

Segal, M. B., Preston, J. E., Collis, C. S. and Zlokovic, B. V. (1990). Kinetics and Na independence of amino acid uptake by blood side of the perfused sheep choroid plexus. *Am. J. Physiol.*, **258**, F1288–F1294.

Shulkin, B. L., Betz, A. L., Koeppe, R. A. and Agranoff, B. W. (1995). Inhibition of neutral amino acid transport across the human blood–brain barrier by phenylalanine. *J. Neurochem.*, **64**, 1252–7.

Smith, Q. R. (1995). Carrier-mediated drug transport at the blood–brain barrier and the potential for drug targeting to the brain. In *New Concepts of a Blood–Brain Barrier*, ed. J. Greenwood *et al.*, pp. 265–76. New York: Plenum Press.

Smith, Q. R. (1996). Brain perfusion systems for studies of drug uptake and metabolism in the central nervous system. In *Models for Assessing Drug Absorption and Metabolism*, eds. R. T. Borchardt *et al.*, pp. 285–307. New York: Plenum Press.

Smith, Q. R. and Cooper, A. J. L. (1992). Amino acid transport into brain. In *Mammalian Amino Acid Transport*, ed. M. S. Kilberg and D. Haussinger, pp. 165–93. New York: Plenum Press.

Smith, Q. R., Momma, S., Aoyagi, M. and Rapoport, S. I. (1987). Kinetics of neutral amino acid transport across the blood–brain barrier. *J. Neurochem.*, **49**, 1651–8.

Stoll, J., Wadhwani, K. C. and Smith, Q. R. (1993). Identification of the cationic amino acid transporter (System y$^+$) of the rat blood–brain barrier. *J. Neurochem.*, **60**, 1956–9.

Takada, Y., Vistica, D. T., Greig, N. H. *et al.* (1992). Rapid high-affinity transport of a chemotherapeutic amino acid across the blood–brain barrier. *Cancer Res.*, **52**, 2191–6.

Takasato, Y., Rapoport, S. I. and Smith, Q. R. (1984). An *in situ* brain perfusion technique to study cerebrovascular transport in the rat. *Am. J. Physiol.*, **247**, H484–H493.

Tamai, I., Senmaru, M., Terasaki, T. and Tsuji, A. (1995). Na$^+$ and Cl$^-$-dependent transport of taurine at the blood–brain barrier. *Biochem. Pharmacol.*, **50**, 1783–93.

Tate, S. H., Yan, N. and Udenfriend, S. (1992). Expression cloning of a Na$^+$-independent neutral amino acid transporter from rat kidney. *Proc. Natl. Acad. Sci., USA*, **89**, 1–5.

Tayarani, I., Lefauconnier, J. M., Roux, F. and Bourre, J. M. (1987). Evidence for an alanine, serine and cysteine system of transport in isolated brain capillaries. *J. Cereb. Blood Flow Metab.*, **7**, 585–91.

Tayarani, I., Clöez, I., Lefauconnier, J. M. and Bourre, J. M. (1989). Sodium-dependent high affinity uptake of taurine by isolated rat brain capillaries. *Biochim. Biophys. Acta*, **985**, 168–72.

Tovar, A., Tews, J. K., Torres, N. and Harper, A. E. (1988). Some characteristics of threonine transport across the blood–brain barrier of the rat. *J. Neurochem.*, **51**, 1285–93.

Uchida, S., Kwon, H. M., Yamauchi, A. *et al.* (1992). Molecular cloning of the cDNA for an MDCK cell Na$^+$– and Cl$^-$ dependent taurine transporter that is regulated by hypertonicity. *Proc. Natl. Acad. Sci., USA*, **89**, 8230–4.

Wade, L. A. and Brady, H. M. (1981). Cysteine and cystine transport at the blood–brain barrier. *J. Neurochem.*, **37**, 730–4.

Wang, H., Kavanaugh, M. P., North, R. A. and Kabat, D. (1992). Cell-surface receptor for ecotropic murine retroviruses is a basic amino acid transporter. *Nature (Lond.)*, **352**, 729–31.

Wells, R. G. and Hediger, M. A. (1992). Cloning of a rat kidney cDNA that stimulates dibasic and neutral amino acid transport and has sequence similarity to glucosidases. *Proc. Natl. Acad. Sci., USA*, **89**, 5596–600.

Yoshimoto, T., Yoshimoto, E. and Meruelo, D. (1992). Enhanced gene expression of the murine ecotropic retroviral receptor and its human homolog in proliferating cells. *J. Virol.*, **66**, 4377–81.

21 P-glycoprotein, a guardian of the brain

P. BORST and A. H. SCHINKEL

- Introduction
- P-glycoprotein is present in the blood–brain barrier
- Mice without P-gp in their blood–brain barrier
- Ivermectin and the blood–brain barrier
- Studies on P-gp mediated drug transport by monolayers of isolated capillary endothelium; potential and pitfalls
- How important is P-gp function in the blood–brain barrier with inhibitors
- Blocking P-gp function in the blood–brain barrier with inhibitors
- Consequences of brain P-gp for drug use and drug design
- Concluding remarks

Introduction

A drug-transporting P-glycoprotein (P-gp) is present in the blood–brain barrier of all mammals investigated, including humans. The P-gp is present in the apical membrane of the endothelial cells lining brain capillaries and optimally placed to extrude drugs from the endothelial cells into the blood. The generation of knockout mice, completely lacking P-gp in their brain capillaries, has provided a model system to test the ability of P-gp to guard the brain against intrusion of compounds that are lipophilic enough to diffuse readily across the blood–brain barrier. Drugs transported by P-gp accumulate to a much higher extent in the brains of the knockout mice than in those of wild-type mice. For drugs such as vinblastine, ivermectin or digoxin, the difference is one to two orders of magnitude. This shows that P-gp is an important component of the blood–brain barrier and that active extrusion of drugs by P-gp explains many, if not all, examples of lipophilic drugs entering the brain at a much lower rate than expected on the basis of their lipophilicity.

The presence of P-gp in the blood–brain barrier has potential consequences for drug use and drug design. Following the development of potent inhibitors of P-gp (so-called reversal agents) with relatively low toxicity, clinical trials have been started in which these inhibitors are used to overcome multidrug resistance in tumors. Obviously, this may lead to serious toxicity as drugs, normally excluded from the brain by P-gp, now gain access. On the positive side, however, knowledge of P-gp activity in the blood–brain barrier might be used to increase access of drugs to the brain, either by drug modification or by combining drugs with P-gp inhibitors.

P-glycoprotein is present in the blood–brain barrier

P-glycoproteins (P-gps) are plasma membrane glycoproteins of about 170 kDa that belong to the superfamily of ATP-binding cassette (ABC) transporters, also called traffic ATPases (Higgins, 1992;

198

Doige and Ferro-Luzzi Ames, 1993). They were discovered by Juliano and Ling (1976) in multidrug resistant (MDR) cancer cells and they cause resistance by the active extrusion of a wide range of large amphipathic natural product drugs used to treat cancer. In 1989, two groups independently demonstrated the presence of P-gp in human brain capillaries (Cordon-Cardo *et al.*, 1989; Thiebaut *et al.*, 1989). P-gp was also detected in rat brain capillaries (Thiebaut *et al.*, 1989), suggesting that the presence of P-gp might be a more general property of the mammalian blood–brain barrier. No P-gp was seen in the choroid plexus, meninges, peripheral nerves or sympathetic ganglia, or in capillaries of most tissues other than brain (Cordon-Cardo *et al.*, 1989). However, P-gp was also found in the capillaries of the testes, raising the possibility that P-gp has a general function in guarding blood–tissue barrier sites.

Subsequent work confirmed the presence of P-gp in capillaries of human brain and primary brain tumors (Sugawara, 1990; Van der Valk *et al.*, 1990; Becker *et al.*, 1991; Nabors *et al.*, 1991; Tanaka *et al.*, 1994; Tóth *et al.*, 1996) and in isolated capillary endothelium of humans (Biegel *et al.*, 1995), rats (Barrand *et al.*, 1995; Jetté *et al.*, 1995a), mice (Hegmann *et al.*, 1992; Shirai *et al.*, 1994; Jetté *et al.*, 1995b), pigs (Hegmann *et al.*, 1992) and cattle (Tsuji *et al.*, 1992; Tsuji *et al.*, 1993). By immunoelectronmicroscopy P-gp was localized in the apical (luminal surface) membrane of endothelial cells in direct contact with blood (Sugawara, 1990; Tsuji *et al.*, 1992; Shirai *et al.*, 1994; Tanaka *et al.*, 1994; Biegel *et al.*, 1995).

To test whether the P-gp in brain capillaries restricts access of amphipathic drugs to the brain, several groups tested the effect of P-gp inhibitors on drug accumulation. (These inhibitors are also known as 'reversal agents', because of their ability to reverse multidrug resistance of tumor cells). When the P-gp inhibitor quinidine was coadministered with Cyclosporin A (CsA), (a P-gp substrate and inhibitor), through a microdialysis probe implanted in the brain, it increased the extravascular extraction of CsA 2.5-fold (Sakata *et al.*, 1994). In another microdialysis study CsA was shown to increase the distribution to the brain of rhodamine-123, also a P-gp substrate (Wang *et al.*, 1995). Finally, Chikhale *et al.* (1995) showed that

the P-gp inhibitor verapamil markedly increases the influx of some hydrophobic peptides into the rat brain. Although these inhibitor studies suggested that P-gp is present in all brain capillaries and is able to protect the entire brain, the experiments were not conclusive. Drugs have side effects, and even the most potent and specific inhibitors of P-gp also inhibit some other transporters (see e.g. Böhme *et al.*, 1994). How important P-gp really is in the blood–brain barrier only became clear when mice were generated with a targeted disruption of the P-gp gene expressed in the blood–brain barrier.

Mice without P-gp in their blood–brain barrier

Mice have three P-gp genes, one for a phosphatidylcholine translocator (Smit *et al.*, 1993), called *mdr2*, and two for drug transporting P-gps, called *mdr1a* (or *mdr3*) and *mdr1b* (or *mdr1*). The *mdr1a* and *1b* P-gps differ in tissue distribution (Croop *et al.*, 1989; Borst *et al.*, 1993), but together they are represented in all tissues in which the single human MDR1 P-gp is present. In the past four years, mice have been generated with defective *mdr* genes. Such knockout mice carry disrupted genes in their germline and in all somatic cells and are designated *mdr* (−/−) mice, to distinguish them from wild-type (+/+) and heterozygotes (+/−). Each of the three mouse *mdr* genes has been disrupted, and also both genes for drug transporting P-gps. The results obtained with the *mdr2* (−/−) mice (Smit *et al.*, 1993), the *mdr1a* (−/−) mice (Schinkel *et al.*, 1994, 1995b; Van Asperen *et al.*, 1996; Schinkel *et al.*, 1996; Mayer *et al.*, 1996), the *mdr1b* (−/−) and *mdr1a/1b* (−/−) mice (Schinkel *et al.*, 1997) have been published in detail. A brief summary can be found in a recent review (Borst and Schinkel, 1996).

The *mdr1a* (−/−) mice have been very useful for dissecting the contribution of P-gp to the blood–brain barrier, because these mice have completely lost the immunochemically detectable P-gp in their brain capillaries (Schinkel *et al.*, 1994). Apparently, the *mdr1b* and *mdr2* genes are not expressed in normal mouse brain endothelial cells.

Mdr1a (−/−) mice are completely normal, if not

Table 21.1. *Drug accumulation in the mouse brain; a comparison of* mdr1a *(−/−) and wild-type (+/+) mice*

Drug	Transport by P-gp*	Accumulation of drug** Relative concentration [ratio (−/−)/(+/+)]		Method of analysis
		Plasma	Brain	
Vinblastine	+++	2	22	Vinblastine
[³H]Ivermectin	+++	3	87	Radioactivity
[³H]Digoxin	+++	4	66	Radioactivity
[³H]Cyclosporin A	+++	1	17	Radioactivity
[³H]Dexamethasone	+++	1	2	Radioactivity
[³H]Morphine	+	1	2	Radioactivity
[³H]Domperidone	+++	1	1***	Radioactivity
[³H]Haloperidol	±	1	1	Radioactivity
[³H]Clozapine	±	1	1	Radioactivity
[¹⁴H]Phenytoin	+	1	1	Radioactivity
[¹⁴H]Ondansetron	++	1	4	Radioactivity
[³H]Loperamide	+++	2	13	Radioactivity

*Transport by P-gp was assessed semi-quantitatively by determining the drug flux through a monolayer of pig kidney cells transfected with cDNA constructs containing either the human *MDR1* or the murine *mdr1a* gene. The P-gps encoded by these genes localize in the apical membrane and this results in vectorial transport through the monolayer from basal to apical (see Schinkel *et al.*, 1995).
**Most values were obtained 4 hours after a single i.v. injection of drug.
***Lack of effect on apparent accumulation probably due to rapid metabolism (see text).
(Based on data in Schinkel *et al.*, 1994, 1995, 1996; Mayer *et al.*, 1996). See text for caveats.

challenged with drugs. They lack morphological abnormalities, they are fertile and their life-span is unaltered. However, they are hypersensitive to a range of drugs known to be transported by P-gp. Accumulation of these drugs in the brain of *mdr1a* (−/−) mice is often highly increased relative to wild-type (+/+) mice.

Table 21.1 summarizes some of the main results obtained thus far. To avoid misinterpretation, some of the limitations in these analyses should be stressed. With the exception of vinblastine, all drugs were followed by radioactivity and the accumulation data here presented represent the sum of unaltered drug and drug metabolites. As the metabolites may not be transported by P-gp and as metabolism may be fast, the values in Table 21.1 may grossly underestimate the real difference

in accumulation of parent drug between the *mdr1a* (−/−) and (+/+) brain. This is the case for domperidone (see below), but probably also for dexamethasone (Schinkel *et al.*, 1995*b*). A second complication is that most of these drugs were studied only at a single time point, 4 hours after an i.v. injection. Especially when a drug is rapidly metabolized, a 4 hour time point may largely miss the effect of the absence of P-gp in the blood–brain barrier. The only drugs studied in detail thus far are vinblastine (Van Asperen *et al.*, 1996) and digoxin (Mayer *et al.*, 1996). These caveats emphasize that the data in Table 21.1 must not be taken too literally. Nevertheless it is already clear from this limited survey that drugs transported by P-gp tend to accumulate to a higher extent in the brain when P-gp is absent from the blood–brain barrier.

The increased penetration of drugs into the brain of *mdr1a* (−/−) mice is often accompanied by increased toxicity. The most dramatic example is ivermectin, where a 100-fold increase in brain accumulation is accompanied by a 100-fold decrease in the lethal dose (Schinkel *et al.*, 1994). Increased CNS toxicity has also been seen, however, for domperidone and loperamide (Schinkel *et al.*, 1996). In fact, even though domperidone is so rapidly metabolized that the increased brain uptake in *mdr1a* (−/−) mice could not be detected (Table 21.1), even 30 min after i.v. administration, a substantial increase in CNS toxicity was observed in the *mdr1a* (−/−) mice (Schinkel *et al.*, 1996), indicating that the absence of P-gp in the blood–brain barrier allows better access of domperidone to the brain, as expected from the high rate at which domperidone is transported by P-gp (Table 21.1).

Another interesting example of increased and altered toxicity is provided by loperamide. This is an opioid drug that does not pass the blood–brain barrier of normal mammals. It has hardly any known opiate-like CNS effect. Loperamide is a good substrate for P-gp, however (Table 21.1); it accumulates in the brain of *mdr1a* (−/−) mice and accumulation is accompanied by pronounced opiate-like CNS toxicity (Schinkel *et al.*, 1996). Inactivation of P-gp therefore unmasks the strong central activity of this relatively innocuous antidiarrheal drug, which only has peripheral actions in normal animals.

Ivermectin and the blood–brain barrier

The removal of P-gp from the mammalian blood–brain barrier turns this widely used anthelmintic, acaricidal and insecticidal agent into a deadly drug. This was accidentally discovered by the killing of *mdr1a* (−/−) mice, but not their (+/−) littermates, during a routine treatment of mice for a mite infection (Schinkel *et al.*, 1994). Sadly, this result has unintentionally been reproduced in another laboratory (personal communication), showing that routine spraying with ivermectin is sufficient for killing mice, if they are not protected by P-gp. Ivermectin is a neurotransmitter agonist with a high safety margin in vertebrates. Clearly, P-gp

is an essential determinant of this safety margin.

Interestingly, an inbred strain of collie dogs is known to be extremely sensitive to ivermectin, the lethal dose being 200-fold lower than in normal dogs. Hypersensitivity is associated with increased brain accumulation of ivermectin (see discussion in Schinkel *et al.*, 1994). It is likely that the inbred collies lack a functional P-gp in the blood–brain barrier, but the exact nature of the defect has not been verified. If they are indeed P-gp (−/−), these collies would provide a large animal model for testing the effect of P-gp on drug accumulation in the brain.

It is intriguing that more than 10 million people have been treated with ivermectin for river blindness (onchocerciasis) without reported untoward effect (discussed in Schinkel *et al.*, 1994). This suggests that a severe deficiency of MDR1 P-gp is very rare in the treated African population. This may mean that humans homozygous for *MDR1* null alleles do not survive *in utero* or as infants in Africa. It is also possible, however, that deadly incidents with ivermectin due to P-gp deficiency did occur, but were misinterpreted, or that humans have more ways to deal with ivermectin than mice.

Studies on P-gp mediated drug transport by monolayers of isolated capillary endothelium; potential and pitfalls

Several groups have demonstrated the presence of P-gp in cultured brain capillary endothelial cells from several mammals. This P-gp could be labeled by substrate analogues and its functional significance was shown by restricted uptake of MDR drugs in these cells, reversed by MDR reversal agents (Hegmann *et al.*, 1992; Tatsuta *et al.*, 1992; Tsuji *et al.*, 1992, 1993; Barrand *et al.*, 1995; Biegel *et al.*, 1995; Jetté *et al.*, 1995*a,b*). Relatively tight polarized monolayers can be formed by these endothelial cells allowing the analysis of P-gp mediated transport of drugs from basal side to apical side (Tatsuta *et al.*, 1992; Biegel *et al.*, 1995).

Tatsuta *et al.* (1992) reported that their cultured mouse brain endothelial cells expressed the *mdr1b* gene, as judged from hybridization experiments using gene-specific probes. Analysis of the *mdr1a* (−/−) mice subsequently demonstrated, however, that only the *mdr1a* gene is expressed in the capillaries of intact mouse brain (Schinkel *et al.*, 1994) and the same result was obtained with freshly isolated mouse brain capillaries by Jetté *et al.* (1995*b*). The discrepancy was resolved by Barrand *et al.* (1995) using cultured rat brain endothelial cells. Whereas the intact capillaries only contained the rat equivalent of the mouse mdr1a P-gp, cells in culture gradually lost mdr1a P-gp and replaced it by the mdr1b P-gp. This interesting result provides a striking illustration of the tendency of brain endothelial cells to dedifferentiate *in vitro* and lose the specific properties characteristic of brain capillaries. These may depend on intimate contact with astrocytes (discussed in Biegel *et al.*, 1995). One should therefore be cautious in extrapolating results obtained with cultured brain endothelium to the intact blood–brain barrier *in vivo*.

How important is P-gp for the barrier function of the blood–brain barrier?

Until very recently, the blood–brain barrier was described in reviews and textbooks as a lipid wall without specific doors for hydrophobic customers. Specialized entries were known to be available for hydrophilic molecules – transporters for small ones, receptor-mediated transcytosis for proteins – but hydrophobic molecules were thought to pass the barrier by passive diffusion (see Levin, 1980; Bradbury, 1985). As a first approximation, the octanol–H_2O partition coefficient divided by the square root of the molecular weight of the drug was indeed found to predict the ability of hydrophobic drugs to enter the brain. Exceptions were noted, however, and these gave rise to increasingly sophisticated physicochemical refinements of the octanol–H_2O partition approach (Seelig *et al.*, 1994).

It is now clear that many of these exceptions are P-gp substrates and that the anomalously low brain accumulation of these compounds is not due to their sluggish diffusion through membranes, but to interception and active extrusion by P-gp. Some of the early exceptions studied (Levin, 1980), the

carcinostatic agents doxorubicin, vincristine and etoposide, are now known to be excellent P-gp substrates. These drugs are included in the multidrug resistance spectrum caused by raised P-gp levels in cancer cells. The presence of P-gp in the blood–brain barrier also provides a simple explanation for the inability of hydrophobic compounds >700 kDa to enter the brain at significant rates. Apparently these compounds are good substrates for P-gp, as shown by the examples tested: digoxin (M_r 781), vinblastine (811), paclitaxel (854), ivermectin (874), and Cyclosporin A (1203). The rate at which these drugs diffuse through a tight monolayer of pig kidney cells is not lower than that of morphine; they are only better substrates for P-gp than morphine (Schinkel *et al.*, 1996).

Two recent studies further illustrate the importance of P-gp as a guardian of the brain. The first of these was carried out by Seelig *et al.* (1994) who studied 28 drugs varying in hydrophobicity and found six very hydrophobic compounds that entered the brain poorly. They suggested that these are trapped in the membrane interior and are unable 'to reprotonate at the CNS side of the membrane in order to leave for the brain fluid'. Trapping was found to correlate with the surface activity of the drug. A low concentration at surface activity onset and a low critical micelle concentration at which the surface pressure reaches a limiting value was found to result in poor brain penetration.

Two of the anomalous hydrophobic CNS negative drugs studied by Seelig *et al.* (1994) are domperidone and loperamide, compounds also listed in our Table 21.1. Both compounds are excellent P-gp substrates. Moreover, both compounds diffuse through a kidney monolayer at substantial rate, 3–4 times as fast as morphine (Schinkel *et al.*, 1996). Obviously, these drugs have no problem in passing membranes; they just have difficulty in getting past P-gp. A third hydrophobic CNS negative drug studied by Seelig *et al.* (1994), terfenadine, is a known reversal agent of multidrug resistance caused by P-gp (Hait *et al.*, 1993). It must therefore interact with P-gp and is probably transported by P-gp, like many reversal agents. The other three hydrophobic CNS negative drugs studied by Seelig *et al.* (1994) have not been tested as P-gp substrates, but we would be surprised if they are not.

The second illuminating study was done with a

series of D-phenylalanine peptides with blocked termini (Chikhale *et al.*, 1994). The ability of these peptides to move through the brain capillary wall did not correlate well with their ability to partition into octanol. A better correlation was found, however, with the number of potential hydrogen bonds that these peptides could make with water (more H bonds, lower permeability). In a subsequent study, Chikhale *et al.* (1995) found, however, that the P-gp inhibitor verapamil drastically increased the permeability coefficient of the peptides with high hydrogen bonding potential. It seems therefore that the anomalously low coefficient of these peptides can also be explained by the presence of P-gp in the blood–brain barrier.

The results of Seelig *et al.* (1994) and Chikhale *et al.* (1994; 1995) are of interest because they may help to define drug properties important for transport by P-gp. Notwithstanding considerable work, these properties remain ill-defined (Ecker and Chiba, 1995).

The examples discussed in this section show that P-gp is an important impediment for the entry of hydrophobic drugs into the brain. Although only a limited number of hydrophobic CNS negative drugs have been studied thus far, it is noteworthy that every single one of these proved to be a P-gp substrate. Although sweeping generalizations are usually incorrect, we nevertheless think that the presence of P-gp in the blood–brain barrier is responsible for the inability of most, if not all, hydrophobic, membrane-permeant drugs to pass this barrier.

Blocking P-gp function in the blood–brain barrier with inhibitors

The contribution of P-gp to multidrug resistance in cancer cells has stimulated efforts to develop inhibitors of P-gp that could reverse resistance in patients. Since Tsuruo and coworkers (see Watanabe *et al.*, 1995) discovered the first of these reversal agents, verapamil, a large range of compounds with reversal activity have been described (Ford, 1995). Most of these compounds are actually transported by P-gp, but as they are less cytotoxic than the anti-cancer drugs used to kill cells, they can be used to inhibit P-gp without cell kill. A number of

these inhibitors are being tested in clinical trials to reverse multidrug resistance (Fisher and Sikic, 1995; Goldstein, 1995).

Reversal agents inhibit P-gp in isolated brain capillaries as effectively as P-gp in tumors or other tissues. This is not surprising as there are no indications for brain-specific modifications of P-gp that could affect its interaction with drugs or inhibitors. Few studies have looked at the inhibition of brain P-gp in intact organisms and a weak point in all these studies is the lack of a suitable reference point to assess how completely brain P-gp had been inhibited. The *mdr1a* (−/−) and *mdr1a/1b* (−/−) mice provide this point of reference and these mice have been used to study the effect of P-gp inhibitors on the accumulation of radioactive digoxin in the brain, as this is a convenient test system. The accumulation of digoxin in the brain of *mdr1a* (−/−) mice is at least two orders of magnitude higher than in wild-type mice and toxicity is minimal, as mice are resistant to digoxin (Mayer *et al.*, 1996). Studies with PSC 833, a Cyclosporin A analogue without immunosuppressive effect and one of the most potent reversal agents now in clinical trial, showed that the maximal dose of PSC 833 tolerated by mice is unable to completely block brain P-gp. Although the digoxin accumulation in the brains of PSC 833 treated wild-type mice is 10-fold higher than in untreated wild-type mice, it remains 5-fold below the level in the *mdr1a/1b* (−/−) mice (Mayer *et al.*, 1997). This proves that PSC 833 does not completely inhibit brain P-gp under these experimental conditions, probably because binding to plasma proteins lowers its availability, a problem also encountered with other reversal agents (Lehnert *et al.*, 1996). These results illustrate the usefulness of the *mdr1a* (−/−) mice as gold standard for testing the effectiveness of the new P-gp inhibitors being developed by several pharmaceutical firms.

This unexpected result prompts a check on the effect of 100% serum on the efficacy of PSC 833 as a P-gp inhibitor. In recent experiments with kidney cell monolayers (Schinkel *et al.*, 1995*b*, 1996) it has been found that serum strongly inhibits the effect of PSC 833 on P-gp-mediated transport through these monolayers (A. J. Smith and P. Borst, unpublished). It is assumed that this is due to binding of PSC 833 to serum proteins.

The maximal plasma levels of PSC 833 tolerated by the mice gave only a partial inhibition of digoxin or daunorubicin transport through the monolayers providing a simple explanation for the incomplete inhibition of P-gp in the blood–brain barrier.

These experiments underline the need for realistic *in vivo* and *in vitro* models for the evaluation of P-gp inhibitors.

Consequences of brain P-gp for drug use and drug design

The consequences of an active P-gp in the blood–brain barrier for drug use and drug design are fairly obvious:

1. Many natural product drugs used to treat cancer are good P-gp substrates. If these drugs are combined with P-gp inhibitors to overcome multidrug resistance, increased toxicity can be expected. Fortunately, most anticancer drugs are relatively non-toxic to the brain. For instance, the 20-fold increase of vinblastine caused by P-gp deficiency in *mdr1a* (−/−) mice (Table 21.1) is not associated with specific CNS toxicity. However, cancer patients get other drugs than anticancer drugs, such as the anti-emetic ondansetron or the cardiac glycoside digoxin. The results presented in Table 21.1 suggest that these drugs might cause serious toxicity if co-administered with P-gp inhibitors. Knowledge of P-gp in the blood–brain barrier and its effect on drug entry should help to avoid such mishaps.

2. As P-gp is an important impediment to the influx of hydrophobic drugs into the brain, it would seem wise to take this parameter into account in drug design. It is possible that surface activity or hydrogen-bonding potential of a drug can indicate whether it is transported by P-gp (see preceding section), but as it has proven difficult to predict which molecules are good P-gp substrates, it is more sensible to test transport of a new drug directly in cells overproducing P-gp. The knowledge obtained in such systems could help to design drug analogs that enter the brain better (or less well, whatever is desired). We note in passing that P-gp in the gut epithelium limits the oral availability of some hydrophobic drugs (see Sparreboom *et al.*, 1997) and knowledge of a drug's interaction with P-gp is therefore also useful for assessing its potential oral availability.

3. With the advent of relatively non-toxic P-gp inhibitors it may become possible to block brain P-gp for short periods with a short-acting inhibitor to promote entry of drugs normally kept out of the brain by P-gp. If structure–function studies of a drug of interest indicate that its pharmacological effects on brain are linked to structural features that make it a good P-gp substrate, blocking P-gp may be the only way to get the drug to its target tissue.

4. Whereas metastatic brain tumors induce the formation of neo-vasculature without blood–brain barrier characteristics, primary brain tumors of the glioma type may have a largely intact blood–brain barrier with conspicuous P-gp. Moreover, some gliomas contain P-gp in the tumor cells (Becker *et al.*, 1991; Nabors *et al.*, 1991; Tanaka *et al.*, 1994; Tóth *et al.*, 1996). This suggests that P-gp may limit the effectiveness of cancer chemotherapy in gliomas. In line with this suggestion, metastatic brain tumors are as sensitive to chemotherapy as the primary tumors (Boogerd *et al.*, 1993), whereas gliomas are generally resistant (see Fine, 1994; Glantz *et al.*, 1995; Williams *et al.*, 1995). It seems therefore worthwhile to test whether P-gp inhibitors could make the chemotherapy of gliomas more effective.

Concluding remarks

In our experience pharmacologists tend to rely on chemistry, biochemistry, and pharmacokinetics to decipher the disposition of drugs and they tend to underestimate the potential of genetic approaches. The work on P-gp knockout mice may serve to illustrate the power of a genetic dissection of complex metabolic pathways by gene disruption. Mouse genes are being disrupted at exponentially increasing rate. It will be possible by simple genetic crossing to assemble multiple gene disruptions in a single mouse. These mice can not only be used for metabolic studies in intact animals, but also for the generation of cell lines with specific defects. With a mouse genome project well underway, even such a highly specialized field as research on the blood–brain barrier could benefit from an increased attention to the potential of genetically modified mice, even though we admit that mice have small veins and small brains.

Acknowledgments

We thank our colleagues Sander Smith, Judith van Asperen and Drs Ulrich Mayer, Alex Sparreboom, Olaf van Tellingen and Jos Beijnen for permission to quote unpublished results on digoxin and paclitaxel metabolism in *mdr1a* (−/−) and *mdr1a/1b* (−/−) mice. We are indebted to Drs E.C.M. de Lange and D. Breimer (Center for Bio-Pharmaceutical Sciences, University Leiden) for helpful comments on the manuscript. The experimental work in our laboratory is supported in part by grant NKI 92-41 of the Dutch Cancer Society.

References

Barrand, M. A., Robertson, K. J. and Von Weikersthal, S. F. (1995). Comparisons of P-glycoprotein expression in isolated rat brain microvessels and in primary cultures of endothelial cells derived from microvasculature of rat brain, epididymal fat pad and from aorta. *FEBS Lett.*, **374**, 179–83.

Becker, K., Becker, K.-F., Meyermann, R. and Höllt, V. (1991). The multidrug-resistance gene MDR1 is expressed in human glial tumors. *Acta Neuropathol.*, **82**, 516–19.

Biegel, D., Spencer, D. D. and Pachter, J. S. (1995). Isolation and culture of human brain microvessel endothelial cells for the study of blood–brain barrier properties in vitro. *Brain Res.*, **692**, 183–9.

Böhme, M., Jedlitschky, G., Leier, I. *et al.* (1994). ATP-Dependent export pumps and their inhibition by cyclosporins. *Adv. Enz. Regul.*, **34**, 371–80.

Boogerd, W., Vos, V. W., Hart, A. A. M. and Baris, G. (1993). Brain metastases in breast cancer; natural history, prognostic factors and outcome. *J. Neuro-Oncol.*, **15**, 165–74.

Borst, P. and Schinkel, A. H. (1996). What have we learnt thus far from mice with disrupted P-glycoprotein genes? *Eur. J. Cancer*, **32A**, 985–90.

Borst, P., Schinkel, A. H., Smit, J. J. M. *et al.* (1993). Classical and novel forms of multidrug resistance and the physiological functions of P-glycoproteins in mammals. *Pharmacol. Ther.*, **60**, 289–99.

Bradbury, M. W. B. (1985). The blood–brain barrier. *Circ. Res.*, **57**, 213–22.

Chikhale, E. G., Ng, K., Burton, P. S. and Borchardt, R. T. (1994). Hydrogen bonding potential as a determinant of the in vitro and in situ blood–brain barrier permeability of peptides. *Pharmaceut. Res.*, **11**, 412–19.

Chikhale, E. G., Burton, P. S. and Borchardt, R. T. (1995). The effect of verapamil on the transport of peptides across the blood brain barrier in rats: kinetic evidence for an apically polarized efflux mechanism. *J. Pharmacol. Exp. Ther.*, **273**, 298–303.

Cordon-Cardo, C., O'Brien, J. P., Casals, D. *et al.* (1989). Multidrug-resistance gene (P-glycoprotein) is expressed by endothelial cells at blood–brain barrier sites. *Proc. Natl. Acad. Sci. USA*, **86**, 695–8.

Croop, J. M., Raymond, M., Haber, D. *et al.* (1989). The three mouse multidrug resistance (*mdr*) genes are expressed in a tissue-specific manner in normal mouse tissues. *Mol. Cell. Biol.*, **9**, 1346–50.

Doige, C. A. and Ferro-Luzzi Ames, G. (1993). ATP-dependent transport systems in bacteria and humans: relevance to cystic fibrosis and multidrug resistance. *Annu. Rev. Microbiol.*, **47**, 291–319.

Ecker, G. and Chiba, P. (1995). Structure–activity relationship studies on modulators of the multidrug transporter P-glycoprotein – an overview. *Wien. Klin. Wochenschr.*, **107/22**, 681–6.

Fine, H. A. (1994). Brain tumor chemotherapy trials: slow start, but quickly gaining. *J. Clin. Oncol.*, **12**, 2003–4.

Fisher, G. A. and Sikic, B. I. (1995). Clinical studies with modulators of multidrug resistance. *Hematol. Oncol. Clin. N. Am.*, **9**, 363–82.

Ford, J. M. (1995). Modulators of multidrug resistance. Preclinical studies. *Hematol. Oncol. Clin. N. Am.*, **9**, 337–61.

Glantz, M. J., Choy, H., Kearns, C. M. *et al.* (1995). Paclitaxel disposition in plasma and central nervous systems of humans and rats with brain tumors. *J. N. C. I.*, **87**, 1077–81.

Goldstein, L. (1995). Clinical reversal of drug resistance. *Curr. Probl. Cancer*, **XIX**, 67–124.

Hait, W. N., Gesmonde, J. F., Murren, J. R. *et al.* (1993). Terfenadine (Seldane®): a new drug for restoring sensitivity to multidrug resistant cancer cells. *Biochem. Pharmacol.*, **45**, 401–6.

Hegmann, E. J., Bauer, H. C. and Kerbel, R. S. (1992). Expression and functional activity of P-glycoprotein in cultured cerebral capillary endothelial cells. *Cancer Res.*, **52**, 6969–75.

Higgins, C. F. (1992). ABC transporters: from microorganisms to man. *Annu. Rev. Cell Biol.*, **8**, 67–113.

Jetté, L., Murphy, G. F., Leclerc, J. and Béliveau, R. (1995a). Interaction of drugs with P-glycoprotein in brain capillaries. *Biochem. Pharmacol.*, **50**, 1701–9.

Jetté, L., Pouliot, J., Murphy, G. F. and Béliveau, R. (1995*b*). Isoform I (mdr3) is the major form of P-glycoprotein expressed in mouse brain capillaries. Evidence for cross-reactivity of antibody C219 with an unrelated protein. *Biochem. J.*, **305**, 761–6.

Juliano, R. L. and Ling, V. (1976). A surface glycoprotein modulating drug permeability in Chinese hamster ovary cell mutants. *Biochim. Biophys. Acta*, **455**, 152–62.

Lehnert, M., De Giuli, R., Kunke, K. *et al.* (1996). Serum can inhibit reversal of multidrug resistance by chemosensitisers. *Eur. J. Cancer*, **32A**, 862–7.

Levin, V. A. (1980). Relationship of octanol/water partition coefficient and molecular weight to rat brain capillary permeability. *J. Med. Chem.*, **23**, 682–4.

Mayer, U., Wagenaar, E., Beijnen, J. H. *et al.* (1996). Substantial excretion of digoxin via the intestinal mucosa and prevention of long-term digoxin accumulation in the brain by the mdr1a P-glycoprotein. *Br. J. Pharmacol.*, **119**, 1038–44.

Mayer, U., Wagenaar, E., Dorobek, B. *et al.* (1997). Full blockade of intestinal P-glycoprotein and extensive inhibition of blood–brain barrier P-glycoprotein by oral treatment of mice with PSC833. *J. Clin. Invest.*, **100**, 2430–6.

Nabors, M. W., Griffin, C. A., Zehnbauer, B. A. *et al.* (1991). Multidrug resistance gene (MDR1) expression in human brain tumors. *J. Neurosurg.*, **75**, 941–6.

Sakata, A., Tamai, I., Kawazu, K. *et al.* (1994). *In vivo* evidence for ATP-dependent and P-glycoprotein-mediated transport of cyclosporin A at the blood–brain barrier. *Biochem. Pharmacol.*, **48**, 1989–92.

Schinkel, A. H., Smit, J. J. M., Van Tellingen, O. *et al.* (1994). Disruption of the mouse *mdr*1a P-glycoprotein gene leads to a deficiency in the blood–brain barrier and to increased sensitivity to drugs. *Cell*, **77**, 491–502.

Schinkel, A. H., Mol, C. A. A. M., Wagenaar, E. *et al.* (1995*a*). Multidrug resistance and the role of P-glycoprotein knockout mice. *Eur. J. Cancer*, **31A**, 1295–8.

Schinkel, A. H., Wagenaar, E., Van Deemter, L. *et al.* (1995*b*). Absence of the mdr1a P-glycoprotein in mice affects tissue distribution and pharmacokinetics of dexamethasone, digoxin and cyclosporin A. *J. Clin. Invest.*, **96**, 1698–705.

Schinkel, A. H., Wagenaar, E., Mol, C. A. A. M. and Van Deemter, L. (1996). P-glycoprotein in blood–brain barrier of mice influences the brain penetration and pharmacological activity of many drugs. *J. Clin. Invest.*, **97**, 2517–24.

Schinkel, A. H., Mayer, U., Wagenaar, E. *et al.* (1997). Normal viability and altered pharmacokinetics in mice lacking mdr1-type (drug-transporting) P-glycoproteins. *Proc. Natl. Acad. Sci. USA*, **94**, 4028–33.

Seelig, A., Gottschlich, R. and Devant, R. M. (1994). A method to determine the ability of drugs to diffuse through the blood–brain barrier. *Proc. Natl. Acad. Sci. USA*, **91**, 68–72.

Shirai, A., Naito, M., Tatsuta, T. *et al.* (1994). Transport of cyclosporin A across the brain capillary endothelial cell monolayer by P-glycoprotein. *Biochim. Biophys. Acta*, **1222**, 400–4.

Smit, J. J. M., Schinkel, A. H., Oude Elferink, R. P. J. *et al.* (1993). Homozygous disruption of the murine *mdr*2 P-glycoprotein gene leads to a complete absence of phospholipid from bile and to liver disease. *Cell*, **75**, 451–62.

Sparreboom, A., Van Asperen, J., Mayer, U. *et al.* (1997). Limited oral bio-availability and active epithelial excretion of paclitaxel (taxol) caused by P-glycoprotein in the intestine. *Proc. Natl. Acad. Sci. USA*, **94**, 2031–5.

Sugawara, I. (1990). Expression and functions of P-glycoprotein (*mdr*1 gene product) in normal and malignant tissues. *Acta Pathol. Jpn.*, **40**, 545–53.

Tanaka, Y., Abe, Y., Tsugu, A. *et al.* (1994). Ultrastructural localization of P-glycoprotein on capillary endothelial cells in human gliomas. *Virchows Arch.*, **425**, 133–8.

Tatsuta, T., Naito, M., Oh-hara, T. *et al.* (1992). Functional involvement of P-glycoprotein in blood–brain barrier. *J. Biol. Chem.*, **267**, 20383–91.

Thiebaut, F., Tsuruo, T., Hamada, H. *et al.* (1989). Immunohistochemical localization in normal tissues of different epitopes in the multidrug transport protein P170: Evidence for localization in brain capillaries and crossreactivity of one antibody with a muscle protein. *J. Histochem. Cytochem.*, **37**, 159–64.

Tóth, K., Vaughan, M. M., Peress, N. S. *et al.* (1996). *MDR1* P-glycoprotein is expressed by endothelial cells of newly formed capillaries in human gliomas but is not expressed in the neovasculature of other primary tumors. *Am. J. Pathol.*, **149**, 853–8.

Tsuji, A., Terasaki, T., Takabatake, Y. *et al.* (1992). P-glycoprotein as the drug efflux pump in primary cultured bovine brain capillary endothelial cells. *Life Sci.*, **51**, 1427–37.

Tsuji, A., Tamai, I., Sakata, A. *et al.* (1993). Restricted transport of cyclosporin A across the blood–brain by a multidrug transporter, P-glycoprotein. *Biochem. Pharmacol.*, **46**, 1096–9.

Van Asperen, J., Schinkel, A. H., Beijnen, J. H. *et al.* (1996). Altered pharmacokinetics of vinblastine in mdr1a P-glycoprotein deficient mice. *J. Natl. Cancer Inst.*, **88**, 994–9.

Van der Valk, P., van Kalken, C. K., Ketelaars, H. *et al.* (1990). Distribution of multi-drug resistance-associated P-glycoprotein in normal and neoplastic human tissues. *Ann. Oncol.*, **1**, 56–64.

Wang, Q., Yang, H., Miller, D. W. and Elmquist, W. F. (1995). Effect of the P-glycoprotein inhibitor, cyclosporin A, on the distribution of rhodamine-123 to the brain: an in vivo microdialysis study in freely moving rats. *Biochem. Biophys. Res. Comm.*, **211**, 719–26.

Watanabe, T., Tsuge, H., Oh-hara, T. *et al.* (1995). Comparative study on reversal efficacy of SDZ PSC 833, cyclosporin A and verapamil on multidrug resistance in vitro and in vivo. *Acta Oncol.*, **34**, 235–41.

Williams, P. C., Henner, W. D., Roman-Goldstein, S. *et al.* (1995). Toxicity and efficacy of carboplatin and etoposide in conjunction with disruption of the blood–brain tumor barrier in the treatment of intracranial neoplasms. *Neurosurg.*, **37**, 17–27.

22 Blood–brain barrier ion transport

RICHARD F. KEEP, STEVEN R. ENNIS and A. LORRIS BETZ

- Introduction
- Methodology
- Biology
- Conclusion

Introduction

The blood–brain barrier (BBB), formed by the cerebral endothelial cells and their connecting tight junctions, has a very low permeability to ions unless specific transporters are present. The endothelial movement of ions, via either ion transporters or ion channels, has a number of important functions. It is involved in the regulation of several key ion concentrations in the brain (e.g. K^+, Ca^{2+}, H^+), the uptake and extrusion of trace metals, fluid secretion and, by linkage to the endothelial sodium gradient, nutrient transport. Ion transport is also important in regulating BBB function. For example, changes in endothelial cell $[Ca^{2+}]$ and volume modulate BBB integrity (Rapoport et al., 1980; Olesen and Crone, 1986).

Understanding ion transport at the BBB may aid in the treatment of a number of disease states, particularly those such as stroke where edema formation results from a net accumulation of ions and thus water in the brain (Betz et al., 1994). However, despite the importance of BBB ion transport in normal and pathophysiological conditions and its potential for modulating BBB function, our knowledge of ion transport and its regulation is still far from complete. This particularly reflects the limitations of in vivo BBB experimentation and deficiencies in current in vitro preparations. Although

such difficulties apply to all studies of the BBB, they are particularly pertinent to ion transport because of the low rate of transport.

Methodology

Preparations

Blood–brain barrier ion transport has been studied using in vitro preparations, isolated capillaries, cultured endothelium and endothelial cell membrane vesicles. Data generated in vivo, with the animal perfusing its own brain, is the most cogent to understanding BBB function. However, the experimental manipulations required to study ion transport (such as ion substitution) are often impossible in vivo, thus limiting the information that has been generated from that type of preparation.

Two preparations that allow the investigator to modify greatly the brain perfusate are the brain uptake index (BUI) and the in situ brain perfusion techniques (Oldendorf and Szabo, 1976; Takasato et al., 1984). In the former, isotope uptake is measured from a bolus of fluid injected into the carotid artery, while in the latter the carotid circulation is perfused by an artificial perfusate. Although these preparations have the advantage of allowing greater control of the brain perfusate (e.g. the removal of Na^+ and the inclusion of inhibitors that might have profound systemic effects: Ennis *et al.*, 1996), they are limited to measurements of transport in the blood to brain direction.

Isolated tissues, cells and vesicles allow the greatest control of the external or even internal milieu and the best access for measurements of different end points. Of the available preparations, isolated capillaries have the advantage of speed of preparation (about 2 hours) and may, therefore, more closely reflect *in vivo* ion transport. There are, however, concerns over purity, access to the luminal membrane and energy status (Keep *et al.*, 1993). This preparation can not be used for transendothelial measurements and may best be used to examine what transporters are present at the BBB (if it is possible to overcome purity concerns) and their potential regulation. Due to impaired metabolic function resulting from the isolation procedure (Sussman *et al.*, 1988), absolute rates of transport are questionable.

Cultured endothelial cells (freshly isolated or immortalized) have provided much information on ion transport. Unlike isolated microvessels, these cultures consist of a single cell type with access to all membranes. There are, however, concerns over whether the cells dedifferentiate and cease to express all BBB ion transporters or start to express transporters that are not present *in vivo*. Furthermore, monolayers of these endothelial cells have an electrical resistance at least an order of magnitude less than the BBB *in vitro* (Rutten *et al.*, 1987; Butt and Jones 1992). They are, therefore, of limited use in the study of transendothelial ion transport since paracellular diffusion may exceed transcellular transport. Nevertheless, they might be used to examine the polarity (luminal versus abluminal membranes *in vivo*) of inhibitor binding (Sun *et al.*, 1995) if the inhibitor has a limited paracellular permeability and if polarity is maintained *in vitro*.

Because the BBB exhibits polarity (Betz 1985), efforts have been made to isolate vesicles from the luminal or abluminal membrane of the endothelium (Betz *et al.*, 1980; Sanchez del Pino *et al.*, 1995a). This system requires markers for the respective membranes. As yet, System-A amino acid transport is the best available marker since it is absent from the luminal membrane (Betz and Goldstein, 1978; Sanchez del Pino *et al.*, 1995b).

However, these vesicles are derived from isolated capillaries, and there is concern that the presence of System-A transport may not only reflect abluminal membrane vesicles but also contamination from other cell types.

Apart from the preparations described above, ion transporter localization can be examined in fixed brain sections using a variety of techniques including histochemistry (Betz *et al.*, 1980; Vorbrodt, 1988), immunohistochemistry (Gragera, *et al.*, 1993) and, potentially, *in situ* hybridization. The same techniques can also be used in isolated capillaries to facilitate localization.

Techniques

Three broad methods have been used to examine BBB ion transport. The first, measurements based on physiology, investigates ion transport by examining whether ion concentrations, electrical potential or isotopic ion fluxes are affected by ion substitutions or transport inhibitors. Such experiments are difficult *in vivo* because plasma concentrations of most ions can only be manipulated within a narrow range and ion transport inhibitors may have systemic or cerebral as well as direct BBB effects. Furthermore, of the endpoints, it is impossible to measure endothelial cell ion concentrations or potential *in vivo* and it is uncertain whether transendothelial measurements reflect changes in BBB or brain parenchymal function. Thus, almost all data *in vivo* reflect measurements of isotopic fluxes. Although such experiments have provided data on the overall rates of ion transport and have demonstrated changes in ion transport under conditions such as hyperosmolality and altered plasma $[K^+]$ (Bradbury and Kleeman, 1967; Cserr *et al.*, 1987; Stummer *et al.*, 1994), they have provided little information on which ion transporters are involved. Much greater manipulations of ion gradients are possible with *in situ* brain perfusion and BUI techniques (Betz, 1983a; Ennis *et al.*, 1996). Furthermore, transport inhibitors can be used at concentrations that would have marked systemic effects. In combination with isotopic flux measurement, they have proven useful in examining BBB Na^+ transport (Betz, 1983a; Ennis, *et al.*, 1996).

In contrast to *in vivo*, *in vitro* the investigator has almost total control of the external milieu. Of the endpoints, most work has examined the effects of ion substitution and transport inhibitors on isotopic fluxes since the thinness of the cerebral endothelial cell tends to preclude the use of conventional electrodes to record membrane potential or intracellular ion concentrations. However, ion- and potential-sensitive fluorescent dyes, such as Fura-2 for $[Ca^{2+}]$ (Revest *et al.*, 1991), can be used to circumvent that problem and it is also possible to record membrane potential with whole-cell patch clamp.

The second methodology involves anatomical studies to localize ion transport. Transporters, for ions or other substances, can be localized using histochemistry (Betz *et al.*, 1980; Vorbrodt, 1988), immunohistochemistry (Cornford *et al.*, 1993; Gragera, *et al.*, 1993) or *in situ* hybridization (Pardridge *et al.*, 1990). Because the cerebral endothelial cells are very thin (about 0.2 μm), such studies require electron microscopy if distribution on the luminal or abluminal membranes is to be determined.

The third type of methodology uses similar techniques to the second but in combination with isolated tissues. Thus, for example, Na^+/K^+ ATPase can be examined in isolated microvessels, endothelial cells or membranes using biochemical assays (Betz *et al.*, 1980), ouabain binding (Harik *et al.*, 1985) and Western blots (Mooradian and Bastani, 1993; Zlokovic *et al.*, 1993). Although as yet unpublished for ion transporters, it is also possible to use cDNA probes and Northern blotting as shown by studies of the BBB glucose transporter (Boado and Pardridge, 1994).

Biology

Distribution of ion transporters

For the major monovalent ions, Na^+, Cl^- and K^+, the BBB permeabilities are low, being about 1, 1 and 10×10^{-7} cm s^{-1} respectively (Smith and Rapoport, 1986). The disparity in the permeability for K^+ reflects greater transport since the rate of free diffusion for this ion is similar to that of Na^+ (Smith and Rapoport, 1986). For Na^+ and Cl^- the permeabilities are two orders of magnitude less than at the choroid plexus epithelium, reflecting the greater role of the choroid plexus in CSF secretion.

There is evidence for a variety of ion transporters at the BBB. For Na^+, there is evidence for Na^+/K^+ ATPase both *in vivo* and *in vitro* (Betz 1983b; Bradbury and Stulcova, 1970). This enzyme appears to possess a predominantly abluminal distribution (Betz *et al.*, 1980). All known isoforms (α_1, α_2, α_3, β_1, β_2) are present in isolated microvessels (Zlokovic *et al.*, 1993) but whether this reflects preparation contamination has yet to be fully elucidated. There is also evidence for Na^+/H^+ antiporter *in vivo* and *in vitro* (Betz, 1983b; Ennis *et al.*, 1996) and the observation that amiloride analogs inhibit Na^+ influx into brain suggests that this transporter is present on the luminal membrane at least. $Na^+/K^+/Cl^-$ has been found *in vitro* (O'Donnell *et al.*, 1995) and proposed to have a luminal distribution (Sun *et al.*, 1995). However, *in vivo* evidence for the transporter is lacking (Ennis *et al.*, 1996). There is also evidence for at least two non-selective cation channels (Chapter 23). For K^+, there is evidence for a number of K^+ channels (Chapter 23) as well as the Na^+/K^+ ATPase and the $Na^+/K^+/Cl^-$ co-transporter. Recent evidence using Western blots suggests that H^+/K^+ ATPase is absent at the BBB (Mooradian and Bastani 1993).

Two proton transporters are present at the BBB. In addition to the Na^+/H^+ antiporter, a H^+ ATPase is present (Mooradian and Bastani, 1993). This latter transporter is present in vacuoles in other tissues and it may not play a role in transendothelial proton transport.

Little is known about the Ca^{2+} and Mg^{2+} transport mechanisms at the BBB. Ca^{2+}- and Mg^{2+}-dependent ATPases have been demonstrated histochemically (Vorbrodt, 1988). It should be noted, however, that such studies do not indicate whether these ATPases transport Ca^{2+} and Mg^{2+} or are just dependent on their presence. Whether Na^+/Ca^{2+} exchange occurs has not been examined, although it is present at the choroid plexus (Johanson 1989). There is also a paucity of studies on the mechanisms of anion (Cl^-, HCO_3^- or SO_4^{2-}) transport at the BBB but the results of Smith and Rapoport (Smith and Rapoport, 1984) indicate that Cl^- uptake into brain is saturable.

For trace metals, there appears to be two types of transport across the BBB. There may be specific transporters for trace metals as with iron which, when complexed to transferrin, undergoes endocytosis after it binds to the transferrin receptor (Fishman *et al.*, 1987). Since transferrin binds aluminium, manganese, gallium and indium, this mechanism may also play a role in the uptake of these trace metals as well (Smith, 1990). Some other metals do not appear to have specific transporters but instead complex with amino acids (e.g. methylmercury–L-cysteine and zinc–histidine) and these complexes are transported by BBB amino acid carriers (Bradbury, 1995; Smith, 1990).

Function

A major question in BBB ion transport is the extent to which any transporter is involved in the transendothelial movement of ions and thus potentially brain rather than endothelial cell ion regulation. This section, as an example, examines the evidence about the ion transporters that may be involved in fluid secretion (Fig. 22.1).

Unlike K^+, the concentrations of Na^+ and Cl^- in the brain extracellular space are not regulated. This reflects the inability, long-term, of the brain to maintain an osmotic gradient between itself and blood and means that any net movement of Na^+ and Cl^- across the BBB results in net water movement. Like the choroid plexus, the BBB has an antiluminal distribution of Na^+/K^+ ATPase (Betz *et al.*, 1980) that might produce local osmotic gradients resulting in a movement of fluid into the brain (Bradbury, 1985) and the extrachoroidal production of CSF (e.g. Milhorat *et al.*, 1971).

For abluminal Na^+/K^+ ATPase to be involved in fluid secretion there must be a Na^+ entry mechanism at the luminal membrane (Fig. 22.1). At present, there is evidence for three, a Na^+/H^+ antiporter (Betz, 1983*a*; Ennis *et al.*, 1996), a Na^+ channel sensitive to amiloride analogs (Ennis *et al.*, 1996; Vigne *et al.*, 1989) and a $Na^+/K^+/Cl^-$ cotransporter (O'Donnell *et al.*, 1995). The evidence concerning the latter is, however, controversial (Lin, 1985; Keep *et al.*, 1993; O'Donnell, *et al.*, 1995; Ennis *et al.*, 1996) and it may be that the transporter is upregulated *in vitro*.

Fluid secretion also requires the movement of Cl^-. Whether that movement is transendothelial or paracellular has not been determined although BBB Cl^- transport is saturable (Smith and Rapo-

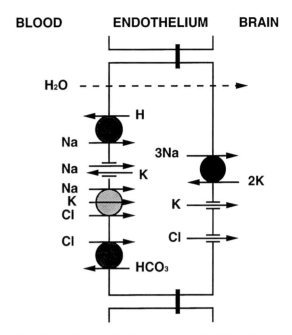

Fig. 22.1. Model of fluid transport at the BBB. There is *in vivo* evidence for this distribution of Na^+/K^+ ATPase (Bradbury and Stulcova, 1970), the Na^+/H^+ exchanger and the Na^+ channel (Ennis *et al.*, 1996). There is *in vitro* evidence for the $Na^+/K^+/Cl^-$ cotransporter (Sun *et al.*, 1995) and the K^+ channel (Hoyer *et al.*, 1991). The Cl^-/HCO_3^- exchanger and Cl^- channel are hypothetical.

port, 1984). In the choroid plexus, Cl^- entry from blood is via a Cl^-/HCO_3^- exchanger (Lindsey *et al.*, 1990) with production of HCO_3^- and H^+ by carbonic anhydrase providing the exchanging ion for both Cl^- and Na^+ entry (Johanson, 1989). Carbonic anhydrase is also present at the BBB although the isozyme is different from that at the choroid plexus (Ghandour *et al.*, 1992).

Epithelia that transport fluid by a similar mechanism also have a K^+ channel on the same membrane as the Na^+/K^+ ATPase to recycle K^+. A number of K^+ and non-selective cation channels are present in cerebral microvessels (Vigne *et al.*, 1989; Hoyer *et al.*, 1991; Popp and Gogelein, 1992; Popp *et al.*, 1992; Janigro *et al.*, 1994). In particular, Hoyer *et al.* (1991) have identified a channel that is inactivated by depolarization as would occur during Na^+/K^+ ATPase inactivation. At the BBB, such channels may also play a role in brain K^+ homeostasis.

Regulation of ion transport

The previous sections, and most of the literature, has dealt with which transporters are present at the BBB and their possible functions. It should be noted that several transporters have been proposed to fulfill more than one function. This is most obvious in the case of Na^+/K^+ ATPase. It has been suggested that this transporter is involved in $[K^+]$ regulation (Bradbury and Stulcova, 1970; Stummer *et al.*, 1995), fluid secretion (Bradbury, 1985) and providing a Na^+ gradient to drive nutrient transport such as the amino acid System-A (Betz and Goldstein, 1978). How a transporter could fulfill several functions that might need to be independently regulated is a major unanswered question. In the case of Na^+/K^+ ATPase, there are several different isoforms (Zlokovic *et al.*, 1993) that might be regulated independently or ion channels could be opened to short circuit either K^+ or Na^+ transport. It is also possible that the BBB might consist of more than one cell type possessing different functions (e.g. ion regulation versus nutrient transport).

The system of transporters at the BBB is not static. For example, regulation of K^+ influx into brain during variations in plasma $[K^+]$ does not appear to result from the saturation kinetics of K^+ transport, but rather a change in the number or activity of K^+ transporters (Stummer *et al.*, 1994). Another factor that alters BBB K^+ transport *in vivo* is acute hyperosmolality, which results in a very pronounced stimulation in the absence of changes in plasma $[K^+]$ (Cserr *et al.*, 1987).

Factors such as plasma $[K^+]$ and osmolality that influence BBB ion transport may act directly on the barrier. However, there is also evidence of regulation by the nervous system or hormonal release. The BBB receives adrenergic innervation from the locus ceruleus and there is reduced ouabain binding in brain microvessels isolated from rats with lesions to that area (Harik, 1986). In isolated brain microvessels, atrial natriuretic peptide inhibits amiloride-sensitive $^{22}Na^+$ uptake (Ibaragi *et al.*,

1989) while endothelins activate Na^+/H^+ exchange (Vigne *et al.*, 1991). In cultured endothelial cells, a wide variety of vasoactive agents have been shown to modulate $Na^+/K^+/Cl^-$ cotransport (O'Donnell *et al.*, 1995). Bradykinin and histamine both increase endothelial cell intracellular $[Ca^{2+}]$ and although part of this increase is due to release from intracellular stores, these agents also appear to alter Ca^{2+} transport (Revest *et al.*, 1991). Regulation of BBB ion transport may also occur by modulation of ion channels (Vigne *et al.*, 1989; Hoyer *et al.*, 1991; Janigro *et al.*, 1994).

In vivo results suggest that neuronal or hormonal modulation of BBB ion transport occurs but proof is lacking. For example, vasopressin increases Na^+ ($Na^+/K^+/Cl^-$) transport *in vitro* (O'Donnell *et al.*, 1995) and the Brattleboro rat that lacks vasopressin has smaller increases in brain Na^+ content in response to hyperosmotic or ischemic stress (DePasquale *et al.*, 1989; Dickinson and Betz 1992), but experiments designed to examine the intermediate step, that vasopressin increases BBB Na^+ transport from blood-to-brain, have proven negative or difficult to interpret (DePasquale *et al.*, 1989; Dickinson and Betz, 1992).

Conclusion

An array of ion transporters are present at the BBB that contribute to brain (and endothelial) ion and volume regulation. A full understanding of the precise function, interaction and regulation of these transporters, however, awaits the development of new or improved experimental techniques. Such an understanding may be of great therapeutic value in a number of neurological disorders.

Acknowledgments

This work was supported by grants NS-23870 (A.L.B.), NS-34709 (R.F.K.) and HL-18575 (A.L.B.) from the National Institutes of Health.

References

Betz, A. L. (1983*a*). Sodium transport from blood to brain: inhibition by furosemide and amiloride. *J. Neurochem.*, **41**, 1158–64.

Betz, A. L. (1983*b*). Sodium transport in capillaries isolated from rat brain. *J. Neurochem.*, **41**, 1150–7.

Betz, A. L. (1985). Epithelial properties of brain capillary endothelium. *Fed. Proc.*, **44**, 2614–15.

Betz, A. L. and Goldstein, G. W. (1978). Polarity of the blood–brain barrier: neutral amino acid transport into isolated brain capillaries. *Science*, **202**, 225–7.

Betz, A. L., Firth, J. A. and Goldstein, G. W. (1980). Polarity of the blood–brain barrier: distribution of enzymes between the luminal and antiluminal membranes of brain capillary endothelial cells. *Brain Res.*, **192**, 17–28.

Betz, A. L., Keep, R. F., Beer, M. E. and Ren, X.-D. (1994). Blood–brain barrier permeability and brain concentration of sodium, potassium, and chloride during focal ischemia. *J. Cereb. Blood Flow Metab.*, **14**, 29–37.

Boado, R. J. and Pardridge, W. M. (1994). Measurement of blood–brain barrier GLUT1 glucose transporter and actin mRNA by a quantitative polymerase chain reaction assay. *J. Neurochem.*, **62**, 2085–90.

Bradbury, M. W. B. (1985). The blood–brain barrier. Transport across the cerebral endothelium. *Circ. Res.*, **57**, 213–22.

Bradbury, M. W. B. (1995). Developing views of the blood–brain barrier. In *New Concepts of a Blood-Brain Barrier*, ed. J. Greenwood, D. J. Begley and M. B. Segal, pp. 1–9. New York: Plenum.

Bradbury, M. W. B. and Kleeman, C. R. (1967). Stability of the potassium content of cerebrospinal fluid and brain. *Am. J. Physiol.*, **213**, 519–28.

Bradbury, M. W. B. and Stulcova, B. (1970). Efflux mechanism contributing to the stability of the potassium concentration in cerebrospinal fluid. *J. Physiol.*, **208**, 415–30.

Butt, A. M. and Jones, H. C. (1992). Effect of histamine and antagonists on electrical resistance across the blood–brain barrier in rat brain-surface microvessels. *Brain Res.*, **569**, 100–5.

Cornford, E. M., Hyman, S. and Pardridge, W. M. (1993). An electron microscopic immunogold analysis of developmental up-regulation of the blood–brain barrier GLUT-1 glucose transporter. *J. Cereb. Blood Flow Metab.*, **13**, 841–54.

Cserr, H. F., DePasquale, M. and Patlak, C. S. (1987). Volume regulatory influx of electrolytes from plasma to brain during acute hyperosmolality. *Am. J. Physiol.*, **253**, F530–F537.

DePasquale, M., Patlak, C. S. and Cserr, H. F. (1989). Brain ion and volume regulation during acute hypernatremia in Brattleboro rats. *Am. J. Physiol.*, **256**, F1059–F1066.

Dickinson, L. D. and Betz, A. L. (1992). Attenuated development of ischemic brain edema in vasopressin-deficient rats. *J. Cereb. Blood Flow Metab.*, **12**, 681–90.

Ennis, S. R., Ren, X.-D. and Betz, A. L. (1996). Mechanisms of sodium transport at the blood–brain barrier studied with in situ perfusion of the rat brain. *J. Neurochem.*, **66**, 756–63.

Fishman, J. B., Rubin, J. B., Handrahan, J. V. *et al.* (1987). Receptor-mediated transcytosis of transferrin across the blood–brain barrier. *J. Neurosci. Res.*, **18**, 299–304.

Ghandour, M. S., Langley, O. K., Zhu, X. L. *et al.* (1992). Carbonic anhydrase IV on brain capillary endothelial cells: a marker associated with the blood–brain barrier. *Proc. Natl. Acad. Sci. USA*, **89**, 6823–7.

Gragera, R. R., Muniz, E. and Martinez-Rodriguez, R. (1993). Molecular and ultrastructural basis of blood–brain barrier function. Immunohistochemical demonstration of Na+/K+ ATPase, alpha-actin, phosphocreatine and clathrin in the capillary wall and its microenvironment. *Cell. Mol. Biol.*, **39**, 819–28.

Harik, S. I. (1986). Blood–brain barrier sodium/potassium pump: modulation by central noradrenergic innervation. *Proc. Natl. Acad. Sci. USA*, **83**, 4067–70.

Harik, S. I., Doull, G. H. and Dick, A. P. K. (1985). Specific ouabain binding to brain microvessels and choroid plexus. *J. Cereb. Blood Flow Metab.*, **5**, 156–60.

Hoyer, J., Popp, R., Meyer, J. *et al.* (1991). Angiotensin II, vasopressin and GTP[γ-S] inhibit inward-rectifying K+ channels in porcine cerebral capillary endothelial cells. *J Membrane Biol*, **123**, 55–62.

Ibaragi, M.-A., Niwa, M. and Ozaki, M. (1989). Atrial natriuretic peptide modulates amiloride-sensitive Na+ transport across the blood–brain barrier. *J Neurochem*, **53**, 1802–6.

Janigro, D., West, G. A., Nguyen, T.-S. and Winn, H. R. (1994). Regulation of blood–brain barrier endothelial cells by nitric oxide. *Circ. Res.*, **75**, 528–38.

Johanson, C. E. (1989). Potential for pharmacologic manipulation of the blood-cerebrospinal fluid barrier. In *Implications of the Blood-Brain Barrier and its Manipulation*, ed. E. A. Neuwelt, pp. 223–60. New York: Plenum.

Keep, R. F., Xiang, J. and Betz, A. L. (1993). Potassium transport at the blood–brain and blood–CSF barriers. *Adv. Exp. Med. Biol.*, **331**, 43–54.

Lin, J. D. (1985). Potassium transport in isolated cerebral microvessels from rat. *Jap. J. Physiol*, **35**, 817–30.

Lindsey, A. E., Schneider, K., Simmons, D. M. *et al.* (1990). Functional expression and subcellular localization of an anion exchanger cloned from choroid plexus. *Proc. Natl. Acad. Sci. USA*, **87**, 5278–82.

Milhorat, T. H., Hammock, M. K., Fenstermacher, J. D. *et al.* (1971). Cerebrospinal fluid production by the choroid plexus and brain. *Science*, **173**, 330–2.

Mooradian, A. D. and Bastani, B. (1993). Identification of proton-translocating adenosine triphosphatases in rat cerebral microvessels. *Brain Res.*, **629**, 128–32.

O'Donnell, M. E., Martinez, A. and Sun, D. (1995). Cerebral microvascular endothelial cell Na–K–Cl cotransport: regulation by astrocyte-conditioned medium. *Am. J. Physiol.*, **268**, C747–C754.

Oldendorf, W. H. and Szabo, J. (1976). Amino acid assignment to one of three blood–brain barrier amino acid carriers. *Am. J. Physiol.*, **230**, 94–8.

Olesen, S.-P. and Crone, C. (1986). Substances that rapidly augment ionic conductance of endothelium in cerebral venules. *Acta Physiol Scand*, **127**, 233–41.

Pardridge, W. M., Boado, R. J. and Farrell, C. R. (1990). Brain-type glucose transporter (GLUT-1) is selectively localized to the blood–brain barrier. Studies with quantitative western blotting and in situ hybridization. *J. Biol. Chem.*, **265**, 18035–40.

Popp, R. and Gogelein, H. (1992). A calcium and ATP sensitive nonselective cation channel in the antiluminal membrane of rat cerebral capillary endothelial cells. *Biochim. Biophys. Acta*, **1108**, 59–66.

Popp, R., Hoyer, J., Meyer, J. *et al.* (1992). Stretch-activated non-selective cation channels in the antiluminal membrane of porcine cerebral capillaries. *J. Physiol.*, **454**, 435–49.

Rapoport, S. I., Fredericks, W. R., Ohno, K. and Pettigrew, K. D. (1980). Quantitative aspects of reversible osmotic opening of the blood–brain barrier. *Am. J. Physiol.*, **238**, R421–R431.

Revest, P. A., Abbott, N. J. and Gillespie, J. I. (1991). Receptor-mediated changes in intracellular [Ca^{2+}] in cultured rat brain capillary endothelial cells. *Brain Res*, **549**, 159–61.

Rutten, M. J., Hoover, R. L. and Karnovsky, M. J. (1987). Electrical resistance and macromolecular permeability of brain endothelial monolayer cultures. *Brain Res.*, **425**, 301–10.

Sanchez del Pino, M. M., Hawkins, R. A. and Peterson, D. R. (1995a). Biochemical discrimination between luminal and abluminal enzyme and transport activities of the blood–brain barrier. *J. Biol. Chem.*, **270**, 14907–12.

Sanchez del Pino, M. M., Peterson, D. R. and Hawkins, R. A. (1995b). Neutral amino acid transport characterization of isolated luminal and abluminal membranes of the blood–brain barrier. *J. Biol. Chem.*, **270**, 14913–18.

Smith, Q. R. (1990). Regulation of metal uptake and distribution within brain. In *Nutrition and the Brain*, ed. R. J. Wurtmann and J. J. Wurtmann, pp. 25–74. New York: Raven Press.

Smith, Q. R. and Rapoport, S. I. (1984). Carrier-mediated transport of chloride across the blood–brain barrier. *J. Neurochem.*, **42**, 754–63.

Smith, Q. R. and Rapoport, S. I. (1986). Cerebrovascular permeability coefficients to sodium, potassium, and chloride. *J Neurochem*, **46**, 1732–42.

Stummer, W., Keep, R. F. and Betz, A. L. (1994). Rubidium entry into brain and cerebrospinal fluid during acute and chronic alterations in plasma potassium. *Am. J. Physiol.*, **266**, H2239–H2246.

Stummer, W., Betz, A. L. and Keep, R. F. (1995). Mechanisms of brain ion homeostasis during acute and chronic variations of plasma potassium. *J. Cereb. Blood Flow Metab.*, **15**, 336–44.

Sun, D., Lytle, C. and O'Donnel, M. E. (1995). Astroglial cell-induced expression of Na–K–Cl cotransporter in brain microvascular endothelial cells. *Am. J. Physiol.*, **269**, C1506–C1512.

Sussman, I., Carson, M. P., McCall, A. L. *et al.* (1988). Energy state of bovine cerebral microvessels: comparison of isolation methods. *Microvasc. Res.*, **35**, 167–78.

Takasato, Y., Rapoport, S. I. and Smith, Q. R. (1984). An in situ brain perfusion technique to study cerebrovascular transport in the rat. *Am. J. Physiol.*, **247**, H484–H493.

Vigne, P., Champigny, G., Marsault *et al.* (1989). A new type of amiloride-sensitive cationic channel in endothelial cells of brain microvessels. *J. Biol. Chem.*, **264**, 7663–8.

Vigne, P., Ladoux, A. and Frelin, C. (1991). Endothelins activate Na+/H+ exchange in brain capillary endothelial cells via a high affinity endothelin-3 receptor that is not coupled to phospholipase C. *J. Biol. Chem.*, **266**, 5925–8.

Vorbrodt, A. W. (1988). Ultrastructural cytochemistry of blood–brain barrier endothelia. In *Progress in Histochemistry and Cytochemistry*, ed. W. Graumann, Z. Lojda, A. G. E. Pearse and T. H. Schiebler, pp. 1–99. Gustave Fischer Verlag.

Zlokovic, B. V., Wang, L., Mackic, J. B. *et al.* (1993). Expression of Na,K-ATPase at the blood–brain interface. *Adv. Exp. Med. Biol.*, **331**, 55–60.

23 Ion channels in endothelial cells

CHRISTIAN FRELIN and PAUL VIGNE

- Introduction
- Na$^+$ channels
- K$^+$ channels
- Nonselective cationic channels
- Ca^{2+} channels
- Other channels
- The blood–cardiac barrier paradigm
- Polarized expression of ion channel
- Conclusion

Introduction

Voltage gated channels are essential for determining membrane excitability, for instance in neurons. A large body of evidence indicates that voltage gated channels are not the only forms of channels expressed by mammalian cells and that expression of ion channels is not restricted to excitable cells. Voltage independent channels do not open in response to a change in the membrane potential. They open (or close) in response to phosphorylation, to intracellular ligands (ATP, H$^+$, etc.) and signalling molecules (Ca^{2+}, G proteins, etc.), to extracellular ligands (acetylcholine, serotonine, ATP, GABA, excitatory amino acids) and to physical stimuli (shear stress, osmolarity, etc.). Increasing evidence also suggests that vascular endothelial cells from peripheral vessels express ion channels and that these channels play an important role for modulating endothelial cell functions (Adams, 1994; Takeda and Klepper, 1990). This chapter reviews the properties, regulations and possible functions of ion channels expressed by brain capillary endothelial cells (BCEC).

Expression of ion channels is best analyzed using patch clamp techniques. Channels are characterized by their voltage dependence, ionic selectivity, unit conductance and in some favorable cases by unique pharmacological properties. Ion channel activity can sometimes be analyzed by ion flux techniques (e.g. Van Renterghem et al., 1995) or by ligand binding techniques (e.g. Vigne et al., 1989). Molecular data are available for many voltage gated channels (Catterall, 1995).

Most of our knowledge about ion channel expression by BCEC comes from studies using cells cultured in vitro. It should be stressed however that expression of ion channels may be altered during long term cultivation of the cells and that the properties of cultured cells are not necessarily identical to those of cells in situ. This can be circumvented by using freshly isolated cells (e.g. Popp et al., 1992). Ion channels of the abluminal face (brain side) of intact microvessels are easily accessible to patch electrodes (e.g. Popp et al., 1992). Channels of the luminal face are not. This severely limits the analysis of the role of ion channels at the blood–brain barrier (BBB).

Na⁺ channels

Voltage gated Na⁺ channels are responsible for the ascending phase of action potentials in excitable cells. They comprise a family of structures related to voltage gated Ca^{2+} and K⁺ channels (Catterall, 1995). They are not present in vascular endothelial cells.

Voltage independent, Na⁺ selective, channels are mainly found in water reabsorbing epithelia such as the frog skin, renal, intestinal and pulmonary epithelia. They are inhibited by the diuretic drug amiloride and by its guanidino-substituted derivatives (benzamil and phenamil). Epithelial Na⁺ channels are oligomeric structures composed of at least three different subunits. They are regulated by glucocorticoids, mineralocorticoids and by cAMP dependent phosphorylation mechanisms (Barbry, 1996).

Rat BCEC express an amiloride sensitive channel (Vigne *et al.*, 1989). The mean unit channel conductance at 140 mM Na⁺ is 23 picosiemens (pS). The channel is different from the epithelial Na⁺ channel in that it is not Na⁺ selective. It is permeable to K⁺ (PNa⁺/PK⁺ = 1.5/1), but not to Ca^{2+}. It is less sensitive to amiloride than the epithelial Na⁺ channel. Its molecular structure is probably different from that of the epithelial Na⁺ channel. It is present at the blood side of the BBB (Ennis *et al.*, 1996).

K⁺ channels

K⁺ channels constitute a vast and heterogenous family of ion channels. They are important for maintaining the membrane potential, membrane excitability and for K⁺ secretion. At least 35 different genes encoding K⁺ channels have been identified (Chandy and Gutman, 1993).

Inward rectifying K⁺ channels have been identified in rat and pig BCEC (Hoyer *et al.*, 1991; Van Renterghem *et al.*, 1995). In isolated pig cells, two conductance states (7 and 35 pS) have been recorded. Cell-attached recording performed at the abluminal membrane of freshly isolated porcine microvessels only recorded the 30 pS channel. Inward rectifiers in pig cells are inhibited by angiotensin II and arginine vasopressin (Hoyer *et al.*, 1991).

K⁺(ATP) channels control insulin secretion from β cells in the pancreas. They are present in the cardiovascular system and probably play an important role during hypoxic episodes. They are targets for a new class of vasodilators, the K⁺ channel openers and are inhibited by antidiabetic drugs of the class of sulfonylureas (Lazdunski, 1994). Under physiological conditions, K⁺(ATP) channels are blocked by intracellular ATP. They are activated by ATP depletion, for instance consecutive to metabolic inhibition and to hypoxia/ischemia. ATP sensitive K⁺ channels have been identified in rat BCEC using electrophysiological techniques (Janigro *et al.*, 1993) but not by biochemical techniques using [³H]glibenclamide binding assays (Sullivan and Harik, 1993).

Different forms of Ca^{2+} activated K⁺ channels are recognized. They differ in their unit conductance, in voltage and Ca^{2+} sensitivity and in their pharmacology. SK channels are specifically inhibited by the bee venom toxin apamin. They have a small unitary conductance (6–22 pS) and little voltage sensitivity. BK channels have a larger conductance (100–250 pS) and are activated by smaller variations in intracellular Ca^{2+} and by depolarization. They are inhibited by charybdotoxin (Kolb, 1990).

Cultured rat BCEC express a K⁺(Ca^{2+}) channel, which like SK channels has a small conductance (10–40 pS) but which like BK channels is sensitive to charybdotoxin (Van Renterghem *et al.*, 1995). K⁺(Ca^{2+}) channels are activated by agonists of phospholipase C such as endothelins, bombesin like peptides, and nucleotides (Van Renterghem *et al.*, 1995; Vigne *et al.*, 1995). These actions are mediated by ETA receptors, neuromedin B preferring receptor and P2Y2 purinergic receptors. Bovine aortic endothelial cells express a similar K⁺(Ca^{2+}) channel that is activated by bradykinin via a G protein mediated increase in the sensitivity of the channel for activator Ca^{2+} (Vaca *et al.*, 1992).

In vascular smooth muscle cells, charybdotoxin-sensitive K⁺(Ca^{2+}) channels are activated by cGMP dependent protein kinase and are thus targets for nitrovasodilators (Archer *et al.*, 1994). Cultured rat BCEC respond to NO donor molecules and to natriuretic peptides by the formation of cGMP (Marsault and Frelin, 1992; Vigne and Frelin,

1992). This action is not accompanied by an activation of K⁺(Ca²⁺) channels (Van Renterghem *et al.*, 1995).

Large conductance $K^+(Ca^{2+})$ channels have occasionally been observed in rat and pig BCEC (Popp *et al.*, 1992; Van Renterghem *et al.*, 1995).

Nonselective cationic channels

Stretch activated nonselective cation channels (SA channels) have been identified in isolated porcine BCEC and in the abluminal membrane of isolated microvessels (Popp *et al.*, 1992). They are permeable to Na^+, K^+ and Ca^{2+}. They are activated during cell swelling. In endothelial cells from large vessels, SA channels act as mechanotransducers for hemodynamic (shear) stress (Lansman *et al.*, 1987). They adjust smooth muscle tone to hemodynamic stimuli, via a production of nitric oxide and prostacyclin. They also play a role in the regulation of the cell volume.

A Ca^{2+} and ATP sensitive nonselective cation channel has been identified at the abluminal membrane of freshly isolated rat brain capillaries. The channel is equally permeable to Na^+ and K^+ but not to Ca^{2+}. It is activated by cytosolic Ca^{2+} and inhibited by intracellular ATP (Popp and Gögelein, 1992). The channel is inhibited by derivatives of diphenylamine-2-carboxylate, by flufenamic acid and by gadolinium (Popp *et al.*, 1993).

Ca²⁺ channels

Voltage gated Ca^{2+} channels have been described in endothelial cells freshly dissociated from bovine adrenals but their functional role is not clear (Bossu *et al.*, 1992). No evidence for the presence of voltage gated Ca^{2+} channels has been obtained in cultured bovine aortic endothelial cells (Takeda *et al.*, 1987) or in BCEC of various origins.

Changes in the cytosolic Ca^{2+} concentration play an important signalling role in capillary endothelial cells (Frelin and Vigne, 1993). Vasoactive agents such as endothelins (Vigne *et al.*, 1990), neuromedin B (Vigne *et al.*, 1995), bradykinin (Frelin and Vigne, 1993) and purines (Frelin *et al.*, 1993) are potent agonists of phospholipase C in rat

BCEC. They increase cytosolic Ca^{2+} via an inositol (1,4,5)trisphosphate mediated mobilization of intracellular Ca^{2+} stores and the opening of a capacitative Ca^{2+} entry mechanism in the plasma membrane.

Other channels

Ion channels gated by extracellular ligands such as nicotinic receptors, GABA A receptors, P2X purinoceptors and ionotropic receptors for excitatory aminoacids have not been detected in BCEC.

Voltage dependent, cAMP activatable and Ca^{2+} activatable Cl^- channels have been identified in endothelial cells from peripheral vessels (Adams, 1994). Opening of Cl^- channels produces either an inward or and outward current (i.e. a depolarization or a hyperpolarization of the membrane) depending on the driving force for Cl^- movement. Cl^- channels are probably expressed at the BBB but they have not yet been characterized. It is also worth noting that MDR, the multidrug resistance protein, whose expression is essential for the function of the BBB, probably acts as a regulator of different membrane conductances.

The blood–cardiac barrier paradigm

Endocardial cells line the cardiac cavities. They have been suggested to play a role similar to cells of the BBB. Endocardial cells pump K^+ to the blood and prevent an accumulation of interstitial K^+, which is critical in maintaining the function of cardiac myocytes (Brutsaert and Andries, 1992). Endocardial cells and BCEC express similar forms of channels: nonselective channels, $K^+(Ca^{2+})$ channels and inward rectifying K^+ channels (Manabe *et al.*, 1995). One advantage of the endocardium is that both its abluminal and luminal faces can be easily patched. Manabe *et al.* (1995) showed that only nonselective cationic channels are asymmetrically distributed and are preferentially located in the luminal membrane of the endothelium. All other channels are present on both luminal and abluminal faces of the endocardial cells. They suggested that nonselective cationic channels play an important role in K⁺ secretion by the endo-cardium.

Polarized expression of ion channel

It is well recognized that the BBB mediates net transport of NaCl and water from the blood to the brain (Betz, 1983). It is also well recognized that K⁺ transport is mainly directed from the brain to the blood (Hansen *et al.*, 1977) and that one function of the BBB is to control homeostasis of brain K⁺ concentration by actively secreting K⁺ into the blood (Bradbury and Stulcova, 1970; Katzman, 1976; Goldstein, 1979).

An asymmetrical distribution of ion channels between the luminal and abluminal membranes supplemented by that of the (Na⁺,K⁺)ATPase is considered to provide a basis for ion transport through epithelia (the pump-leak arrangement) (Gögelein, 1990). A similar mechanism probably accounts for polarized ion transport across the BBB. There is clear evidence that the (Na⁺,K⁺)ATPase is preferentially located on the abluminal side of the BBB (Betz *et al.*, 1980; Harik, 1986). An asymmetric distribution of ion channels has not yet been clearly demonstrated.

A model for constitutive K⁺ secretion

Figure 23.1 shows that a selective expression of nonselective, amiloride sensitive channels and of the (Na⁺,K⁺)ATPase at the luminal and abluminal faces of the BCEC respectively can favor Na⁺ uptake and K⁺ secretion by the BBB. Our original model (Vigne *et al.*, 1989) was modified to take into account the presence of abluminal inward rectifying K⁺ channels (Hoyer *et al.*, 1991). These channels probably limit K⁺ secretion by recycling K⁺ to the brain. Partial evidence that this model applies to *in vivo* situations is provided by the observation that inhibitors of amiloride sensitive channels reduce brain uptake of Na⁺ (Ennis *et al.*, 1996).

A model for K⁺ secretion during short-term ischemia

Cerebral disorders, like ischemia, often result in cytotoxic brain edema. During ischemia, brain

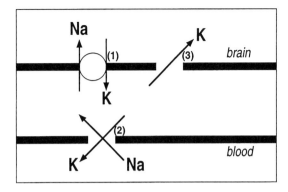

Fig. 23.1. A model for K⁺ secretion by the BBB. Under resting conditions, (Na⁺,K⁺)ATPase activity (1) is limited by intracellular Na⁺. Na⁺ is provided by luminal, amiloride sensitive, nonselective channels (2). K⁺ pumped by the (Na⁺,K⁺)ATPase in exchange for Na⁺ flows into the blood by nonselective channels or is recycled to the brain by inward rectifying K⁺ channels (3).

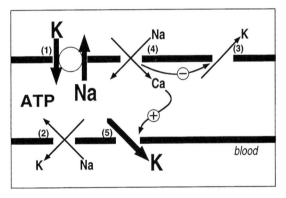

Fig. 23.2. A model for K⁺ secretion by the BBB during short-term hypoxia/ischemia. Under hypoxic/ischemic conditions and provided that endothelial cells have enough ATP to fuel the (Na⁺,K⁺)ATPase (1), activity of the pump is stimulated by the rise in extracellular K⁺ (released by neurons) and a rise in intracellular Na⁺ (consecutive to the osmotic activation of SA channels (4)). K⁺ is secreted into the blood by amiloride sensitive channels (2) and by K⁺(Ca²⁺) channels (5) that have been opened by Ca²⁺ flowing through SA channels. Closing inward rectifying K⁺ channels (3) by the membrane depolarization induced by the opening of SA channels further promotes vectorial K⁺ secretion to the blood. This mechanism can protect the brain during short ischemic episodes. Upon prolonged ischemia, decreasing endothelial cell ATP concentrations and collapsing of membrane ionic gradients prevent endothelial cells pumping K⁺.

cells take up Na$^+$, release K$^+$ and interstitial K$^+$ concentrations raise. It has been proposed that during ischemia, an osmotic activation of SA channels could favor K$^+$ secretion to the blood and hence protect neuronal cells (Popp *et al.*, 1992). Figure 23.2 illustrates the essential features of this model. It requires however that enough ATP is still present to fuel the (Na$^+$,K$^+$)ATPase. BCEC, like neurons, strongly rely on oxygen for synthesizing ATP and upon prolonged ischemia, ATP levels in endothelial cells may fall, thus limiting (Na$^+$,K$^+$)ATPase activity and hence K$^+$ secretion. ATP depletion may have other consequences such as the opening of Ca^{2+} and ATP-sensitive nonselective channels (Popp and Gögelein, 1992) and of K$^+$(ATP) channels (Janigro *et al.*, 1993).

When intracellular ATP concentrations are too low to fuel the (Na$^+$,K$^+$)ATPase and in the presence of unaltered transmembrane ionic gradients, the only abluminal mechanism that could pump brain K$^+$ is the Na$^+$,K$^+$,Cl$^-$ co-transporter. It is of interest that BCEC express a Na$^+$,K$^+$,Cl$^-$ cotransport activity that is sensitive to osmolarity (Vigne *et al.*, 1994). It should be noted however that while SA channels are activated by a cell swelling (i.e. by

hypoosmolar solutions), the Na$^+$,K$^+$,Cl$^-$ cotransporter is activated by a cell shrinking (i.e. by hyperosmolar solutions).

Distinct alterations of ion transport may occur during reperfusion of ischemic zones. These may involve changes in the activity of the Na$^+$/H$^+$ antiport as described during the myocardial oxygen paradox (Lazdunski *et al.*, 1985) and the production of reactive oxygen species that have selective actions on K$^+$ channels (Duprat *et al.*, 1995).

Activated K$^+$ secretion

Ion transport pathways are highly regulated mechanisms. Inward rectifying K$^+$ channels are inhibited by angiotensin II and arginine vasopressin (Hoyer *et al.*, 1991). The Na$^+$,K$^+$,Cl$^-$ cotransporter and K$^+$(Ca^{2+}) channels are activated by endothelins, neuromedin B and purines (Vigne *et al.*, 1994, 1995; Van Renterghem *et al.*, 1995). Finally, the Na$^+$/H$^+$ antiporter is activated by endothelins (Vigne *et al.*, 1991) and by neuromedin B (Vigne *et al.*, 1995). Figure 23.3 proposes a model by which activation of phospholipase C can promote K$^+$ secretion by the BBB. This model is heavily

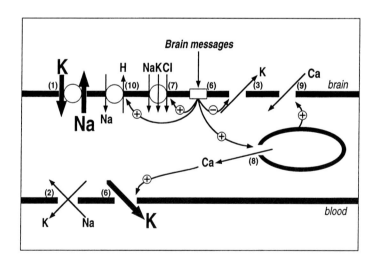

Fig. 23.3. A model for K$^+$ secretion by activated BBB.
Agonists of phospholipase C, acting via abluminal receptors stimulate abluminal Na$^+$,K$^+$,Cl$^-$ cotransporters (7) and Na$^+$/H$^+$ antiporters (10), thus resulting in net uptakes of Na$^+$ and K$^+$ and in a secondary activation of the (Na$^+$,K$^+$)ATPase (1). Ca^{2+} mobilized from intracellular stores (8) and that entered cells via the capacitative entry mechanism (9) opens luminal K$^+$(Ca2$^+$) channels (6). G protein mediated inhibition of abluminal inward rectifying K$^+$ channels (3) closes the abluminal K$^+$ shunt pathway and further promotes vectorial K$^+$ transport.

dependent upon assumptions about the distributions of ion transport mechanisms and of receptors that have still to be documented. As an hypothesis we further propose that agonists of phospholipase C originating from brain cells could signal endothelial cells to pump K^+ to the blood. By this mechanism K^+ secretion could be adjusted to neuronal activity.

Conclusion

Available evidence suggests that BCEC express a variety of ion channels, mainly nonselective cationic channels, $K^+(Ca^{2+})$ channels and inward rectifying K^+ channels. Increasing evidence also suggests that activity of these channels is controlled by intracellular signals generated by the phospholipase C signalling cascade. This regulation is more conspicious than regulations by cAMP or cGMP-dependent signalling pathways that are well known to control the permeability of the BBB (Rubin *et al.*, 1991) and salt secretion/reabsorption by tight epithelia.

Although there is little doubt that ion channels observed in BCEC participate in Na^+ uptake to the brain and most importantly in K^+ efflux from the brain, the mechanisms involved are still conjectural. The availability of *in vitro* models of BBB that develop large transendothelial electrical resistances (Meresse *et al.*, 1989; Rubin *et al.*, 1991) will be useful to define the polarity of expression of ion channels at the BBB and of the receptors that control their activities.

References

Adams, D. J. (1994). Ionic channels in vascular endothelial cells. *Trends Cardiovasc. Med.*, **4**, 18–26.

Archer, S. L., Huang, J. M. C., Hampl, V., Nelson, D. P., Shultz, P. J. and Weir, E. K. (1994). Nitric oxide and cGMP cause vasodilatation by activation of a charybdotoxin sensitive K^+ channel by cGMP dependent protein kinase. *Proc. Natl. Acad. Sci. USA*, **91**, 7583–7.

Barbry, P. (1996). Structure and regulation of the amiloride sensitive epithelial Na^+ channel. In *Ion Channels*, Vol 4, ed. T. Narahashi (in press).

Betz, L. (1983). Sodium transport from blood to brain: Inhibition by furosemide and amiloride. *J. Neurochem.*, **41**, 1158–64.

Betz, A. L., Firth, J. A. and Goldstein, G. W. (1980). Polarity of the blood brain barrier: distribution of enzymes between the luminal and antiluminal membranes of brain capillary endothelial cells. *Brain Res.*, **192**, 17–28.

Bossu, J. L., Elhamdani, A., Feltz, A. *et al.* (1992). Voltage gated Ca^{2+} entry in isolated bovine capillary endothelial cells: evidence of a new type of Bay K 8644 sensitive channel. *Pflügers Archiv.*, **420**, 200–7.

Bradbury, M. W. B. and Stulcova, B. (1970). Efflux mechanism contributing to the stability of the potassium concentration in cerebrospinal fluid. *J. Physiol.*, **208**, 415–30.

Brutsaert, D. L. and Andries, L. J. (1992). The endocardial endothelium. *Am. J. Physiol.*, **263**, H985–H1002.

Catterall, W. A. (1995). Structure and function of voltage gated ion channels. *Annual Review of Biochemistry*, **64**, 493–531.

Chandy, K. G. and Gutman, G. A. (1993). Nomenclature of mammalian potassium channel genes. *Trends Pharmacol. Sci.*, **14**, 434.

Duprat, F., Guillemare, E., Romey, G. *et al.* (1995). Susceptibility of cloned K^+ channels to reactive oxygen species. *Proc. Natl. Acad. Sci. USA*, **92**, 11796–800.

Ennis, S. R., Ren, X. D. and Betz, A. L. (1996). Mechanisms of sodium transport at the blood brain barrier studied with *in situ* perfusion of rat brain. *J. Neurochem.*, **66**, 756–63.

Frelin, C. and Vigne, P. (1993). Brain microvascular vasoactive agents: receptors and mechanisms of action. In *The Blood Brain Barrier. Cellular and Molecular Biology*. ed. W. M. Pardridge, pp. 249–65. New York: Raven Press.

Frelin, C., Breittmayer, J. P. and Vigne, P. (1993). ADP induces inositol phosphate independent intracellular Ca^{2+} mobilization in brain capillary endothelial cells. *J. Biol. Chem.*, **268**, 8787–92.

Gögelein, H. (1990). Ion channels in mammalian proximal renal tubules. *Renal Physiol. Biochem.*, **13**, 8–25.

Goldstein, G. W. (1979). Relation of potassium transport to oxidative metabolism in isolated brain capillaries. *J. Physiol.*, **286**, 185–95.

Hansen, A. J., Lund-Andersen, H. and Crone, C. (1977). K^+ permeability of the blood brain barrier, investigated by aid of a K^+ sensitive microelectrode. *Acta Physiol. Scand.*, **101**, 438–45.

Harik, S. I. (1986). Blood brain barrier sodium/potassium pump: modulation by central noradrenergic innervation. *Proc. Natl. Acad. Sci. USA*, **83**, 4067–70.

Hoyer, J., Popp, R., Meyer, J. *et al.* (1991). Angiotensin II, vasopressin and GTP[γS] inhibit inward rectifying K^+ channels in porcine cerebral capillary endothelial cells. *J. Memb. Biol.*, **123**, 55–62.

Janigro, D., West, G. A., Gordon, E. L. and Winn, H. R. (1993). ATP sensitive K^+ channels in rat aorta and brain microvascular endothelial cells. *Am. J. Physiol.*, **265**, C812–C821.

Katzman, R. (1976). Maintenance of a constant brain extracellular potassium. *Fed. Proc.*, **35**, 1244–7.

Kolb, H. A. (1990). Potassium channels in excitable and non excitable cells. *Rev. Physiol. Biochem. Pharmacol.*, **115**, 51–91.

Lansman, J. B., Hallam, T. J. and Rink, T. J. (1987). Single stretch activated ion channels in vascular endothelial cells as mechanotransducers? *Nature*, **325**, 811–13.

Lazdunski, M. (1994). ATP sensitive potassium channels: an overview. *J. Cardiovasc. Pharmacol.*, **24**, S1–S5.

Lazdunski, M., Frelin, C. and Vigne, P. (1985). The sodium/hydrogen exchange system in cardiac cells: its biochemical and pharmacological properties and its role in regulating internal concentrations of sodium and internal pH. *J. Molec. Cell. Cardiol.*, **17**, 1029–42.

Manabe, K., Ito, H., Matsuda *et al.* (1995). Classification of ion channels in the luminal and abluminal membranes of guinea pig endocardial endothelial cells. *J. Physiol.*, **484**, 41–52.

Marsault, R. and Frelin, C. (1992). Activation by nitric oxide of guanylate cyclase in endothelial cells from brain capillaries. *J. Neurochem.*, **59**, 942–5.

Meresse, S., Dehouck, M. P., Delorme, P. *et al.* (1989). Bovine brain endothelial cells express tight junctions and monoamine oxidase activity in long term culture. *J. Neurochem.*, **53**, 1363–71.

Popp, R. and Gögelein, H. (1992). A calcium and ATP sensitive non selective cation channel in the antiluminal membrane of rat cerebral capillary endothelial cells. *Biochim. Biophys. Acta*, **1108**, 59–66.

Popp, R., Hoyer, J., Meyer, J. *et al.* (1992). Stretch-activated non selective cation channels in the antiluminal membrane of porcine cerebral capillaries. *J. Physiol.*, **454**, 435–49.

Popp, R., Englert, H. C., Lang, H. J. and Gögelein, H. (1993). Inhibitors of non selective cation channels in cells of the blood brain barrier. In *Non Selective Cation Channels: Pharmacology, Physiology and Biophysics*, ed D. Siemen and J. Hescheler, pp. 213–18. Basel: Birkhaüser Verlag.

Rubin, L. L., Hall, D. E., Porter, S. *et al.* (1991). A cell culture model of the blood brain barrier. *J. Cell Biol.*, **115**, 1725–35.

Sullivan, H. C. and Harik, S. I. (1993). ATP-sensitive potassium channels are not expressed in brain microvessels. *Brain Res.*, **612**, 336–8.

Takeda, K. and Klepper, M. (1990). Voltage dependent and agonist activated ionic currents in vascular endothelial cells: a review. *Blood Vessels*, **27**, 169–83.

Takeda, K., Schini, V. and Stoeckel, H. (1987). Voltage activated potassium, but not calcium currents in cultured bovine aortic endothelial cells. *Pflügers Arch.*, **410**, 385–93.

Vaca, L., Schilling, W. P. and Kunze, D. L. (1992). G-protein mediated regulation of a Ca^{2+} dependent K^+ channel in cultured vascular endothelial cells. *Pflügers Arch.*, **422**, 66–74.

Van Renterghem, C., Vigne, P. and Frelin, C. (1995). A charybdotoxin sensitive Ca^{2+} activated K^+ channel with inward rectifying properties in brain microvascular endothelial cells. Properties and activation by endothelins. *J. Neurochem.*, **65**, 1274–81.

Vigne, P. and Frelin, C. (1992). C-type natriuretic peptide is a potent activator of guanylate cyclase in endothelial cells from brain microvessels. *Biochem. Biophys. Res. Comm.*, **183**, 640–4.

Vigne, P., Champigny, G., Marsault, R. *et al.* (1989). A new type of amiloride sensitive cationic channel in endothelial cells of brain microvessels. *J. Biol. Chem.*, **264**, 7663–8.

Vigne, P., Marsault, R., Breittmayer, J. P. and Frelin, C. (1990). Endothelin stimulates phosphatidylinositol hydrolysis and DNA synthesis in brain capillary endothelial cells. *Biochem. J.*, **266**, 415–20.

Vigne, P., Ladoux, A. and Frelin, C. (1991). Endothelins activate Na/H exchange in brain capillary endothelial cells via a high affinity endothelin-3 receptor that is not coupled to phospholipase C. *J. Biol. Chem.*, **266**, 5925–8.

Vigne, P., Lopez Farré, A. and Frelin, C. (1994). The Na^+–K^+–Cl^- cotransporter of brain capillary endothelial cells. Properties and regulation by endothelins, hyperosmolar solutions, calyculin A and interleukin-1. *J. Biol. Chem.*, **269**, 19925–30.

Vigne, P., Feolde, E., Van Renterghem, C. *et al.* (1995). Properties and functions of a neuromedin B preferring bombesin receptor in brain microvascular endothelial cells. *Eur. J. Biochem.*, **233**, 414–18.

24 Interactions of lipoproteins with the blood–brain barrier

LAURENCE FENART, BÉNÉDICTE DEHOUCK, MARIE-PIERRE DEHOUCK, GÉRARD TORPIER and ROMÉO CECCHELLI

- Introduction
- Occurence of an LDL receptor at the BBB
- Function of the LDL receptor at the BBB

Introduction

A model for cholesterol transport and homeostasis within the central nervous system has been proposed by Pitas *et al.* (1987) after the visualization by immunocytochemistry in rat and monkey brains of the presence of a low-density lipoprotein (LDL) receptor. Apolipoprotein (apo) E and apoAI-containing particles were also detected in human cerebrospinal fluid (Pitas *et al.*, 1987). Furthermore, enzymes involved in lipid metabolism have been located within the brain: LCAT mRNA has been shown to be expressed in rat brains, cholesteryl ester transfer protein which plays a key role in cholesterol homeostasis has been detected in human cerebrospinal fluid and seems to be synthesized in the brain (Albers *et al.*, 1992). The distribution of the low-density lipoprotein receptor-related protein (LRP), a multifunctional receptor that binds apoE, is highly restricted and limited to the grey matter, primarily associated with neuronal cell population (Wolf *et al.*, 1992). The difference in cellular expression of ligand (apoE) and receptor (LRP) may provide a pathway for intracellular transport of apoE-containing lipoproteins in the central nervous system. All these data leave little doubt that the brain is equipped with a relatively self-sufficient transport system for cholesterol.

Cholesterol could be derived from *de novo* synthesis within the brain and from plasma via the blood–brain barrier (BBB). Malavolti *et al.* (1991) have indicated the presence of unexpectedly close communications between extracerebral and brain cholesterol. Changes in the extracerebral cholesterol levels are readily sensed by the LDL receptor in the brain and promptly provoke appropriate modifications in its activity. Furthermore, the fact that enzymes involved in the lipoprotein metabolism are present in the brain microvasculature (Brecher and Kuan, 1979), and that the entire fraction of the drug bound to lipoproteins is available for entry into the brain strongly suggest that this cerebral endothelial receptor plays a role in the interaction of plasma lipoproteins with brain capillaries. These results pinpoint the critical importance of the interactions between brain capillary endothelial cells (ECs) and lipoproteins.

Carrier-mediated transport systems that facilitate the uptake of hexoses, amino acids, purine compounds and mono-carboxylic acids have been revealed in the cerebral endothelium (Betz and Goldstein, 1978), but until now little information has come to light regarding the cerebral uptake of lipids.

To determine whether LDL, the major carrier of cholesterol, is involved in the delivery of lipids through the BBB, Méresse *et al.* (1989) injected radioactive LDL in the absence or in the presence of an excess of unlabelled LDL immediately post-mortem into bovine brain circulation. The total amount of radioactivity that remained associated with the capillaries in the presence of excess unlabelled LDL was only 15% of the radioactivity recovered in the capillaries when LDL was injected alone. This result suggests that LDL binds to a specific receptor on the endothelium of brain capillaries.

In order to confirm this possibility, the binding of LDL on isolated brain capillaries showed that irrespective of the incubation medium, incubation time or concentration of LDL, no difference was observed between the binding in the presence or in the absence of excess unlabelled LDL, suggesting the absence of a high affinity binding process for LDL. However these results could probably be explained by the high nonspecific binding of LDL (approximately 20-fold higher than non-specific binding on purified endothelial membranes), probably due to the large amount of connective tissue attached to the basement membrane. So, it was of interest to test the efficiency of the binding of both purified endothelial and basement membranes of brain capillaries. The endothelial and basement membranes of freshly isolated brain capillaries were separated according to Lidinsky and Drewes (1983) and their own LDL binding capacity recorded. The LDL bound with a saturation kinetic only in the presence of endothelial membranes. The saturability of this binding emphasized the concept that the interaction of LDL with a specific receptor has been detected. When transformed to Scatchard plots, the total binding data show evidence for a single binding site with an apparent dissociation constant (K_d) of 16 nM. The estimate of the affinity is similar to the K_d reported on human fibroblasts (Mahley and Innerarity, 1983). The specificity of the binding was confirmed by the lack of competition with methyl-LDL, which is known not to abolish the specific binding (Weisgraber et al., 1978). This receptor exhibits the same characteristic properties as the LDL receptor on human fibroblasts (Goldstein and Brown, 1977) and steroid-secreting cells (Kovanen et al., 1979): (1) it binds human LDL; (2) HDL3 is a poor competitor; (3) it fails to bind LDL whose lysine residues have been methylated; (4) it requires a divalent cation; (5) it is extremely sensitive to destruction by proteolytic enzymes. The molecular weight determined for bovine capillary receptor by ligand blotting is

132 000 in unreduced SDS-polyacrylamide gel. It is very similar to the 130–132 000 of the LDL receptor detected in bovine adrenal cortex by the same method (Soutar et al., 1986; Kroon et al., 1984).

A separate 'scavenger' pathway of LDL uptake in macrophages and ECs that differs from the LDL receptor in terms of specificity and biochemical properties has been described (Goldstein et al., 1979; Stein and Stein, 1980). This scavenger pathway recognizes only some chemically modified forms of LDL (derivatized by acetylation, acetoacetylation or treatment with malondialdehyde) and biologically modified LDL (incubated with cultured human ECs). The requirement of Ca^{2+} argues against the possibility of a scavenger receptor (Goldstein et al., 1979; Dresel et al., 1984). In addition, the molecular weight determined for the receptor on brain capillary ECs (132 000) is very far from the molecular weight of the scavenger receptor (220–250 000) determined by Dresel et al. (1984). Moreover, the presence of a scavenger receptor on brain capillary ECs is very uncertain. It seems that these cells fail to take up acetylated LDL in vivo (Pitas et al., 1985), whereas in vitro the results are very conflicting (Gaffney et al., 1985; Carson and Haudenschild, 1986).

All these results demonstrate that in vivo brain capillary ECs express an LDL receptor.

The occurrence of an LDL receptor at the BBB addresses two questions :

1. How can we explain, that in contrast to peripheral ECs, brain capillary ECs express, at confluence and in the presence of large quantities of lipoproteins, an LDL receptor?
2. Are lipoproteins, after binding, degraded by the cerebral microvasculature and is the subsequent metabolism of LDL restricted to the vasculature or can it occur in the underlying nervous tissue?

Occurrence of an LDL receptor at the BBB

In recent years, the manner in which capillary ECs in the brain become different from those in the periphery has been examined and the crucial role

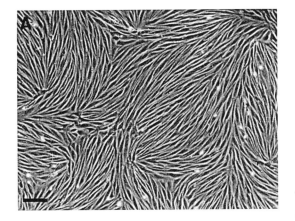

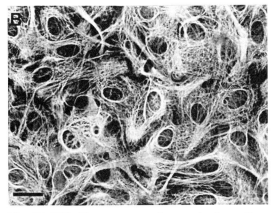

Fig. 24.1(A). Phase contrast micrograph of a confluent brain capillary endothelial cell monolayer. Bar, 100 μm. (B). Immunofluorescent labeling of astrocyte enriched culture with an anti-GFAP (glial fibrillary acidic protein) serum. Bar, 50 μm.

of the environment in which they grow has been demonstrated (Stewart and Wiley, 1981). Astrocytes, the nearest neighbour of brain capillaries, have been shown to induce some of the specialized properties of ECs (Janzer and Raff, 1987).

In attempts to investigate such interactions, the development of *in vitro* models of the BBB enables the reconstruction of some of the complexities of the cellular environment that exist *in vivo* while retaining the experimental advantages associated with tissue culture (Joó, 1993).

By culturing brain capillary ECs and astrocytes on opposite sides of a filter, Dehouck *et al.* (1990) have developed a BBB model that closely mimics the *in vivo* situation (Fig.24.1). Thus, the culture medium is shared by both cell populations, allow-

ing humoral interchange without direct cell contact.

In contrast to what was observed on ECs from large vessels, labeled LDL bound specifically to brain capillary ECs (Volpe *et al.*, 1978). These data revealed the presence on brain capillary ECs of a single class of high-affinity LDL binding sites with a K_d of the order of nM. Our findings also showed that the capacity of ECs to bind LDL is greater when co-cultured with astrocytes than in their absence. It is well-known that astrocytes are capable of influencing the differentiation of brain ECs in culture, as they are *in vivo*. Like other cells in the body, astrocytes possess an apo(B, E) receptor, and at the cellular level, this receptor provides a regulated mechanism for supplying cells with cholesterol (Pitas *et al.*, 1987; Tao-Cheng *et al.*, 1990). As demonstrated by HPLC analysis, when a complete serum containing medium was changed to a medium containing 10% lipoprotein-deficient serum (LPDS) for 36 hours, the cholesterol content of the astrocytes was depleted. When these cells were co-cultured again with brain capillary ECs a six-fold increase in the binding of LDL to ECs was observed (Dehouck *et al.*, 1994). This result indicates that the lipid requirement of astrocytes modulates the expression of endothelial cell LDL receptors. Furthermore, the same experiments performed with smooth muscle cells plated instead of astrocytes, or with aortic ECs instead of brain capillary ECs, did not enhance LDL receptor expression on ECs. Thus, the two close neighbours *in vivo*, brain endothelium and astrocytes, interact specifically *in vitro* to induce the expression of the LDL receptor at the luminal side of brain capillary ECs. Furthermore, astrocytes cultured 'in solo' during the co-culture phase do not upregulate LDL receptors on brain capillary ECs, during the induction phase. This indicates that a cross-talk takes place between brain capillary ECs and astrocytes during the co-culture. The previous observations (Estrada *et al.*, 1990) that brain ECs can increase the incidence of intramembranous particle arrays in astrocytes, are in agreement with these results showing that ECs can in turn induce changes in associated glia. The nature of the signal is not known, but Estrada *et al.* (1990) have shown that a peptide, with a molecular weight greater than 50 000, derived from cerebral capillary ECs could be involved in the local signaling between cell types that control new vessel formation in development (i.e., brain capillary ECs and astrocytes). These results could explain why with this co-culture model, a conditioned medium of astrocytes cultured 'in solo' did not increase the γ-glutamyl-transpeptidase activity and the electrical resistance of the brain capillary endothelial cell monolayer (Dehouck *et al.*, 1990).

Furthermore, although brain capillary ECs bind specifically acetylated LDL (Volpe *et al.*, 1978; Hofmann *et al.*, 1987), astrocytes co-cultured with brain capillary ECs for 12 days and fed with LPDS, cannot upregulate scavenger receptor expression on brain capillary ECs surface. Therefore, the astrocyte-regulating LDL receptor factor seems to regulate LDL receptor expression specifically.

Since these effects were mediated through a filter that prevents direct cell-to-cell contact, the possible involvement of a soluble factor(s) in this phenomenon was suspected. The involvement of a soluble factor(s) in the upregulation mechanism was demonstrated using conditioned medium from cholesterol-depleted astrocytes. The fact that the upregulation is lower when the astrocyte conditioned medium was used could be explained by the secretion of an unstable molecule(s) by astrocytes. The secretion of this factor requires co-cultured cells, indicating that the reciprocal differentiation of both cell types might happen. The experiments using dialysis bags allowed only factor(s) with molecular weights between 3500 and 14000 to diffuse to the brain capillary ECs. Since these EC–astrocyte effects are cross-species (bovine–rat), it is likely to be a fundamental property of the two cell types. Astrocyte-regulating factor liberation is specific and occurs only with co-cultured brain capillary ECs and astrocytes.

In conclusion, taken together, these experiments indicate that the occurrence of the LDL receptor on brain capillary ECs at confluence and in the presence of a high concentration of lipoproteins could be explained not only by the originality of the cell type used, brain capillary ECs, but also by the local control of astrocytes. These results confirm the notion that ECs in general do not express their final destination-specific differentiated features until these features are induced by local environment-produced conditions. Therefore, the expression of

the LDL receptor could be considered as another special feature of brain capillary ECs.

Function of the LDL receptor at the BBB.

In contrast to acetylated LDL, which do not cross the BBB, LDL is specifically transcytosed across the monolayer. The C7 monoclonal antibody, known to interact with the LDL receptor binding domain, totally blocked the transcytosis of LDL, while control of irrelevant IgG had no effect, suggesting that the transcytosis is mediated by the receptor. Furthermore, radiolabeled LDL was not degraded during the transcytosis, indicating that the transcytotic pathway in brain capillary ECs is different from the LDL receptor classical pathway. Owing to the fact that the lipid requirement of astrocytes increases the number of LDL receptors at the luminal side of brain capillary endothelial cells, Dehouck *et al.* (1997) investigated the capacity of astrocytes to modulate LDL transcytosis. When the astrocytes were preincubated in LPDS prior to co-culture, the rate of LDL transcytosis was increased (Fig. 24.2) compared to that observed when ECs co-cultured with astrocytes were pre-incubated in complete media. These preliminary results confirm that the transcytosis of LDL through the BBB is receptor mediated. These results integrated into the model proposed by Pitas *et al.* (1987), a model for cholesterol transport and homeostasis within the central nervous system and strongly suggest that the cerebral endothelial receptor plays a role in cholesterol transport across the BBB (Fig. 24.3). ApoE, secreted by astrocytes within the brain, transports and redistributes cholesterol via brain interstitial fluid to cells that require cholesterol and express apo(B,E) LDL receptors (Hofmann *et al.*, 1987). Furthermore, the influence of astrocytes on the expression of the LDL receptor and the rate of LDL transcytosis suggests the existence of focal differences in lipoprotein influx, which may depend on the lipid state of glial cells. The BBB cannot be considered as a rigid and impermeable structure protecting the brain, but as a dynamic interface able to modify its permeability to the specific needs of certain areas of the brain.

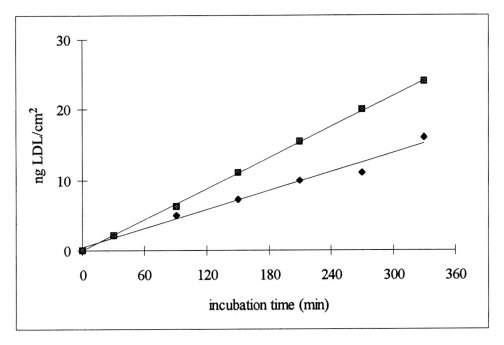

Fig. 24.2. Specific transport of LDL through brain capillary EC monolayer. The experiment was performed with ECs co-cultured with astrocytes (◆) or with cholesterol-depleted astrocytes (▩).

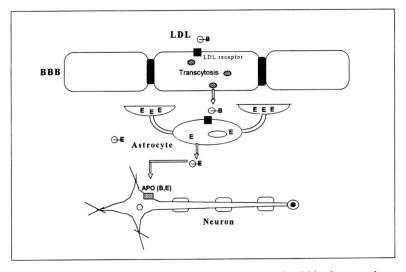

Fig. 24.3. Model for cholesterol transport and homeostasis within the central nervous system.

References

Albers, J. J., Tollefson, J. H., Wolfbauer, G. and Albright, R. E. (1992). Cholesteryl ester transfer protein in human brain. *Int. J. Clin. Lab. Res.*, **21**, 264–6.

Betz, L. and Goldstein, G. W. (1978). Polarity of the blood–brain barrier: neutral amino-acid transport into isolated brain capillaries. *Science*, **202**, 225–7.

Brecher, P. and Kuan, H. T. (1979). Lipoprotein lipase and acid lipase activity in rabbit brain microvessels. *J. Lipid. Res.*, **20**, 464–71.

Carson, M. P. and Haudenschild, C. C. (1986) Microvascular endothelium and pericytes : high yield, low passage cultures. *In Vitro Cell. Dev. Biol.*, **22**, 344–54.

Dehouck, B., Dehouck, M. P., Fruchart, J. C. and Cecchelli, R. (1994). Upregulation of the low density lipoprotein receptor at the blood-brain barrier : intercommunications between brain capillary endothelial cells and astrocytes. *J. Cell. Biol.*, **126**, 465–73.

Dehouck, B., Fenart, L., Dehouck, M. P. *et al.* (1997). A new function for the LDL receptor: transcytosis of LDL across the blood–brain barrier. *J. Cell. Biol.*, **138**, 877–89.

Dehouck, M. P., Méresse, S, Delorme, P *et al.* (1990). An easier, reproducible and mass-production method to study the blood–brain barrier in vitro. *J . Neurochem.*, **54**, 1798–801.

Dehouck, M. P., Dehouck, B., Schluep, C. *et al.* (1995). Drug transport to the brain: comparison between in vitro and in vivo models of the blood–brain barrier. *Eur. J Pharmacol. Sci.*, **3**, 357–65.

Dresel, H. A., Otto, I., Weigel, H. *et al.* (1984). A simple and rapid anti-ligand enzyme immunoassay for visualization of low-density lipoprotein membrane receptors. *Biochim. Biophys. Acta.*, **795**, 452–7.

Estrada, C., Bready, J. V., Berliner, J. A. *et al.* (1990). Astrocyte growth stimulation by a soluble factor produced by cerebral endothelial cells 'in vitro'. *J. Neuropathol. Exp. Neurol.*, **49**, 539–49.

Gaffney, J., West, D., Arnould F. *et al.* (1985). Differences in the uptake of modified low density lipoproteins by tissue cultured endothelial cells. *J. Cell. Sci.*, **79**, 317–25.

Goldstein, J. L. and. Brown, M. S. (1977). The low-density lipoprotein pathway and its relation to atherosclerosis. *Annu. Rev. Biochem.*, **46**, 897–930.

Goldstein, J. L., Ho, Y. K., Basu, S. K. and Brown, M. S. (1979). Binding site on macrophages that mediates uptake and degradation of acetylated low-density lipoprotein, producing massive cholesterol deposition. *Proc. Natl. Acad. Sci. USA*, **76**, 333–7.

Hofmann, S. L., Russel, D. W., Goldstein, J. L. and Brown, M. S. (1987). mRNA for low-density lipoprotein receptor in brain and spinal cord of immature and mature rabbits. *Proc. Natl. Acad. Sci. USA*, **84**, 6312–16.

Janzer, R. C. and Raff, M. C. (1987). Astrocytes induce blood–brain barrier properties in endothelial cells. *Nature (Lond.)*, **325**, 253–7.

Joó, F. (1993). The blood–brain barrier in vitro: the second decade. *Neurochem. Int.*, **23**, 499–521.

Kovanen, P. T., Faust, J. R., Brown, M. S. and Goldstein, J. L. (1979). Low-density lipoprotein receptors in bovine adrenal crotex. I. Receptor mediated uptake of low density lipoprotein and utilization of its cholesterol for steroid synthesis in cultured adrenocortical cells. *Endocrinology*, **104**, 599–609.

Kroon, P. A, Thompson, G. M. and Chao, Y. S. (1984). A comparison of the LDL receptor from bovine adrenal cortex, rabbit and rat liver and adrenal gland by lipoprotein blotting. *Biochem. J.*, **223**, 329–35.

Lidinsky, W. A. and Drewes, L. R. (1983). Characterization of the blood–brain barrier: protein composition of the capillary endothelial cell membrane. *J. Neurochem.*, **41**, 1341–8.

Mahley, R. W. and Innerarity, T. L. (1983). Lipoprotein receptors and cholesterol homeostasis. *Biochim. Biophys. Acta*, **737**, 197–222.

Malavolti, M., Fromm, H., Ceryak, S. and Shehan, K. L. . (1991). Cerebral low-density lipoprotein (LDL) uptake is stimulated by acute bile drainage. *Biochem. Biophys. Acta*, **1081**, 106–8.

Méresse, S., Delbart, C., Fruchart, J. C. and Cecchelli, R. (1989). Low-density lipoprotein receptor on endothelium of brain capillaries. *J. Neurochem.*, **53**, 340–5.

Pitas, R. E., Boyles, J. K., Lee, S. H. *et al.* (1985). Uptake of chemically modified low density lipoproteins in vivo is mediated by specific endothelial cells. *J. Cell. Biol.*, **100**, 103–17.

Pitas, R. E., Boyles, J. K., Lee, S. H. *et al.* (1987). Lipoproteins and their receptors in the central nervous system. Characterization of the lipoproteins in cerebrospinal fluid and identification of apolipoprotein B, E (LDL) receptors in the brain. *J. Biol. Chem.*, **262**, 14352–60.

Soutar, A. K., Hardes-Spengel, K., Wade, D. P. and Knight, B. L. (1986). Detection and quantitation of LDL receptors in human liver by ligand blotting, immunoblotting and radioimmunoassay. *J. Biol. Chem.*, **261**, 17123–7.

Stein, O. and Stein, Y. (1980). Bovine aortic endothelial cells display macrophage-like properties towards acetylated ^{125}I-labelled low-density lipoprotein. *Biochim. Biophys. Acta.*, **620**, 631–5.

Stewart, P. A. and Wiley, M. J. (1981). Developing nervous tissue induces formation of blood–brain barrier characteristics in invading endothelial cells; a study using quail-chick transplantation chimeras. *Dev. Biol.*, **84**, 183–92.

Tao-Cheng, J. M., Nagy, Z. and Brightman, M. W. (1990). Astrocytic orthogonal arrays of intramembranous particle assemblies are modulated by brain endothelial cells in vitro. *J. Cell. Biol.*, **96**, 1677–89.

Volpe, J. J., Hennesy, S. W. and Wong, T. (1978). Regulation of cholesterol ester synthesis in cultured glia and neuronal cells. Relation to control of cholesterol synthesis. *Biochim. Biophys. Acta.*, **528**, 424–35.

Weisgraber, K. H., Innerarity, T. L. and Mahley, R. W. (1978). Role of lysine residues of plasma lipoproteins in high affinity binding to cell surface receptors on human fibroblasts. *J. Biol. Chem.*, **253**, 9053–62.

Wolf, B. B., Lopez, M. B. S., VandenBerg, S. R. and Gonias, S. L. (1992). Characterization and immunohisto-chemical localization of alpha 2-macroglobulin receptor (low-density lipoprotein receptor-related protein) in human brain. *Am. J. Path.*, **141**, 37–42.

25 Fatty acid and lipid intermediate transport

MARIO ALBERGHINA

- Introduction
- Fatty acid and lysoPtdCho transport studies
- Overview of the transport properties
- Effect of aging and peroxidation
- Future directions

Introduction

Palmitate, docosahexaenoate and arachidonate

The knowledge about the fatty acid (FA) transport through microcapillary barriers is increasing nowadays. The basis upon which studies are built is the assumption that FAs enter the brain across blood–brain barrier (BBB) from blood circulation (Pardridge and Mietus, 1980; Spector, 1992). They are also distributed to the posterior segment tissues through the blood–retina barrier (BRB) via the retinal or choroidal vessels and pigment epithelium (RPE) (Li *et al.*, 1992). In the plasma, there are many vehicles that deliver FAs to cells. Endocytosed lipoproteins are the major source, and free fatty acids (FFA) bound to albumin constitute a much smaller pool. At first sight, the process of cellular FA uptake and sorting from this pool should include release from albumin complexes at the luminal endothelial surface and transport to intracellular organelles or abluminal membrane. The last step might be facilitated by cytosolic fatty acid-binding proteins (Schoentgen *et al.*, 1989). However, we are still lacking strong evidence for or against the idea that one integral protein might serve either as receptor for FA–albumin complexes or carrier for unbound fatty acids at BRB and BBB level. More controversial is whether or not there is a saturable, energy-independent endothelial transporter or simply transendothelial passive exchange (Kimes *et al.*, 1985).

Transport of palmitate (PA), the most prominent FA in nervous tissue, has been the first process to be investigated (Pardridge and Mietus, 1980; Kimes *et al.*, 1985). However, observations that the brain receives very little of its saturated FAs and cholesterol from the circulation, meeting its needs instead by *de novo* biosynthesis (Marbois *et al.*, 1992), are still considered to be valid.

Until now, little has been known about the transport of polyunsaturated fatty acids (PUFA) across BBB or BRB. Docosahexaenoic acid (DHA) is an essential fatty acid highly enriched in the brain lipids and photoreceptor cell phospholipids. The physiological mechanism of this enrichment remains unclear. DHA is normally produced in the liver, and then released by blood circulation to the brain tissue (Anderson *et al.*, 1993) which does not seem to be an important site of DHA formation (Scott and Bazan, 1989). A number of experiments in which the incorporation of saturated and polyunsaturated fatty acids into the brain was compared showed higher uptake of PUFA than PA (Anderson and Connor, 1988; DeGeorge *et al.*, 1989; Thiès *et al.*, 1992). These findings would suggest that PUFA might be transferred through BBB in a preferential manner compared to PA.

Arachidonic acid (AA) is continually required for renewing cell membrane structures. Its metabolites, eicosanoids, have important roles in CNS physiology and pathology. AA is found enriched in phosphatidylinositol, phosphatidylcholine (PtdCho) and phosphatidylethanolamine of nerve endings (Strosznajder *et al.*, 1983), and in a wide range of cell types, including endothelial cells (ECs) (Spector *et al.*, 1980; Vossen *et al.*, 1993). In the brain, AA is synthesized from plasma-derived precursor fatty acids or taken up intact from blood (Moore *et al.*, 1990; Robinson *et al.*, 1992). In rat plasma, 99% of unesterified AA is bound to albumin in charged form (Hamilton and Cistola, 1986).

Lysophosphatidylcholine

Lysophosphatidylcholine (lysoPtdCho) is a normal plasma constituent (5–20% of total phospholipids). In the rat, it is the second most prevalent plasma phospholipid with a concentration of 0.20–0.25 mM (Thiès *et al.*, 1992). In the blood, lysoPtdCho is complexed to albumin and lipoproteins (Mangiapane and Brindley, 1986; Thiès *et al.*, 1992), and originates from two metabolic pathways (Brindley, 1993). It is a prominent component of atherogenic, oxidatively modified lipoproteins. Plasma lysoPtdCho has been considered to be a transport form to tissues of both choline and unsaturated fatty acids (Illingworth and Portman, 1972; Ansell and Spanner, 1982; Thiès *et al.*, 1992; Brindley, 1993). Labeled lysoPtdCho injected into the bloodstream rapidly disappeared from the circulation and was mainly recovered in: (a) PtdCho isolated from several organs, including the brain (Illingworth and Portman, 1972; Morash *et al.*, 1989); (b) fatty acid fraction because of hydrolysis catalyzed by tissue lysophospholipase activity, or (c) water-soluble degradation intermediates (choline, P-choline and betaine) because of extensive enzymatic fragmentation (Illingworth and Portman, 1972). Pardridge and coworkers (1979) have questioned whether lysoPtdCho is able to cross BBB.

Metabolic role of the microvascular endothelium

Much evidence supports the hypothesis that cerebral and retinal endothelium plays a key role in the FA transfer to brain parenchyma and retina. Indeed, isolated microcapillaries are able to metabolize palmitate, and possess lipoprotein lipase activity which may contribute to the influx of FFA into the nervous tissue (Brecher and Kuan, 1979). In addition, microvessels isolated from bovine brain are endowed with the expected enzyme set committed to *de novo* synthesis, reacylation and degradation of PtdCho (Sipione *et al.*, 1996).

Cultured cerebromicrovascular ECs are able to take up linoleic and linolenic acid, and elongate/desaturate essential fatty acids (Moore *et al.*, 1990, 1991, 1993). Neurons, incapable of producing 22:6(*n*-3), could avidly take up DHA from the extracellular medium (Vossen *et al.*, 1993), where it is released from glial cells or capillary endothelium (Moore *et al.*, 1990). An alternative source might be transport through BBB of fatty acids derived from albumin complexes and plasma lipoproteins (Li *et al.*, 1992; Anderson *et al.*, 1993). In fact, retina rods and cones maintain high levels of DHA for phospholipid biosynthesis after accumulation of DHA in RPE triacylglycerols as a consequence of the shedding and phagocytosis process (Gordon *et al.*, 1992). In addition, RPE is able to take up DHA from plasma lipoproteins within choriocapillaries after FA crossing through BRB (Li *et al.*, 1992; Wang and Anderson, 1993), and synthesizes this fatty acid from 18:3(*n*-3) or 22:5(*n*-3) precursors. Retinal tissue is incapable of carrying out this synthesis. ECs do not synthesize an appreciable amount of AA from 18:2(*n*-6) and possess a specific arachidonoyl-CoA synthetase responsible for the high affinity esterification of AA (Morand *et al.*, 1987).

Fatty acid and lysoPtdCho transport studies

In this scenario, work has been done to determine the mechanism by which lipid substances were transported through BBB or BRB. Specific experiments were performed to investigate whether:

Table 25.1. *Retinal and cerebrovascular capillary permeability-surface area* (PS) *products for [1-^{14}C]fatty acid and [1-^{14}C]lysoPtdCho in nervous system regions of the rat.*

Regions	PS (s$^{-1} \cdot 10^{-4}$)				
	PA (*n*=8)	DHA (*n*=7)	AA (*n*=8)	LysoPtdCho (*n*=3)	PL:LA-OOH[b] (*n*=10)
Retina	12.2±2.8	8.45±1.3*[a]	5.76±2.6*[a]	12.7±3.7	16.7±2.3*
Optic nerve	9.03±2.4	9.20±2.3	14.2±5.9	12.8±3.9	29.8±6.3*[a]
Optic tract	12.1±4.1	18.8±5.2	10.5±3.4	26.1±8.8*[a]	31.2±4.9*[a]
Lateral geniculate	7.78±1.9	6.26±2.3	17.6±7.5*[a]	25.1±7.4*[a]	36.3±8.3*[a]
Superior colliculus	7.46±1.6	6.55±1.9	21.3±9.0*[a]	23.5±6.3*[a]	35.2±8.9*[a]
Olfactory bulb	3.19±0.8	2.47±0.5	6.80±2.3*[a]	6.80±2.3*[a]	31.1±7.5*[a]
Visual cortex	22.8±7.1	5.12±0.8*[a]	19.2±8.0	19.2±8.0	32.1±7.8*
Frontal cortex	17.5±4.5	9.42±2.1*[a]	18.4±8.4	25.3±6.4	28.8±4.1*
Parietal cortex	22.6±6.6	10.7±3.5*[a]	15.9±5.3	20.8±7.2	62.4±9.5*[a]
Striatum	7.53±2.2	4.32±1.2	11.4±4.3	12.1±4.0*[a]	28.1±5.2*[a]
Hippocampus	8.18±2.7	5.46±1.7	3.41±1.9*[a]	13.0±2.0	27.5±7.7*[a]

Source: adapted from Alberghina *et al.* (1994a,b,c); Strosznajder *et al.* (1996).
Data are means ±SEM, with the number of rats in parentheses. The *PS* products were determined with 40 μM [1-^{14}C]palmitate, [1-^{14}C]docosahexaenoate, [1-^{14}C]arachidonate, or 1-acyl-L-1-([1-^{14}C]palmitoyl)-2-lyso-*sn*-glycero-3-phosphocholine (LysoPtdCho), 14 μM albumin and 40 μg/ml [^{3}H]inulin in the perfusate, at 20 s after internal carotid perfusion, using the standard assumptions and Eqn (9) of Takasato *et al.* (1984). The perfusion rate was 83 μl/s. Statistical significance of differences between PA and other groups was compared by Student's *t* test, (*) $P<0.05$. One way analysis of variance was also done, followed by Duncan's or Newman–Keuls multiple comparison tests; ([a]) $P<0.05$. ([b]) Sonicated emulsion of peroxidized mixture of phospholipids : linoleate (4:1, w/w; 250 mg in saline, 300–400 nmol hydroperoxides/mg lipid); *PS* values were determined with [1-^{14}C]palmitate as tracer.

(i) 22:6(*n*-3) or 20:4(*n*-6) were transported preferentially to 16:0; (ii) 1-palmitoyl-lysoPtdCho (PamlysoPtdCho) could be transported across BBB and BRB more or less efficiently than unesterified fatty acids (Alberghina *et al.*, 1994a,b,c). The *in situ* brain perfusion technique of Takasato *et al.* (1984) was used to measure transport of [1-^{14}C]palmitate, [1-^{14}C]docosahexaenoate, [1-^{14}C]arachidonate or 1-acyl-L-1-([1-^{14}C]palmitoyl)-2-lyso-*sn*-glycero-3-phosphocholine across the capillaries of the retina, optic nerve, intracranial structures of the visual system and the main brain regions of the rat. Short transit time following arterial injection (single pass) minimizes fatty acid oxidation and abolishes precursor recycling, channelling the transported substrate into direct incorporation into complex lipids.

Table 25.1 shows that the permeability–surface area products (*PSs*) of blood-to-CNS palmitate and DHA transport were higher for the retina, optic tract and parietal cortex than for other white or gray matter areas. This differentiated profile in the FA transport discloses a partial parallelism with the perfusate flow values. For retina and cortex, the uptake of 22:6(*n*-3) was unexpectedly lower than that for palmitate. In other brain regions, DHA *PS* products did not significantly differ from the PA group. Table 25.1 shows that *PS* index of blood-to-CNS arachidonate transport was a little higher for the superior colliculus, visual and frontal cortex than for the retina and other white or gray matter areas. This profile did not resemble data for PA and DHA, which instead showed a parallelism with perfusate flow values. Thus the interpretation was that AA uptake was directly related to metabolic activity of ECs, pericytes, astrocytes and neurons, and fast kinetics of plasma membrane acylation and oxidation enzymes. Furthermore, in all regions except retina, optic tract and hippocampus, *PS* values were higher than those for DHA and PA.

Table 25.1 shows that the *PS* index of Pam-lysoPtdCho transport was higher for the optic nerve and tract, cortex, hippocampus and olfactory bulb than for other areas. In all CNS regions, Pam-lysoPtdCho uptake was not inhibited by probenecid (Alberghina *et al.*, 1994c). In the presence of 14 μM albumin, *PS* products in the retina, optic nerve and tract, visual cortex and prosencephalic structures showed higher values than those for PA or DHA. The results demonstrate that Pam-lysoPtdCho was able to cross retinal and cerebral microvasculature, and that the uptake was inhibited in a dose-dependent fashion by the presence of albumin in the perfusate (Alberghina *et al.*, 1994c). This inhibition may be due to the lysoPtdCho binding to albumin, leading to a decrease in free lysocompound concentration. The results are similar to those of Pardridge and Mietus (1980), who found that the PA uptake by the brain was a function of FA to albumin ratio, and apparently of the unbound FA concentration.

Overview of the transport properties

Saturated against unsaturated fatty acid transport across blood barriers in the nervous system

From the data mentioned above, two conclusions can be drawn: (a) DHA and PA are differently transported through BBB and BRB. The essential, polyunsaturated fatty acid is transported at a lower rate or capacity than the saturated one; (b) the preferential PUFA incorporation into whole brain lipids in intact rat, observed in numerous experiments, does not seem to be a mirror image of their preferential uptake through BRB and BBB. For instance, low transport capacity, especially from brain to blood, and recycling processes may instead explain the retention of the precious DHA in the retina and other nervous system regions. Besides, palmitate may have: (i) a larger intracellular pool, which dilutes its specific radioactivity in endothelial, astroglial and neuronal cells, and (ii) easier transendothelial exchange (from abluminal to lumi-

nal side and reverse direction) mediated by intracellular fatty acid binding protein (FABP) (Schoentgen *et al.*, 1989) showing higher affinity for PA than DHA. Even at an uptake rate higher than DHA, PA net extraction from the blood during passages through BBB and BRB would be lower than that of DHA.

In any kind of cells, the extent of FA transport is critically affected by plasma protein and membrane binding. In plasma, FAs are transported largely in association with albumin, whereas in endothelial cell membrane it is controversial as to whether or not there is: (i) saturable, transendothelial passive exchange (Kimes *et al.*, 1985; Noy *et al.*, 1986), i.e. transbilayer rapid movement via unionized lipophilic form (Kamp and Hamilton, 1993); (ii) saturable, energy-independent endothelial transporter of uncharged FAs (Stremmel and Berk, 1986). In the first case, one would expect the fatty acid permeability to be dependent on partition coefficients between membrane bilayer and albumin-rich aqueous phase. Even if this specific partition coefficient has not been determined for most PUFA, it is known that DHA displays a partition coefficient lower than PA (Anel *et al.*, 1993), and albumin binding stronger compared to that of PA (Savu *et al.*, 1981). Under physiological conditions, the affinities of AA and PA for serum albumin are quite similar (Bojesen and Bojesen, 1994), even though much lower than that of oleic acid. These findings are expected to be according to the greater hydrophobicity of 18:1 compared to those of 16:0 and 20:4. DHA is able to compete strongly for the same albumin binding sites to which AA links (Savu *et al.*, 1981). These properties would fully explain the differential uptakes through microvascular barriers ($PS_{AA} = PS_{PA} > PS_{DHA}$) found. In the second case, the dependence on partition coefficients seems much less evident (see next section).

Two other contributive factors, i.e. the rate of dissociation from albumin, which does not limit the rapid kinetics (within seconds) of the unionized fatty acid uptake (passive diffusion) by ECs (Weisiger *et al.*, 1981) (expected $PS_{AA} = PS_{PA} = PS_{DHA}$), and the metabolic flux and recycling processes in which different FAs are involved inside the blood barrier cells and beyond (expected $PS_{AA} > PS_{PA}$), consolidates the phenomenon. Neither PA nor

DHA is metabolically inert, being rapidly incorporated into the metabolic pools of cell membranes and cytosolic compartments (Alberghina *et al.*, 1994*a*; Strosznajder *et al.*, 1996). AA can be effectively activated and rapidly transferred to the lysophospholipid within the membrane domain of ECs and pericytes.

Retinal and cerebrovascular Pam-lysoPtdCho transport, from the albumin-complex to inside the ECs and glia–neuron network, can be described quantitatively by a model that in principle includes a saturable and non-saturable diffusion component (Alberghina *et al.*, 1994*c*). Substrate transport across the luminal surface membrane implies dissociation from albumin in solution, translocation, partial metabolic utilization across ECs, transport through the abluminal membrane and extracellular matrix, and finally uptake by the glia-neuron plasma membrane prior to undergoing terminal, intracellular acylation–deacylation reactions. Data obtained so far (Alberghina *et al.*, 1994*c*) cannot discriminate which step(s) of the long sequence the kinetic constants measured refer to. However, considering the very small pool size of retinal and cerebral lysoPtdCho, its slight non-saturable component of uptake, and its fast metabolic transformations, the idea that simple membrane diffusion governs Pam-lysoPtdCho exchange across the endothelium seems to be favored.

Saturable transport across the capillary wall: an array of theories

In a survey of recent advances in the transport studies with a wide variety of cellular and perfused organ systems, at least five processes (routes) may be hypothesized to explain transfer of membrane-soluble fatty acids through cells and microvascular endothelium. Theories here reviewed range from highly specific receptor-mediated mechanisms to simple diffusion. They are as follows: (a) transcellular, saturable process mediated by receptor binding of albumin-FA complex (Weisiger *et al.*, 1981; Bassingthwaighte *et al.*, 1989); (b) transcellular, saturable process consequent to spontaneous partitioning of albumin–FA complex into membranes (physical-chemical model) (Noy *et al.*, 1986; Burczynski *et al.*, 1995); (c) transcellular, saturable process mediated by carrier for free fatty acid

(Sorrentino *et al.*, 1996; Abumrad *et al.*, 1984; Stremmel and Berk, 1986); (d) transcellular crossing by simple diffusion (unsaturable, physical process) (De Grella and Light, 1980); (e) lateral diffusion in the plasmalemma (unsaturable process). Thus far, a body of data has been accumulated in order to distinguish these possibilities from each other, even if the probability, for instance, of passive diffusional flux of fatty acid in free form in addition to one saturable process should be always firmly considered.

Contrary to the FA transport across the capillary wall of fenestrated microvessels in tissues other than nervous system, unbound FA penetration via clefts or lateral diffusion (route e) among ECs forming selective blood barriers is obviously unlikely, given the presence of tight junctions. At first sight, only the routes (a) and (b) (facilitated diffusion) seem quantitatively much more relevant, since in the bloodstream, at near equimolar total fatty acid and albumin, about 0.01% of fatty acid is free (Wosilait and Soler-Argilaga, 1975). A simplified illustration of the postulated models of FA transport is depicted in Fig. 25.1.

Route (a) (albumin receptor model) appears to be sustained by solitary data (Bassingthwaighte *et al.*, 1989). In rabbit perfused heart, the PA transport process has been indicated to be saturable in agreement with the 6-fold reduction of *PS* when the PA/albumin ratio was held constant at 0.91, raising the concentration of PA/albumin complex over the range of 0.0048 to 0.88 mM albumin (Bassingthwaighte *et al.*, 1989). Assuming that the complex is too large to diffuse quickly through the endothelial cell membrane as such, and that the rate of dissociation of PA from albumin is too slow to preclude PA transcapillary passage by instantaneous buffering of the free concentration, the inference was that the PA/albumin complex on the endothelial membrane must bind to a surface receptor/translocator. Indeed, the idea of an albumin receptor catalyzing FA uptake on liver cell surface has been reconsidered by the earlier proponents (Weisiger and Ma, 1987) who has suggested a dissociation-limited model to explain the kinetic behavior of FFA uptake by liver sinusoids. The model predicts that removal of bound ligand cannot exceed the rate of its spontaneous dissociation from albumin (see route b).

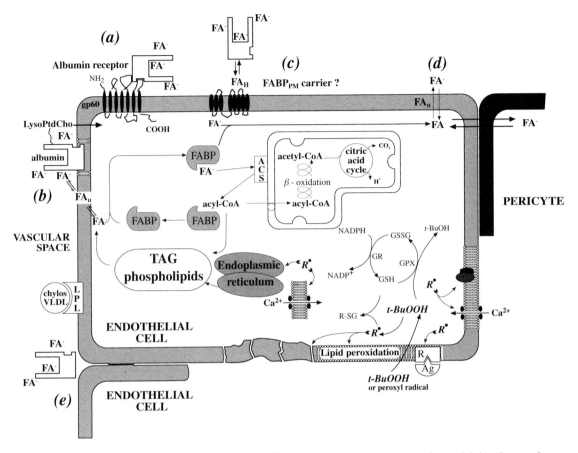

Fig. 25.1. Schematic representation of the various theories considered for explaining data on fatty acid (FA) transport in several cell types. The models refer to an endothelial cell in which some theories have a putative role and some have no experimental evidence (see text). Routes (a), (b), (c), (d), (e) described in the text in principle may be sites of entry for FA. FA$^-$, ionized fatty acid; FA$_H$, protonated fatty acid; FABP, cytosolic fatty acid binding protein; FABP$_{PM}$, plasma membrane fatty acid binding protein; LysoPtdCho, 1-acyl-2-lyso-*sn*-glycero-3-phosphocholine; LPL, lipoprotein lipase; GPX, glutathione peroxidase.

Simplified pathways for postulated mechanisms of the effect of prooxidants on the endothelial cell properties are shown below right. The schema indicates that oxidants may cause altered Ca^{2+} influx–efflux, altered membrane permeability, lipid and protein peroxidation and barrier dysfunction. Free radical-mediated endothelial cell injury may participate in the inflammatory state and/or in the development of atherosclerosis. t-BuOOH, the membrane-permeant organic *tert*-butylhydroperoxide; $R\bullet$, potential radical metabolites.

On the other hand, route (d) (unfacilitated diffusion) undoubtedly could play a role only for neutral, protonated species possibly present at plasma pH or near cell surface, and rapidly metabolized by intracellular enzymes.

Studies in model systems show that variation to pH could be an important factor in regulating FA transfer to phospholipid bilayer from albumin (Hamilton and Cistola, 1986). Unionized fatty acids move quickly across protein-free bilayers (route b), suggesting that a membrane carrier protein may not be required for FA uptake (Kamp and Hamilton, 1993). Many data with perfused liver validate this conclusion. FA uptake is not limited by kinetic factors but is determined instead by the equilibrium distribution of fatty acids between albumin in plasma and membrane phospholipids (Noy *et al.*, 1986). Local acidic environment in the cell plasma membranes may increase the unbound ligand concentration through a conformational change of the albumin molecule (Bos *et al.*, 1989). Incidentally, the notion of uncatalyzed reaction governing transbilayer movement could be instrumental in explaining the fast lysoPtdCho uptake (see above) for which a carrier-facilitated uptake mechanism seems to us very unlikely (Alberghina *et al.*, 1994c).

However, ECs lining the microvasculature of many tissues, except the brain, express a binding protein (gp60) which mediates the adsorptive transcytosis of free, native albumin via plasmalemma vesicles (Ghinea *et al.*, 1989; Schintzer *et al.*, 1992; Tiruppathi *et al.*, 1996). This protein has the ability to bind more readily circulating FA–albumin complexes. Additional data suggest that transport sites for long-chain FAs might be protein-determined microdomains of phospholipids (Bojesen and Bojesen, 1995). Therefore, in addition to the strict process of albumin transcytosis, it could be possible that this cell surface receptor cooperates by accident in a nonspecific, saturable fashion in delivering fatty acid either into the lipid bilayer of the luminal surface or directly to the other side of the endothelial plasmalemma (Weisiger *et al.*, 1981; Bassingthwaighte *et al.*, 1989; Burczynski *et al.*, 1995) where it may became associated with cytosolic FABP. There are currently no data to distinguish these mechanistic possibilities from each other. It must be emphasized that attachment of FA–albumin complex to a membrane receptor/translocator on the luminal surface requires the presence of the same process on the cell abluminal side allowing the transit from inside to out of FAs in bulk, since ECs consume little fatty acid (Burczynski *et al.*, 1995). Interestingly, all the above considerations tend to integrate conceptually the primitive diffusion-reaction model of FA uptake with protein elements of an uncatalytic, facilitation mechanism through the albumin, particularly useful, for instance, in explaining data obtained with adipocytes (Trigatti and Gerber, 1995), hepatocytes but not myocytes (Burczynski *et al.*, 1995). Indeed, as compelling studies were progressed, routes (a) and (b) seem to share common features and approximate each other.

Along these lines, it is conceivable that the complex environment of plasma membrane of a living cell could also foresee the presence of fatty acid binding proteins able to promote FA transendothelial uptake. This opposite hypothesis (route c) is supported by a number of reports demonstrating that the rapid, saturable uptake of FAs observed with perfused liver and isolated myocytes and adipocytes could be explained at least in part by the presence of a receptor for FA rather than for FA–albumin complex. However, the observations confirmed by *in vitro* and *in vivo* experiments (Sorrentino *et al.*, 1996; Abumrad *et al.*, 1984; Stremmel and Berk *et al.*, 1986) do not allow the drawing of unequivocal conclusions. Contrary to what is claimed, findings may be interpreted as not dependent on the concentration of unbound fatty acid. The main concern raised is that the interpretation of data is particularly based on the inhibitory effect on FA transport of either protein modifying agents or antibodies against FA binding protein. At once, doubt arises that the effect, while not specific, could simultaneously be accompanied by alteration of processes such as FA partitioning into cell membranes, functioning of any albumin binding protein, and even the rapid, plasmalemmal FA metabolism (acylation reactions). All of them might contribute per se to FA transport impairment. Furthermore, the proposed interpretations seemed strongly affected by bias, given that factors such as (i) intrinsic permeability of lipid bilayer to lipophilic substrates, (ii) presence of albumin–FA complex binding proteins in EC plasma membrane, (iii) low concentration of FA protonated species at pH 7.4, and (iv) long-chain FA metabolic conversion, even during the short-time incubations with living cells, were all disregarded. The latter factor might be indeed true for adipocytes or hepatocytes, but not for myocytes and cerebral endothelium. In fact, radioactive FAs reach steady-state concentration in cerebral parenchyma, within seconds (Pardridge and Mietus, 1980; Spector, 1992).

In the last decade, reports have appeared describing isolation and characterization of specific, plasma membrane proteins that may facilitate and regulate the transmembrane translocation of long-chain fatty acids (FABP$_{PM}$s of 22, 40–43, 60, 71 or 88 kDa) in rat liver, jejunal microvillous

(Burczynski *et al.*, 1995; Stremmel *et al.*, 1995), adipocyte (Zhou *et al.*, 1992; Schaffer and Lodish, 1994; Poirier *et al.*, 1996) and sarcolemmal membranes (Fuji *et al.*, 1987). Disappointingly, in mammalian tissues purified proteins bind at high affinity FAs solely in ionized form, and the striking differences in their apparent molecular weight do not reconcile easily with a unitary model of the FA transport process. Furthermore, in the endothelium the presence of such proteins has not been demonstrated until now.

The notion of a $FABP_{PM}$ mediating saturable FA uptake in hepatocytes and adipocytes has been recently refined by proponents who suggest a mixed model of transport (Zhou *et al.*, 1992). Thus uptake kinetics can be explained by the sum of a saturable (facilitated) and a non-saturable component, with $FABP_{PM}$ as part of the saturable transport mechanism for long-chain FA. On the other hand, two independent studies (Richieri *et al.*, 1993; Rose *et al.*, 1994) have recently demonstrated that unbound FA levels in equilibrium with BSA were markedly lower than those currently used (Sorrentino *et al.*, 1996; Abumrad *et al.*, 1984; Stremmel and Berk *et al.*, 1986). This means that published kinetic parameters (K_m and V_{max}) for saturable FA uptake by a variety of cells (Sorrentino *et al.*, 1996; Stremmel and Berk *et al.*, 1986; Stremmel, 1988) must be all recalculated, with obvious consequences on the percentage distribution of saturable and nonsaturable component of FA transport.

Effect of aging and peroxidation

Some evidence indicates that senescence is associated with slight though significant region-specific changes in metabolic substrate transport through the capillary endothelium (Banks and Kastin, 1985; Mooradian, 1994; Rapaport, 1994). Since the lipid composition of cerebrovascular endothelium membranes may play a role in the transport properties of BBB, especially for non carrier-mediated transport systems, and since the content of conjugated dienes in the cerebral microvessels of aged rats seems to be increased (see Chapter 33), the hypothesis of age-dependent alterations in the blood–ocular, blood–nerve and blood–brain bar-

rier function using rats aged 4, 14, and 28 months has been tested (Strosznajder *et al.*, 1996). PA and AA were used as tracers for transport. Palmitate *PS* products in the retina, optic nerve and tract, lateral geniculate, visual and parietal cortex did not significantly differ between age groups. For superior colliculus, frontal cortex, striatum, hippocampus and olfactory bulb, a slight but statistically significant *PS* increase with aging was observed. Similarly, in retina and brain regions PS products for AA were not negatively affected by aging (Strosnajder *et al.*, 1996). This confirmed invariance is in line with the idea that most metabolic and functional parameters, in absence of disease, do not decline with age (Tabata *et al.*, 1988).

In light of these findings, two main conclusions were drawn: (i) in many CNS regions of senescent animals, the absence of measurable changes of vascular permeability to poorly penetrating tracers such as sucrose, albumin, horseradish peroxidase was confirmed (see references in Banks and Kastin, 1985; Mooradian, 1994; Rapaport, 1994); (ii) the data did not agree with age-related decline in carrier-mediated transport of peptides, choline, glucose and thyroid hormones in Fischer-344 rats or amino acids in mice (see Banks and Kastin, 1985; Mooradian, 1994; Rapaport, 1994; Strosznajder *et al.*, 1996). Thus, parameters of carrier function (K_m or V_{max}) in ECs might be the target of an effect due to age. Transport properties of substrates, for which a carrier involvement has not been demonstrated while a transmembrane diffusion is at present postulated, might not be negatively affected by aging. In addition, these data underline the fact that, for some brain areas, a modest capillary leakiness was apparent. Such a change could be involved in the CNS dysfunctions found in aging and age-related diseases.

FA hydroperoxides appear as agents capable of increasing the transfer of albumin and low-density lipoprotein across endothelial monolayers in culture (Henning and Chow, 1988), and cause morphological changes of aortic intima when intravenously administered (Yagi *et al.*, 1981). Since highly polyunsaturated phospholipids of endothelium membranes are susceptible to being extensively peroxidized, the question whether BRB and BBB could have been influenced by a peroxidative stress was raised (Alberghina *et al.*,

1994*c*). Table 25.1 clearly shows that intravenous treatment for one week with a peroxidized mixture of phospholipids:linoleate (Anfuso *et al.*, 1994) soon increased significantly the palmitate *PS* values, particularly in the optic pathway structures, striatum and olfactory bulb (Alberghina *et al.*, 1994*c*). The easier PA transport could be ascribed to changes in the content of membrane PUFA, partial loss of asymmetric distribution of amino-phospholipids and to a consequent decrease of luminal and abluminal membrane fluidity. Oxidation of the membrane protein -SH groups or amino acid and protein peroxide adducts might also contribute to membrane damage (see Fig. 25.1). It is conceivable that a disarray of cytoskeletal elements of ECs could influence selective, carrier-mediated as well as diffusion-sustained membrane transport processes.

Future directions

Even if FA transfer across plasma membranes has been extensively studied, and a theory could interpret experimental data better than another, no consistent proposal for unitary mechanism of FA transport has emerged. Given that cultures or co-cultures of microcapillary ECs from brain and retina can be easily established, it would appear particularly important to characterize FA transport in those specific preparations. The studies, together with *in vivo* experiments in perfused brain, should allow dissection of the role of these front-line cells in the transfer of blood-borne FAs from the wide variety of their own vehicles to second-line cells (astrocytes and neurons). So far, FA transport properties of brain microvascular EC are untested. It should be noted that findings in one cell cannot always be broadly extrapolated to another.

Acknowledgments

I am grateful to the members of my laboratory Drs G. Lupo, C. D. Anfuso and S. Sipione, and Mr. A. Giacchetto for their critical comments and significant experimental contributions. This work was supported in part by CNR-Italy and MURST grants.

References

Abumrad, N. A., Park, J. H. and Park, C. R. (1984). Permeation of long-chain fatty acid into adipocytes. Kinetics, specificity, and evidence for involvement of a membrane protein. *J. Biol. Chem.*, **259**, 8945–53.

Alberghina, M., Lupo, G., Anfuso, C. D. and Infarinato, S. (1994*a*). Differential transport of docosahexaenoate and palmitate through the blood-retina and blood–brain barrier of the rat. *Neurosci. Lett.*, **171**, 133–6.

Alberghina, M., Infarinato, S., Anfuso, C. D. *et al.* (1994*b*). Lipid hydroperoxides induce changes in palmitate uptake across the rat blood–retina and blood–brain barrier. *Neurosci. Lett.*, **176**, 247–50.

Alberghina, M., Infarinato, S., Anfuso, C. D. and Lupo, G. (1994*c*). 1-Acyl-2-lysophosphatidylcholine transport acrosss the rat blood–retina and blood–brain barrier. *FEBS Lett.*, **351**, 181–5.

Anderson, G. J. and Connor, W. E. (1988). Uptake of fatty acids by the developing rat brain. *Lipids*, **23**, 286–90.

Anderson, G. J., Hohimer, A. R. and Willeke, G. B. (1993). Uptake of docosahexaenoic acid by microvessels from developing rat brain. *Life Sci.*, **53**, 1089–98.

Anel, A., Richieri, G. V. and Kleinfeld, A. M. (1993). Membrane partition of fatty acids and inhibition of T cell function. *Biochemistry*, **32**, 530–6.

Anfuso, C. D., Lupo, G., Sipione, S. and Alberghina, M. (1994). Susceptibility of rat retina acyl-CoA:1-acyl-sn-glycero-3-phosphocholine *O*-acyltransferase and CTP:phosphocholine cytidylyltransferase activity to lipid peroxidation and hydroperoxide treatment. *FEBS Lett.*, **347**, 123–7.

Ansell, G. B. and Spanner, S. (1982). Choline transport and metabolism in the brain. In *Phospholipids in the Nervous System*, vol 1, ed. L. A. Horrocks, G. B. Ansell and G. Porcellati, pp. 137–44. New York: Raven Press.

Banks, W. A. and Kastin, A. J. (1985). Aging and the blood–brain barrier: changes in the carrier-mediated transport of peptides in rats. *Neurosci. Lett.*, **61**, 171–5.

Bassingthwaighte, J. B., Noodleman, L., van der Vusse, G. and Glatz, J. F. C. (1989). Modeling of palmitate transport in the heart. *Mol. Cell. Biochem.*, **88**, 51–8.

Bojesen, I. N. and Bojesen, E. (1994). Binding of arachidonate and oleate to bovine serum albumin. *J. Lipid Res.*, **35**, 770–8.

Bojesen, I. N. and Bojesen, E. (1995). Specificity of red cell membrane sites transporting three long chain fatty acids. *J. Membrane Biol.*, **149**, 257–67.

Bos, O. J. M., Labro, J. F. A., Fischer, M. J. E. *et al.* (1989). The molecular mechanism of the neutral-to-base transition of human serum albumin. *J. Biol. Chem.*, **264**, 953–9.

Brecher, P. and Kuan, H.-T. (1979). Lipoprotein lipase and acid lipase activity in rabbit brain microvessels. *J. Lipid Res.*, **20**, 464–71.

Brindley, D. N. (1993). Hepatic secretion of lysophosphatidylcholine: a novel transport system for polyunsaturated fatty acids and choline. *J. Nutr. Biochem.*, **18**, 442–9.

Burczynski, F. J., Cai, Z.-S., Moran, J. B. *et al.* (1995). Palmitate uptake by cardiac myocytes and endothelial cells. *Am. J. Physiol.*, **268**, H1659–66.

DeGeorge, J. J., Noronha, J. G., Bell *et al.* (1989). Intravenous injection of [1–^{14}C]arachidonate to examine regional brain lipid metabolism in unanesthetized rats. *J. Neurosci. Res.*, **24**, 413–23.

De Grella, R. F. and Light, R. J. (1980). Uptake and metabolism of fatty acids by dispersed adult rat heart myocytes. II. Inhibition by albumin and fatty acid homologues, and the effect of temperature and metabolic reagents. *J. Biol. Chem.*, **255**, 9739–45.

Fuji, S., Kawaguchi, H. and Yasuda, H. (1987). Purification of high affinity fatty acid receptors in rat myocardial sarcolemmal membranes. *Lipids*, **22**, 544–6.

Ghinea N., Eskenasy, M., Simionescu, M. and Simionescu, N. (1989). Endothelial albumin binding proteins are membrane-associated components exposed on the cell surface. *J. Biol. Chem.*, **264**, 4755–8.

Gordon, W. C., Rodriguez de Turco, E. B. and Bazan, N. G. (1992). Retinal pigment epithelial cells play a central role in the conservation of docosahexaenoic acid by photoreceptor cells after shedding and phagocytosis. *Curr. Eye Res.*, **11**, 73–83.

Hamilton, J. A. and Cistola, D. P. (1986). Transfer of oleic acid between albumin and phospholipid vesicles. *Proc. Natl. Acad. Sci. USA*, **83**, 82–6.

Henning, B. and Chow, C. K. (1988). Lipid peroxidation and endothelial cell injury: implications in atherosclerosis. *Free Rad. Biol. Med.*, **4**, 99–106.

Illingworth, D. R. and Portman, O. W. (1972). The uptake and metabolism of plasma lysophosphatidylcholine in vivo by the brain of squirrel monkey. *Biochem. J.*, **130**, 557–67.

Kamp, F. and Hamilton, J. A. (1993). Movement of fatty acids, fatty acid analogues, and bile acids across phospholipid bilayers. *Biochemistry*, **32**, 11074–86.

Kimes, A. S., Sweeney, D. and Rapoport, S. I. (1985). Brain palmitate incorporation in awake and anesthetized rats. *Brain Res.*, **341**, 164–70.

Li, J., Wetzel, M. G. and O'Brien, P. J. (1992). Transport of n-3 fatty acids from the intestine to the retina in rats. *J. Lipid Res.*, **33**, 539–48.

Mangiapane, E. H. and Brindley, D. N. (1986). Effects of dexamethasone and insulin on the synthesis of triacylglycerols and phosphatidylcholine and the secretion of very-low-density lipoproteins and lysophosphatidylcholine by monolayer cultures of rat hepatocytes. *Biochem. J.*, **233**, 151–60.

Marbois, B. N., Ajie H. O., Korsak, R. A. *et al.* (1992). The origin of palmitic acid in brain of the developing rat. *Lipids*, **27**, 587–92.

Mooradian, A. D. (1994). Potential mechanisms of age-related changes in the blood–brain barrier. *Neurobiol. Aging*, **15**, 751–6.

Moore, S. A., Yoder, E. and Spector, A. A. (1990). Role of the blood–brain barrier in the formation of long-chain ω-3 and ω-6 fatty acids from essential fatty acid precursors. *J. Neurochem.*, **53**, 391–402.

Moore, S. A., Yoder, E., Murphy, S. *et al.* (1991). Astrocytes, not neurons, produce docosahexaenoic acid (22:6ω-3) and arachidonic acid (20:4ω-6). *J. Neurochem.*, **56**, 518–24.

Moore, S. A., Sprecher, H. and Spector, A. A. (1993). Cerebral endothelium synthesizes docosahexaenoic acid (22:6ω-6) from 24-carbon precursors. *ISSFAL Int. Congress, Abstract Book*, 93.

Morand, O., Carré, J. B., Homayoun, P. *et al.* (1987). Arachidonoyl-coenzyme A synthetase and nonspecific acyl-Coenzyme A synthetase activities in purified rat brain microvessels. *J. Neurochem.*, **48**, 1150–6.

Morash, S. C., Cook, H. W. and Spence, M. W. (1989). Lysophosphatidylcholine as an intermediate in phosphatidylcholine metabolism and glycerophosphocholine synthesis in cultured cells: an evaluation of the roles of 1-acyl and 2-acyl-lysophosphatidylcholine. *Biochim. Biophys. Acta*, **1004**, 221–9.

Noy, N., Donnelly, T. M. and Zakim, D. (1986). Physical-chemical model for the entry of water-insoluble compounds into cells. Studies of fatty acid uptake by the liver. *Biochemistry*, **25**, 2013–21.

Pardridge, W. M. and Mietus, L. J. (1980). Palmitate and cholesterol transport through the blood–brain barrier. *J. Neurochem.*, **34**, 463–6.

Pardridge, W. M., Cornford, E. M., Braun, L. D. and Oldendorf, W. H. (1979). Choline and lecithin in brain disorders. In *Nutrition and the Brain*, vol. 5, ed. A. Barbeau, J. H. Growdon and R. J. Wurtman, pp. 25–34. New York: Raven Press.

Poirier, H., Degrace, P., Niot, I. *et al.* (1996). Localization and regulation of the putative membrane fatty-acid transporter (FAT) in the small intestine. Comparison with fatty acid-binding proteins (FABP). *Eur. J. Biochem.*, **238**, 368–73.

Rapoport, S. I. (1994). Aging and the blood–brain barrier. *Neurobiol. Aging*, **15**, 759–60.

Richieri, G. V., Anel, A. and Kleinfeld, A. M. (1993). Interaction of long-chain fatty acids and albumin: determination of free fatty acid levels using the fluorescent probe ADIFAB. *Biochemistry*, **32**, 7574–80.

Robinson, P. J., Noronha, J., DeGeorge, J. J. *et al.* (1992). A quantitative method for measuring regional in vivo fatty-acid incorporation into and turnover within brain phospholipids: review and critical analysis. *Brain Res. Rev.*, **17**, 187–214.

Rose, H., Conventz, M., Fischer, Y. *et al.* (1994). Long-chain fatty acid-binding to albumin: re-evaluation with directly measured concentrations. *Biochim. Biophys. Acta*, **1215**, 321–6.

Savu, L., Benassayag, C., Vallette, G. *et al.* (1981). Mouse α_1-fetoprotein and albumin. A comparision of their binding properties with estrogen and fatty acid ligands. *J. Biol. Chem.*, **256** , 9414–18.

Schaffer, J. E. and Lodish, H. F. (1994). Expression cloning and characterization of a novel adipocyte long chain fatty acid transport protein. *Cell*, **79**, 427–36.

Schnitzer, J. E., Sung, A., Horvat, R. and Bravo, J. (1992). Preferential interaction of albumin-binding proteins, gp30 and gp18, with conformationally modified albumins. Presence in many cells and tissues with a possible role in catabolism. *J. Biol. Chem.*, **267**, 24544–53.

Schoentgen, F., Pignède, G., Bonanno, L. M. and Jollès, P. (1989). Fatty-acid-binding protein from bovine brain. Amino acid sequence and some properties. *Eur. J. Biochem.*, **185**, 35–40.

Scott, B. L. and Bazan, N. C. (1989). Membrane docosahexaenoate is supplied to the developing brain and retina by the liver. *Proc. Natl. Acad. Sci. USA*, **86**, 2903–7.

Sipione S., Lupo G., Anfuso C. D. *et al.* (1996). Phosphatidylcholine synthesis-related enzyme activities of bovine brain microvessels exhibits susceptibility to peroxidation. *FEBS Lett.*, **384**, 19–24.

Sorrentino, D., Stump, D. D., Van Ness *et al.* (1996). Oleate uptake by isolated hepatocytes and the perfused rat liver is competitively inhibited by palmitate. *Am. J. Physiol.*, **270**, G385–92.

Spector, R. (1992). Fatty acid transport through the blood–brain barrier. *J. Neurochem.*, **50**, 639–43.

Spector, A. A., Hoak, J. C., Fry, G. L. *et al.* (1980). Effect of fatty acid modification on prostacyclin production by cultured human endothelial cells. *J. Clin. Invest.*, **65**, 1003–12.

Stremmel, W. (1988). Fatty acid uptake by isolated rat heart myocytes represents a carrier-mediated transport process. *J. Clin. Invest.*, **81**, 844–52.

Stremmel, W. and Berk, P. D. (1986) Hepatocellular influx of oleate reflects membrane transport rather than intracellular metabolism or binding. *Proc. Natl. Acad. Sci. USA*, **83**, 3086–90.

Stremmel, W., Lotz, G., Strohmeyer, G. and Berk, P. D. (1995). Identification, isolation, and partial characterization of a fatty acid binding protein from rat jejunal microvillous membranes. *J. Clin. Invest.*, **75**, 1068–76.

Strosznajder, J., Foudin, L., Tang, W. and Sun, G. Y. (1983). Serum albumin washing specifically enhances arachidonate incorporation into synaptosomal phosphatidylinositols. *J. Neurochem.*, **40**, 84–90.

Strosznajder J., Chalimoniuk M., Strosznajder R. P. *et al.* (1996). Arachidonate transport through the blood–retina and blood–brain barrier of the rat during aging. *Neurosci. Lett.*, **209**, 145–8.

Tabata, H., Kimes, A. S., Robinson, P. J. and Rapoport, S. I. (1988). Stability of brain incorporation of plasma palmitate in unanesthetized rats of different ages, with appendix on palmitate model. *Exp. Neurol.*, **102**, 221–9.

Takasato, Y., Rapoport, S. I. and Smith, Q. R. (1984). An in situ brain perfusion technique to study cerebrovascular transport in the rat. *Am. J. Physiol.*, **247**, H484–93.

Thiès, F., Delachambre, M. C., Bentejac, M. *et al.* (1992). Unsaturated fatty acids esterified in 2-acyl-1-lysophosphatidyl-choline bound to albumin are more efficiently taken up by the young rat brain than the unesterified form. *J. Neurochem.*, **59**, 1110–16.

Tiruppathi, C., Finnegan, A. and Malik, A. B. (1996). Isolation and characterization of a cell surface albumin-binding protein from vascular endothelial cells. *Proc. Natl. Acad. Sci. USA*, **93**, 250–4.

Trigatti, B. L. and Gerber, G. E. (1995). A direct role for serum albumin in the cellular uptake of long-chain fatty acids. *Biochem. J.*, **308**, 155–9.

Vossen, R. C. R. M., Feijge, M. A. H., Heemskerk, J. W. M. *et al.* (1993). Long-term fatty acid modification of endothelial cells: implication for arachidonic acid distribution in phospholipid classes. *J. Lipid Res.*, **34**, 409–20.

Wang, N. and Anderson, R. E. (1993). Transport of 22:6n-3 in the plasma and uptake into retinal pigment epithelium and retina. *Exp. Eye Res.*, **57**, 225–33.

Weisiger, R. A. and Ma, W. (1987) Uptake of oleate from albumin solutions by rat liver. Failure to detect catalysis of the dissociation of oleate from albumin by an albumin receptor. *J. Clin. Invest.*, **79**, 1070–7.

Weisiger, R., Gollan, J. and Ockner, R. (1981). Receptor for albumin on the liver cell surface may mediate uptake of fatty acids and other albumin-bound substances. *Science*, **211**, 1048–50.

Wosilait, W. D. and Soler-Argilaga, C. (1975). A theoretical analysis of the multiple binding of palmitate by bovine serum albumin: the relationship to uptake of free fatty acids by tissues. *Life Sci.*, **17**, 159–66.

Yagi, K., Ohkawa, H., Ohishi, N. *et al.* (1981). Lesion of aortic intima caused by intravenous administration of linoleic acid hydroperoxide. *J. Appl. Biochem.*, **3**, 58–65.

Zhou, S-L., Stump, D., Sorrentino, D. *et al.* (1992). Adipocytes differentiation of 3T3-L1 cells involves augmented expression of a 43-kDa plasma membrane fatty acid-binding protein. *J. Biol. Chem.*, **267**, 14456–61.

237

26 Blood–brain barrier transport of drugs

AKIRA TSUJI and IKUMI TAMAI

- Introduction
- Lipid-mediated BBB transport of drugs
- Plasma protein binding affects the BBB transport of drugs
- Is there a molecular weight limit for BBB transport of drugs?
- Is P-glycoprotein an active efflux pump functioning at the BBB?
- Carrier-mediated BBB transport of drugs
- Transport of peptides across the BBB
- Conclusion

Introduction

The ability to permeate across the blood–brain barrier (BBB) is essential for drugs acting on the central nervous system (CNS), whereas for peripherally acting drugs negligible penetration across the BBB is preferable to avoid CNS side-effects. Transfers of compounds from the circulating blood into the brain interstitial fluid are strictly regulated by the function of brain capillary endothelial cells, which are lined by tight intercellular junctions, lacking fenestrae, and make up the BBB *in vivo*.

This chapter summarizes the mechanisms regulating the influx and efflux processes of drugs, including large peptides, at the BBB in order to understand the net drug transport into the brain, and describes possible strategies to regulate drug entry into the brain, not by lipid-mediated transport, but by utilizing specific transport systems expressed at the brain capillary endothelial cell membrane. This is not intended to be a comprehensive review of the literature on drug delivery into the brain: readers are referred to recent review articles for more detailed information (Cornford, 1985; Pardridge, 1991, 1995*a,b*; Banks

et al., 1992; Terasaki and Tsuji, 1994, 1995; Bergley, 1996; Border and Prokai, 1995; Zlokovic, 1995; Tamai and Tsuji, 1996; Tsuji and Tamai, 1997).

Lipid-mediated BBB transport of drugs

Drugs in blood passing through the BBB may enter the brain compartment by passively diffusing across or being solubilized into the lipid-bilayer membrane of the brain capillary endothelial cells. Therefore, there should be a good relationship between the rate of passage of these drug molecules through the BBB and the octanol/buffer partition coefficient (P or log P) as an *in vitro* measure of relative lipophilic character. As shown in Fig. 26.1, Levin (1980) has established such a relationship in the absence of plasma protein binding of compounds in the rat brain. Very similar correlations were reported in earlier *in vivo* brain uptake studies in rats and rabbits (Cornford, 1985).

It has been suggested that delta log P, defined as the log $P_{\text{octanol/buffer}}$ minus log $P_{\text{cyclohexane/buffer}}$ is a better predictor of brain uptake of a substrate.

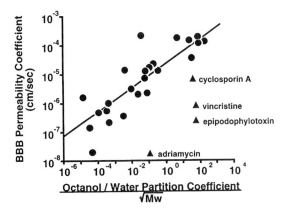

Fig. 26.1. Correlation between BBB permeability coefficient and the octanol/water partition coefficient divided by the square root of molecular weight for various drugs.

Delta log *P* reflects the hydrogen-bonding capacity of the substrate (Bergley, 1996). The less the degree of hydrogen bonding with water, the greater the possibility of partitioning of the drugs to the membrane, and this approach has been applied to interpret the passive diffusion rates of anticonvulsant drugs (Cornford, 1985) and steroid hormones (Pardridge, 1995a) at the BBB.

Plasma protein binding affects the BBB transport of drugs

It has been believed that plasma protein-bound drugs are not available for transport through the BBB. Although this has been confirmed to be valid for several drugs such as propranolol, some plasma-bound drugs are transported into the brain. For example, although tryptophol, which is highly lipid-soluble and has an octanol/water partition coefficient of 30, is bound by plasma albumin to the extent of more than 95% *in vitro*, albumin-bound tryptophol is available for transport through the BBB *in vivo* (Cornford *et al.*, 1979). This is attributed to enhanced dissociation owing to conformational changes near the albumin-ligand binding site *in vivo*. Such conformational changes may be induced by (a) non-specific adsorption at surfaces such as the glycocalyx of the brain capillary endothelium or (b) local pH effects at the cell surface (Pardridge, 1995a).

Is there a molecular weight limit for BBB transport of drugs?

Levin (1980) and Pardridge (1995a) have claimed that the use of log *P* as an index of BBB transport is valid only when the molecular weight is less than approximately 400–600 Da. As shown in Fig. 26.1, the BBB transport of doxorubicin, epipodophylotoxin, vincristine and cyclosporin A, which have molecular weights of 800–1200 Da, was found to be several log orders of magnitude lower than that predicted from the log *P* for these compounds. Pardridge (1995a) has explained the existence of a molecular weight threshold on the basis that kinks or holes in the membrane phospholipid bilayer are generated by rotations about carbon–carbon bonds, and the presence of such kinks creates a kind of pore through which small molecules may permeate through the membrane. This hypothesis implies that the size of the pore may define the molecular weight limit, resulting in poor permeability of the BBB to compounds of molecular weight larger than 800 Da. According to this hypothesis, if a drug has a molecular weight in excess of 400–600 Da, then the drug, even if it has high lipophilicity, may not be transported through the BBB in pharmacologically significant amounts (Pardridge, 1995a).

Is P-glycoprotein an active efflux pump functioning at the BBB?

In contrast to the above hypothesis (Levin, 1980; Pardridge, 1995a), a new concept that active efflux of drugs by P-glycoprotein (P-gp) expressed at the luminal membrane of the brain capillary endothelial cells accounts for the apparently poor BBB permeability to certain drugs was proposed (Tatsuta *et al.*, 1992; Tsuji *et al.*, 1992, 1993b; Sakata *et al.*, 1994; Ohnishi *et al.*, 1995; Tamai and Tsuji, 1996; Tsujij and Tamai, 1997). This idea was based on the observations (a) that P-gp, which pumps out several anticancer agents such as *Vinca* alkaloids or anthracyclines from multidrug-resistant (MDR) tumor cells, was expressed at the BBB of humans as well as animals (Cordon-Cardo *et al.*, 1989; Thiebault *et al.*, 1989) and (b) the finding of an immunosuppressive agent, cyclosporin A, to be

239

Table 26.1. *Effect of brain ischemia on the BBB transport function and ATP content in brain*

Post-ischemia	Control	0 min	30 min	24 h
ATP content (nmol/g brain)	1.43±0.21	0.04±0.017*	1.73±0.31	1.50±0.090
	Permeability coefficient (µL/min/g brain)			
[^{14}C]Sucrose	19.0±1.0	20.0±1.0	24.0±1.0	23.0±3.0
[^{14}C]Antipyrine	930±117	909±69	N.D.	N.D.
[^{3}H]3-*O*-methyl-glucose	313±34	138±13*	N.D.	349±27
[^{3}H]Cyclosporin A	100±21.0	315±42.0*	N.D.	N.D.
Doxorubicin	14.0±2.0	243±25.0*	14.0±5.0	18.4±2.3

Cerebrovascular permeability was measured at the perfusion rate of 4.98 mL/min for 30 s and was corrected with that of sucrose as the vascular space.
ATP content was measured with luciferin–luciferase method.
Each result represents the mean±SEM ($n = 3$–6). N.D., not determined
*Significantly different from the control value ($p < 0.05$).

a substrate for P-gp by means of competitive binding with *Vinca* alkaloid to P-gp using a photo-affinity labeling technique (Tamai and Safa, 1990).

It has been observed that the uptakes of [^{3}H]vincristine and [^{3}H]cyclosporin A were reduced in primary cultured bovine brain capillary endothelial cells expressing P-gp at the luminal side and that these compounds underwent active efflux from the cells (Tsuji *et al.*, 1992, 1993). The steady-state uptakes were significantly increased in the presence of MDR-reversing agents such as verapamil and the anti-P-gp antibody, MRK16. Although the expression of 170 kD P-gp is markedly down-regulated in primary-cultured BCECs (Pardridge, 1995*a*), sufficient P-gp activity remains to function as an active efflux system for drugs. Attempts have been made to establish immortalized brain capillary endothelial cell line from mice, resulting in high-level expression of P-gp and uni-directional transport of [3H]vincristine from the basal side to the apical side (Tatsuta *et al.*, 1992).

P-gp is an ATP-dependent pump. When the ATP content was decreased in primary cultured BCECs by metabolic inhibitors, the uptake of doxorubicin was increased, and upon recovery of the ATP content the drug uptake decreased again to the normal level (Ohnishi *et al.*, 1995). *In vivo* evidence for ATP-dependent and P-gp-mediated transport was demonstrated by using a brain

ischemic rat model as shown in Table 26.1 (Sakata *et al.*, 1994; Ohnishi *et al.*, 1995). The changes of permeation of doxorubicin and cyclosporin A measured by the *in situ* brain perfusion method were inversely correlated with the change in brain ATP content, whereas the permeation of [^{14}C]sucrose, a cerebrovascular space marker, was essentially constant. Strikingly large increases of approximately 17-fold and 3-fold of doxorubicin and cyclosporin A permeation, respectively, across the BBB were observed in forebrain ischemia (Sakata *et al.*, 1994; Ohnishi *et al.*, 1995). These *in vitro* and *in vivo* observations suggest the significance of brain ATP content for doxorubicin and cyclosporin A transport, presumably by P-gp.

Recent studies have also succeeded in demonstrating the physiological significance of P-gp at the BBB *in vivo*. The brain AUC of rhodamine-123 was increased more than three-fold on co-administration of a P-gp inhibitor, cyclosporin A, as evaluated by using a brain microdialysis technique to quantitate rhodamine-123 in the brain extracellular fluid, whereas no significant change in the treated/control plasma AUC ratio of cyclosporin A of 0.96 was observed in rats (Wang *et al.*, 1995). The results provide further evidence that the reduced brain accumulation of rhodamine-123 was due to the efflux function of P-gp at the BBB. The most convincing evidence for involvement of P-gp in BBB function in the physiological state has come from the generation of a mouse strain which lacks P-gp encoded by the *mdr*1a gene (Schinkel *et al.*, 1994). The details are described in Chapter 21.

At present, only P-gp has been confirmed to function for the extrusion of drugs from the brain, thereby decreasing the apparent BBB permeability. By the brain efflux index method, efflux of *para*-aminohippuric acid, taurocholic acid, valproic acid, etc. from brain to blood was also demonstrated, as described in Chapter 3. These lines of study are likely to lead to the discovery of novel BBB efflux transporters. Furthermore, it should become possible to enhance the efficacy of drugs or to reduce side-effects in the CNS by modulating the function of P-gp and the other efflux transporters to increase or decrease the apparent BBB permeability to the drugs, respectively.

Carrier-mediated BBB transport of drugs

The brain capillary endothelial cells have several transport systems regulating entry into the brain across the BBB for nutrients and endogenous compounds such as amino acids, monocarboxylic acids, amines, hexoses, thyroid hormones, purine bases, and nucleosides (Terasaki and Tsuji, 1994; Pardridge, 1995*a*; Bergley, 1996; Joo, 1996; Tamai and Tsuji, 1996). In the small intestine, there are several kinds of carrier-mediated transport systems of endogenous substances, such as monocarboxylic acids, oligopeptides, and phosphoric acids and these transporters are also responsible for the absorption of hydrophilic drugs (Tsuji and Tamai, 1996). Some of the evidence for carrier-mediated brain transport of certain drugs is summarized below.

a) Transport of monocarboxylic acids

The monocarboxylic acid carrier(s) at the BBB transports short-chain monocarboxylic acids (MCAs) such as acetate, lactate and pyruvate and ketone bodies such as β-hydroxybutyrate and acetoacetate, which are essential for brain metabolism (Pardridge, 1995*a*). Using the *in vivo* carotid artery injection technique and an *in vitro* transport experimental system of primary cultured bovine BCECs, a significant competitive inhibitory effect of salicylic acid and valproic acid was observed on the transport of [^{3}H]acetic acid, whereas di- and tricarboxylic acids, amino acids and choline were not inhibitory (Terasaki *et al.*, 1991; Tamai and Tsuji, 1996). These results suggest that acidic drugs bearing a monocarboxylic acid moiety can cross the BBB via the monocarboxylic acid specific transporter(s). Pharmacologically active forms of 3-hydroxy-3-methylglutaryl Coenzyme A (HMG-CoA) reductase inhibitors such as simvastatin acid (the most lipophilic derivative), lovastatin acid and pravastatin, all of which contain a carboxylic acid moiety, have been shown, by measuring transcellular transport and luminal uptake of lipophilic [^{14}C]simvastatin acid in primary cultured BCECs, to be transported by proton/monocarboxylic acid co-transporter(s) at the BBB (Tsuji *et al.*, 1993*a*; Saheki *et al.*, 1994). Less lipophilic pravastatin showed comparable permeability to that of [14C]sucrose and had a low affinity for the simvastatin acid transporter, as evaluated from its inhibitory effect on the uptake of [^{14}C]simvastatin acid. Simvastatin, a prodrug of simvastatin acid, is known to cause sleep disturbance, whereas pravastatin apparently does not, which suggests that these drugs may differ in ability to permeate through the BBB (Tamai and Tsuji, 1996). The absence of CNS side-effects of pravastatin may be ascribed to its very low affinity for the transporter. Therefore, one way to avoid an undesirable side-effect may be to reduce the affinity of drugs for the transporter functioning at the BBB.

It is of interest to identify and clone the gene(s) for the MCA-transporter at the BBB. Recently, the proton-coupled MCA-transporter, MCT1, was cloned from rat small intestinal epithelial cells; the cDNA was 3320 base pairs long and encodes a putative protein of 494 amino acids with a molecular mass of 53 235, having 12 membrane-spanning regions (Takanaga *et al.*, 1995; Tsuji and Tamai, 1996). By northern blot hybridization, MCT1 was identified in various tissues, including whole brain (Garcia *et al.*, 1994; Takanaga *et al.*, 1995). In order to examine whether MCT1 is present at the BBB or not, RT-PCR was performed by using poly(A)$^+$ RNA isolated from rat brain capillary as the template for RT and a set of PCR primers based on the nucleotide sequences of rat MCT1. The nucleotide sequence of the PCR product was confirmed to be identical with a part of rat MCT1 gene (Takanaga *et al.*, 1995). The result indicates that MCT1 is present at the BBB and functions for the transport of lactic acid and other monocarboxylic acid compounds. Lactic acid transport across the BBB seems to be bi-directional (Tamai and Tsuji, 1996). Since the precise localization of MCT1 at the BBB has not been elucidated yet, it is not clear whether MCT1 operates for uptake from blood, efflux from brain, or both. After completion of this review, it was established that MCT1 is localized at luminal and abluminal membranes (Gerhart *et al.*, 1997).

b) Transport of amine compounds

The transport mechanisms for amine drugs have not yet been well elucidated, but passive diffusion and participation of carrier-mediated transport have been suggested for several drugs. An endogenous hydrophilic amine, choline, has been demonstrated to be taken up by a carrier-mediated transport mechanism (Pardridge, 1995a; Joo, 1996; Tamai and Tsuji, 1996; Tsuji and Tamai, 1996). When evaluated by the BUI method, uptake of [³H]choline was inhibited by amine compounds (eperisone, scopolamine, thiamine, isoproterenol, and hemicholinium-3), whereas zwitterionic or anionic compounds were not inhibitory (Kang *et al.*, 1990).

The observations previously reported for the BBB transport of amine compounds suggest that there are at least two different carrier-mediated transport mechanisms specific to choline and amine drugs. For example, carrier-mediated transport of H_1-antagonists was demonstrated (Yamazaki *et al.*, 1994a). Clarifying the BBB transport mechanism for H_1-antagonists is important, since H_1-antagonists often exhibit a significant sedative side effect, presumably caused by H_1-receptor blockade in the CNS. By uptake and transport studies using monolayers of primary cultured BCEC, saturable uptake of a classical H_1-antagonist, [³H]mepyramine, into the brain was observed (Yamazaki *et al.*, 1994a). The uptake was inhibited by amine drugs such as chlorpheniramine, diphenhydramine, and others, but not by

choline, hemicholinium-3 or anionic drugs. Several H_1-antagonists, azelastine, ketotifen, cyproheptadine, emedastine, and cetirizine, competitively inhibited the uptake of [³H]mepyramine by monolayers of primary cultured BCEC to 8.6, 15.1, 15.8, 28.5, and 75.1% of the control, respectively, which suggests that they share common transport mechanisms with mepyramine (Yamazaki *et al.*, 1994b). Among them, the weakest inhibitory effect was observed with cetirizine, which has a carboxylated side chain. Accordingly, introduction of an anionic moiety within the molecule may decrease affinity for the transporters, which would be desirable for drugs with CNS side-effects.

c) Amphoteric drugs and glycoside-conjugated drugs

Among nutrient transport systems at the BBB, the neutral amino acid transport system (system L) has the highest maximum permeability rate evaluated in terms of V_{max}/K_m (Pardridge, 1995a; Bergley,

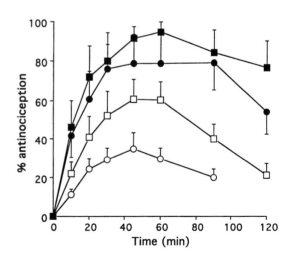

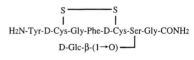

Designed Glycopeptide

Fig. 26.2. The i.p. administration of glycopeptide to mice led to dose-related antinociception in the 55 °C hot-plate test. Glycopeptide doses (i.p.): 30 mg/kg (○), 45 mg/kg (□), 60 mg/kg (●), and 75 mg/kg (■).

1996), where V_{max} and K_m represent the maximum rate and the Michaelis constant, respectively. The drug design of neutral amino acid analogues could be useful in developing strategies to deliver amphoteric drugs to the brain. Several amino acid-mimetic drugs such as L-dopa, α-methyl-dopa, α-methyltyrosine, baclofen, gabapentin (neurontin) and phenylalanine mustard are suspected to be taken up by the neutral amino acid transport system (Pardridge, 1995a; Bergley, 1996). Orally ingested taurine is taken up by a secondary active β-alanine transporter (Komura *et al.*, 1996) utilizing gradients of both Na^+ and Cl^- as the driving force (Tamai *et al.*, 1995).

The brain-type hexose transporter, GLUT-1, has a very large V_{max} value. Some L-serinyl-β-D-glycoside analogues of Met^{5}enkephalin have been shown to be transported across the BBB and to produce a marked and long-lasting analgesia after intraperitoneal administration in mice (Polt *et al.*, 1994). The result is shown in Fig. 26.2. This result implies that GLUT-1 is responsible for transporting these glycopeptides into the CNS, and indicates that glycosylation might be a promising way to deliver into the brain drugs with CNS activity but low permeability across the BBB.

Transport of peptides across the BBB

There are many biologically active peptides in the CNS, so it is important to develop delivery systems for neuropharmaceutical peptides across the BBB. Since peptides are in general relatively large, hydrophilic and unstable, efficient permeation into the brain cannot be expected unless a specific delivery strategy is employed. Such strategies for peptides have been well documented and reviewed (Pardridge, 1991; 1995a,b; Banks *et al.*, 1992; Terasaki and Tsuji, 1994, 1995; Bodor and Prokai, 1995; Zlokovic, 1995; Bergley, 1996; Tamai and Tsuji, 1996). One approach is a physiologically based strategy involving the use of carrier-mediated transport mechanisms for relatively small di- or tripeptides, and adsorptive-mediated endocytosis (AME) or receptor-mediated endocytosis (RME) for larger peptides. Another approach is the pharmacologically based strategy of converting water-soluble peptides into lipid-soluble ones.

The physiologically based strategy to manipulate large peptides to enhance their permeation into the brain involves the synthesis of chimeric peptides. These are formed by the covalent attachment of a nonpermeant but pharmacologically effective peptide to an appropriate vector that can drive transport across the BBB. Pardridge (1991) proposed a novel strategy for the delivery of chimeric peptides through the BBB. First, the chimeric peptide is transported into brain endothelial cytoplasm by AME or RME. Secondly, the intact chimeric peptide is transferred into the brain interstitial space by absorptive-mediated or receptor-mediated exocytosis. Thirdly, the linkage between the vector and the pharmacologically active peptide is cleaved. Finally, the released peptide exerts its pharmacological effect in the CNS. Cationized albumin and histone as targets of AME, and monoclonal antibodies with specific affinity to receptors present at the luminal surface of the BCECs, such as transferrin receptor and insulin receptor, are potential candidates as delivery vehicles.

Examples of delivery of peptides into the brain by means of the above-mentioned strategies are described below.

a) Carrier-mediated transport of peptides.

Some transport systems for small peptides have been suggested to exist at the BBB (Banks *et al.*, 1992; Bergley, 1996). Enkephalins were demonstrated to be taken up efficiently into the brain, and the involvement of a saturable mechanism for the transport of leucine enkephalin was shown by the *in situ* vascular brain perfusion technique. Several other peptides, thyrotropin releasing hormone, arginine–vasopressin, Peptide-T, alpha-melanocyte stimulating hormone, luteinizing hormone-releasing hormone, delta sleep-inducing peptide and interleukin 1, have been shown to cross the BBB and some of them showed saturable uptake, suggesting participation of carrier-mediated transport. The peptide transport mechanisms involved are classified as peptide transport systems PTS-1 to -5 (Banks *et al.*, 1992; Bergley, 1996). When the transport of the reduced form of glutathione across the BBB was examined by using the BUI method, the uptake of ^{35}S-labeled GSH was saturable with a K_m value of 5.8 mM and the surprisingly high maximal extraction of 30%

(Kannan *et al.*, 1990). From the study of functional expression in *Xenopus laevis* oocytes of RNA obtained from bovine brain capillary, a presence of a sodium dependent GSH transporter, which is distinct from the rat canalicular GSH transporter or γ-glutamyl transpeptidase, was demonstrated as the novel BBB GSH transporter (Kannan *et al.*, 1996).

Whether these peptide transporters existing at the BBB can be useful for the specific brain delivery of small peptides or peptide-mimetic drugs remains to be fully investigated.

b) Adsorptive-mediated endocytosis

Utilization of the transcytosis mechanism for enhancement of the brain delivery of peptides seems promising because of its applicability to a wide range of peptides, including synthetic ones. Adsorptive-mediated endocytosis (AME) is triggered by an electrostatic interaction between a positively charged moiety of the peptide and a negatively charged plasma membrane surface region. Lower affinity and higher capacity of AME compared with that of receptor-mediated endocytosis (RME) should be favorable for delivery of peptides to the brain (Pardridge, 1991, 1995*a,b*; Tamai and Tsuji, 1996; Tamai *et al.*, 1997).

Several studies have been done on AME of neuropharmaceutical peptides that have the characteristics of stability to enzymes and cationic charge as a consequence of suitable chemical modifications of the native peptides. Ebiratide, a synthetic peptide analogous to adrenocorticotropic hormone, that is used to treat Alzheimer's disease, is positively charged with an isoelectric point of 10 and its resistance to metabolism has been enhanced by chemical modifications of the constituent natural amino acids. The internalization of [^{125}I]ebiratide was saturable in primary cultures of bovine BCECs. Furthermore, the characteristics of its internalization were consistent with AME in various respects, including energy-dependence and the inhibitory effects of polycationic peptides and endocytosis inhibitors (Terasaki *et al.*, 1992; Terasaki and Tsuji, 1995; Tamai and Tsuji, 1996). Similar AME has been demonstrated for E-2078, an analogue of dynorphin (Cornford, 1985; Pardridge, 1991, 1995*a,b*; Banks *et al.*, 1992; Terasaki

and Tsuji, 1994, 1995; Bodor and Prokai, 1995), which has a high affinity for opioid receptor and has an analgesic activity after systemic administration (Terasaki *et al.*, 1989; Terasaki and Tsuji, 1995; Tamai and Tsuji, 1996).

c) Receptor-mediated endocytosis.

Transferrin receptor is present at relatively high concentration on the vascular endothelium of the brain capillaries. The OX-26 antibody, which is a mouse IgG2a monoclonal antibody to rat transferrin receptor, binds to an extracellular epitope on the transferrin receptor that is distinct from the transferrin ligand binding site, so binding of the OX-26 monoclonal antibody to the receptor does not interfere with transferrin binding. By using the capillary depletion technique to estimate the extent of transport into brain parenchyma, it was established that the OX-26 monoclonal antibody is transported across the BBB and is effective as a drug delivery vehicle (Pardridge, 1991, 1995*b*). Saito et al. (1995) used OX-26 monoclonal antibody to enhance the BBB permeation of β-amyloid peptide, A β which binds to preexisting amyloid plaques in Alzheimer's disease. Since the dementia in Alzheimer's disease is correlated with amyloid deposition in the brain, the peptide could be useful for the diagnostic assay of Alzheimer's disease, if it can be delivered to the brain.

The utilization of insulin receptor existing at the BBB is also effective. As shown in Fig. 26.3, after mice received an i.v. injection of horseradish peroxidase (HRP, M_r 40 000) conjugated with insulin, the HRP activity in the brain was significantly higher than that after HRP injection (Fukuta *et al.*, 1994). A fragment of insulin obtained by trypsin digestion showed high insulin receptor binding activity and scarcely any hypoglycemic activity in mice, suggesting that this fragment may be useful as a carrier to transport therapeutic peptides across the BBB via RME.

d) Lipid-mediated delivery of chemically designed peptides

Another promising approach to the delivery of peptides to the brain is to increase the lipophilicity

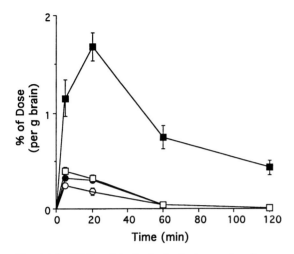

Fig. 26.3. HRP activity in the brain (squares) and blood (circles) of mice after i.v. administration of HRP (230 μg) and INS-HRP (213 μg: closed symbols), respectively. HRP activity in blood represents the results obtained in 5.76 μl of blood.

Conclusion

Recent advances in studies on the BBB transport of xenobiotics, as well as of nutrients and neuroactive agents, have led to a change in our concept of the BBB. It is no longer regarded as a static lipoidal membrane barrier of endothelial cells that have tight junctions without fenestrations. The BBB is now considered to be a dynamic interface that has physiological functions of specific and selective membrane transport from blood to brain and active efflux from brain to blood for many compounds, as well as degradative enzymatic activities. From the viewpoint of drug delivery, designing drugs (including peptides) with greater lipophilicity to enhance the BBB permeability seems to be an easy approach. However, such a strategy would not only increase the permeation into tissues other than brain, but also decrease the bioavailability due to the hepatic first-pass metabolism in the case of oral administration. Accordingly, for the development of brain-specific drug delivery systems for neuroactive drugs, it may be most effective to utilize the specific transport mechanisms at the BBB. Designing drugs that mimic the substrates to be taken up by particular transporters or receptors existing at the BBB appears to have great promise. Further studies on the various structural requirements of specific transport or receptor systems of the BBB and peripheral tissues could help to provide a more rational basis for brain-specific drug delivery.

by introducing a lipid-soluble moiety (Border and Prokai, 1995). To enhance the permeability of hydrophilic leucine enkephalin (log $P = 0.60$), the carboxyl terminal was esterified with 1-adamantanol, producing a lipophilicity increase to log P of 2.12. This derivative showed analgesic activity *in vivo* (Tsuzuki *et al.*, 1991). So-called packaged enkephalin is also a lipophilic derivative of enkephalin. It has a peptidase-cleavable L-alanyl spacer, and is expected to be cleaved to the active form in the brain (Bodor and Prokai, 1995).

References

Banks, W. A., Audus, K. and Davis, T. P. (1992). Permeability of the blood–brain barrier to peptides: an approach to the development of therapeutically useful analogs. *Peptides*, **13**, 1289–94.

Bergley, D. J. (1996). The blood–brain barrier: principles for targeting peptides and drugs to the central nervous system. *J. Pharm. Pharmacol.*, **48**, 136–46.

Bodor, N. and Prokai, L. (1995). Molecular packaging, peptide delivery to the central nervous system by sequential metabolism. In *Peptide-Based Drug Design* ed. M. D. Taylor and G. L. Amidon, pp. 317–16.

Cordon-Cardo, C., O'Brien, J. P., Casals *et al.* (1989). Multidrug-resistance gene (P-glycoprotein) is expressed by endothelial cells at blood–brain barrier sites. *Proc. Natl. Acad. Sci. USA*, **86**, 695–8.

Cornford, E. M. (1985). The blood–brain barrier, a dynamic regulatory interface. *Mol. Physiol.*, **7**, 219–60.

Cornfold, E. M., Bocash, W. D., Braun, L. D. *et al.* (1979). Rapid distribution of tryptophol (3-indole ethanol) to the brain and other tissues. *J. Clin. Invest.*, 63, 1241–8.

Fukuta, M., Okada, H., Iinuma, S. *et al.* (1994). Insulin fragments as a carrier for peptide delivery across the blood–brain barrier. *Pharm. Res.*, **11**, 1681–8.

Garcia, C. K., Li, X., Luna, J. and Francket, U. (1994). cDNA cloning of the human monocarboxylate transporter 1 and chromosomal localization of the SLC16A1 locus to 1p13. 2-p12. *Genomics*, 23, 500–3.

Gerhart, D. Z., Enerson, B. E., Zhdankina, O. Y. *et al.* (1997). Expression of moncarboxylate transporter MCT1 by brain endothelium and glia in adult and suckling rats. *Am. J. Physiol.*, **273**, E207–13.

Joo, F. (1996). Endothelial cells of the brain and other organ systems: some similarities and differences. *Prog. Neurobiol.*, **48**, 255–73.

Kang, Y. S., Terasaki, T., Ohnishi, T. and Tsuji, A. (1990). In vivo and in vitro evidence for a common carrier-mediated transport of choline and basic drugs through the blood–brain barrier. *J. Pharmacobio-Dyn.*, **13**, 353–60.

Kannan, R., Kuhlenkamp, J. F., Jeandidier, E. *et al.* (1990). Evidence for carrier-mediated transport of glutathione across the blood–brain barrier in the rat. *J. Clin. Invest.*, **85**, 2009–13.

Kannan, R., Yi, J. R., Tang, D. *et al.* (1996). Evidence for the existence of a sodium-dependent glutathione (GSH) transporter. Expression of bovine brain capillary mRNA and size fractions in *Xenopus laevis* oocytes and dissociation from gamma-glutamyltranspeptidase and facilitative GSH transporters. *J. Biol. Chem.*, **271**, 9754–8.

Komura, J., Tamai, I., Senmaru, M. *et al.* (1996). Sodium and cloride ion-dependent transport of β-alanine across the blood–brain barrier. *J. Neurochem.*, **67**, 330–5.

Levin, V. A. (1980). Relationship of octanol/water partition coefficient and molecular weight to rat brain capillary permeability. *J. Med. Chem.*, **23**, 682–4.

Ohnishi, T., Tamai, I., Sakanaka, K. *et al.* (1995). In vivo and in vitro evidence for ATP-dependency of P-glycoprotein-mediated efflux of doxorubicin at the blood–brain barrier. *Biochem. Pharmacol.*, **49**, 1541–4.

Pardridge, W. M. (1991). *Peptide Drug Delivery to the Brain*. New York: Raven Press.

Pardridge, W. M. (1995a). Transport of small molecules through the blood–brain barrier: biology and methodology. *Adv. Drug Delivery Rev.*, **15**, 5–36.

Pardridge, W. M. (1995b). Blood–brain barrier peptide transport and peptide drug delivery to the brain. In *Peptide-Based Drug Design*, ed. by M. D. Taylor and G. L. Amidon, pp. 265–96.

Polt, B., Porreca, F., Szabo, L. Z. *et al.* (1994). Glycopeptide enkephalin analogues produce analgesia in mice: Evidence for penetration of the blood–brain barrier. *Proc. Natl. Acad. Sci. USA*, **91**, 7114–18.

Saheki, A., Terasaki, T., Tamai, I. and Tsuji, A. (1994). In vivo and in vitro blood–brain barrier transport of 3-hydroxy-3-methylglutaryl coenzyme A (HMG-CoA) reductase inhibitors. *Pharm. Res.*, **11**, 305–11.

Saito, Y., Buciak, J., Yang, J. and Pardridge, W. M. (1995). Vector-mediated delivery of ^{125}I-labeled beta-amyloid peptide A-beta1–40 through the blood–brain barrier and binding to Alzheimer disease amyloid of the A-beta1–40/vector complex. *Proc. Natl. Acad. Sci. USA*, **92**, 10227–31.

Sakata, A., Tamai, I., Kawazu, K. *et al.* (1994). In vivo evidence for ATP-dependent and P-glycoprotein-mediated transport of cyclosporin A at the blood–brain barrier. *Biochem. Pharmacol.*, **48**, 1989–92.

Schinkel, A. H., Smit, J. J. M., van Tellingen, O. *et al.* (1994). Disruption of the mouse mdr1a P-glycoprotein gene leads to a deficiency in the blood–brain barrier and to increased sensitivity to drugs. *Cell*, **77**, 491–502.

Takanaga, H., Tamai, I., Inaba, S. *et al.* (1995). cDNA cloning and functional characterization of rat intestinal monocarboxylate transporter. *Biochem. Biophys. Res. Commun.*, **217**, 370–7.

Tamai, I. and Safa, A. R. (1990). Competitive interaction of cyclosporins with the Vinca alkaloid-binding site of P-glycoprotein in multidrug resistant cells. *J. Biol. Chem.*, **265**, 16509–13.

Tamai, I. and Tsuji, A. (1996). Drug delivery through the blood–brain barrier. *Adv. Drug Deliv. Rev.*, **19**, 401–24.

Tamai, I., Senmaru, M., Terasaki T. and Tsuji, A. (1995). Na$^+$ and Cl$^-$-dependent transport of taurine at the blood–brain barrier. *Biochem. Pharmacol.*, **50**, 1783–93.

Tamai, I., Sai, Y., Kobayashi, H. *et al.* (1997). Structure-internalization relationship for adsorptive-mediated endocytosis of basic peptides at the blood–brain barrier. *J. Pharmacol. Exp. Ther.*, **280**, 410–15.

Tatsuta, T., Naito, M., Oh-hara, K. *et al.* (1992). Functional involvement of P-glycoprotein in blood–brain barrier. *J. Biol. Chem.*, **267**, 20383–91.

Terasaki, T. and Tsuji, A. (1994). Drug delivery to the brain utilizing blood–brain barrier transport systems. *J. Controll. Rel.*, **29**, 163–9.

Terasaki, T. and Tsuji, A. (1995). Oligopeptide drug delivery to the brain, importance of absorptive-mediated endocytosis and P-glycoprotein associated active efflux transport at the blood–brain barrier. In *Peptide-Based Drug Design*, ed. by M. D. Taylor and G. L. Amidon, pp. 297–316.

Terasaki, T., Hirai, K., Sato, H. *et al.* (1989). Absorptive-mediated endocytosis of a dynorphin-like analgesic peptide, E-2078, into the blood–brain barrier. *J. Pharmacol. Exp. Ther.*, **251**, 351–7.

Terasaki, T., Takakuwa, S., Moritani, S. and Tsuji, A. (1991). Transport of monocarboxylic acids at the blood–brain barrier: studies with monolayers of primary cultured bovine brain capillary endothelial cells. *J. Pharmacol. Exp. Ther.*, **258**, 932–7.

Terasaki, T., Takakuwa, S., Saheki, A. *et al.* (1992). Absorptive-mediated endocytosis of an adrenocorticotropic hormone (ACTH) analogue, ebiratide, into the blood–brain barrier: Studies with monolayers of primary cultured bovine brain capillary endothelial cells. *Pharm. Res.*, **9**, 529–34.

Thiebaut, F., Tsuruo, T., Hamada, H. *et al.* (1989). Immunohistochemical localization in normal tissues of different epitopes in the multidrug transport protein P170: evidence for localization in brain capillaries and crossreactivity of one antibody with a muscle protein. *J. Histochem. Cytochem.*, **37**, 159–64.

Tsuji, A. and Tamai, I. (1997). Blood–brain barrier function of P-glycoprotein. *Adv. Drug Deliv. Rev.*, **25**, 287–98.

Tsuji, A. and Tamai, I. (1996). Carrier-mediated intestinal transport of drugs. *Pharm. Res.*, **13**, 963–77.

Tsuji, A., Terasaki, T., Takabatake, Y., *et al.* (1992). P-Glycoprotein as the drug efflux pump in primary cultured brain capillary endothelial cells. *Life Sci.*, **51**, 1427–37.

Tsuji, A., Saheki, A., Tamai, I. and Terasaki, T. (1993*a*). Transport mechanism of 3-hydroxy-3-methylglutaryl coenzyme A reductase inhibitors at the blood–brain barrier. *J. Pharmacol. Exp. Ther.*, **267**, 1085–90.

Tsuji, A., Tamai, I., Sakata, A. *et al.* (1993*b*). Restricted transport of cyclosporin A across the blood–brain barrier by a multidrug transporter, P-glycoprotein. *Biochem. Pharmacol.*, 46, 1096–9.

Tsuzuki, N., Hama, T., Hibi, T. *et al.* (1991). Adamantanes as a brain-directed drug carrier for poorly absorbed drug: antinociceptive effects of [D-ala²]leu-enkephalin derivatives conjugated with the 1-adamantane moiety. *Biochem. Pharmacol.*, **41**, R5–8.

Wang, Q., Yang, H., Miller, D. W. and Elmquist, W. F. (1995). Effect of the P-glycoprotein inhibitor, cyclosporin A, on the distribution of rhodamine-123 to the brain: an in vivo microdialysis study in freely moving rats. *Biochem. Biophys. Res. Commun.*, **211**, 719–26.

Yamazaki, M., Terasaki, T., Yoshioka, K. *et al.* (1994*a*). Mepyramine uptake into bovine brain capillary endothelial cells in primary monolayer cultures. *Pharm. Res.*, **11**, 975–8.

Yamazaki, M., Terasaki, T., Yoshioka, K., *et al.* (1994*b*). Carrier-mediated transport of H_1-antagonist at the blood–brain barrier: a common transport system of H_1-antagonists and lipophilic basic drugs. *Pharm. Res.*, **11**, 1516–18.

Zlokovic, B. V. (1995). Cerebrovascular permeability to peptides: Manipulations of transport systems at the blood–brain barrier. *Pharm. Res.*, **12**, 1395–406.

PART III

General aspects of CNS transport

27 The blood–CSF barrier and the choroid plexus

MALCOLM SEGAL

- Introduction
- Methods of study
- Mechanism of CSF secretion
- The role of the choroid plexus
- References

Introduction

The environment of the neurons, the brain interstitial fluid (ISF), is protected from fluctuations in the composition of the blood by two barriers. The first and largest interface is that of the blood–brain barrier (BBB) located at the cell walls and the tight junctions between the cells of the cerebral endothelium, i.e. 'tight' capillaries. The second is a composite barrier, the blood–cerebrospinal fluid barrier (BCSFB) and is made up of the choroid plexuses, the arachnoid membrane and the circumventricular organs. These tissues have fenestrated 'leaky' capillaries and their barrier function is provided by the tight junctions between the cells of their modified ependymal layer (Davson and Segal, 1996).

The choroid plexuses (CP) are located in the two lateral ventricles and the third ventricle with a further CP in the fourth ventricle as a single sheet of tissue that forms the roof of this cavity. The external covering (CSF side) of these structures is modified ependymal cells that closely resemble a transporting epithelium such as found in the nephron. The cell walls on the CSF or apical side of these cells are covered with microvilli, which greatly expands the surface area at the interface between the cytoplasm and CSF (Fig. 27.1). The

cells of the CP are joined together by an occluding band of tight junctions (TJs) close to the CSF side of the cells. These junctions are made up of multiple strands yet are slightly more permeable than those of the BBB (Møllgård et al., 1976; Meller, 1985). The TJs do permit the flow of water and some salts between the cells – the paracellular pathway – yet restrict the passage of small molecules such as mannitol (Fig. 27.2). The cell walls of the baso-lateral sides of CP cells are highly convoluted, which also greatly expands the surface area between the cytoplasm and the extracellular fluid (ECF) of the CP, and have a different repertoire of ion channels and pumps compared to the apical (CSF) side. The large CPs of the lateral ventricles are leaflike in structure and float in the ventricular CSF. Inside these tissues there is a complex, mainly venular, capillary network which being fenestrated is highly permeable and supplies the blood gases and nutrients needed to support the active secretion of CSF and the transport process between blood and CSF.

Methods of study

The study of the mechanism of secretion of CSF has presented a variety of technical problems since

251

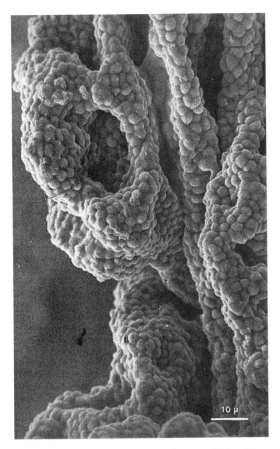

Fig. 27.1. A scanning electron micrograph showing the surface features of the choroid plexus of the cat. The figure clearly illustrates the convoluted structure of the CSF side of this tissue. (Clementi and Marini, 1972.)

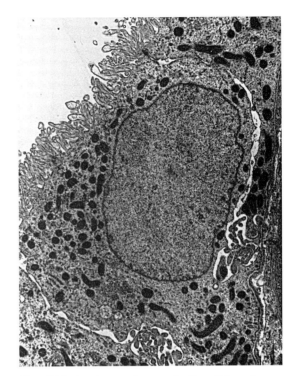

Fig. 27.2. An electonmicrograph of a cell from the rabbit choroid plexus. On the upper left is the cerebrospinal fluid, and on this side of the cell there are prominent microvilli with a tight junction between the cells. The cell cytoplasm contains many mitochondria. On the basal (blood) side of the cell and the lateral intercellular spaces there are prominent interdigitations between the cells. The space between the cells is larger than normal as the secretion of CSF was inhibited in this animal by ouabain in the CSF (Segal and Burgess, 1974).

these tissues are buried deep within the brain and are extremely delicate due to the lack of connective tissue in the CNS. The earliest attempt to measure the rate of CSF secretion was to place a catheter in the spinal sac and allow the fluid to drain until a steady-state was reached. This technique upsets the normal pressure relations within the ventricular system and has to use a negative pressure to maintain flow, so is now considered to be a poor method for the measurement of the rate of CSF secretion (Riser, 1929). In 1950 Leusen developed the technique of ventriculo-cisternal perfusion (VC) by placing needle catheters in the lateral ventricle and in the cisterna magna then perfusing the ventricular system with a mock CSF. If a large molecular weight dye, such as Blue Dextran, is included in the perfusate, the dilution of this marker can be used to measure the steady-state secretion rate of CSF (Davson and Segal, 1970). This method has been used extensively by many workers in the field to study the rate of CSF secretion in species from rat to cattle and even including man (Davson and Segal, 1996). As can be seen from Table 27.1 the rate of secretion expressed as a fraction of the CSF volume is remarkably constant and suggests a common mechanism of secretion across the species. The VC technique is usually performed in anaesthetized animals but the pioneering work of Pappenheimer *et al.* (1962) in the conscious goat has revealed that anaesthesia does not depress CSF secretion to any marked degree. The technique of VC perfusion has also been used to study the entry from blood

Table 27.1. *Concentrations of various solutes (mEq/kg H$_2$O) in cerebrospinal fluid and plasma of the rabbit, and distribution ratios*

Substance	Plasma	CSF	R_{CSF}	R_{Dial}
Na	148.0	149.0	1.005	0.945
K	4.3	2.19	0.675	0.96
Mg	2.02	1.74	0.92	0.80
Ca	5.60	2.47	0.45	0.65
Cl	106.0	130.0	1.23	1.04
HCO^3	25.0	22.0	0.92	1.04
Glucose	8.3	5.35	0.64	0.97
Amino acids	2.84	0.89	0.31	—
Urea	8.35	6.5	0.78	1.00
Osmolality	298.5	305.2	1.02	0.995
pH	7.46	7.27	—	—

From Davson and Segal (1996).

R_{CSF}=Concn in CSF/Concn in plasma and

R_{Dial}=Concn in dialysate/Concn in plasma.

into CSF of a wide range of endogenous molecules such as ions, sugars, amino acids, thyroid hormones, peptides, etc. but this *in vivo* method will also include an added component of entry across the blood–brain barrier into the brain ISF, which will then drain into the CSF. In addition this method is ideal for the study of the uptake of molecules from ventricular CSF into the brain and blood. (Davson *et al.*, 1982). To eliminate the added route of entry across the BBB and to study the nature of newly formed CSF, a number of other techniques have been used. One of the earliest was that of Ames *et al.* (1964), who exposed the choroid plexus *in situ* and filled the ventricle with oil (Fig. 27.3). The droplets of nascent CSF formed on the surface of the CP were collected under the oil (which was heavier than water), with a fine pipette for micro-analysis. Welch (1963) used a similar technique with the added measurement of CP blood flow by injecting oil drops into the blood and recording their rate of exit from a catheter in the choroidal venous drainage; this gave further proof that the CP was forming CSF since the haematocrit of this venous blood had increased its ratio by 1:15. Later methods included the encapsulation of the choroid plexus within a tiny chamber and the collection of nascent CSF over a

longer period of time (Miner and Reed, 1972) (Fig. 27.3). An alternative technique has been to mount the single-sided choroid plexus of the fourth ventricle in a miniature Ussing chamber *in vitro*. This was described in a series of elegant experiments by Wright (1970) using the large plexus of the American bull frog and has also been used in the cat by Welch and Araki (1975). However although these *in vitro* techniques are ideal for the study of the basic transport mechanisms, the lack of a vascular flow within the tissue can lead to data that are not seen by methods which retain vascular flow (Deane and Segal, 1985). To achieve a situation close to that *in vivo*, Pollay *et al.* (1972) developed the *in situ* isolated perfused choroid plexus of the sheep, which secretes CSF at close to a normal rate but is completely isolated from any entry across the BBB. This method has been modified to include both choroid plexuses and has been used extensively to study the entry of sugars, amino acids and thyroid hormones and recently to study the entry of nucleosides into the choroid plexus (Redžić *et al.*, 1996).

Since the choroid plexus is very thin it can be incubated *in vitro* so remaining viable for several hours and this method has been used by Johanson and his group to study both uptake and efflux from the CP (Johanson *et al.*, 1990). While much useful information has been derived from the *in vitro* technique, the lack of a vascular flow within the cells can lead to accumulation of molecules such as sugars and amino acids within the plexus so that tissue/medium (T/M) ratios of much greater than 1 are found. *In vivo* the vascular flow maintains a steep concentration gradient across the ependymal layer into the blood so T/M ratios of much greater than 1 are not usually found; in fact if the blood flow through the perfused CP is reduced the T/M ratio is raised, which confirms the importance of blood flow to the normal transport processes across these tissues (Deane and Segal, 1979).

Recently the ultimate in reductionist techniques, the patch clamp, has been applied to the apical membrane of the choroid plexus and these studies support the transport of chloride as the principle ion during the secretion of CSF (Garner and Brown, 1992).

Finally there have been recent reports of a cultured choroid plexus model. Earlier attempts at

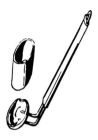

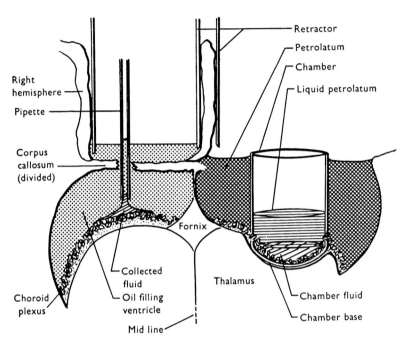

Fig. 27.3. A section through the lateral ventricles of the cat. On the left of the main figure is shown the choroid plexus covered with oil and the method of collection of nascent CSF. On the right is shown the chamber method that was used to enclose the choroid plexus. The upper figure shows the actual form of the chamber. (From Miner and Reed, 1972, with permission.)

this technique were bedevilled by the difficulty of obtaining a pure cell line of CP ependymal cells. This has now been achieved and it appears that these cultured mono-layers may secrete CSF, which will permit the confirmation of whether sodium or chloride is the principle transportation ion responsible for the secretion of CSF (Gath *et al.*, 1996).

Mechanism of CSF secretion

Using the above techniques both *in vitro* and *in vivo*, the secretion of CSF has been shown to be an energy-dependent process. The first clear studies were those of Hugh Davson, when he carefully analysed CSF and plasma sampled at the same time and compared the CSF/plasma ratio of the ions in these fluids to that of dialysate and revealed that there were small but significant differences between these two sets of values (Davson and Segal, 1996). These studies elegantly demonstrated that CSF was a secretion and not an ultrafiltrate, which was the view at this time. The work was based on the fact that the measured CSF/plasma ratios for electrolytes could not be produced by passive ultrafiltration (the dialysate ratio) given the

Table 27.2. *Rates of secretion of CSF by various species estimated by ventriculo-cisternal perfusion*

Species	μl/min	Rate (% per min)	μl/min.mgCP^{-1}
Mouse	0.325	0.89	—
Rat	2.1–5.4	0.72–1.89	—
Guinea-pig	3.5	0.875	—
Rabbit	10.0	0.43	0.43
Cat	20.0–22.0	0.45–0.50	0.50–0.55
Dog	47.0–66.0	0.40	0.625–0.77
Goat	164.0	0.65	0.36
Sheep	118.0	0.83	—
Monkey	28.6–41.0	—	—
Man	350.0–370.0	0.38	—

From Davson and Segal (1996).

magnitude of available pressures within the vascular system (Table 27.2). These finding were an amazing feat of careful chemical analysis since at that time gravimetric techniques were mostly used and the analysis of each ion took over a week!

By the use of the VC technique, often combined with a stepped intravenous infusion, the plasma level of isotopes such as Na$^+$, K$^+$, etc. can be kept constant and the effect of inhibitors of transport studied both on the rate of CSF secretion and on the entry of ions such as Na$^+$ into the VC perfusate (Davson and Segal, 1970). From such studies it was shown that whenever an inhibitor reduced the secretion of CSF a parallel inhibition of sodium entry into CSF also occurred. Acetazoleamide (Diamox), the carbonic anhydrase inhibitor, was shown to cause a 70% reduction in CSF secretion as was DNP (Pollay and Davson, 1963). Ouabain, the Na/K ATPase inhibitor, also caused a similar reduction in CSF secretion and ouabain-binding studies demonstrated that this enzyme was preferentially located to the apical or CSF side of the cell (Quinton *et al.*, 1973). Later studies have shown that in fact there are three ATPases in the choroid plexus by their sensitivity to Na$^+$/K$^+$, Mg^{2+} and HCO$_3^-$, which suggests the active transport of the four ions by this tissue (Miwa *et al.*, 1980). Using the isolated CP *in vitro* Johanson *et al.* (1990) have shown that the loop diuretics frusemide and bumetanide inhibited sodium and chloride uptake by the CP from the CSF side, which

confirmed Davson and Segal (1970) earlier studies showing an inhibition of CSF secretion with frusemide and with amiloride from the blood side *in vivo*. Studies with the stilbene anion inhibitors DIDS and SITS also affected Cl$^-$/HCO$_3^-$ exchange, which also reduced the CSF secretion (Johanson *et al.*, 1985, Deng and Johanson, 1989).

Patch clamp studies have thrown some further light on the channels present in the CP apical membrane and have identified two K$^+$ channels and two Cl$^-$ channels on the CSF side, which may play a key role in the secretory processes and may be 5HT activated (Garner and Brown, 1992; Garner *et al.*, 1993; Kotera and Brown, 1994; Watson *et al.*, 1995). A composite model derived from the findings of the above groups is shown in Fig. 27.4.

Further studies are now necessary to revisit the mechanism of secretion of CSF comparing the data from the *in vitro* culture model with that of the perfused sheep choroid plexus with an intact vascular system and taking into consideration the findings of all the different techniques.

In absorptive epithelia the process of osmotic coupling between salt and water appears to occur in the lateral spaces between the cells (Tormey and Diamond, 1967). In secretory epithelia a major problem is to identify the site where the transport of an ion is coupled to the osmotic movement of water, since morphologically these epithelia have the same structure as those that absorb fluid (Segal

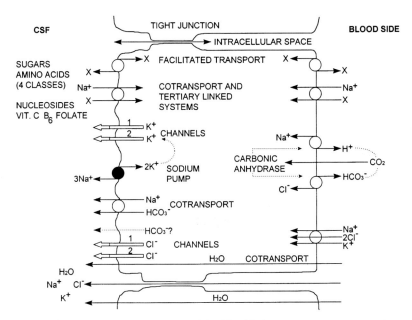

Fig. 27.4. A diagram showing some of the identified transport process occurring across the choroid plexus. The upper part of the figure shows the mechanisms for non-electrolyte transport with both facilitated, co-transport and tertiary transport mechanisms very similar to those found in the nephron. The lower part of the diagram shows the location of the sodium pump and the various ion channels and co-transport mechanisms identified at present.

and Burgess, 1974; Segal and Pollay, 1977). A further problem is that no inhibitor has been found that inhibits CSF secretion by more than 70% *in vivo* and this has led to the suggestion that 10–20% of CSF is being formed by the BBB. Direct evidence for the secretion of brain ECF by the BBB has been hard to obtain since the high resistance offered by the endothelial tight junction of the cerebral capillaries would make such a secretion very small and difficult to measure and its presence has only been deduced from other studies (Curl and Pollay, 1968; Cserr *et al.*, 1981).

The role of the choroid plexus

While the secretion of CSF is the prime role of the CPs these tissues can transport many molecules and ions between blood and CSF, which may be of importance in brain homeostasis or may simply be a reflection of the processes found in all such epithelial like cells and of little functional value. This lack of function can be exemplified by glucose, where it was shown using the isolated incu-bated CP that it accumulates glucose by a Na^+ dependent process which leads to a high T/M ratio. Since bulk phase CSF has 50% of the glucose concentration of plasma, these findings led to the suggestion that the low concentration of glucose in the CSF was produced by an efflux process across the CP of this non-electrolyte out of CSF. However when studies were made on the kinetics of glucose transport from blood to CSF and CSF to blood using the isolated perfused CP, it was revealed that there was always a net entry of glucose from blood to CSF and that the low concentration of glucose in CSF was a consequence of the low rate of entry kinetics from blood to CSF and not on the efflux processes (Deane and Segal, 1985). From these findings it would appear that the efflux of glucose by the CP is of little functional significance. Similarly it has been argued by Spector (1989) that the deoxyribonucleoside thymidine cannot cross the BBB and gains entry to the brain via the CP/CSF route. The lack of BBB transport for thymidine was derived from rapid single pass studies, but when this study was repeated using a modified Zlokovic technique over a longer time course clear evidence of a carrier-mediated transport across the BBB was obtained (Thomas and Segal, (1996); Zlokovic *et al.*, 1986).

In contrast to these findings, when the transport of amino acids was investigated using perfused CP, four carrier types were identified, for large and small neutral, and for basic and acidic amino acids. These carriers were stereospecific with little cross-competition between the types and again there was a net entry of these molecules from blood to CSF (Preston *et al.*, 1989, Preston and Segal, 1992). However, when the level of glycine was increased in CSF an efflux mechanism from CSF was revealed, which caused the net transport to reverse and the transport now occurred from CSF to blood (Preston and Segal, 1990). In this case the CP transport could be of functional significance and aid the 'sink action' of CSF, so contributing to the brain homeostasis for these molecules, some of which have neurotransmitter activity (Davson and Segal, 1996).

The CSF shows a remarkable stability in its ionic composition in the face of wide fluctuations of the plasma values for these ions. This property is a complex of the low permeability of the BBB and the ability of the CP and glia to control the composition of both the CSF and brain ISF. Studies by Bradbury and Davson (1965) showed that when the ventricular system was perfused with both low and high K$^+$ mock CSF, the emerging fluid had been controlled to a value close to that of normal CSF.

Of considerable recent interest have been the findings of Schreiber and his group, who demonstrated that the choroid plexuses can synthesize and secrete transthyretin (TTR), the thyroid hormone transporting protein, into the CSF. In fact this ability of the CP predates that of the liver in evolution, so would appear to be of functional significance (Schreiber *et al.*, 1990, 1993). Studies with the perfused choroid plexus have shown that triodothyronine (T$_3$) and thyroxine (T$_4$) are transported across the CP and it could be that the secretion of TTR explains why T$_4$ crosses from blood into CSF more rapidly than T$_3$ although the latter is a more lipid-soluble molecule than T$_4$ (Hagen and Solberg, 1974; Preston and Segal, 1992).

The CP will also transport many peptides such as delta sleep inducing peptide DSIP (Zlokovic *et al.*, 1988) and vasopressin (Zlokovic *et al.*, 1991) with receptor types for such peptides demonstrated in this tissue *in vivo*. Studies have also shown that a variety of organic bases and acids are removed from the CSF as well as neurogenic amines such as 5HT, etc., all of these process may aid the 'sink action' of the CSF in brain homeostasis; see Davson and Segal (1996) for a review of these processes. Of course such *in vivo* studies include interaction across the blood–brain barrier so it is more reasonable to assume that the BBB and BCSFB work in parallel. From these findings the choroid plexuses not only secrete CSF but appear to have a wide spectrum of transport processes both into and out of CSF, which may play a key role in brain homeostasis.

References

Ames, A., Sakanoue, M. and Endo, S. (1964). Na, K, Ca, Mg, and Cl concentrations in choroid plexus fluid and cisternal fluid compared with plasma ultrafiltrate. *J. Neurophysiol.*, **27**, 672–81.

Bradbury, M. W. B. and Davson, H. (1965). The transport of potassium between blood, cerebrospinal fluid and brain. *J. Physiol.*, **181**, 151–74.

Clementi, F. and Marini, D. (1972). The surface fine structure of the walls of cerebral ventricles and of choroid plexus in the cat. *Z. Zellforsch. Mikroskop. Anat.*, **123**, 82–95.

Cserr, H. F., Cooper, D. N., Suri, P. K. and Patlak, C. S. (1981). Efflux of radiolabeled polyethylene glycols and albumin from rat brain. *Am. J. Physiol.*, **240**, F319–F328.

Curl, F. D. and Pollay, M. (1968). Transport of water and electrolytes between brain and ventricular fluid in the rabbit. *Exp. Neurol.*, **20**, 558–74.

Davson, H. and Segal, M. B. (1970). The effects of some inhibitors and accelerators of sodium transport on the turnover of ^{22}Na in the cerebrospinal fluid and the brain. *J. Physiol.*, **209**, 131–53.

Davson, H. and Segal, M. B. (1996). *Physiology of The CSF and Blood–Brain Barriers*. Boca Raton: CRC Press.

Davson, H., Hollingsworth, J. G., Carey, M. B. and Fenstermacher, J. (1982). Ventriculo-cisternal perfusion of twelve amino acids in the rabbit. *J. Neurobiol.*, **13**, 282–318.

Deane, R. and Segal, M. B. (1979). The effect of vascular perfusion of the choroid plexus on the secretion of cerebrospinal fluid. *J. Physiol.*, **293**, 18–19P.

Deane, R. and Segal, M. B. (1985). The transport of sugars across the perfused choroid plexus of the sheep. *J. Physiol.* **362**, 245–60.

Deng, Q. S. and Johanson, C. E. (1989). Stilbenes inhibit exchange of chloride between blood, choroid plexus and cerebrospinal fluid. *Brain Res.*, **501**, 183–7.

Garner, C. and Brown, P. D. (1992). Two types of chloride channel in the apical membrane of rat choroid plexus epithelial cells. *Brain Res.*, **591**, 137–45.

Garner, C., Feniuk, W. and Brown, P. D. (1993). Serotonin activates Cl⁻ channels in the apical membrane of rat choroid plexus epithelial cells. *Eur. J. Pharmacol.*, **239**, 31–7.

Gath, U., Hakvoort, A., Hellwig, S. and Glalla H.-J. (1996). The blood–CSF barrier *in vitro*. In *Biology of the Blood–Brain Barrier: Transport, Cellular Interactions and Brain Pathologies*, ed. P. O. Conrad and D. Scherman. New York: Plenum.

Hagen, G. A. and Solberg, L. A. (1974). Brain and cerebrospinal fluid permeability to intravenous thyroid hormones. *Endocrinology.*, **95**, 1398–410.

Johanson, C. E., Parandoosh, Z. and Smith, Q. R. (1985). Cl⁻-HCO₃⁻ exchange in choroid plexus: analysis by the DMO method for cell pH. *Am. J. Physiol.*, **249**, F478–F484.

Johanson, C. E., Sweeney, S. M., Parmelee, J. T. and Epstein, M. H. (1990). Cotransport of sodium and chloride by the adult mammalian choroid plexus. *Am. J. Physiol.*, **258**, C211–C216.

Kotera, T. and Brown, P. D. (1994). Evidence for two types of potassium current in rat choroid plexus epithelial cells. *Pflügers Archiv. – Eur. J. Physiol.*, **427**, 317–24.

Leusen, I. (1950). The influence of calcium, potassium and magnesium ions in cerebrospinal fluid on vasomotor system. *J. Physiol.*, **110**, 319–29.

Meller, K. (1985). Ultrastructural aspects of the choroid plexus epithelium as revealed by the rapid-freezing and deep-etching techniques. *Cell Tiss. Res.*, **239**, 189–201.

Miner, L. and Reed, D. J. (1972). Composition of fluid obtained from choroid plexus tissue isolated in a chamber *in situ*. *J. Physiol.*, **227**, 127–39.

Miwa, S., Inagaki, C., Fujiwara, M. and Takaori, S. (1980). Na⁺, K⁺, Mg²⁺ and HCO₃⁻-adenosine triphosphatases in the rabbit brain choroid plexus. *Jap. J. Pharmacol.*, **30**, 337–45.

Møllgård, K., Malinowska, D. H. and Saunders, N. R. (1976). Lack of correlation between tight junction morphology and permeability properties in developing choroid plexus. *Nature*, **264**, 292–4.

Pappenheimer, J. R., Heisey, S. R., Jordan, E. F. and Downer, J. de C. (1962). Perfusion of the cerebral ventricular system in unanesthetized goats. *Am. J. Physiol.*, **203**, 763–74.

Pollay, M. and Davson, H. (1963). The passage of certain substances out of the cerebrospinal fluid. *Brain*, **86**, 137–50.

Pollay, M., Stevens, A., Estrada, E. and Kaplan, R. (1972). Extracorporeal perfusion of choroid plexus. *J. Appl. Physiol.*, **32**, 612–17.

Preston, J. E. and Segal, M. B. (1990). The steady-state amino acid fluxes across the perfused choroid plexus of the sheep. *Brain Res.*, **525**, 275–9.

Preston, J. E. and Segal, M. B. (1992). Saturable uptake of [¹²⁵I]L-triiothyronine at the basolateral (blood) and apical (cerebrospinal fluid) sides of the isolated perfused sheep choroid plexus. *Brain Res.*, **592**, 84–90.

Preston, J. E., Segal, M. B., Walley, G. J. and Zlokovic, B. V. (1989). Neutral amino acid uptake by the isolated perfused sheep choroid plexus. *J. Physiol.*, **408**, 31–43.

Quinton, P. M., Wright, E. M. and Tormey J. Mc. D. (1973). Localization of sodium pumps in the choroid plexus epithelium. *J. Cell Biol.*, **58**, 724–30.

Redžić, Z. B., Segal, M. B., Marković, I. V. *et al.* (1997). The characteristics of basolateral nucleoside transport in the perfused sheep choroid plexus and the effect of NO inhibition on these processes. *Brain Res.*, in press.

Riser, P. (1929). *Le Liquide Céphalo-Rachidien.* Paris: Masson.

Schreiber, G., Aldred, A. R., Jaworowski, A. *et al.* (1990). Thyroxine transport from blood to brain via transthyretin synthesis in choroid plexus. *Am. J. Physiol.*, **258**, R338–R345.

Schreiber, G., Pettersson, T. M., Southwell, B. R. *et al.* (1993). Transthyretin expression evolved more recently in liver than in brain. *Comp. Biochem. Physiol.*, **105B**, 317–25.

Segal, M. B. and Burgess, A. M. C. (1974). A combined physiological and morphological study of the secretory process in the rabbit choroid plexus. *J. Cell Sci.*, **14**, 339–50.

Segal, M. B. and Pollay, M. (1977). The secretion of cerebrospinal fluid. *Exp. Eye Res.*, Suppl. **25**, 127–48.

Spector, R. (1989). Micronutrient homeostasis in mammalian brain and cerebrospinal fluid. *J. Neurochem.*, **53**, 1667–74.

Thomas, S. A. and Segal, M. B. (1996). Identification of a saturable uptake system for deoxyribonucleosides at the blood–brain and blood–cerebrospinal fluid barriers. *Brain Res.*, **741**, 230–9.

Tormey, J. McD. and Diamond, J. M. (1967). The ultrastructural route of fluid transport in rabbit gall bladder. *J. Gen. Physiol.*, **50**, 2031–60.

Watson, J. A., Elliot, A. C. and Brown, P. D. (1995). Seretonin elevates intracellular Ca²⁺ in rat choroid plexus epithelial cells acting on 5-HT₂C receptors. *Cell Calcium*, **17**, 120–8.

Welch, K. (1963). Secretion of cerebrospinal fluid by choroid plexus of the rabbit. *Am. J. Physiol.*, **205**, 617–24.

Welch, K. and Araki, H. (1975). Features of the choroid plexus of the cat, studied *in vitro*. In *Fluid Environment of the Brain*, ed. H. F. Cserr, J. D. Fenstermacher and V. Fencl, pp. 157–65. New York: Academic Press.

Wright, E. M. (1970). Ion transport across the frog posterior choroid plexus. *Brain Res.*, **23**, 302–4.

Zlokovic, B. V., Begley, D. J., Djuricic, B. M. and Mitrovic, D. M. (1986). Measurement of solute transport across the blood–brain barrier in the perfused guinea-pig: method and application of N-methyl-α-aminoisobutyric acid. *J. Neurochem.*, **46**, 1444–51.

Zlokovic, B. V., Segal, M. B., Davson, H. and Jankov, R. M. (1988). Delta sleep-inducing peptide (DSIP) across the blood–cerebrospinal fluid barrier. *Peptides*, **9**, 533–8.

Zlokovic, B. V., Segal, M. B., McComb, J. G. *et al.* (1991). Kinetics of circulating vasopressin uptake by choroid plexus. *Am. J. Physiol.*, **260**, F216–F224.

28 Arachnoid membrane, subarachnoid CSF and pia–glia

CONRAD E. JOHANSON

- Introduction
- Background
- Anatomic considerations
- Functions of leptomeningeal cells
- Subarachnoid space and cerebrospinal fluid dynamics
- CSF homeostasis: permeability and transport functions of the arachnoid membrane
- Expression of proteins in the arachnoid membrane
- Volume transmission of secreted substances
- Involvement of meninges and choroid plexus in CNS volume/pressure regulation?
- Volume and pockets of subarachnoid CSF
- Involvement of meninges and CSF in infections and immunologic responses
- Meningeal drug metabolism and detoxification
- Leptomeningeal cultures for studying arachnoidal functions
- Opportunities/needs for future research on the leptomeninges and subarachnoid space

Introduction

Well-ordered neuronal activity requires regulated extracellular milieu. To provide such micro-environmental stability for neurons, the blood–brain and blood–CSF barriers work together to maintain extracellular fluid. Blood–CSF barrier is comprised not only of choroid plexus but also of arachnoid membrane. Choroid and arachnoid cells are intimately associated with ventricular and subarachnoid CSF, respectively, in anatomically 'interior' and 'exterior' aspects of the brain. Thus, CSF in the ventricles and subarachnoid space contributes substantially to the volume and hydrodynamics of CNS extracellular fluid (Johanson, 1995).

Subarachnoidal CSF, together with the arachnoid and pia mater that enclose it (Fig. 28.1), have been analyzed less than the ventricular CSF with its surrounding choroidal/ependymal cells (Johan-

son, 1988). However, there has been a recent upswing in interest in the subarachnoid space and its encompassing leptomeninges. Secretion, transport and convective distribution of solutes and water (fluid) throughout the subarachnoid CSF system impacts CNS pharmacokinetics (Bacher *et al.*, 1994), the spread of infections, neuroimmunologic phenomena, edema resolution (Groger *et al.*, 1994), bleedings, and metastases/chemotherapy. Bulk flow of substances in subarachnoid CSF also contributes to modulation of brain development.

The paucity of literature reviews on functional aspects of subarachnoid CSF and leptomeninges reflects limited research in this area. Therefore, the aims of this chapter are: to summarize knowledge of arachnoid and pial membranes; to relate functions in the subarachnoid CSF system to those in the ventricles; and to identify 'knowledge gaps' that need to be filled.

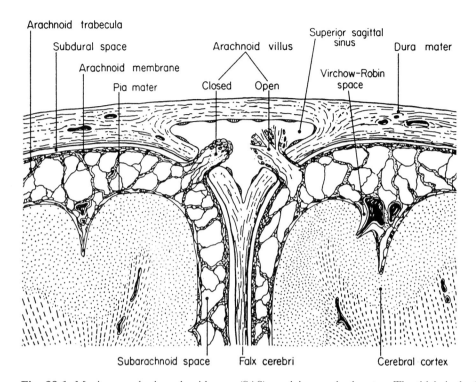

Fig. 28.1. Meninges and subarachnoid space (SAS) overlying cerebral cortex. The thick, inelastic dura covers the leptomeninges (arachnoid membrane and pia mater). In mammals, the very thin subdural space is not part of the CSF system. Arachnoid and pia are supported by a trabecular framework that criss-crosses SAS and produces a 'latticework' through which CSF percolates. Subarachnoid space contains CSF, received from the 4th ventricle. SAS also receives interstitial (CSF-like) fluid from the underlying cortex, because the pia mater is permeable and thus permits exchange of water and solutes across its pia–glial membranes. Perivascular spaces (otherwise known as Virchow–Robin) exist where veins or arteries penetrate cortical tissue (Broadwell and Sofroniew, 1993); each such entry site is sealed by a reflection of pia that ends as a blind cul-de-sac (Greenberg *et al.*, 1994). Arachnoid villi represent the most distal part of the SAS CSF system. Each villus, a fist-like evagination of arachnoid into dura, is covered by endothelium lining the venous sinus. Arachnoid villi function like one-way valves, closing when CSF pressure becomes less than central venous pressure, to prevent blood regurgitation into CSF. Larger, more complex versions of arachnoid villi called Pacchionian granulations are not present in humans until a year or more after birth. Drawing from Rapoport (1976) reproduced with permission of S. Rapoport and Raven Press.

Background

The arachnoid membrane, 'sandwiched' between pia and dura maters (Fig. 28.1), has long 'struggled' for its anatomical and functional identity. Up to the Renaissance, 'arachnoid' referred to inner eye parts. Oribasius used *arachnid* for the ciliary process, the tissue that secretes aqueous humor like the choroid plexus elaborates CSF. In 1665, however, the Amsterdam Anatomic Society coined the term *arachnoidea cerebri* for the soft outer layer of

brain; at the same time, the term *arachnoidea oculis* was abandoned. 'Pia mater' was introduced by Galen in 1127; in his Arabic translation, 'pia' (devoted) connoted a soft tissue protecting and nourishing the brain as a mother would her child (Bakay, 1991).

Arachnoid has not always been viewed separately from pia mater; in the Middle Ages, they were not distinguished. Resembling a spider (arachnid) web, the arachnoid was eventually delineated by the 17th century. Thus, the arachnoid membrane stretched over gyri, but unlike pia mater, did not dip into sulci. By 1850, it was still not appreciated that CSF was present between the two membranes. Even today, knowledge of arachnoid and pia mater lags that of choroid plexus and blood–brain barrier (Johanson, 1988).

Anatomic considerations

Together, the arachnoid membrane and underlying pia mater are known as the leptomeninges, or *thin membranes*. Derived from ectoderm, the arachnoid is multilayered, about a dozen cells thick. Two or three layers are distinctive leptomeningeal (LM) cells: large in size, having plentiful mitochondria, and containing long, interdigitating pseudopodia. Innermost layers of arachnoid contain cells that are loosely associated by gap junctions and desmosomes (Nabeshima *et al.*, 1975). Outer layers, close to the dura, are fastened by tight junctions between arachnoid cells; this 'tight barrier' effectively isolates subarachnoid CSF from overlying dural circulation (Balin *et al.*, 1986). This is the blood–CSF barrier in the arachnoid, a common feature among vertebrates, even in those that have a glial rather than an endothelial blood–brain barrier (Brightman and Tao-Cheng, 1993).

On the other hand, subarachnoid CSF communicates freely with underlying brain interstitial fluid, due to discontinuous gap junctions between LM cells in pia mater. As the inner lining of subarachnoid space (SAS), the pia has a layer or two of LM cells set upon a subpial layer of astrocytes. A basement membrane separates pial cells from subjacent glia. This permeable pial–glial membrane blankets most of the external surface of brain and spinal cord.

Functions of leptomeningeal cells

Capabilities of arachnoidal and pial cells include: (i) structural support and protection of CNS, (ii) production of extracellular matrix, (iii) CSF flow regulation, (iv) secretion of proteins for modulating brain function and development, (v) immunologic and phagocytic activity, (vi) drug-metabolizing and detoxifying enzymatic activity,

and (vii) synthesis and secretion of factors and cytokines capable of promoting or attenuating brain tumors and other pathologic disorders.

Subarachnoid space and cerebrospinal fluid dynamics

Is subarachnoid space a site for extrachoroidal formation of CSF? SAS surrounding brain and spinal cord lacks choroid plexus tissue. However, this does not necessarily preclude formation of CSF, or a CSF-like fluid, in SAS. Earlier investigators considered that major blood vessels coursing through the SAS were sites for fluid formation, based on extravasation of dyes into CSF. Yet, it is difficult to see mechanistically how arteries or veins could contribute to fluid production within SAS.

Another site implicated in fluid elaboration is the arachnoid, for which blood flow data are needed. Tissues that form fluid at a relatively high rate, e.g. choroid plexus, have a brisk blood flow. Choroidal flows of 4–5 ml/min/g have been established for adult mammals (Faraci *et al.*, 1988; Williams *et al.*, 1991; Szmydynger-Chodobska *et al.*, 1994). Ample vascularization of amphibian arachnoid led Perez-Gomez *et al.* (1976) to advocate a role for the arachnoid in frog CSF dynamics. Further information for blood flow in mammalian arachnoid would help to evaluate its potential for 'turning over' fluid into subarachnoid cavities.

Pial cells on the 'floor' of the SAS are histologically analogous to ependymal cells lining the ventricles. Ultrastructural analysis of organelle profiles does not suggest that pia and ependyma are likely sites of vigorous CSF formation. Moreover, gap junctions present between adjacent pial, and ependymal, cells can be permeated by large molecules. Thus, there is adequate permeability in the pia–glial membrane to allow bulk flow of interstitial fluid (secreted by capillary endothelium of blood–brain barrier) from brain interstitium into the subarachnoid compartment. However, this bulk flow of 0.2 µl/min/g brain (Cserr and Knopf, 1992), driven by a gradient of hydrostatic pressure, is about a thousand-fold less than the rate of generation of CSF by choroid plexus. Experimental perfusion of spinal SAS, which could theoretically detect significant contributions from arachnoid as well as pia–glial cells, found negligible fluid forming capacity (Lux and Fenstermacher, 1975). Thus, fluid accretion into SAS is normally much slower than fluid generation by choroid tissues within the ventricles.

When normal hydrodynamic balance obtains, CSF 'downstream' drains across arachnoid villi at the same rate as it is formed 'upstream' in the ventriculo-subarachnoid spaces. Such CSF clearance from brain by bulk flow is dependent upon a positive hydrostatic pressure gradient between CSF and cerebral venous blood. Arachnoid villi represent a pivotal site in CSF flow. Subarachnoid hemorrhages (Butler, 1989) lead to trapping of erythrocytes and blood clots in the villi, which can interfere with CSF drainage and lead to fluid retention or hydrocephalus. There are new insights that an excess, in CNS, of growth factors like TGFbeta and bFGF causes fibrosis near the arachnoid cells in the villi, which increases resistance to outflow; this causes a backing-up of CSF with resulting ventriculomegaly (Mittler *et al.*, 1996). Collagen content of arachnoid villi (like choroid plexus) is high, and this can interfere with IR spectroscopic analyses (Jackson *et al.*, 1995)

CSF is also reabsorbed from SAS in specific regions of spinal cord. In the meningeal 'angle region', the multilayered arachnoid membrane is only 3–4 cells thick with gap junctions between LM cells; in this region, cytoplasmic fenestrations, intercellular discontinuities and vesiculations promote direct communication of SAS with cisterns of the arachnoid reticular layer. Cationized ferritin marker injected into the rat SAS passed through the arachnoid to reach blood vessels and lymphatics in the dura mater; the ferritin also moved in the other direction, i.e. across pial cell layers for eventual reabsorption by pial vessels (Zenker *et al.*, 1994). Thus, there are multiple CSF reabsorption sites in mammalian cord and brain.

CSF homeostasis: permeability and transport functions of the arachnoid membrane

The marked impermeability in most areas of the arachnoid is in contrast to the more permeable pia–glial membrane. Arachnoid cells in middle and outer layers are joined by extensive tight junctions, as revealed by electron microscopy (Dermietzel, 1975). Whereas choroid plexus is composed of a single layer of epithelia linked by tight junctions, the arachnoid generally has 12–15 layers of flattened epithelia. Bullfrog arachnoid, mounted in an Ussing-type chamber, has an electrical resistance of about 2000 ohm cm^2, comparable to very tight epithelia like urinary bladder. Thus, plasma ion fluctuations are not readily transmitted to SAS CSF, because permeability coefficients for Cl^-, K^+ and Na^+ are relatively low, i.e. about 10-fold smaller in arachnoid than in choroid plexus. A steady-state transmembrane potential difference of up to 45 mV, CSF positive to plasma, can be maintained; this is consistent with the arachnoid's high electrical resistance. Such membrane tightness promotes CSF homeostasis by preventing leakage (back diffusion) of actively transported substances.

Mitochondrial abundance, occurring in arachnoid cells as well as in choroid plexus epithelium and cerebral endothelium (Bradbury, 1979), is the hallmark of cells busily engaged in reabsorption and secretion. Amino acid concentrations in SAS CSF as well as ventricular CSF are held at levels well below those in plasma. Secondary active transporters in epithelial membranes of the barriers remove amino acids from CSF. Leucine and glycine are examples of amino acids concentrated by arachnoid tissue, or transported across it, from CSF to blood (Wright *et al.*, 1971; O'Tuama *et al.*, 1973; Wright, 1974). There is active transport of Na^+ (Johanson and Murphy, 1992), Cl^- (Johanson *et al.*, 1992), ascorbate, vitamins B and other micronutrients (Spector and Ells, 1984) across plexus, as part of CSF homeostatic mechanisms (Spector and Johanson, 1989); evidence for similar reabsorptive and secretory transporters in arachnoid needs to be sought. Nevertheless, the available evidence indicates that leptomeningeal and choroidal epithelia work integratively with blood–brain barrier to insure a stable and specialized extracellular environment for neurons.

Expression of proteins in the arachnoid membrane

Arachnoidal synthesis and secretion of proteins into SAS is an important area of developmental neurobiology, and it probably has a bearing on CNS repair mechanisms following injury. Certain proteins are expressed in choroid plexus epithelium and in arachnoid cells. Thus, mRNA for Beta-trace protein or prostaglandin D synthase (Blodorn *et al.*, 1996), as well as for protein phosphatase 1 and phosphatase inhibitor 1 (Sakagami *et al.*, 1994), has been localized to both the plexus and leptomeninges. Beta-trace protein is secreted into CSF. Retinoic acid and IGF-II (with its binding protein) are also secreted by choroid plexus and arachnoid cells (Ocrant *et al.*, 1992; Ishikawa *et al.*, 1995; Yamamoto *et al.*, 1996). Retinoic acid and IGF-II are important modulators of brain growth and development. A dual source of secretion of proteins and growth factors, i.e. by choroidal and arachnoidal tissues, supplies the interior (ventricles) and exterior (SAS) of the brain with these trophic molecules during ontogeny and for repair. These and other molecules can be distributed throughout brain by diffusion (Ohata and Marmarou, 1992) and by volume transmission or convective transport (see below).

Volume transmission of secreted substances

Upon secretion into CSF, by arachnoid or choroidal epithelium, a protein or other 'informational substance' can be conveyed by bulk flow to a distant target cell, e.g. neuron. CSF sweeps down the cranial neuraxis, driven by the pressure head of the choroid plexus generation of fluid, carrying with it entrained molecules. This convective flow of proteins and peptides is an endocrine-like process, but involves the 'third circulation' (Milhorat, 1987), i.e. CSF flow, rather than the vascular system (Fig. 28.3). Bulk flow is a much faster mode of distribution of materials, compared to diffusion, especially when macromolecules are involved. Thus, the CSF can be used as a transportation system to move signal molecules, protease inhibitors (Palm *et al.*, 1995) or trophic factors through CNS.

Choroid plexus is a 'hotbed' of growth factor synthesis and secretion, and it likely contributes to repair of injured brain (Knuckey *et al.*, 1996). Retinoic acid, secreted by 4th ventricle plexus, promotes neurite outgrowth and development of

cerebellum (Yamamoto *et al.*, 1996). In view of the growing interest in recovery processes following CNS trauma and ischemia, arachnoid expression and secretion is an area deserving more research attention (Bidmon and Stumpf, 1992; Ikegaki *et al.*, 1994; Kiningham *et al.*, 1995).

Involvement of meninges and choroid plexus in CNS volume/pressure regulation?

Neuropeptides such as angiotensin II (Ang II), arginine vasopressin (AVP) and atrial natriuretic peptide (ANP) are part of a neuroendocrine system, involving barrier tissues, that can regulate CSF dynamics (Faraci *et al.*, 1988; Chodobski *et al.*, 1994; 1995). These three peptides are synthesized in CNS (hypothalamus and choroid plexus) and have receptors in meninges, choroid plexus and the cerebral capillary wall. Neuropeptide receptor density and K_D are altered in response to changes in CSF pressure and volume; for example, K_D values for ANP in the meninges are increased after spaceflight (Herbute *et al.*, 1994). Barrier tissues involved in neuroendocrine control, like the arachnoid and plexus, may be both a source and a target (Fig. 28.3) for Ang II, AVP and ANP transported by CSF volume transmission (Nilsson *et al.*, 1992).

Volume and pockets of subarachnoid CSF

Because pia tightly hugs the contour of nervous tissue, while the arachnoid membrane forms bridges over the sulci of the brain and cord, quite large pockets of CSF are established between the leptomeninges. Where the bridging over the gaps is substantial, large cisterns are formed, particularly at the base of the brain. Consequently, the volume of subarachnoid fluid is much greater than the CSF in the four ventricles combined. Thus, over 80% of human CSF is in SAS, while less than 20% is in ventricles. Although regional brain volumes change with age, the central and subarachnoid CSF volumes do not (DeCarli *et al.*, 1992), except in rare cases (Prassopoulos *et al.*, 1995).

263

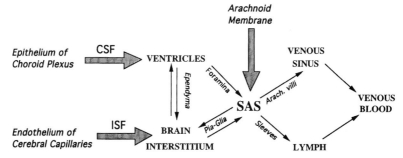

Fig. 28.2. Centrality of the subarachnoid space (SAS) in CNS extracellular fluid dynamics. Most of the large-cavity CSF in humans, about 80%, is contained within the subarachnoid system. CSF, or CSF-like fluid, in the SAS is derived from several sources, mainly from the upstream ventricular choroid plexuses (Johanson, 1989), but also from the arachnoid membrane (the other component of the blood–CSF barrier) and cerebral endothelium (blood–brain barrier). An important interface between the ventricular and subarachnoid spaces are the foramina or small openings in the walls of the 4th ventricle. CSF is cleared from the SAS to venous blood by bulk flow mechanisms, at two major drainage sites: the arachnoid villi valves in the cranial dural venous sinuses, and along sleeves of subarachnoid space surrounding nerves (e.g. olfactory nerve to the nasal mucosa). Of immunological significance is the fact that some of the draining CSF contacts lymph glands prior to reaching venous blood.

VOLUME TRANSMISSION INVOLVING CSF AND SURROUNDING TISSUES

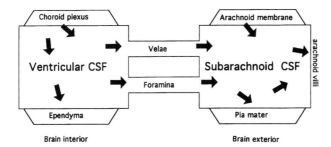

Fig. 28.3. The medium that enables volume transmission (VT) is the extracellular fluid or CSF (Johanson, 1993). Ventricular and subarachnoid CSF are the two major compartments of CSF, and they are contiguous via foramina in the 4th ventricle (Luschka and Magendie) and by velum pathways in the 3rd and 4th ventricles. Choroid plexus-secreted molecules are distributed through the ventricles, making contact with, and perhaps moving across, the ependyma; molecules gaining access to brain tissue can move by bulk flow through narrow channels in the interstitium. Not depicted is the reverse pathway, i.e. release of a substance in the ependymal wall (e.g. serotonin) with subsequent convection to 5-HT receptors in choroid plexus (Hartig, 1989). An alternate pathway for choroidal secretions is from large-cavity ventricular CSF to the velar SAS in 3rd or 4th ventricles, a distribution that can occur in several minutes (Ghersi-Egea *et al.*,1996). Arachnoid-secreted substances distribute through SAS CSF, and can interact with the underlying pia. Except in pathologic states, the general flow of CSF is from ventricle to SAS, not in the reverse direction (as may occur in a retrograde CSF ventricular infection in meningitis). VT is the transport of a molecule in extracellular fluid over a distance of microns, or greater (Zoli and Agnati, 1996), thus VT is more like paracrine than autocrine transmission. Once a substance is in the CSF, the potential distance for transport by convection may be substantial, i.e. several mm or cm, thereby mimicking endocrine distribution. Ventricular CSF, via choroid plexus and ependyma, helps to modulate periventricular tissues (except circumventricular organs) and the interior of the brain, while SAS CSF furnishes substances (both choroidally- and arachnoidally-derived) to exterior regions of brain tissue.

Because subarachnoid CSF comprises a relatively large volume of extracellular fluid in CNS, it is worthwhile to pursue implications of these CSF cisterns or 'reservoirs' in the context of sequestration of drugs, vectors, lymphocytes, platelets (as sequelae of subarachnoid hemorrhage), and the displacement of CSF by blood. An example is a recent CT analysis of subarachnoid hemorrhage in various cisterns, with the finding that for predicting delayed ischemic deficits, the best correlation was obtained with a score formed by the sum of the individual cisternal grades for amount (volume) of subarachnoid blood (Forssell *et al.*, 1995).

Involvement of meninges and CSF in infections and immunologic responses

The blood–CSF barrier and CSF system have a substantial role in CNS infections and central immune responses. Choroid plexus is a 'port of entry' for many pathogens into brain (Levine, 1987). Microbes that invade the CSF system infect both the plexus and leptomeninges, sometimes differentially (Lagace-Simard *et al.*, 1982). Virus infection can lead to hydrocephalus (Wolinsky *et al.*, 1974). In hydrocephalic states, arachnoidal cells are less likely to slough into CSF than are choroid and ependymal cells (Wilkins and Odom, 1974). Some exfoliated cells, cellular debris and released proteins (antigens) drain from CSF into lymph glands (Fig. 28.2). Such lymphatic drainage pathways have immunologic implications for CNS.

Immune surveillance of CNS is mediated in part by convective flow pathways, which promote widespread distribution of lymphocytes and macrophages (Cserr and Knopf, 1992). In addition to CSF routes, bulk flow of extracellular fluid occurs along subependymal myelinated fibers (white matter) and along vessel walls (Virchow-Robin spaces) (Fig. 28.1). Antigen-presenting cells are present in choroid plexus (Nathanson and Chun, 1990), and probably also in arachnoid. Arachnoid cells may have antigen-presenting capabilities because they phagocytize foreign tissue and have IgG and complement receptors (Frank, 1995).

In early stages of experimental autoimmune encephalomyelitis (EAE), inflammatory cells initially appear in the SAS and infiltrate the subpial region (Shin *et al.*, 1995). In EAE, the leptomeninges constitutively express ICAM-1 and fibronectin. Regulation of immune function in CNS also involves expression of exoglycoproteins in leptomeningeal and choroidal tissues (Lakos *et al.*, 1994), and expression of class II MHC antigens in ependyma (Steiniger and van der Meide, 1988).

CNS tumor spread can be facilitated by CSF bulk flow. Mammary carcinoma cells injected into the cisterna magna of rats distribute over the entire CSF system, interior and exterior, in brain and spinal cord (Sagar and Price, 1995). The leptomeningeal metastases elicit immune response. Thus, these tumor cells are extensively infiltrated by macrophages and suppressor T cells. Intrathecal delivery of monoclonal antibodies to treat CNS malignancies has been more effective when dose regimens are targeted to tumor cells in CSF as compared to brain tissue (Papanasiassiou *et al.*, 1995).

Meningeal drug metabolism and detoxification

Several enzymes in hepatic drug metabolism are present in choroid plexus, arachnoid and pia. The enzymes are inducible and can act at these transport interfaces as enzymatic barriers to influx. The protective role of these enzymes in the blood–CSF barrier tissues has been reviewed by Ghersi-Egea *et al.* (1995).

There is widespread expression of metallothionein (MT), a metal-binding protein, in pia-arachnoid, ependyma and choroid plexus. MTs are low molecular weight, inducible proteins that protect against toxic insults, including heavy metals. Fetal brain (21 wk) shows no MT expression, but 35-wk-old fetal CNS begins to have MT (Suzuki *et al.*, 1994*a*). In aged human, MT immunostaining occurs in pia mater, ependyma and astrocytes (Suzuki *et al.*, 1994*b*). MT exists in isoforms I, II and III. MT-I mRNA signal is high in ependyma and plexus (Choudhuri *et al.*, 1995). In rats, polyclonal antibody against MT stains pia-arachnoid, ependyma and capillary endothelium

(Kiningham et al., 1995). Blaauwgeers and colleagues (1994) reviewed the abundant expression of MT in meninges and plexus/ependyma cells, and its role in supplying metals to neurons while protecting the latter against toxic ions.

Leptomeningeal cultures for studying arachnoidal functions

Initial development of in vitro pia arachnoid research was with organotypic cultures (Spatz et al., 1975; Hervonen et al., 1981). More recently, primary cultures of human leptomeningeal cells (LM) have been shown to grow in serum-free medium (Motohashi et al., 1994). Maintenance of LM cells in culture devoid of serum allows analysis of effects of growth factors, which may be associated with LM fibrosis seen in various CNS disorders, e.g. arachnoiditis. Cytokeratin, a specific marker for human arachnoid cells in vitro (Frank et al., 1983), is useful because its positive staining rules out fibroblasts (which lack cytokeratin).

Rutka and colleagues (1986) used three cell lines derived from normal human LM to demonstrate arachnoidal synthesis of several collagen subtypes presumably responsible for the 'fibrous' response of LM to infection, trauma and tumors. Similarities between meningiomas and arachnoid cells in culture suggest that the former derive from the latter. Meningiomas also release factors that promote growth of neurites (Matthiessen et al., 1991) and neuroblasts (Gensburger et al., 1986) in culture. A canine LM organ culture is being utilized for modeling cerebrovascular B-amyloidosis (Prior et al., 1996).

Opportunities/needs for future research on the leptomeninges and subarachnoid space

Molecular and immunocytochemical studies (Ikegaki et al., 1994) have revealed that arachnoid cells express many proteins synthesized also by choroid epithelia and ependyma. Similar patterns of expression point to comparable functions of these membranes. An important difference is the hydrodynamic capabilities: the plexus has a greater

capacity to form CSF, while some leptomeningeal cells are specialized to reabsorb CSF. Nevertheless, in terms of barrier exclusion (tight junctions), immunologic functions, drug metabolizing and detoxifying activities, secretion of proteins to promote brain development/repair, etc., the choroid/ependyma system shares much in common with the leptomeninges. Whereas the plexus serves the interior of the brain, the pia-arachnoid help to modulate function in the exterior portions of the CNS.

Developmental neurobiologists will likely have increasing interest in the arachnoid, now that it is understood that LM cells secrete growth factors, cytokines, and extracellular matrix proteins integral to the orderly flow of ontogenetic processes in brain. At the other end of the age spectrum, those investigating aging phenomena need to explore the functional significance of the 'cloudiness' of leptomeninges, as a consequence of connective tissue proliferation with advancing age. Similar degenerative changes occur in choroid plexus (Johanson, 1997), and may hamper the ability of the choroid plexus–CSF system to maintain 'sink action'.

Neurosurgeons, neurologists, and neuroimmunologists are continually concerned with intrathecal fluid instillations (Välfors et al., 1983), subarachnoid hemorrhage, leptomeningeal tumors, meningitis and autoimmune disorders. Increasing popularity with arachnoid cell and meningioma cultures, as well as implants (Kaplan et al., 1996) and transplants (Joseph et al., 1994; Franklin and Blakemore, 1995; Kyoshima et al., 1995) will almost certainly shed more light on the development and treatment of leptomeningeal tumors, and on the role of the meninges and subarachnoid CSF in various immune responses.

Finally, gene therapy approaches for a variety of CNS disorders may well be able to take advantage of unique properties of the meninges, plexus epithelium and ependyma. Studies with adenovirus vectors have demonstrated that transgene expression is particularly strong in ependymal cells (Akli et al., 1993; Betz et al., 1995). Moreover, in retrovirus investigations, it has been found that retroviral vectors survive in CSF, retain their infectivity, and effectively transduce tumor cells (Ram et al., 1994). Thus, in the treatment of certain brain cancers, and with ischemia problems (Betz *et al.*, 1995), the CSF and the cells that line its

cavities, show considerable promise as an access route for gene therapy.

References

Akli, S., Caillaud, C., Vigne, E. *et al.* (1993). Transfer of a foreign gene into the brain using adenovirus vectors. *Nature Genet.*, **3**, 224–8.

Bacher, J. D., Balis, F. M., McCully, C. L. and Godwin, K. S. (1994). Cerebral subarachnoid sampling of cerebrospinal fluid in the rhesus monkey. *Lab. Anim. Sci.*, **44**(2), 148–52.

Bakay, L. (1991). Discovery of the arachnoid membrane. *Surg. Neurol.*, **36**, 63–8.

Balin, B. J., Broadwell, R. D., Salcman, M. and El-Kalliny, M. (1986). Avenues for entry of peripherally administered protein to the central nervous system in mouse, rat, and squirrel monkey. *J. Comp. Neurol.*, **251**, 260–80.

Betz, A. L., Yang, G.-Y. and Davidson, B. L. (1995). Attenuation of stroke size in rats using an adenoviral vector to induce overexpression of interleukin-1 receptor antagonist in brain. *J. Cereb. Blood Flow Metab.*, **15**, 547–51.

Bidmon, H. J. and Stumpf, W. E. (1992). Choroid plexus, ependyma and arachnoidea express receptors for vitamin D: differences between 'seasonal' and 'non-seasonal' breeders. *Prog. Brain Res.*, **91**, 279–83.

Blaauwgeers, H. G., Sillevis Smitt, P. A., de Jong, J. M. and Troost, D. (1994). Localization of metallothionein in the mammalian central nervous system. *Biol. Signals*, **3**(4), 181–7.

Blodorn, B., Mader, M., Yoshihiro, U. *et al.* (1996). Choroid plexus: the major site of mRNA expression for the B-trace protein (prostaglandin D synthase) in human brain. *Neurosci. Lett.*, **209**(2), 117–20.

Bradbury, M. (1979). Energy-dependent transport at the barriers. In *The Concept of a Blood–Brain Barrier*, 465 pp., New York: John Wiley.

Brightman, M. W. and Tao-Cheng, J. H. (1993). Tight junctions of brain endothelium and epithelium. In *The Blood–Brain Barrier*, ed. W. M. Pardridge, pp. 165–80. New York: Raven Press.

Broadwell, R. D. and Sofroniew, M. V. (1993). Serum proteins bypass the blood–brain fluid barriers for extracellular entry to the central nervous system. *Exp. Neurol.*, **120**, 245–63.

Butler, A. B. (1989) Alteration of CSF Outflow in Experimental Acute Subarachnoid Hemorrhage. In *Outflow of Cerebrospinal Fluid*, ed. F. Gjerris, S. E. Borgesen, and P. S. Sorensen, pp. 69–75. Copenhagen: Munksgaard.

Chodobski, A., Szmydynger-Chodobska, J., Vannorsdall, M. D. *et al.* (1994). AT₁ receptor subtype mediates the inhibitory effect of central angiotensin II on cerebrospinal fluid formation in the rat. *Regulat. Peptides*, **53**(2), 123–9.

Chodobski, A., Szmydynger-Chodobska, J., Epstein, M. H. and Johanson, C. E. (1995). The role of angiotensin II in the regulation of blood flow to choroid plexuses and cerebrospinal fluid formation in the rat. *J. Cereb. Blood Flow Metab.*, **15**, 143–51.

Choudhuri, S., Kramer, K. K., Berman, N. E. *et al.* (1995). Constitutive expression of metallothionein genes in mouse brain. *Toxicol. Appl. Pharmacol.*, **131**, 144–54.

Cserr, H. F. and Knopf, P. M. (1992). Cervical lymphatics, the blood–brain barrier and the immunoreactivity of the brain: a new view. *Immunol. Today*, **13**, 507–12.

DeCarli, C., Maisog, J., Murphy, D. G. *et al.* (1992). Method for quantification of brain, ventricular, and subarachnoid CSF volumes from MR images. *J. Comput. Assist. Tomogr.*, **16**(2), 274–84.

Dermietzel, R. (1975). Junctions in the central nervous system of the cat. V. The junctional complex of the pia-arachnoid membrane. *Cell. Tissue Res.*, **164**, 309–29.

Faraci, F. M., Mayhan, W. G., Farrell, W. J. and Heistad, D. D. (1988). Humoral regulation of blood flow to choroid plexus: role of arginine vasopressin. *Circ. Res.*, **63**, 373–9.

Forssell, A., Larsson, C., Ronneberg, J. and Fodstad, H. (1995). CT assessment of subarachnoid haemorrhage. A comparison between different CT methods of grading subarachnoid haemorrhage. *Br. J. Neurosurg.*, **9**, 21–7.

Frank, E. (1995). HLA-DR expression on arachnoid cells. A role in the fibrotic inflammation surrounding nerve roots in spondylotic cervical myelopathy. *Spine*, **20**(19), 2093–6.

Frank, E. H., Burge, B. W., Liwnicz, B. H. *et al.* (1983). Cytokeratin provides a specific marker for human arachnoid cells grown in vitro. *Exp. Cell Res.*, **146**, 371–6.

Franklin, R. J. and Blakemore, W. F. (1995) Reconstruction of the glia limitans by sub-arachnoid transplantation of astrocyte-enriched cultures. *Microsc. Res. Tech.*, **32**, 295–301.

Gensburger, C., Labourdette, G. and Sensenbrenner, M. (1986). Influence of meningeal cells on the proliferation and maturation of rat neuroblasts in culture. *Exp. Brain Res.*, **63**, 321–30.

Ghersi-Egea, J. F., Leininger-Muller, B., Cecchelli, R. and Fenstermacher, J. D. (1995). Blood–brain interfaces: relevance to cerebral drug metabolism. *Toxicol. Lett.*, 82–3, 645–53.

Ghersi-Egea, J.-F., Finnegan, W., Chen, J.-L. and Fenstermacher, J. D. (1996). Rapid distribution of intraventricularly administered sucrose into cerebrospinal fluid cisterns via subarachnoid velae in rat. *Neuroscience*, **75**, 1271–88.

Greenberg, R. W., Lane, E. L., Cinnamon, J. *et al.* (1994). The cranial meninges: anatomic considerations. *Semin. Ultrasound, CT & MRI*, **15**(6), 454–65.

Groger, U., Huber, P. and Reulen, H. J. (1994). Formation and resolution of human peritumoral brain edema. *Acta Neurochir.* (Wien), **60**, 373–4.

Hartig, P. R. (1989) Serotonin 5-HT 1c receptors: What do they do? In *Serotonin Actions, Receptors, Pathophysiology*, ed. E. J. Mylecharane, J. A. Angus and I. S. de la Lande, pp 180–7. Macmillan Press.

267

Herbute, S., Oliver, J., Davet, J. *et al.* (1994). ANP binding sites are increased in choroid plexus of SLS-1 rats after 9 days of spaceflight. *Aviat., Space Environ. Med.*, **65**, 134–8.

Hervonen, H., Spatz, M., Bembry, J. and Murray, M. R. (1981). Studies related to the blood–brain barrier to monoamines and protein in pia-arachnoid cultures. *Brain Res.*, **210**, 449–54.

Ikegaki, N., Saito, N., Hashima, M. and Tanaka, C. (1994). Production of specific antibodies against GABA transporter subtypes (GAT1, GAT2, GAT3) and their application to immunocytochemistry. *Brain Res. Mol. Brain Res.* **26**(1–2), 47–54.

Ishikawa, K., Ohe, Y. and Tatemoto, K. (1995). Synthesis and secretion of insulin-like growth factor (IGF)-II and IGF binding protein-2 by cultivated brain meningeal cells. *Brain Res.*, **697**(1–2), 122–9.

Jackson, M., Choo, L. P., Watson, P. H. *et al.* (1995). Beware of connective tissue proteins: assignment and implications of collagen absorptions in infrared spectra of human tissues. *Biochim. Biophys. Acta*, **1270**(1), 1–6.

Johanson, C. E. (1988). The choroid plexus–arachnoid membrane–cerebrospinal fluid system. In *Neuromethods, Vol. 9: Neuronal Microenvironment-Electrolytes and Water Spaces*, ed. A. Boulton, G. Baker and W. Walz, pp. 33–104. Humana Press.

Johanson, C. E. (1989). Potential for pharmacologic manipulation of the blood–cerebrospinal fluid barrier. In *Implications of the Blood–Brain Barrier and Its Manipulation, Vol. 1: Basic Science Aspects*, ed. E. A. Neuwelt, pp. 223–60. New York: Plenum Press.

Johanson, C. E. (1993). Diffusion, bulk flow, and volume transmission of proteins and peptides within the brain. In *Tissue Barriers*, ed. K. L. Audus and T. R. Raub. pp. 467–86. New York: Plenum Press.

Johanson, C. E. (1995). Ventricles and Cerebrospinal Fluid. In *Neuroscience in Medicine*, ed. P. M. Conn, pp. 171–96. Philadelphia: J. B. Lippincott Co.

Johanson, C. E. (1997). The choroid plexus. In *Encyclopedia for Neuroscience*, Vol. I, ed. G. Adelman, pp. 236–9 (and on CD-ROM). Boston: Birkhauser.

Johanson, C. E. and Murphy, V. A. (1992). Acetazolamide and insulin alter choroid plexus epithelial cell [Na⁺], pH, and volume. *Am. J. Physiol.*, **258**, F1538–F1546.

Johanson, C. E., Palm, D. E., Dyas, M. L. and Knuckey, N. W. (1992). Microdialysis analysis of effects of loop diuretics and acetazolamide on chloride transport from blood to CSF. *Brain Res.*, **641**, 121–6.

Joseph, J. M., Goddard, M. B., Mills, J. *et al.* (1994). Transplantation of encapsulated bovine chromaffin cells in the sheep subarachnoid space: a preclinical study for the treatment of cancer pain. *Cell Transplant*, **3**(5), 355–64.

Kaplan, F. A., Krueger, P. M., Harvey, J. and Goddard, M. B. (1996) Peripheral xenogenic immunological response to encapsulated bovine adrenal chromaffin cells implanted within the sheep lumbar intrathecal space. *Transplantation*, **61**, 1215–21.

Kiningham, K., Bi, X. and Kasarskis, E. J. (1995). Neuronal localization of metallothioneins in rat and human spinal cord. *Neurochem. Int.* **27**(1), 105–9.

Knuckey, N. W., Finch, P., Palm, D. E. *et al.* (1996) Differential neuronal and astrocytic expression of transforming growth factor beta isoforms in rat hippocampus following transient forebrain ischemia. *Brain Res. Mol. Brain Res.*, **40**, 1–14.

Kyoshima, K., Matsuda, M. and Handa, J. (1995) Transplantation of basal forebrain cells of foetal rats into the subarachnoid space: improvement of disturbance of passive avoidance memory due to injury of nucleus basalis magnocellularis. *Acta Neurochir.* (Wien), **133**, 68–72.

Lagace-Simard, J., Descoteaux, J. and Lussier, G. (1982). Experimental pneumovirus infections 2. Hydrocephalus of hamsters and mice due to infection with human respiratory syncytial virus (RS). *Am. J. Pathol.*, **107**, 36–40.

Lakos, S. F., Thormodsson, F. R. and Grafstein, B. (1994). Immunolocalization of exoglycoproteins ('ependymins') in the goldfish brain. *Neurochem. Res.*, **19**(11), 1401–12.

Levine, S. (1987). Choroid plexus: target for systemic disease and pathway to the brain. *Lab. Invest.*, **56**, 231.

Lux, W. E. Jr and Fenstermacher, J. D. (1975). Cerebrospinal fluid formation in ventricles and spinal subarachnoid space of the rhesus monkey. *J. Neurosurg.*, **42**, 674–8.

Matthiessen, H. P., Schmalenbach, C. and Muller, H. W. (1991). Identification of meningeal cell released neurite promoting activities for embryonic hippocampal neurons. *J. Neurochem.*, **56**, 759–68.

Milhorat, T. H. (1987). *Cerebrospinal Fluid and the Brain Edemas*, pp. 1–161. Neuroscience Society of New York.

Mittler, M. A., Lebow, M. H., Stopa, E. G. *et al.* (1996). Ventriculomegaly after chronic infusion of FGF-2 into the lateral ventricles of adult rats. *Soc. Neurosci. Abstr.*, **22**, 1958.

Motohashi, O., Suzuki, M., Yanai, N. *et al.* (1994). Primary culture of human leptomeningeal cells in serum-free medium. *Neurosci. Lett.*, **165**, 122–4.

Nabeshima, S., Reese, T. S., Landis, D. M. D. and Brightman, M. W. (1975). Junctions in the meninges and marginal glia. *J. Comp. Neurol.*, **164**, 127–70.

Nathanson, J. A. and Chun, L. L. Y. (1990). Possible role of the choroid plexus in immunological communication between the brain and periphery. In *Pathophysiology of the Blood–Brain Barrier*. ed. B. B. Johansson, Ch. Owman and H. Widner, pp. 501–7. Elsevier Science Publishers.

Nilsson, C., Lindvall-Axelsson, M. and Owman, C. (1992). Neuroendocrine regulatory mechanisms in the choroid plexus-cerebrospinal fluid system. *Brain Res. Brain Res. Rev.* **17**, 109–38.

Ocrant, I., Fay, C. T. and Parmelee, J. T. (1990). Characterization of insulin-like growth factor binding proteins produced in the rat central nervous system. *Endocrinology*, **127**, 1260–7.

Ohata, K. and Marmarou, A. (1992). Clearance of brain edema and macromolecules through the cortical extracellular space. *J. Neurosurg.*, **77**(3), 387–96.

O'Tuama, L. A., Remler, M. P. and Nichols, H. N. (1973). Accumulation of radiolabelled neutral amino acids by canine dura-arachnoid. *Soc. Neurosci. Abstr., 3rd Ann. Meet.*, 374.

Palm, D., Knuckey, M. W., Primiano, M. J. *et al.* (1995). Cystatin C, a protease inhibitor, in degenerating rat hippocampal neurons following transient forebrain ischemia. *Brain Res.*, **691**, 1–8.

Papanasiassiou, V., Pizer, B. L. and Chandler, C. L. (1995). Pharmacokinetics and dose estimates following intrathecal administration of 131-monoclonal antibodies for the treatment of central nervous system malignancies. *Physics*, **31**(3), 541 -52.

Perez-Gomez, J., Bindslev, N., Orkand, P. M. and Wright, E. M. (1976). Electrical properties and structure of the frog arachnoid membrane. *J. Neurobiol.*, **7**, 259–70.

Prassopoulos, P., Cavouras, D., Golfinopoulos, S. and Nezi, M. (1995). The size of the intra- and extraventricular cerebrospinal fluid compartments in children with idiopathic benign widening of the frontal subarachnoid space. *Neuroradiology*, **37**(5), 418–21.

Prior, R., D'Urso, D., Frank, R. *et al.* (1996). Canine leptomeningeal organ culture: an new experimental model for cerebrovascular B-amyloidosis. *J. Neurosci. Meth.*, **68**(2), 143–8.

Ram, Z., Walbridge, S., Oshiro, E. M. *et al.* (1994) Intrathecal gene therapy for malignant leptomeningeal neoplasia. *Cancer Res.*, **54**(5), 2141–5.

Rapoport, S. I. (1976). *Blood–Brain Barrier in Physiology and Medicine*, pp. 1–316. New York: Raven Press.

Rutka, J. T., Giblin, J., Dougherty, D. V. *et al.* (1986). An ultrastructural and immunocytochemical analysis of leptomeningeal and meningioma cultures. *J. Neuropathol. Exp. Neurol.*, **45**, 285–303.

Sagar, S. M. and Price, K. J. (1995). An experimental model of leptomeningeal metastases employing rat mammary carcinoma cells. *J. Neurooncol.*, **23**(1), 15–21.

Sakagami, H., Ebina, K. and Kondo, H. (1994). Localization of phosphatase inhibitor-1 mRNA in the developing and adult rat brain in comparison with that of protein phosphatase-1 mRNAs. *Brain Res. Mol. Brain Res.*, **25**, 7–18.

Shin, T., Kojima, T., Tanuma, N. *et al.* (1995). The subarachnoid space as a site for precursor T cell proliferation and effector T cell selection in experimental autoimmune encephalomyelitis. *J. Neuroimmunol.*, **56**(2), 171–8.

Spatz, M., Rankawek, K., Murray, M. R. and Klatzo, I. (1975). Uptake of radiolabeled glucose analogues by organotypic pia arachnoid cultures. *Brain Res.*, **100**, 710–15.

Spector, R. and Ells, J. (1984). Deoxynucleoside and vitamin transport into the central nervous system. *Fed. Proc.*, **43**, 196–200.

Spector, R. and Johanson, C. E. (1989). The mammalian choroid plexus. *Sci. American*, **261**, 68–74.

Steiniger, B. and van der Meide, P. H. (1988). Rat ependyma and microglia cells express class II MHC antigens after intravenous infusion of recombinant gamma interferon. *J. Neuroimmunol.*, **19**, 111–18.

Suzuki, K., Nakajima, K., Otaki, N. and Kimura, M. (1994*a*) Metallothionein in developing human brain. *Biol. Signals*, **3**, 188–92.

Suzuki, K., Nakajima, K., Otaki, N. *et al.* (1994*b*). Localization of metallothionein in aged human brain. *Pathol. Internat.*, **44**, 20–6.

Szmydynger-Chodobska, J., Chodobski, A. and Johanson, C. E. (1994). Postnatal developmental changes in blood flow to choroid plexuses and cerebral cortex of the rat. *Am. J. Physiol.*, **266**, R1488–R1492.

Vällfors, B., Hansson, H. A. and Belghmaidi, M. (1983). Mesothelial cell integrity of the subdural and arachnoid surfaces of the cat brain after exposure to neurosurgical irrigation fluids and air: A scanning electron microscopic study. *Neurosurgery.*, **12**, 35–9.

Wilkins, R. H. and Odom, G. L. (1974). Ependymal-choroidal cells in cerebrospinal fluid. Increased incidence in hydrocephalic infants. *J. Neurosurg.*, **41**, 555–60.

Williams, J. L., Jones, S. C., Page, R. B. and Bryan, R. M., Jr. (1991). Vascular responses of choroid plexus during hypercapnia in rats. *Am. J. Physiol.*, **260**, R1066–R1070.

Wolinsky, J. S., Baringer, R., Margolis, G. and Kilham, L. (1974). Ultrastructure of mumps virus replication in newborn hamster central nervous system. *Lab. Invest.*, **31**(4), 403–12.

Wright, E. M. (1974). Active transport of glycine across the frog arachnoid membrane. *Brain Res.*, **76**, 354–8.

Wright, P. M., Nogueira, G. J. and Levin, E. (1971). Role of the pia mater in the transfer of substances in and out of the cerebrospinal fluid. *Exp. Brain Res.*, **13**, 294–305.

Yamamoto, M., McCaffery, P. and Drager, U. C. (1996). Influence of the choroid plexus on cerebellar development: analysis of retinoic acid synthesis. *Brain Res. Dev. Brain Res.*, **93**, 182–90.

Zenker, W., Bankoul, S. and Braun, J. B. (1994). Morphological indications for considerable diffuse reabsorption of cerebrospinal fluid in spinal meninges particularly in the areas of meningeal funnels. An electronmicroscopical study including tracing experiments in rats. *Anat. Embryol.* (Berl.), **189**(3), 243–58.

Zoli, M and Agnati, L. F. (1996). Wiring and volume transmission in the central nervous system: the concept of closed and open synapses. *Prog. Neurobiol.*, **49**(4), 363–80.

29 Circumventricular organs of the brain

LISE PRESCOTT and MILTON W. BRIGHTMAN

- Introduction
- Fenestrated vessels
- Blood circulation through CVO
- Ependyma
- CVO as portals into brain
- Plasticity
- CVO connections

Introduction

Seven small aggregates of tissue, that together account for less than 0.5% of the brain's volume (Gross and Weindl, 1987), have the vital role of transducing blood-borne, humoral signals into neural responses that maintain systemic homeostasis. Their location at the mid-sagittal surface of the cerebral ventricles suggests that the aggregates,

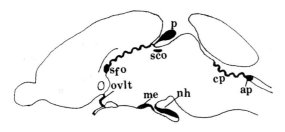

Fig. 29.1. Location of the circumventricular organs (CVO). Median sagittal section through a rodent brain. The choroid plexus, the vessels and stroma of which are continuous with those of the area postrema, has also been considered by some as a CVO. (After Weindl and Schinko, 1975.) ap, area postrema; cp, choroid plexus; me, median eminence; nh, neurohypophysis; ovlt, organum vasculosum of lamina terminalis; p, pineal gland; sco, subcommissural organ; sfo, subfornical organ.

designated as circumventricular organs (CVO), are in a position to participate in the exchange of substances between blood and the cerebrospinal fluid (CSF) (Fig. 29.1). They are able to receive solutes from blood and to release their secretory material into blood because they lie outside of the blood–brain barrier. The morphological basis of the vessels' permeability is like that for the capillaries of endocrine glands: a fenestrated endothelium, a constant feature of all but one CVO, the subcommissural organ. Accordingly, the structure, induction and physiology of fenestrated endothelium will be considered at length.

Fenestrated vessels

The endothelium of fenestrated vessels (FV) is passively permeable to hydrophilic solutes. FV are highly attentuated and perforated by clusters of holes or fenestrae, about 40–60 nm wide (Fig. 29.3), each spanned by a thin diaphragm, about 5 nm thick (Figs. 29.2 and 29.5). The diaphragms, although tenuous, are, nevertheless, impervious to protein (Pino and Essner, 1981) which, presumably, traverses the endothelium by either a vesi-

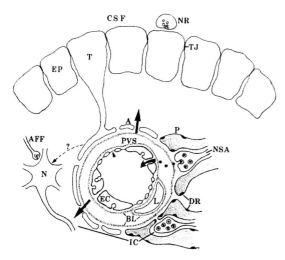

Fig. 29.2. Humoral and neural components of CVO. CVO consist of a connective tissue stroma containing vessels with permeable endothelial cells (EC) bearing fenestrae (arrowhead), neurons (N), neurites and astrocytes (A), all covered by special ependymal cells (EP) adjacent, in places, to intraventricular neurons and their neurites (NR). CVO receives signals from blood, afferent neurites (AFF) and, perhaps, from CSF via NR. Blood-borne solute leaves the capillaries to reach intrinsic neurons, which are activated as part of a neuroendocrine response to the solute. The left side of the capillary represents various CVO. In the neural lobe (right side), neurosecretory axon (NSA) terminals release peptides that pass through basal lamina (BL) into the perivascular space (PVS), which is part of the interstitial compartment (IC), across EC into blood. The role of pituicytes (P), distinguished from astrocytes by their dynorphin receptors (DR) (Bicknell *et al.*, 1989), is discussed above. Some solutes may reach the overlying ependymal cells joined by tight junctions (TJ), which leak (Fig. 29.4) but still impede the extracellular exchange of CSF and interstitial fluid. It is questionable whether exchange is by way of special ependyma: tanycytes (T). L is a leptomeningeal cell.

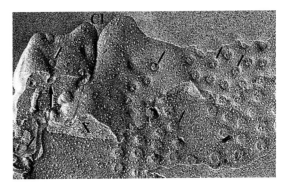

Fig. 29.3. Freeze-fractured plasma membranes of two endothelial cells with intervening extracellular cleft (Cl). Fenestrae and many pits or caveolae (lines), some omega-shaped (arrow), indent the cell membrane. The cytoplasm has also been cross-fractured (X) ($\times 60\,000$).

culo-tubular route or through patent intercellular clefts (Fig. 29.2). The FV of, for example, the area postrema and subfornical organ have about 44% more junctions and, therefore, intercellular clefts than do barrier capillaries (Coomber and Stewart, 1985). If even one of these junctions were patent at one moment, then a route of passage would be transiently available for solute transfer. Additional structural features may also enhance the permeability of the FV in these two CVOs; their endo-

thelium is over a third thinner with several fold more pits or vesicles than barrier capillaries (Coomber and Stewart, 1985). Whatever the path taken by substances across fenestrated endothelium, FV are associated with permeability. A constant, additional feature of these CVO microvessels, are wide perivascular space containing collagen fibrils and pericytes and bounded by fibroblastic, leptomeningeal cells (Fig. 29.2).

Although a perivascular position around FV is the usual location of neuroendocrine terminals, there does not appear to be a tropic factor on the surface of FV that specifically attracts these axonal endings. The adrenal medulla, pineal gland or neural lobe are normally supplied by FV. When fragments of these glands are grafted to the hypothalamus, they become abnormal targets of neurosecretory axons that have been damaged. The axons regenerate and come to lie at variable distances from FV regardless of the grafts' origin (Kadota *et al.*, 1990). Solute penetration, as discussed below, does not depend so much on length of the diffusion path from axon terminal to capillary as it does on the intervention of astrocytes between them.

What brings about the development of fenestrae and the accompanying attributes that make an endothelium permeable, is unknown. Astrocytes have been implicated in the induction or maintenance of barrier properties but there is accumulating evidence against this supposition (Brightman, 1991; Holash *et al.*, 1993; Krum and Rosenstein, 1993). Although fenestrae may be constitutively expressed by CVO endothelium, they are labile under certain environmental conditions. Vessels with a continuous endothelium, like that of brain or muscle, can be changed to FV in fetal muscle grafted to choroid plexus of a mature recipient. The change might be effected by a hypothetical conversion factor present in fetal muscle up to an age of E14 or 15 (E is embryonic day) (Naito et al., 1995). The opposite conversion, from FV to continuous capillaries, happens during normal development in brain. The brain is initially vascularized by sprouts from a pericerebral plexus containing many FV. By E18, only continuous endothelium is apparent in rat brain except for the CVO (Yoshida et al., 1988). Perhaps a factor, comparable to that of fetal muscle, is present in brain and converts the FV of fetal brain to the continuous endothelium of mature barrier capillaries. Whether or not the FV phenotype of CVO is sustained by glial presence can best be tested *in vitro* with co-cultures of astrocytes and endothelial cells dissociated from FV.

The permeability of fenestrated capillaries of most CVO is, however, only one of several attributes that account for neuroendocrine responses to signals carried by blood as well as by way of neural afferents. Properties such as capillary surface area, rates of blood flow and transit time have also been measured by quantitative autoradiography, an approach that has placed considerations of CVO on a quantitative footing by Gross and associates.

Blood circulation through CVO

Although the summed surface area of the capillaries of all seven CVO, each approximately 1 mm³ in volume, 'comprise only 1% of that for the entire brain' (Gross and Weindl, 1987), these tissue entities have widespread physiological effects. Peculiarities of the rate of blood flow and transit time: the time that a blood constituent is in contact with the luminal face of the blood vessel, as well as the vessels' permeability, permit the CVO to act as sensors and as information conduits between brain and other organs. These parameters not only differ between CVO (Gross, et al., 1986), but regionally, within a given CVO, as well (Shaver et al., 1990; Gross et al., 1991).

One striking peculiarity is that the soma and dendrites of an individual neurosecretory neuron in the supraoptic or paraventricular nucleus are supplied by an extremely rich bed of barrier vessels while their terminals abut permeable, fenestrated capillaries. Osmoreception appears to reside primarily in the organum vasculosum lamina terminalis (evidence summarized by Johnson and Gross, 1993). However, the semi-permeability of the extremely rich skein of capillaries around neurosecretory neurons enables them to act, perhaps, as osmometers transducing osmotic forces to signals for the release of neurosecretory peptides vasopressin and dynorphin from their axon terminals. The fenestrated capillaries at their axon tips, being permeable, can transfer the released peptides to blood. The high permeability of CVO capillaries is illustrated by the small, neutral amino acid α-amino isobutyric acid, which is transferred about 200 to 700 times more quickly across CVO vessels than it is across barrier vessels (Gross et al., 1987).

A more informative expression that takes the surface area (S) of the capillary bed into account, is the *PS* product. The hypothalamo-neurohypophyseal system again provides an instructive example of how useful this factor is in comparing capillaries among CVO and with barrier vessels of brain. The *PS* product for α-amino isobutyric acid is 260 times greater in the neural lobe than in its origin, the supraoptic nuclei (Gross et al., 1986). Although the S is about 30 mm²/mm³ and the same for the supraoptic nucleus and neural lobe, the much larger *PS* product of the neural lobe indicates that the permeability of the neural lobe's capillary bed is greater than that of its nucleus of origin (Gross et al., 1986). The most relevant factor that accounts for this difference is a fenestrated endothelium, compared with the continuous, barrier type. Among CVO, the *PS* product has been ranked pineal gland > neural lobe > subfornical organ > median eminence (Gross et al., 1987), an order correlatable with vessel type and functional properties (Gross, 1992; Gross et al., 1991).

Other properties that enhance the degree to which a CVO can sense a plasma solute is its transit time through a vessel and the rate of blood flow through that capillary. The transit time for serum albumin through the microcirculation of the subfornical organ is as high as 3 seconds or 2–12 fold

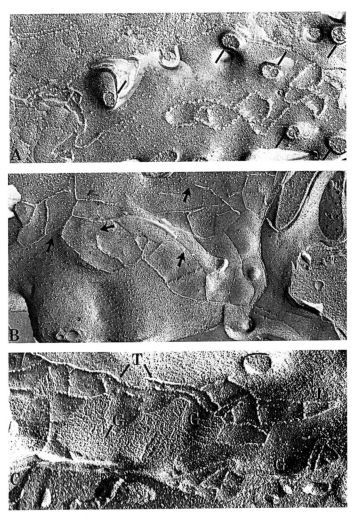

Fig. 29.4. Ependymal tight junctions of mouse median eminence: freeze-fractured.
(A) Discontinuous junctional strands between ependymal cells. The strands course among microvilli (lines) at the ventricular surface (×20 000).
(B) Discontinuities (arrows) among tight junction strands may partly account for the leakiness of these junctions (×50 000).
(C) Intercalation of non-circumferential gap junctions (G) among the strands of tight junctions (T), may also account for junctional leakiness (×110 000).

slower than in brain. The second property, circulation time, is also very low compared with barrier regions of brain (Gross, 1992). Long transit time, high permeability (Gross and Weindl, 1987) and low flow rate are features that ensure that messengers circulating through CVO have longer periods of contact with the permeable vessel wall and higher rates of transfer across it than in the barrier vessels of brain (Gross, 1992; Johnson and Gross, 1993).

Ependyma

Access of solutes from CSF to circumventricular organs would appear to be transcellular through tanycytic ependymal cells rather than intercellular. The special ependymal cells overlying CVO are tethered to each other by a complex of gap and tight junctions (Figs. 29.2 and 29.4) that impede the extracellular flow of horseradish peroxidase (Brightman *et al.*, 1975). Accordingly, solutes can reach the CVO parenchyma primarily by being incorporated and transcytosed by these cells. Neurons and neurites within the CVO would be in a position to test only the interstitial fluid of the CVO itself rather than the CSF directly. These junctions would also prevent blood-borne substances that had traversed fenestrated endothelium into the CVO interstitium, from entering the CSF. As a result, the neurons and neurites within the interstitium would have a longer opportunity to sample substances derived from blood.

A curious feature of CVO ependyma in vertebrates, including primates, is that free neurons and neurites consistently lie upon its ventricular surface. The supraependymal neurons and neurites are especially numerous on the free, ependymal surface of the hamster's median eminence where they form a ganglion-like aggregate with an organized neuropil that includes axosomatic and axodendritic synaptic contacts (Card and Mitchell, 1978). The tanycytes lack cilia so that the abutment of neurons, neurites and ependymal cells is undisturbed. Individual neurites and even a thick fascicle of them pass between ependymal cells to reach the parenchyma of the underlying median eminence.

The connections of the supraependymal neurons can be traced only by retrograde means. Attempts to label the neurons' terminals anterogradely by injecting tracer into their somata would be confounded by diffusion of the label into the CSF, thence between common ependymal cells with subsequent labeling of the hypothalamic neuropil. Retrograde labeling by injecting the pituitary gland target indicates that the intermediate and neural lobes, but not the anterior lobe, receive an input from the supraependymal neurons over the median eminence (Michael et al., 1989). The functional significance of this connection has not been determined.

CVO as portals into brain

Although such probe molecules as Evans blue–serum albumin (MW ~69 000), or the glycoprotein horseradish peroxidase (HRP; M_r 40 000), freely enter CVO, their penetration into the adjacent brain is minimal after a single bolus of the probe is injected intravascularly. If the plasma concentration of the probe is maintained at a high level, the probe spreads further but it is still confined to the adjacent brain. Although the neuropil beyond the CVO remains free of detectable probe, certain brain stem nuclei can, nevertheless, be labeled from the blood. The probe may enter the nuclei by diffusing extracellularly from an adjacent CVO or from the periphery. Axon branches from the nucleus solitarius that terminate in the organum vasculosum lamina terminalis and area postrema, are labeled from the extracellular spaces of these CVO (Broadwell and Brightman, 1976). A crude imitation of a CVO has been made with isogeneic or allogeneic grafts of skeletal muscle placed on the choroid plexus of the medulla's IV ventricle; as do CVO, the grafts act as a focal port for the entry of circulating protein (Wakai et al., 1986). The graft, in contrast, permits more circulating probe, injected intravenously as a single bolus, to penetrate farther into the underlying medulla than from the nearby area postrema (Wakai et al., 1986).

It is doubtful that virions, agents much larger than protein, enter brain from the CVO. Appreciable titers of inactivated, circulating, herpes-1 virus have been recovered from brain only when the blood–brain barrier has been osmotically breached. This breach is a diffuse one made by the intracarotid infusion of hyperosmotic saccharide at about the time that a bolus of the virus is injected (Neuwelt et al., 1991). If the endothelium itself is intact and not penetrated by virus, it is likely that even when high titers of virus are sustained, no appreciable amount would enter brain by passing directly across the fenestrated endothelium of CVO.

Plasticity

The spatial relationship between the neurohemal axon terminals of neurosecretory cells and specialized astrocytes, the pituicytes, of the neurohypophysis is a striking example of structural plasticity. This dynamic property of pituicytes was first discerned by electron microscopy. The neurosecretory axons of the supraoptic and paraventricular nuclei of the hypothalamus terminate in the pars nervosa, also referred to as the neural lobe of the

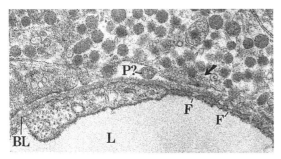

Fig. 29.5. Endothelial cell with fenestrae (F) is separated by a basal lamina (BL) and the tip of a process that might be a pituicyte (P?), from axon terminals. The terminals contain large neurosecretory granules and clusters of small spheres (arrow), the size of synaptic vesicles. Capillary lumen (L) is at the bottom of the figure (×40 000).

pituitary gland (Figs. 29.1 and 29.2). The 'quiesent' terminals of normally hydrated animals are partially covered by pituicyte processes which, accordingly, intervene between terminal and the basal lamina of the fenestrated endothelium (Figs. 29.2 and 29.5). A variety of stimuli, including prolonged water deprivation, stimulate the neurosecretory cells to release peptide hormone: vasopressin and dynorphin, from their axon terminals within this CVO. During stimulation, the pituicytes retract their processes, thus laying bare the terminals (Tweedle and Hatton, 1980). Their hormones can then be discharged directly into the perivascular interstitial fluid and thence across permeable FV into blood, which flows very rapidly through the neural lobe. The peptides ultimately reach target receptors on cells of the kidney or brain, including other CVOs. When stimulation ceases, the pituicyte processes once again move into the extracellular space between axon terminal and the perivascular basal lamina of FV (Fig. 29.2) (Tweedle and Hatton, 1980). Astroglial processes around the hypothalamic magnocellular neurons, from which the axons emanate, behave as do pituicytes. The release of oxytocin at parturition or of vasopressin during prolonged osmotic stress is accompanied by the retraction of these astrocytic processes. Neurons and dendrites, no longer separated from each other by intervening astrocytic

processes, become synaptically apposed (Theodosis *et al.*, 1986).

CVO connections

The CVO participate in achieving systemic homeostasis by making widespread neural connections, primarily throughout the brain stem (summarized by Johnson and Gross, 1993). Neurons of the CVO act as sensors and transducers of chemical signals and as relays in complex reflex arcs. Their neurons are usually small. Those of the subfornical organ may, for example, be cholinergic, GABAergic and have receptors for glycine (Weindl *et al.*, 1992). These neurons receive afferents from the septum and other regions and synapse reciprocally with another CVO, the organum vasculosum lamina terminalis. Subfornical circuits are involved in the regulation of fluid balance, respiration and cardiovascular activity (summarized by Weindl *et al.*, 1992). Neurons of the solitary tract nucleus synapse with more than one CVO, so that cranial nerves are brought into the circuits of the area postrema as well as the subfornical organ.

The area postrema subserves the complex reflex of emesis, initiated by the detection of circulating noxious substances that cross the fenestrated vessels of this CVO. Here, chemical signals are transduced to neural activity by small interstitial neurons that project to the adjacent nucleus of the solitary tract. This nucleus may, in turn, act as the initial part of a final common path subserving a variety of emetic signals that elicit vomiting (Miller and Leslie, 1994).

The structural basis for solute entry from blood and CSF into the CVO is understood to a degree but how humoral signals are transduced into neural responses has yet to be resolved. The functional relationship between supraependymal neurons and the median eminence has also proved elusive, but even when these aspects and the precise interactions of neural and endocrine components of extensive neural circuits have been delineated, the wonder remains that so paltry a mass of neurohumoral tissue can have such powerful, prevalent effects.

References

Bicknell, R. J., Luckman, S. M., Inenaga, K. *et al.* (1989). β-adrenergic and opoid receptors on pituicytes cultured from adult rat neurohypophysis: regulation of cell morphology. *Brain Res. Bull.*, **22**, 379–88.

Brightman, M. W. (1991). Implication of astroglia in the blood–brain barrier. In Glial–neuronal interaction. *Annals of the New York Academy of Science*, **633**, 343–7.

Brightman, M. W. and Reese, T. S. (1969). Junctions between intimately apposed cell membranes in the vertebrate brain. *J. Cell Biol.*, **40**, 648–77.

Brightman, M. W., Prescott, L. and Reese, T. S. (1975). Intercellular junctions of special ependyma. In *Brain – Endocrine Interaction*. II. *The Ventricular System in Neuroendocrine Mechanisms*, ed. K. M. Knigge, pp. 146–65. Basle: Karger.

Broadwell, R. D. and Brightman, M. W. (1976). Entry of peroxidase into neurons of the central nervous system from extracerebral and cerebral blood. *J. Comp. Neurol.*, **166**, 257–83.

Card, J. and Mitchell, J. (1978). Electron-microscopic demonstration of a supraependymal cluster of neuronal cells and processes in the hamster third ventricle. *J. Comp. Neurol.*, **180**, 43–58.

Coomber, B. L. and Stewart, P. A. (1985). Morphometric analysis of CNS micro-vascular endothelium. *Microvasc. Res.*, **30**, 99–115.

Gross, P. M. (1992). Circumventricular organ capillaries. *Prog. Brain Res.*, **91**, 219–33.

Gross, P. M., and Weindl, A. (1987). Peering through the windows of the brain. *J. Cereb. Blood Flow Metab.*, **7**, 663–72.

Gross, P. M., Sposito, N. M., Pettersen, S. E and Fenstermacher, J. D (1986). Differences in function and structure of the capillary endothelium in the supra-optic nucleus and pituitary neural lobe of rats. *Neuroendocrinol.*, **44**, 401–7.

Gross, P. M., Blasberg, R. G., Fenstermacher, J. D. and Patlack, C. S. (1987). The microcirculation of rat circumventricular organs and pituitary gland. *Brain Res. Bull.*, **18**, 73–85.

Gross, P. M., Wall, K. M., Wainman, D. S. and Shaver, S. W. (1991). Subregional topography of capillaries in the dorsal vagal complex of rats: II. Physiological properties. *J. Comparative Neurology*, **306**, 83–94.

Holash, H. A., Noden, D. M. and Stewart, P. A. (1993). Re-evaluating the role of astrocytes in blood–brain barrier induction. *Dev. Dyn.*, **197**, 14–25.

Johnson, A. M. and Gross, P. M. (1993). Sensory circumventricular organs and brain homeostatic pathways. *FASEB J.*, **7**, 678–86.

Kadota, Y., Pettigrew, K. and Brightman, M. W. (1990). Regrowth of damaged neurosecretory axons to fenestrated vessels of implanted peripheral tissues. *Synapse*, **5**, 12–32.

Krum, J. M. and Rosenstein, J. M. (1993). Effect of astroglial degeneration on the blood-brain barrier to protein in neonatal rats. *Dev. Brain Res.* **74**, 41–50.

Michael, D. B., Hazlett, J. C. and Mitchell, J. A. (1989). Innervation of the pituitary gland by supraependymal neurons. *Brain Res.*, **478**, 227–32.

Miller, A. and Leslie, R. A. (1994). The area postrema and vomiting. *Front. Neuroendocrinol.*, **15**, 301–20.

Naito, S., Chang, L., Pettigrew, W. K. *et al.* (1995). Conditions that may determine blood vessel phenotype in tissues grafted to brain. *Experimental Neurology*, **134**, 230–43.

Neuwelt, E. A., Pagel, M. A. and Dix, R. D. (1991). Delivery of ultraviolet-inactivated ^{35}S-herpes virus across an osmotically modified blood–brain barrier. *J. Neurosurg.*, **74**, 475–9.

Pino, R. M., and Essner, E. (1981). Permeability of rat choriocapillaries to hemeproteins. *J. Histochem. Cytochem.*, **29**, 281–90.

Shaver, S. W., Sposito, N. M. and Gross, P. M. (1990). Quantitative fine structure of capillaries in subregions of the rat subfornical organ. *J. Comp. Neurol.*, **294**, 145–52.

Theodosis, D. T., Montagnese, C., Rodriguez, F. *et al.* (1986). Oxytocin induces morphological plasticity in the adult hypothalamo-neurohypophysial system. *Nature*, **322**, 738–40.

Tweedle, C. D. and Hatton, G. I. (1980). Evidence for dynamic interactions between pituicytes and neurosecretory axons in the rat. *Neuroscience*, **5**, 661–7.

Wakai, S., Meiselman, S. and Brightman, M. W. (1986). Muscle grafts as entries of blood-borne proteins into the extracellular space of the brain. *Neurosurgery*, **18**, 548–54,

Weindl, A. and Schinko, I. (1975). Vascular and ventricular neurosecretion in the organum vasculosum of the lamina terminalis of the golden hamster. In: *Brain Endocrine Interaction II. The Ventricular System*, ed. K. M. Knigge *et al.*, pp. 190–203. Basel: Karger.

Weindl, A., Bufler, J., Winkler, B. *et al.* (1992). Neurotransmitters and receptors in the subfornical organ. Immunohistochemical and electrophysi-ological evidence. *Prog. Brain Res.*, **91**, 261–9.

Yoshida, Y., Yamada, M., Wakabayashi, K. and Ikuta, F. (1988). Endothelial fenestrae in the rat fetal cerebrum. *Dev. Brain Res.*, **44**. 211–9.

30 Transport in the developing brain

N. R. SAUNDERS and K. M. DZIEGIELEWSKA

- Introduction
- Ion/electrolyte transport
- Heavy metals
- Amino acids
- Peptides
- Proteins
- Molecular studies of barrier transport mechanisms in the developing brain

Introduction

General textbooks of physiology still tend to refer to 'the' blood–brain barrier as though it were a single entity (e.g. Ganong, 1995). However, it is quite clear, at least to those in the field, that the term is now used to describe a wide range of physiological mechanisms that control the composition of the internal environment of the brain to an even greater extent than the mechanisms that control the 'milieu interieur' of the organism as a whole. Nevertheless, there is a sense in which there is a single underlying barrier, namely the presence of a diffusion barrier at the blood–brain and blood–CSF (cerebrospinal fluid) interfaces. This takes the form of tight junctions between adjacent endothelial cells in the cerebral vessels (blood–brain barrier) and between the epithelial cells of the choroid plexus (blood–CSF barrier). The barrier at the blood–brain interface prevents almost absolutely the penetration of macromolecules such as proteins and of ligands that bind to proteins (e.g. some dyes and drugs). For small molecules there is a degree of permeability that is directly proportional to molecular weight. For the blood–CSF interface, the range of molecular size that can penetrate into

CSF by diffusion is much greater. Most of the proteins that are present in CSF are at CSF/plasma ratios that reflect their diffusion coefficients or molecular radii (Felgenhuer, 1974) although at only very low concentrations in CSF compared with those in plasma. The low concentrations of protein in CSF in the adult brain are a consequence of a restricted surface area for exchange and the effect of the continuous turnover of CSF ('sink effect', see Davson and Segal, 1996).

In the developing brain, passive exchange across the blood–brain barrier is also restricted to molecules that are smaller in size than proteins, but the level of transfer is greater for these smaller molecules than is the case in the adult. This is probably a reflection of a greater surface area (number of pores) rather than a change in pore size (Dziegielewska et al., 1979; Saunders, 1992). Similarly, at the blood–CSF interface apparent permeability is also greater in the immature brain. However, the explanation is probably more complex than for the blood–brain interface. As in the adult brain, in the developing brain there is passive permeability across the blood–CSF interface over a much greater molecular size range (from at least sucrose to IgG) than across the blood–brain barrier itself, and at a much greater level of permeability than in the adult. In addition, changes in the rate of secretion (turnover) of CSF (sink effect) with age also influence the steady state (CSF/plasma ratio) of more slowly penetrating molecules. There is also evidence for specific transfer of some plasma proteins from blood to CSF across the choroid plexus early in brain development. This, together with greater passive permeability, contributes to a high concentration of protein in CSF of the immature brain, e.g. over 1000 mg/100 ml at E30 in fetal sheep (E is embryonic day) and around 350 mg/100 ml in E15 fetal rats.

In an introduction to barrier/transport mechanisms in the developing brain, it is appropriate to discuss briefly some methodological considerations, particularly as these are poorly understood and often have led to misleading interpretations of experimental data. Most functional studies of barriers and transport in the developing brain have involved injection of foreign materials into fetuses or newborn animals. As discussed in some detail elsewhere (Saunders, 1992), many of these experiments have been grossly unphysiological in that they have involved injections of either large volumes or high concentrations of protein when compared with the circulating volume or plasma protein concentration in immature animals (see Saunders, 1992 for references). The particular transport/barrier mechanism is often not clearly specified and there is a tendency to refer to 'the' blood–brain barrier as though it were a single entity. A further complication is that different animal species are born at very different stages of development of their various organ systems and the relative stages of development of different organ systems may be quite different within a species, depending upon the length of the gestational period. Thus, all species have, of necessity, a functional respiratory system at birth. The parts of the brainstem and spinal cord involved in function in a species born very early, such as a marsupial, will be well developed and much in advance of the rest of the brain or other parts of the body such as the limbs. A rat is born at a stage of neocortical and midbrain development that is considerably greater than a marsupial at birth, but much less than that of a human baby or newborn lamb. These differences are often not taken account of

and it is extremely confusing to talk about 'newborn' as though it were a stage of development that is comparable in all species. Much of the early work, and much current work, on barrier/transport systems in the developing brain has been carried out in neonatal rats and the information often transferred directly to human newborns. Yet the brains of rats and humans at birth are at quite different stages of development and there is clear evidence that the barrier/transport systems in newborn rats are significantly different from those in human newborns, even if premature. One index of the stage of the development of transport/barrier mechanisms in the developing brain is the concentration of protein in cerebrospinal fluid. This has been shown to be high early in brain development in all species so far investigated (Fig. 30.1 and see Dziegielewska and Saunders, 1988). However, the explanation for this high concentration of protein is *not* that the barrier (tight junctions) to proteins at the blood–CSF interface is immature, but that there is a greater transfer of proteins across the cells in the choroid plexus in the immature brain. This will be dealt with in detail in a separate section (below). In newborn rats, cisternal CSF contains approximately 300 mg/100 ml total protein compared with 25 mg/100 ml in the adult (Dziegielewska et al., 1981). In human neonates, CSF protein concentration is about 60–80 mg/100 ml, which is only about twice normal. Even for infants born 8–10 weeks prematurely, it is not more than about 120 mg/100 ml. It is known to be much higher early in gestation (see Saunders, 1977 and Dziegielewska and Saunders, 1988 for references). Clearly, with respect to protein barriers and transfer mechanisms, newborn rats and newborn humans are quite different.

A more human aspect to the interpretation of experimental data is that authors often select the data that fits with their preconceived notions and ignore inconvenient and incompatible data. Worse, some may read into experiments results that are simply not found. For example, Behnsen (1927) is often cited as providing evidence of immaturity of the blood–brain barrier in experiments involving injections of dyes into newborn rats. His evidence is presented as coloured dots on outlines of drawings of sagittal sections of rat brains. However, the drawings for both newborn and adult brains corre-

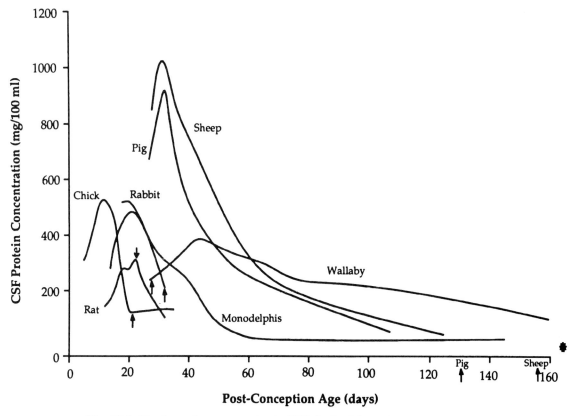

Fig. 30.1. Total protein concentration in CSF obtained from cisterna magna of different species during development. Abscissa: age from day of conception; ordinate: protein concentration (mg/100 ml). Arrows indicate time of birth. Adult CSF protein concentration is indicated by*. Note that peak in protein concentration occurs early in brain development in all species and is not related to time of birth. Redrawn from Saunders (1992).

spond to outlines of adult brains. Since the proportions of different brain regions are quite different in newborn and adult, this gives rise to Behnsen's observation that the areas that in the adult are known to be permeable to dyes are larger in the newborn. More importantly, Behnsen did not describe any staining of the neocortex, which would be expected if the barrier were, indeed, immature; this is because the neocortex is the least mature part of the brain at birth in the rat. This was confirmed by a recent extensive study by Moos and Møllgård (1993) in which they also point out the importance of not injecting so much dye that the binding capacity of albumin in circulating blood is exceeded. A recent paper (Fabian and Hulsebosch, 1993) cites Wislocki (1920) as showing immaturity of the blood–brain barrier to

dyes in fetal guinea pigs. The paper actually shows unequivocally that Trypan Blue injected into midgestation fetal guinea pigs does *not* stain the brain, which is the same result as that obtained if this dye is injected into an adult animal.

There are several other matters/mechanisms that need to be taken account of when interpreting the results from experimental investigations of transport across the blood–brain and blood–CSF barriers during brain development. Unfortunately for the experimenter, molecules that penetrate from blood to brain or CSF by mechanisms other than diffusion are likely to be metabolically important for brain development and function. If the metabolic usage by the brain of a particular molecule or class of molecules, e.g. amino acids, changes during development, then it is likely to be difficult to distinguish changes in transfer due to changes in transport as against changes in brain metabolism. Similarly, molecules penetrating into brain and CSF tend to be cleared back into the circulation by the continuous turnover of CSF ('sink effect' see Davson and Segal, 1996); this is particularly important for more slowly penetrating molecules. Since the turnover of CSF is known to change with age, this needs to be taken account of when interpreting permeability studies.

A further complication is that the extracellular space of brain changes (decreases) during development (e.g. Lehmenküler et al., 1993). Thus, if the material under consideration is confined largely, if not exclusively, to the extracellular space this will influence the apparent transfer of materials from blood to CSF in permeability experiments. Further to be considered is the possibility of protein binding. The concentration of protein in plasma increases considerably during development (e.g. from about 1500 mg/100 ml at E17 in rat fetuses to over 7000 mg/100 ml in the adult, but falls substantially in CSF, e.g. from about 300 mg/100 ml to 25 mg/100 ml over the same period: Dziegielewska et al., 1981; Knott, 1995).

Only two transfer systems have been investigated in any detail in the developing brain, namely that for glucose from blood into brain and CSF and that for proteins from blood into CSF. Glucose transport is dealt with in detail in Chapter 19 and will, therefore, not be considered here. Transfer of protein will be a major part of this review. Before dealing with protein transfer, what is known of other transport systems in the developing brain will be summarized.

Ion/electrolyte transport

This has been studied in the developing brain using two approaches:

1. Concentrations gradients

Analysis of (steady-state, naturally occurring) concentrations of ions such as Na^+, K^+, Mg^{2+}, Ca^{2+} in CSF in whole brain compared with plasma. The presence of a concentration gradient between CSF and plasma has generally been taken to indicate

the presence of an ion pump. However, as indicated in the Introduction, the presence of a gradient also implies that there is a restriction on diffusion, otherwise however hard a pump might work it would not be able to establish a gradient. This means that in the absence of a gradient it is not clear whether the diffusion restraint is not yet developed or that the specific ion pump has yet to start functioning. Most studies of ionic distributions in CSF and plasma during brain development have shown a sequential development of different ion gradients (e.g. Bradbury et al., 1972). Once the gradient for an ion is present, it seems reasonable to suppose that the absence of other ion gradients at a particular stage of brain development is due to an absence or inadequate development of the specific ion pump, but that the overall diffusion restraint is present. In rabbits, a gradient for chloride between CSF and plasma was apparent in the newborn (Åmtorp and Sørensen, 1974). A gradient for potassium (CSF/plasma) was present as early as a week before birth in the rabbit and at birth in the rat (Åmtorp and Sørensen, 1974). In the fetal sheep, some of the first electrolyte gradients to be apparent between CSF and plasma are gradients for Cl^- and Na^+ at around 60 days gestation, E60, (Bradbury et al., 1972); this is a time when a progressive decrease in blood–CSF and blood–brain permeability to small molecular weight non-electrolytes, e.g. sucrose, is occurring (Evans et al., 1974; Dziegielewska et al., 1979). A gradient for Mg^{2+} was apparent even earlier at E45–50 (Bradbury et al., 1972), but the interpretation of this finding is complicated by the fact that CSF protein concentration is high at this age (Dziegielewska and Saunders, 1988) and no measures of ionic as against protein bound Mg^{2+} have yet been made during brain development. Butt et al. (1990) assessed the ion permeability of the blood–brain barrier indirectly by in situ measurement of transendothelial electrical resistance of pial blood vessels on the surface of the brain in rats between E17 and P33. There was a striking increase in electrical resistance just before birth, which was interpreted as a decrease in paracellular ion permeability with increasing maturity of the brain. Butt et al. (1990) have discounted the possibility that there might be a developmentally regulated change in ion transport that might account for the observed increase in electrical resistance. However this does not take account of their own observation that the resistance fell considerably on exposure to metabolic inhibitors or a reduction in temperature.

Studies of steady state distribution of ions between brain and plasma are more difficult to interpret. Most ions have either a predominantly intracellular or predominantly extracellular distribution. But, especially in the case of the latter, as the volume of the extracellular space decreases with age, this may influence the distribution between different compartments and it is not easy to obtain independent measures of intracellular and extracellular ion concentrations, although some studies using ion selective electrodes have been carried out (e.g. Syková *et al.*, 1992; Lehmenkühler *et al.*, 1993).

2. Tracer studies

These have been reviewed by Johanson (1989). One of the earliest such studies was that of Bakay (1953) using ^{32}P. However, interpretation of these results is complicated by the difficulty mentioned in the Introduction of distinguishing between changes in permeability and changes in metabolism during brain development. Several studies have shown that both the rate of uptake and steady-state distribution volume in developing brain for radiolabelled chloride, decline with increasing maturity (see Johanson 1989, for references).

A different barrier mechanism is that which controls iodide levels in the brain. Woodbury (1967) showed that there is an *outward* (brain or CSF to plasma) iodide pump that keeps iodide at a low level in the adult brain. This mechanism is already effective in neonatal rats.

Heavy metals

Iron entry is the only heavy metal to have been much studied in the developing brain, particularly by Morgan and his colleagues (e.g. Taylor and Morgan, 1990; Crowe and Morgan, 1992). This work will be reviewed briefly below as part of the discussion on transferrin.

Amino acids

Amino acid transport systems in the adult brain have been well characterized (see Davson and Segal, 1996 and Chapter 20 in this volume for references). One of the earliest studies in developing animals was that of Korobkin and Cutler (1977), who showed that each of six amino acids studied had a distinctive maturational pattern in their CSF concentrations. From this they concluded that there may be separate amino acid transport mechanisms that mature at different times. Later evidence has shown that amino acid transport in the developing brain is generally high compared with the adult (Banos *et al.* 1978; Braun *et al.*, 1980; Cornford *et al.*, 1982; Brenton and Gardiner, 1988); presumably this is a reflection of the rapid growth of the developing brain. Lefauconnier (1992) has outlined some of the technical problems associated with study of amino acid transport in small immature animals, as well as providing a useful summary of age-related differences. The developing brain appears to have a greater number of amino acid transport systems than in the adult. Thus, in the adult there are three systems, but in the immature animal there appears to be four: the L system, cationic amino acid transport, an ASC system and an A system (see Lefauconnier, 1992, for references).

Peptides

Friden (1993) has reviewed receptor-mediated transport of peptides and proteins across the blood–brain barrier, but deals mainly with the adult. In single pass experiments, insulin uptake was appreciably higher in newborn rabbits than in older animals (Frank *et al.*, 1985). The mechanism of transfer has been suggested to be by transcytosis (Duffy and Pardridge, 1987).

Proteins

It was mentioned in the Introduction to this chapter that CSF in the immature brain is characterized by a high concentration of protein compared to that in the adult (Fig. 30.1). It can be as high as

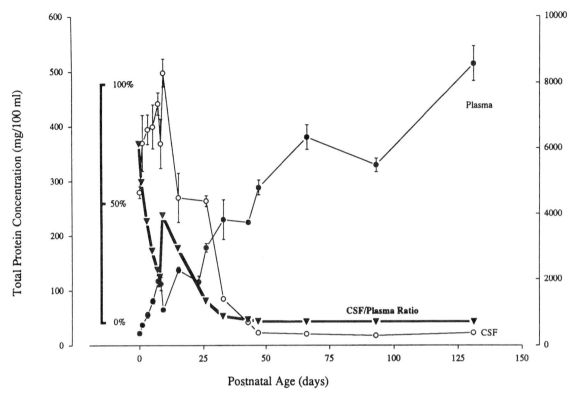

Fig. 30.2. Total protein concentration (mg/100 ml) in plasma (●, right ordinate) and CSF (left ordinate, ○) of postnatal *Monodelphis domestica*. Abscissa, postnatal age in days. Mean ±SEM. CSF/plasma ratio (%, thick line) – concentration in CSF over concentration in plasma × 100. From Dziegielewska *et al.* (1997), with permission of the University of New South Wales Press, Australia.

200 times greater. The change in gradient (CSF/plasma) with age is even more striking as the protein concentration in plasma in the immature fetus or newborn is low compared with that in the adult and increases during development, at a time when the concentration in CSF is falling, as is illustrated in Fig. 30.2. The composition of proteins in fetal and newborn CSF of various species has been reviewed previously (Dziegielewska and Saunders, 1988). It is clear that most of the proteins in immature CSF originate from and are immunologically indistinguishable from those in plasma. Current evidence summarized here suggests that there are two mechanisms that determine the higher concentration of proteins in CSF in the immature brain: (a) greater passive (diffusional) permeability; (b) presence of a developmentally regulated specific protein transfer mechanism.

Evidence for greater passive permeability in the developing brain comes from studies of Evans *et al.* (1974) and Dziegielewska *et al.* (1979) in fetal sheep and of Woodbury and colleagues (e.g. Ferguson and Woodbury, 1969) and of Habgood *et al.* (1993) in fetal and newborn rats. The study of Dziegielewska *et al.* (1979) in particular showed that the passive permeability of a wide range of molecular sizes from blood into CSF is greater in the immature than in the mature sheep fetus. For penetration into brain, there appears to be a molecular size cut-off above inulin (molecular weight 5000, molecular radius 1.3 nm) reflecting the presence of tight junctions between cerebral endothelial cells that are well enough developed to restrict the entry of protein into the brain (see also Saunders, 1992).

Extensive studies by Felgenhauer (1974) based on measurements of proteins in human CSF and serum have shown that the concentrations of almost

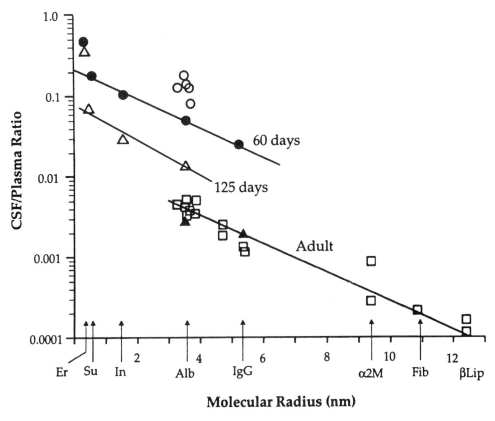

Fig. 30.3. Relation of molecular size to CSF/plasma concentration ratio in fetal sheep and adult humans and sheep for lipid-insoluble molecules of a wide range of molecular radii. Upper line (filled circles) 60 day gestation fetal sheep. Middle line (open triangles) 125 day fetal sheep. Lower line, squares are human data, filled triangles are sheep data.

Protein data are from immunoassays of endogenous proteins in CSF and plasma. Erythritol, sucrose and inulin data are from intravenously injected steady-state experiments.

Note parallel log-linear lines with decreasing CSF/plasma ratios as age increases. This relationship suggests unrestricted diffusion through very large pores with a reduction in the number of pores (rather than in their size) during development. Values for erythritol are above the lines, suggesting that it is small enough to penetrate into cells.

Note points (open circles) above 60 day fetal sheep line. These are ratios for the five main plasma proteins present in fetal sheep CSF (α-fetoprotein, fetuin, α-antitrypsin, transferrin and albumin) that are transported through the choroid plexus epithelial cells early in gestation. Redrawn from Saunders (1992)

all proteins in CSF in the adult can be accounted for on the basis of their molecular radius. A similar approach applied to the data from fetal sheep studies (Saunders, 1992; Saunders and Dziegiel-ewska, 1996) shows that the CSF/plasma ratios of lipid insoluble molecules ranging in size from sucrose (0.51 nm) to *exogenous* IgG (5.3 nm) fits well with the same explanation, namely that the penetration of such molecules from blood to CSF depends upon their concentration in plasma and their molecular radius. However, it is clear that in addition, some of the proteins present in immature CSF have steady-state ratios (CSF/plasma) that are considerably in excess of that which would be expected from their molecular size and plasma concentration (Fig. 30.3). The same is also the case for the rat (Habgood *et al.*, 1992).

In the study of Dziegielewska *et al.* (1980), it was

apparent that several of the proteins, both endogenous and exogenous, attained steady-state CSF/plasma ratios that were higher than would be expected for their molecular size and diffusion coefficients. The proteins concerned included α-fetoprotein, transferrin and albumin. In the case of albumin, there was the unexpected result that human albumin fitted well with entry by diffusion but the natural steady level for endogenous (sheep) albumin was some 2 to 3 times higher. This was investigated in detail by Dziegielewska et al. (1991) who showed that there was a range of CSF/plasma steady-state ratios for albumins from different animal species. Only goat albumin achieved the same steady-state CSF/plasma ratio as sheep albumin. Bovine albumin approached the sheep CSF/plasma ratio but more slowly than that for the goat experiments. Human and chicken albumin gave substantially lower CSF/plasma steady-state ratios. These differences in permeability for albumin from different animal species were shown to be developmentally regulated in that they were demonstrated at E60 and by E75 and later when overall protein permeability is much less, the differences between different albumins were no longer apparent. This phenomenon was further investigated in the rat (Habgood et al., 1992). In addition to confirming that albumins from different species may have different permeabilities between blood and CSF (see Fig. 30.4), Habgood et al. also showed that various chemical modifications of albumin uniformly reduced the penetration of the modified albumin from blood into CSF to a basal level that was consistent with passive diffusion (Fig. 30.4). From these studies it has been proposed that albumin in the developing brain penetrates into CSF by two parallel pathways, one diffusional and the other by specific transfer mechanism, the nature of which still has to be determined. Further support for such a proposition has come from studies of the permeability of different albumins in neonatal opossums (Monodelphis domestica) by Knott et al. (1997). These studies showed that, as in neonatal rats, human albumin penetrates into CSF to achieve approximately the same steady-state ratio as the naturally occurring albumin, whereas bovine albumin reaches a lower steady-state and chemical modification also reduces the penetration of the albumin. This specific transfer of albumins in the opossum also appears to be developmentally regulated in that the differences were most marked in the early postnatal period and had largely disappeared by around postnatal day 30.

Detailed studies of the tight junctions between adjacent choroid plexus epithelial cells have shown that these junctions develop very early and do not change much in their general characteristics during fetal development (Møllgård et al., 1976). Immunocytochemistry has therefore been used to try to define the likely route of penetration of proteins, including albumin, from plasma into cerebrospinal fluid. Several studies have shown that choroid plexus epithelial cells are positive for a range of plasma proteins including albumin, in a number of different species (human, Møllgård et al., 1979; sheep, Jacobson et al., 1983, Dziegielewska et al., 1991; opossum, Knott et al., 1997).

Specific studies of the immunohistochemical distribution of albumin in developing choroid plexus linked to parallel studies of permeability in the developing brain have been carried out in fetal sheep (Dziegielewska et al., 1991) and in postnatal opossums (Knott et al., 1997). These studies show that only a small proportion of choroid plexus epithelial cells are positive for either endogenous or exogenous albumin. The most detailed studies have been carried out in neonatal opossums. These show that there is a good correlation between the maximum number of positive cells and the peak concentration of albumin in cerebrospinal fluid, both, for example, being at their highest at around postnatal day 8 (P8) in this species. In addition, in this species human albumin achieves approximately the same steady-state CSF/plasma ratio as for the naturally occurring Monodelphis albumin and the immunocytochemical studies showed that choroid plexus epithelial cells that were positive for Monodelphis albumin were also always positive for exogenously applied human albumin (Fig. 30.5). However, in the case of chemically modified bovine serum albumin (succinylated), which achieves a much lower steady-state CSF/plasma ratio than either human or Monodelphis albumin, it was found that only a small proportion of the cells that were positive for Monodelphis albumin were also positive for the modified BSA. This was found to be the case at P8. In contrast, by the time the specific

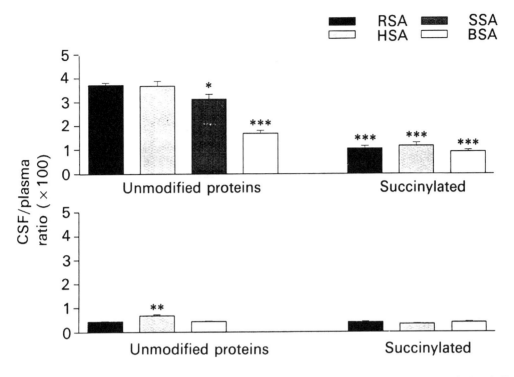

Fig. 30.4. Steady-state CSF/plasma ratios for various species of unmodified and succinylated albumin (rat, RSA; human, HSA; sheep, SSA; bovine, BSA) in 3-day-old rats (upper panel) and 20-day-old rats (lower panel). The data for unmodified RSA are the naturally occuring CSF/plasma ratios, all others are 16–20 h after i.p. injection. Asterisks indicate steady-state CSF/plasma ratios that were significantly different from the endogenous rat albumin ratio (*$P<0.05$, **$P<00.01$, ***$P<0.001$, paired t tests). There were no significant differences between different species of succinylated albumin in the 3-day-old rats, or in the 20-day-old rats. Error bars shown are standard errors of the mean (SEM). From Habgood *et al.* (1992).

transfer of albumin could no longer be detected (P30), up to 90% of the cells that were positive for endogenous *Monodelphis* albumin were also positive for exogenously administered chemically modified BSA.

The mechanism of the specific transfer of albumin from blood to CSF in the developing brain that has now been demonstrated in three species (sheep, Dziegielewska *et al.*, 1991; rat, Habgood *et al.*, 1992; opossum, Knott *et al.*, 1997) is not clear. As long ago as 1964, Klatzo and his colleagues (Smith *et al.*, 1964) demonstrated *in vitro* transfer of albumin from the apical surface of immature choroid plexus cells (chick and rabbit) to the stroma, which was temperature dependent and inhibited by metabolic inhibitors. This transfer was in the opposite direction to that observed in

the *in vivo* experiments described above, but it raises the possibility of a metabolically dependent (and, therefore, active) transport of albumin across the choroid plexus. Indirect evidence for active transport was put forward by Habgood *et al.* (1992) based on a comparison of CSF/plasma concentration ratios for different albumins at different plasma albumin concentrations. Rat albumin (and also human and sheep albumin, which were transferred into the CSF from plasma to about the same extent) did not show any concentration dependence, whereas bovine albumin, which was transferred to a much lesser extent than the other albumins, did show concentration dependence in its transfer from blood to CSF. This was interpreted as suggesting that transfer of endogenous rat albumin (as well as human and sheep albumins)

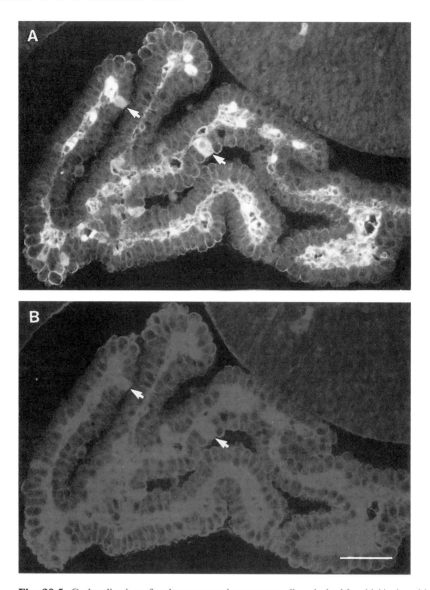

Fig. 30.5. Co-localization of endogenous and exogenous albumin in *Monodelphis* choroid plexus. Double immunohistochemical staining for the localization of *Monodelphis* albumin and human albumin in the lateral ventricular choroid plexus of *Monodelphis* (A, B). All of the epithelial cells that were immunoreactive for *Monodelphis* albumin (A) were also stained by anti-human albumin antiserum (B). Examples of such double-stained cells are indicated by arrows. Bar is 50 μm. Plate kindly prepared by Dr Z. Li.

was by active transport at a level that is already saturated by the high concentration of albumin in plasma. Presumably such a mechanism would be receptor mediated. Bovine serum albumin was suggested to be transported by a separate concentration-dependent mechanism involving diffusion (Habgood *et al.*, 1992). The subcellular route for

the transfer of albumin appears to be via a system of tubuloendoplasmic reticulum (Balslev *et al.*, 1997).

The only other plasma protein that has been studied extensively in the developing brain is transferrin. Since the description of transferrin receptors on endothelial cells of brain capillaries by

Jefferies *et al.* (1984), a substantial amount of work has been carried out by several groups on the transport of transferrin and iron into brain, particularly in the adult. In the adult, the evidence on whether or not transferrin is actually transported into the brain is controversial. Even amongst the same authors, opposing conclusions have been reached (cf. Fishman *et al.*, 1987 and Roberts *et al.*, 1992). Some possible reasons for the differences, based on methodological considerations, have been discussed by Roberts *et al.* (1992) and by Skarlatos *et al.* (1995). On balance, it seems likely that little or no transferrin gets beyond the endothelial cells of cerebral vessels, whereas a substantial amount of the iron carried by the transferrin is transported into the brain and transferred to, as yet, not clearly identified iron-binding proteins. Transferrin is present in the adult brain, particularly within oligodendroglia (Bloch *et al.*, 1985) but is present also in some neurons, for example layer IV pyramidal cortical neurons and anterior horn cells in the spinal cord (Connor and Fine, 1986). In the developing brain there is clear evidence for transfer from blood to cerebrospinal fluid both in the sheep fetus (Dziegielewska *et al.*, 1980) and in newborn rats (Taylor and Morgan, 1990; Crowe and Morgan, 1992). For penetration from blood into brain, as in the adult, the situation seems confused, if not controversial. On balance, the evidence from Morgan and his colleagues suggests that little, if any, transferrin transfers across the cerebral endothelium, in contrast with the very much larger transfer of iron.

The distribution of transferrin has been studied in the immature brain of a number of species. Unlike adults, when transferrin is predominantly located in oligodendroglia, in the fetus and newborn of species born at an immature stage (e.g. rats) transferrin is mainly found in different neuron populations. This has been demonstrated in human fetuses (Møllgård *et al.*, 1979), fetal sheep (Møllgård *et al.*, 1984; Reynolds and Møllgård, 1985) and postnatal rats (Connor and Fine, 1987). Except for the study of Lin and Connor (1989) on the optic nerve of the postnatal rat (which, of course, contains no neurons), no studies of the distribution of transferrin receptors in the developing brain appear to have been carried out, although for the studies of transport of iron and transferrin in the postnatal rat brain, Crowe (1996) has concluded that the density of transferrin receptors on cerebral endothelial cells of developing rat brain may be appreciably higher than in the adult. Evan Morgan's group in Perth, WA has carried out extensive studies of iron and transferrin transfer in the developing (postnatal) rat brain. These have shown unequivocally that the transport of iron greatly exceeds that of transferrin and that most of the transferrin taken up by cerebral endothelial cells is recycled back into the plasma and that at most only a very small percentage reaches the brain side of the cerebral endothelial cells (Taylor and Morgan, 1990; Crowe and Morgan, 1992). These experiments also showed that the rate of iron uptake by the immature (P15) rat brain is greater than in the adult and declines during development.

The thyroxine transporting protein transthyretin has been shown to be expressed in the developing choroid plexuses of a number of species including rat (Thomas *et al.*, 1988) and opossum (Li *et al.*, 1997). Only one report of its transfer from blood to CSF in the immature brain has been published (Dziegielewska *et al.*, 1980). The relation between transthyretin transferred across the choroid plexus and that synthesized and secreted by the plexus remains to be determined.

Molecular studies of barrier transport mechanisms in the developing brain

The only transport mechanism in the developing brain that has been studied at the molecular level is that for glucose (see Chapter 19). Otherwise molecular studies have been aimed at characterizing the developmental sequence of endothelial cell markers, functional significance of which is so far not known although some have been suggested to have a possible transport role (e.g. HT7, Seulberger and Risau, 1993).

Acknowledgements

The authors gratefully acknowledge the support of The Wellcome Trust and The Australian Research Council.

References

Åmtorp, O. and Sørensen, S. C. (1974). The ontogenetic development of concentration differences for protein and ions between plasma and cerebrospinal fluid in rabbits and rats. *J. Physiol.*, **243**, 387–400.

Bakay, L. (1953). Studies on the blood–brain barrier with radioactive phosphorus. III. Embryonic development of the barrier. *Arch. Neurol. Psychiat.*, **70**, 30–9.

Balslev, Y., Dziegielewska, K. M., Møllgård, K. and Saunders, N. R. (1997). Intercellular barriers to and transcellular transfer of protein albumin in the fetal sheep. *Anat. Embryol.*, **195**, 229–36.

Baños, G, Daniel, P. M. and Pratt, O. E. (1978). The effect of age upon the entry of some amino acids into the brain, and their incorporation into cerebral protein. *Dev. Med. Child Neurol.*, **20**, 335–46.

Behnsen, G. (1927). Über die Farbstoffspeicherung im Zentralnervensystem der Weissen Maus in verschiedenen Alterzuständen. *Z. Zellforsch.*, **133**, 231–48.

Bloch, B., Popovici, T., Levin, M. J. *et al.* (1985). Transferrin gene expression visualized in oligodendrocytes of the rat brain by using *in situ* hybridization and immunohistochemistry. *Proc. Natl. Acad. Sci. USA*, **82**, 6706–10.

Bradbury, M. W. B., Crowder, J., Desai, S. *et al.* (1972). Electrolytes and water in the brain and cerebrospinal fluid of the foetal sheep and guinea pig. *J. Physiol.*, **227**, 591–610.

Braun, L. D., Cornford, E. M. and Oldendorf, W. H. (1980). Newborn rabbit blood–brain barrier is selectively permeable and differs substantially from the adult. *J. Neurochem.*, **34**, 147–152.

Brenton, D. P. and Gardiner, R. M. (1988). Transport of L-phenylalanine and related amino acids at the ovine blood–brain barrier. *J. Physiol.*, **402**, 497–514.

Butt, A. M., Jones, H. C. and Abbott, N. J. (1990). Electrical resistance across the blood–brain barrier in anaesthetized rats: a developmental study. *J. Physiol.*, **429**, 47–62.

Connor, J. R. and Fine, R. E. (1986). The distribution of transferrin immunoreactivity in the rat central nervous system. *Brain Res.*, **368**, 319–28.

Connor, J. R. and Fine, R. E. (1987). Development of transferrin-positive oligodendrocytes in the rat central nervous system. *J. Neurosci. Res.*, **17**, 51–9.

Cornford, E. M., Braun, L. D. and Oldendorf, W. H. (1982). Developmental modulations of blood–brain barrier permeability as an indicator of changing nutritional requirements in the brain. *Ped. Res.*, **16**, 324–8.

Crowe, A. P. (1996). The effect of neurotoxic metals on the uptake of iron into the brain and other organs of the developing rat with normal and altered iron status. PhD Thesis, University of Western Australia, 319 pp.

Crowe, A. and Morgan, E. H. (1992). Iron and transferrin uptake by brain and cerebrospinal fluid in the rat. *Brain Res.*, **592**, 8–16.

Davson, H. and Segal, M. B. (1996). *Physiology of the CSF and Blood–Brain Barriers*. Times Mirror International Publishers.

Duffy, K. R. and Pardridge, W. M. (1987). Blood–brain barrier transcytosis of insulin in developing rabbits. *Brain Res.*, **420**, 32–8.

Dziegielewska, K. M. and Saunders, N. R. (1988). The development of the blood–brain barrier: proteins in fetal and neonatal CSF, their nature and origins. In *Handbook of Human Growth and Biological Development*, ed. E. Meisami and P. S. Timiras, pp. 169–91. Boca Raton: CRC Press.

Dziegielewska, K. M., Evans, C. A. N., Malinowska, D. *et al.* (1979). Studies of the development of brain barrier systems to lipid insoluble molecules in foetal sheep. *J. Physiol.*, **292**, 207–31.

Dziegielewska, K. M., Kocsis, G. and Saunders, N. R. (1980). Identification of fetuin and other proteins in cerebrospinal fluid and plasma of fetal pigs during development. *Comp. Biochem Physiol.*, **66B**, 535–41.

Dziegielewska, K. M., Evans, C. A. N., Lai, P. C. W. *et al.* (1981). Proteins in cerebrospinal fluid and plasma of fetal rats during development. *Dev. Biol.*, **83**, 192–200.

Dziegielewska, K. M., Habgood, M. D., Møllgård, K. *et al.* (1991). Species specific transfer of plasma albumin from blood into different cerebrospinal fluid compartments in the immature fetal sheep. *J. Physiol.*, **439**, 215–37.

Dziegielewska, K. M., Knott, G. W. and Saunders, N. R. (1997). Proteins in plasma, cerebrospinal fluid and brain during postnatal development in marsupials. In *Marsupial Biology: Recent Research, New Perspectives*, ed. N. R. Saunders and L. A. Hinds, pp. 346–57. University of NSW Press.

Evans, C. A. N., Reynolds, J. M., Reynolds, M. L. *et al.* (1974). The development of a blood–brain barrier mechanism in foetal sheep. *J. Physiol.*, **238**, 371–86.

Fabian, R. H. and Hulsebosch, C. E. (1993). Plasma nerve growth factor access to the postnatal central nervous system. *Brain Res.*, **611**, 46–52.

Felgenhauer, K. (1974). Protein size and cerebrospinal fluid composition. *Klin. Wochenschr.*, **52**, 1158–64.

Ferguson, R. K. and Woodbury, D. M. (1969). Penetration of C-inulin and C-sucrose into brain, cerebrospinal fluid and skeletal muscle of developing rats. *Exp. Brain Res.*, **7**, 181–94.

Fishman, J. B., Rubin, J. B., Handrahan, J. V. *et al.* (1987). Receptor-mediated transcytosis of transferrin across the blood–brain barrier. *J. Neurosci. Res.*, **18**, 299–304.

Frank, J. H., Jankovic-Vokes, T., Pardridge, W. M. and Morris, W. L. (1985). Enhanced insulin binding to blood–brain barrier *in vivo* and to brain microvessels *in vitro* in newborn rabbits. *Diabetes*, **34**, 728–33.

Friden, P. M. (1993). Receptor-mediated transport of peptides and proteins across the blood–brain barrier. In *The Blood-Brain Barrier. Cellular and Molecular Biology*, ed. W. M. Pardridge, pp 229–47. New York: Raven Press.

Ganong, W. F. (1995). *Review of Medical Physiology*, 15th edn, pp. 754. USA: Prentice-Hall International Inc.

Habgood, M. D., Sedgwick, J. E. C., Dziegielewska, K. M. and Saunders, N. R. (1992). A developmentally regulated blood–cerebrospinal fluid transfer mechanism for albumin-immature rats. *J. Physiol.*, **456**, 181–92.

Habgood, M. D., Knott, G. W., Dziegielewska, K. M. and Saunders, N. R. (1993). The nature of the decrease in blood–CSF barrier exchange during postnatal brain development in the rat. *J. Physiol.*, **468**, 73–83.

Jacobsen, M., Møllgård, K., Reynolds, M. L. and Saunders, N. R. (1983). The choroid plexus in fetal sheep during development with special reference to intracellular plasma proteins. *Dev. Brain Res.*, **8**, 77–88.

Jefferies, W. A., Brandon, M. R., Hunt, S. V. *et al.* (1984). Transferrin receptor on endothelium of brain capillaries. *Nature*, **312**, 162–3.

Johanson, C. E. (1989). Ontogeny and phylogeny of the blood–brain barrier. In *Implications of the Blood–Brain Barrier and its Manipulation*, vol. 1, ed. E. A. Neuwelt, pp. 157–98. Plenum Publishing Corporation.

Knott, G. W. (1995). Barriers of the Developing Brain. PhD Thesis, University of Tasmania, 159 pp.

Knott, G. W., Dziegielewska, K. M., Habgood, M. D. *et al.* (1997). Albumin transfer across the choroid plexus of postnatal South American opossum (*Monodelphis domestica*). *J. Physiol.*, **499**, 179–94.

Korobkin, R. K. and Cutler, R. W. P (1977). Maturational changes of amino acid concentration in cerebrospinal fluid of the rat. *Brain Res.*, **119**, 181–7.

Lefauconnier, J.-M. (1992). Transport of amino acids. In *Physiology and Pharmacology of the Blood-Brain Barrier*, ed. M. W. B. Bradbury, pp. 117–50. Berlin: Springer Verlag.

Lefauconnier, J.-M. and Trouvé, R. (1983). Developmental changes in the pattern of amino acid transport at the blood–brain barrier in rats. *Dev. Brain Res.*, **6**, 175–82.

Lehmenkühler, A., Syková, E., Svoboda, J. *et al.* (1993). Extracellular space parameters in the rat neocortex and subcortical white matter during postnatal development determined by diffusion analysis. *Neuroscience*, **55**, 339–51.

Li, Z., Dziegielewska, K. M. and Saunders, N. R. (1997). Transthyretin distribution in the developing choroid plexus of South American opossum (*Monodelphis domestica*). *Cell Tiss. Res.*, **287**, 621–4.

Lin, H. H. and Connor, J. R. (1989). The development of the transferrin–transferrin receptor system in relation to astrocytes, MBP and galactocerebroside in normal and myelin-deficient rat optic nerves. Dev. Brain Res., **49**, 281–93.

Møllgård, K., Malinowska, D. H. and Saunders, N. R. (1976). Lack of correlation between tight junction morphology and permeability properties in developing choroid plexus. *Nature*, **264**, 293–4.

Møllgård, K., Jacobsen, M., Jacobsen, G. K. *et al.* (1979). Immunohisto-chemical evidence for an intracellular localization of plasma proteins in human foetal choroid plexus and brain. *Neurosci. Lett.*, **14**, 85–90.

Møllgård, K., Reynolds, M. L., Jacobsen, M. *et al.* (1984). Differential immuno-cytochemical staining for fetuin and transferrin in the developing cortical plate. *J. Neurocytol.*, **13**, 497–502.

Moos, T. and Møllgård, K. (1993). Cerebrovascular permeability to azo dyes and plasma proteins in rodents of different ages. *Neuropathol. Appl. Neurobiol.*, **19**, 120–7.

Reynolds, M. L., and Møllgård, K. (1985). The distribution of plasma proteins in the neocortex and early allocortex of the developing sheep brain. *Anatomy and Embryology*, **171**, 41–60.

Roberts, R., Sandra, A., Siek, G. C. *et al.* (1992). Studies of the mechanism of ion transport across the blood–brain barrier. *Ann. Neurol.*, **32**, 43–50.

Saunders, N. R. (1977). Ontogeny of the blood–brain barrier. In *The Ocular and Cerebrospinal Fluids*, ed. L. Z. Bito, H. Davson, and J. D. Fenstermacher, pp. 523–50.

Saunders, N. R. (1992). Ontogenetic development of brain barrier mechanisms. In *Physiology and Pharmacology of the Blood–Brain barrier. Handbook of Experimental Pharmacology*, vol. 103, ed. M. W. B. Bradbury, pp. 327–69. Berlin: Springer-Verlag.

Saunders, N. R. and Dziegielewska, K. M. (1997). Barriers in the developing brain. *News Physiol. Sci.*, **12**, 21–31.

Seulberger, H. and Risau, W. (1993). Molecular cloning of a blood–brain barrier cell surface glycoprotein. In *The Blood-Brain Barrier. Cellular and Molecular Biology*, ed. W. M. Pardridge, pp. 229–47. New York: Raven Press.

Skarlatos, S., Yoshikawa, T. and Pardridge, W. M. (1995). Transport of [^{125}I]transferrin through the rat blood–brain barrier. *Brain Res.*, **683**, 164–71.

Smith, D. E., Streicher, E., Milkovic, K. and Klatzo, I. (1964). Observations on the transport of proteins by the isolated choroid plexus. *Acta Neuropath.*, **3**, 372–86.

Syková, E., Jendelová, P., Simonová, Z. and Chvátal, A. (1992). K^{+} and pH homeostasis in the developing rat spinal cord is impaired by early postnatal X-irradiation. *Brain Res.*, **594**, 19–30.

Taylor, E. M. and Morgan, E. H. (1990). Developmental changes in transferrin and iron uptake by the brain in the rat. *Dev. Brain Res.*, **55**, 35–42.

Thomas, T., Power, B., Hudson, P. *et al.* (1988). The expression of transthyretin mRNA in the developing rat brain. *Dev. Biol.*, **128**, 415–27.

Wislocki, G. B. (1920). Experimental studies on fetal absorption. I. The vitality stained fetus. *Contrib. Embryol. Carnegie Insit.*, **4**, 41–52.

Woodbury, D. M. (1967). Distribution of nonelectrolytes and electrolytes in the brain as affected by alterations in cerebrospinal fluid secretion. *Prog. Brain Res.*, **29**, 294–314.

PART IV

Signal transduction/Biochemical aspects

31 Regulation of brain endothelial cell tight junction permeability

LEE L. RUBIN, LOUISE MORGAN and JAMES M. STADDON

- Introduction
- Cell culture
- Physiological assays
- Biochemistry and immunocytochemistry

Introduction

The blood–brain barrier (BBB) forms when endothelial cells (ECs) that make up brain capillaries adopt the dual features of a low rate of fluid phase endocytosis and high resistance tight junctions. Although the BBB has been studied for more than 100 years and is recognized as being important in establishing an appropriate extracellular environment for cells in the brain, there are a surprising number of fundamental uncertainties concerning the formation and regulation of this barrier. One question concerns the time of formation of the BBB, with estimates ranging, for rodent, from embryonic day 15 or so to postnatal day 14 (Mollgard and Saunders, 1986; Risau and Wolberg, 1990). Further, it is not clear whether the barrier forms all at once – becomes impermeable to proteins and ions simultaneously, or only gradually, with, perhaps, ionic impermeability being achieved after macromolecular impermeability. Another question concerns the induction of BBB formation. It is thought that ECs in brain become different from those in the periphery when exposed to factors found only in the brain environment (Stewart and Wiley, 1981). These factors, however, are still unknown. Until recently, it was thought by most investigators that astrocytes were the source of such factors (Janzer and Raff, 1987), perhaps the

only such source, but this has recently been called into question (Holash and Stewart, 1993). In addition, there have not been any studies that have shown convincingly that astrocyte-derived factors will fully convert a peripheral EC into a brain EC, at least from the perspective of tight junction resistance (see, for example, Rubin et al., 1991).

This chapter will concentrate on an aspect of the BBB that is not debatable. Brain ECs *are* coupled by tight junctions that are of extremely high electrical resistance, greater than 1000 ohm-cm^2. Understanding the molecular basis of tight junction regulation will be of fundamental importance to an understanding of how BBB permeability is regulated under normal and pathological conditions.

The molecular composition of tight junctions is in the process of being elucidated. The major tight junction membrane protein in both ECs and epithelial cells is known as occludin (Furuse et al., 1993; Ando-Akatsuka et al., 1996), and several associated cytoplasmic proteins, such as ZO-1, ZO-2, cingulin and p130, have been identified (reviewed by Staddon and Rubin, 1996). Of course, it could well be that tight junction permeability is regulated by altering levels of occludin or of cytoplasmic tight-junction proteins. This is the topic of much investigation at the current time (Balda et al., 1996; Hirase et al., 1997). Studies in the last few years using epithelial cells and ECs, however, have focused attention on two other aspects of cell–cell interaction that are essential for tight junction formation and regulation. The first is calcium-dependent cell adhesion mediated by members of the cadherin family of adhesion molecules and their cytoplasmic transducers. This was first emphasized by the experiments of Gumbiner and Simons (1986), who found that cultured epithelial cell (MDCK) tight junctions could not form if E-cadherin molecules were prevented from binding to one another (either because calcium was removed from the culture medium or because the cells were maintained in the presence of an anti-E-cadherin antibody). A few years later, it was discovered that the extracellular 'adhesion' domains of E-cadherin alone are not sufficient to mediate proper cell–cell binding and, by implication, tight junction formation (Nagafuchi and Takeichi, 1988). Rather, it is necessary for cadherins also to be able to interact with a set of cytoplasmic proteins called catenins (Ozawa et al., 1989). The cadherin–catenin association is essential for tight junction formation even though none of these molecules is part of the tight junction itself. Conceptually, then, these studies suggest that the process of tight junction formation can be thought of as being initiated by cadherin-mediated cell–cell adhesion, transduced via cytoplasmic reorganization involving the catenins and certain cytoskeletal proteins, and completed by the appearance of occludin and associated proteins at the tight junction. Further, this work suggests that tight junctions can be regulated, at least in part, by changes in cell–cell adhesion achieved via modification of the cadherin/catenin complex.

The second process that appears to be fundamentally important in tight junction regulation is signal transduction. For example, work in our laboratory several years ago showed that elevation of cyclic AMP levels in brain ECs causes a profound structural reorganization of the actin-based cytoskeleton and a striking increase in tight junction resistance (Rubin et al., 1991). More recently, we and others have identified several other cytoplasmic signalling systems that modulate tight junction resistance (e.g. Staddon et al., 1995a; Schulze et al., 1997. One of the more important involves the activity of a set of src-like tyrosine kinases that are

associated with the adherens junction complex in epithelial cells and perhaps in ECs, including those from brain, as well (Tsukita et al., 1991; see also Achen et al., 1995). When these junctional kinases are active or, more exactly, when cellular tyrosine phosphatases (which may also be junctional; Brady-Kalny et al., 1995) are inactive, tight junction resistance is decreased (Staddon et al., 1995a). At the same time, the amount of protein tyrosine phosphorylation at the junctional region increases significantly, becoming obvious when cells are labelled with an anti-phosphotyrosine antibody.

Work in our laboratory is based on the concept that tight junction properties are regulated by signal transduction. Thus, we have concentrated on identifying junctional proteins that are phosphorylated when tight junction resistance is altered by a variety of modulators. This should facilitate a molecular understanding of how tight junctions are regulated. It can be expected that, on a whole cell basis, there will be many proteins phosphorylated by individual protein kinases, and this will significantly complicate any analysis. Therefore, it would be preferable to restrict studies to examining the state of phosphorylation of proteins expected to play some role in regulating tight junctions. Naturally, this would include occludin and its associated proteins, but, based on the above discussion, must also include the adherens junction proteins. In fact, this type of analysis was carried out by Staddon et al. (1995a) to understand how tyrosine phosphorylation affects tight junction resistance. Their studies were based on the observation that mild detergent solubilization can preserve certain molecular complexes, such as epithelial cell cadherin and its associated catenins. Subsequent incubation with an antibody directed against any individual cadherin or catenin results in the isolation of all members of the complex. Experiments revealed, at first, that β-catenin becomes phosphorylated by junctional tyrosine kinases as tight junction resistance decreases and becomes de-phosphorylated when the resistance returns to control levels. Interestingly, these kinds of experiments also revealed a new member of the adherens junction complex. A molecule termed p120, known already to be a major src substrate, was shown by Staddon et al. (1995b) to be linked to E-cadherin and the classical catenins in epithelial cells and ECs. These investigators and others (Reynolds *et al.*, 1994; Shibamoto *et al.*, 1995) found that: (a) antibodies against E-cadherin, or any of the catenins, co-immunoprecipitate p120 (and a variant termed p100); (b) an antibody against p120 co-immunoprecipitates the other adherens junction proteins; (c) this src substrate is present at all epithelial and endothelial (including brain capillary) junctional contacts both *in vitro* and *in vivo*. Thus, src-like tyrosine kinases and their substrates are present at normal adherens junctions and may be major determinants of tight junction properties.

Experiments such as these require cells and techniques that are briefly reviewed in this chapter. A primary requirement for this type of study is the ability to obtain homogeneous cultures of brain ECs that form high-resistance tight junctions and are available in reasonable quantities for biochemical experiments. Also required are techniques to grow these cells under conditions in which they can be characterized physiologically and techniques – i.e. resistance and flux assays – used to ensure that the cells are brain-like when experiments begin and to determine how various pharmacological treatments affect tight junction properties. The focus of our laboratory is on using cells that are already characterized physiologically for biochemical and molecular biological studies. Highly specific antibodies against junctional proteins are required, as are the relatively standard set of procedures needed to carry out biochemical analysis of proteins phosphorylated on tyrosine or serine/threonine residues. Immunocytochemical techniques are also important in examining the distribution of particular proteins in ECs. Carrying out this type of analysis should assist ultimately in providing an understanding of how brain EC tight junctions form and are regulated under normal and pathological conditions.

Cell culture

Pig brain endothelial cells

The procedures that we currently use are based on those described by Rubin *et al.* (1991). Fresh pig brains are dissected free of meninges, cortical tissue (both grey and white matter) is collected, roughly chopped and homogenized in a Dounce tissue grinder. Microvessel fragments are collected by filtration, briefly digested with trypsin and collagenase, and plated in tissue culture dishes coated with collagen and fibronectin. Microvessel fragments attach to the culture substrate in 2 h, and ECs migrate from the fragments and proliferate over the following few days. Plating medium consists of 45% DMEM with 5% plasma derived serum, 50% astrocyte conditioned medium (ACM; see below) and 125 µg/ml heparin. After 6 days, cells are passaged and plated on 0.4 µm collagen-coated polycarbonate Transwells (Costar) at a density of 36 000 cells/cm^2 in the same medium. Typically, after 4 days on Transwells, the medium is changed to 50% ACM, 50% defined medium supplemented with 250 µM 8-(4-chlorophenylthio) adenosine $3':5'$-cyclic monophosphate and 35 µM Ro20–1724 (an inhibitor of type IV phosphodiesterase). Elevation of cyclic AMP levels in brain ECs causes them to achieve much higher electrical resistance (Rubin *et al.*, 1991).

Astrocyte-conditioned medium

Cultures of astrocytes that are over 95% pure are prepared from 1-day-old rat cortex, essentially as described by Lillien and co-workers (1988). Conditioned medium (DMEM containing 10% plasma derived serum) is collected every 2 days from confluent cultures.

Physiological assays

Transcellular electrical resistance (TER) across EC monolayers is determined using an EVOM resistance system available from World Precision Instruments. Resistance values are expressed in ohm-cm^2 following subtraction of the resistance of a cell-free filter. To measure paracellular flux, tracers of varying sizes – radioactive or fluorescent – are added to the apical (upper) chamber, and the culture is gently agitated on an orbital shaker in a 37 °C incubator. Samples are taken from the basal (lower) chamber at various times and rates of flux calculated.

Biochemistry and immunocytochemistry

General considerations

As already stated, our laboratory is particularly interested in the role of signal transduction and protein phosphorylation in modulating brain EC tight junction permeability. Much of our work has involved analysis of junctional proteins phosphorylated on tyrosine residues. However, it should be recognized that proteins are phosphorylated more abundantly on serine and threonine residues. Serine/threonine kinases, therefore, are also likely to be important in regulating brain EC properties. Our general approach is to characterize first the response of cultured brain ECs to particular physiological modulators using electrical resistance and flux assays. These characterized cells are then examined by immunocytochemical and biochemical procedures using specific antibodies, generated by us or commercially available, against various junctional proteins. Immunocytochemistry provides information concerning changes in distribution of particular proteins, while biochemical assays provide information as to amounts, solubility (association with the cytoskeleton), and phosphorylation of these proteins.

Analysis of protein tyrosine phosphorylation

A. Immunocytochemistry
Tyrosine phosphorylated proteins can be revealed by direct immunostaining of cultured cells or tissue sections with antibodies specific for phosphotyrosine (see Maher and Pasquale, 1988). We have mainly used the mouse monoclonal antibodies 4G10 and PY20, although rabbit antisera are also available. Cells, usually on Transwell filters, are fixed in 3% paraformaldehyde made up in PBS containing 0.5 mM $CaCl_2$ and 0.5 mM $MgSO_4$. After 15 min incubation at room temperature, the cells are washed and then permeabilized by incubation for 10 min with 0.5% Triton X-100 in PBS. After washing, the cells are blocked by incubation for 30 min in PBS containing 10% calf serum plus 0.1 M lysine, pH 7.4. Incubation with primary antibody is in PBS containing 10% calf serum for

either 1 h at room temperature or overnight at 4 °C. After washing, the cells are then incubated for 30–60 min at room temperature with an FITC-conjugated goat anti-mouse antibody, in PBS containing 10% calf serum. When required, rhodamine-labelled phalloidin is included with the secondary antibody to label filamentous actin and provide information concerning the integrity of the cell monolayer and cell–cell junctions. After another washing step, the filters are mounted and viewed with a fluorescence microscope. Specificity of staining can be verified by competition for antibody with exogenous phosphorylated tyrosine, serine or threonine. It is often preferable to co-label cells with antibodies against components of known structures, such as cell–cell junctions, (catenins or ZO-1; Rubin et al., 1991; Staddon et al. 1995a), or focal contacts, (vinculin or paxillin; Schulze et al., 1997).

B. Biochemistry

(I) STRATEGIC CONSIDERATIONS A positive effect on staining – for instance, an increase in junctional phosphotyrosine following treatment of cells with particular physiologically active agents – is good motivation to analyze proteins biochemically. However, it should be noted that false-negatives can be obtained, meaning that the phosphotyrosine antibodies do not recognize all tyrosine phosphorylated proteins. A possible next step is to analyze changes in tyrosine phosphorylation of proteins in whole cell lysates. This gives some idea of how many proteins are phosphorylated following a particular manipulation, but it is not really useful in terms of analyzing individual proteins. One obvious reason for this limitation is that an individual protein of interest may not be abundant enough to analyze in this way. Instead, because we have been particularly interested in proteins at adherens and tight junctions, we have analyzed proteins immunoprecipitated with specific antibodies.

(II) SOLUBILIZATION To examine the level of tyrosine phosphorylation of individual proteins, immunoprecipitation with a phosphotyrosine antibody followed by protein-specific blotting can be performed. Or, reciprocally, protein-specific immunoprecipitation followed by phosphotyrosine blotting should provide similar information. Steps

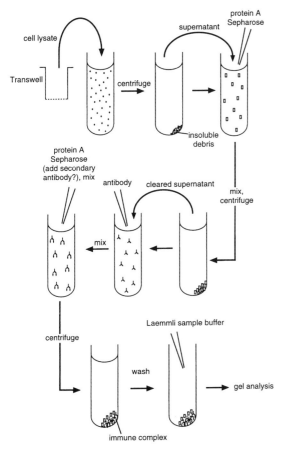

Fig. 31.1. Immunoprecipitation analysis. Cultured cells are lysed at 4 °C in appropriate detergent-containing buffer (except that lysis buffers containing SDS as the only detergent are used hot). The following steps are all at 4 °C. The lysate is collected and transferred to an Eppendorf tube. Insoluble debris is removed by centrifugation and the supernatant is incubated with protein A Sepharose to remove proteins that non-specifically bind to this matrix. Primary antibody is added to the cleared supernatant, and this is mixed (typically head-over-end) for 1 h. Protein A Sepharose is then added to capture the antibody–antigen complex. Rabbit antibodies bind avidly to protein A Sepharose, but, generally, rat and mouse antibodies do not. Rabbit anti-mouse or rat secondary antibodies can be used prior to incubation with protein A Sepharose, or, alternatively, protein G Sepharose can be used (see Harlow and Lane, 1988). After 30–60 min incubation, the Sepharose beads are pelleted by brief centrifugation, washed five times with lysis buffer and, then, immunoprecipitated proteins are eluted with a small volume of Laemmli sample buffer. Proteins are analyzed by gel electrophoresis followed by procedures such as immunoblotting or autoradiography.

involved in a typical immunoprecipitation are depicted in Fig. 31.1. However, many of the proteins that we are interested in exist as complexes with other proteins, which can confuse interpretation.

Consider three proteins, A, B and C of different molecular mass, but associated with one another (see Fig. 31.2). When cells are solubilized under non-denaturing detergent conditions, if A is tyrosine phosphorylated, phosphotyrosine immunoprecipitates will contain A, because of direct recognition by antibody, and also, potentially, B and C by virtue of their association with A, which would be misleading. The reciprocal experiment is more clear-cut. If A is immunoprecipitated, B and C will also appear in the immune complex, but immunoblotting with phosphotyrosine antibody will reveal increased labelling of only A. To overcome these ambiguities, cells can be lysed under denaturing conditions, for example hot SDS, followed by dilution of the lysate into a non-denaturing buffer containing Triton X-100. In this manner, protein complexes are dissociated prior to immunoprecipitation. In general, we have found phosphotyrosine immunoprecipitation followed by protein-specific blotting to be a fairly sensitive method to reveal changes in the amount of phosphorylation of junctional proteins. This can also give some indication of stoichiometry of phosphorylation – the amount of a protein immunoprecipitable with a phosphotyrosine antibody can be compared with the total amount of that protein that is immunoprecipitable. The use of different detergents that we have used to investigate protein phosphorylation is described in the legend to Fig. 31.2.

(III) PROTEIN ANALYSIS Whole cell lysates are prepared by rapidly replacing the culture medium with SDS sample buffer (Laemmli, 1970) followed by heating at 100 °C for 5 min. The 6.5 mm Transwell filters can be conveniently inserted into an Eppendorf tube and heated on a hot block *in situ*. To collect the cell extract quantitatively, the filter, still in the tube, is ripped using a needle and then briefly centrifuged in the Eppendorf tube. Cell extracts or immunoprecipitates in SDS sample buffer are resolved by SDS-PAGE (Laemmli, 1970). Prior to transfer, the slab gels are equilibrated in buffer containing: 48 mM Tris, 39 mM

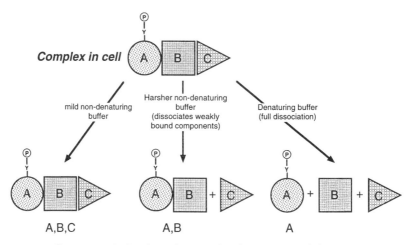

Components in phosphotyrosine immunoprecipitate

Fig. 31.2. Analysis of protein complexes. Adherens junction and tight junction proteins exist as complexes. Schematically shown is what happens when only one protein in a complex of proteins is tyrosine phosphorylated and is subject to immunoprecipitation with phosphotyrosine antibodies. Mild non-denaturing detergents include Triton X-100 and NP-40. Harsher non-denaturing conditions are based on those found in RIPA buffer and might include a mixture of Triton X-100, deoxycholate and SDS at ratios such as 5:2.5:1. Denaturing buffers typically contain only SDS and are heated at 100 °C for 5 min. DNA in these samples makes them viscous, but it can easily be sheared using a 23 G needle. For immunoprecipitation, the SDS must first be diluted into a buffer containing excess Triton X-100. For specific details of buffer composition and procedures, the reader is referred to Gumbiner *et al.* (1991) and Staddon *et al.* (1995*a*,*b*).

glycine, 20% methanol and 0.03% SDS. Proteins are transferred to nitrocellulose filters, stained in Ponceau S, and then blocked in 5% non-fat dried milk in PBS. After being washed in PBS containing 0.05% Tween-20, the filters are probed with primary antibody as required. After washing, antibody is reacted with appropriate horseradish peroxidase-conjugated secondary antibody. The filters are then extensively washed and immunoreactive bands detected by enhanced chemiluminescence.

Analysis of protein serine/threonine phosphorylation

Serine and threonine phosphorylation is also important. Usually, cells are [^{32}P]phosphate-labelled and subject to protein analysis (for example, see Staddon *et al.*, 1990; Meisenhelder and Hunter, 1991; Goeckeler and Wysolmerski, 1995). The phosphoamino acid content of protein can be analyzed by subsequent limited acid hydrolysis fol-

lowed by high voltage electrophoretic separation (Van der Geer and Hunter, 1994). Antibodies recognizing phosphoserine and phosphothreonine are commercially available. These have not been widely evaluated but would permit an isotope-free approach.

Another elegant method to investigate protein phosphorylation exploits the use of phosphopeptide-directed antibodies (for example, see Ginty *et al.*, 1993; Coghlan *et al.*, 1994). A prerequisite is the analysis of phosphorylation sites in the protein of interest. Corresponding phosphopeptides are synthesized and antisera that recognize the phosphorylated, but not the non-phosphorylated, epitope raised. Whereas phosphotyrosine antibodies, in general, recognize phosphotyrosine in protein regardless of sequence, the phosphopeptide-directed antibodies are sequence-specific. This approach allows protein analysis at the cellular or protein level.

References

Achen, M. G., Clauss, M., Schnürch, H. and Risau, W. (1995). The non-receptor tyrosine kinase lyn is localised in the developing murine blood–brain barrier. *Differentiation*, **59**, 15–24.

Ando-Akatsuka, Y., Saitou, M., Hirase, T. *et al.* (1996). Interspecies diversity of the occludin sequence: cDNA cloning of human, mouse, dog, and rat-kangaroo homologues. *J. Cell Biol.*, **133**, 43–7.

Balda, M. S., Whitney, J. A., Flores, C. *et al.* (1996). Functional dissociation of paracellular permeability and transepithelial electrical resistance and disruption of the apical-basolateral intramembrane diffusion barrier by expression of a mutant tight junction membrane protein. *J. Cell Biol.*, **134**, 1031–49.

Brady-Kalnay, S.M., Rimm, D. L. and Tonks, N. K. (1995). Receptor protein tryosine phosphatase PTPμ associates with cadherins and catenins *in vivo*. *J. Cell Biol.*, **130**, 977–86.

Coghlan, M. P., Pillay, T. S., Tavare, J. M. and Siddle, K. (1994). Site-specific anti-phosphopeptide antibodies: use in assessing insulin receptor serine/threonine phophorylation state and identification of serine-1327 as a novel site of phorbol ester-induced phosphorylation. *Biochem. J.*, **303**, 893–9.

Furuse, M., Hirase, T., Itoh, M. *et al.* (1993). Occludin: a novel integral membrane protein localizing at tight junctions. *J. Cell Biol.*, **123**, 1777–88.

Ginty, D. D., Kornhauser, J. M., Thompson, M. A. *et al.* (1993). Regulation of CREB phosphorylation in the suprachiasmatic nucleus by light and a circadian clock. *Science*, **260**, 238–41.

Goeckeler, Z. M. and Wysolmerski, R. B. (1995). Myosin light chain kinase-regulated endothelial cell contraction: the relationship between isometric tension, actin polymerization, and myosin phosphorylation. *J. Cell Biol.*, **130**, 613–27.

Gumbiner, B. and Simons, K. (1986). A functional assay for proteins involved in establishing an epithelial occluding barrier: identification of a uvomorulin-like polypeptide. *J. Cell Biol.*, **102**, 457–68.

Gumbiner, B., Lowenkopf, T., and Apatira, D. (1991). Identification of a 160-kDa polypeptide that binds to the tight junction protein ZO-1. *Proc. Natl. Acad. Sci. USA*, **88**, 3460–4.

Harlow, E. and Lane, D. (1988). *Antibodies: a Laboratory Manual*. Cold Spring Harbour Laboratory.

Hirase, T., Staddon, J.M., Saitou, M. *et al.* (1997). Occludin as a possible determinant of tight junction permeability in endothelial cells. *J. Cell Sci.*, **110**, 1603–13.

Holash, J. A. and Stewart, P. A. (1993). Chorioallantoic membrane (CAM) vessels do not respond to blood–brain barrier (BBB) induction. *Adv. Exp. Med. Biol.*, **331**, 223–8.

Janzer, R. C. and Raff, M.C. (1987). Astrocytes induce blood–brain barrier properties in endothelial cells. *Nature*, **325**, 253–7.

Laemmli, U. K. (1970). Cleavage of structural proteins during the assembly of the head of bacteriophage T4. *Nature*, **227**, 680–85.

Lillien, L. E., Sendtner, M., Rohrer, H. *et al.* (1988). Type-2 astrocyte development in rat brain cultures is initiated by a CNTF-like protein produced by type-1 astrocytes. *Neuron*, **1**, 485–94.

Maher, P. A. and Pasquale, E. B. (1988). Tyrosine phosphorylated tissues in different tissues during chick embryo development. *J. Cell Biol.*, **106**, 1747–55.

Meisenhelder, J. and Hunter, T. (1991). Phosphorylation of phospholipase C *in vivo* and *in vitro*. In *Methods in Enzymology*, Vol. 197, ed E. A. Dennis, pp. 288–305. San Diego, New York, Boston, London, Sydney, Tokyo, Toronto: Academic Press, Inc.

Mollgard, K. and Saunders, N. R. (1986). The development of the human blood–brain and blood–CSF barriers. *Neuropathol. Appl. Neurobiol.*, **12**, 337–58.

Nagafuchi, A. and Takeichi, M. (1988). Cell binding function of E-cadherin is regulated by the cytoplasmic domain. *EMBO J.*, **7**, 3679–84.

Ozawa, M., Baribault, H. and Kemler, R. (1989). The cytoplasmic domain of the cell adhesion molecule uvomorulin associates with three independent proteins structurally related in different species. *EMBO J.*, **8**, 1711–7.

Reynolds, A. B., Daniel, J., McCrea, P. *et al.* (1994). Identification of a new catenin: the tyrosine kinase substrate p120^{cas} associates with E-cadherin complexes. *Mol. Cell. Biol.*, **14**, 8333–42.

Risau, W. and Wolburg, H. (1990). Development of the blood–brain barrier. *Trends Neurosci.*, **13,** 174–8.

Rubin, L. L., Hall, D. E., Porter, S. *et al.* (1991). A cell culture model of the blood–brain barrier. *J. Cell Biol.*, **115**, 1725–35.

Schulze, C., Smales, C., Rubin, L. L. and Staddon, J. M. (1997). Lysophosphatidic acid increases tight junction permeability in cultured brain endothelial cells. *J. Neurochem.*, **68**, 991–1000.

Shibamoto, S., Hayakawa, M., Takeuchi, K. *et al.* (1995). Association of p120, a tyrosine kinase substrate, with E-cadherin/catenin complexes. *J. Cell Biol.*, **128**, 949–57.

Staddon, J. M. and Rubin, L. L. (1996). Cell adhesion, cell junctions and the blood–brain barrier. *Curr. Opin. Neurobiol.*, **6**, 622–7.

Staddon, J. M., Chanter, N., Lax A. J. *et al.* (1990). *Pasteurella multocida* toxin, a potent mitogen, stimulates protein kinase C-dependent and -independent protein phosphorylation in Swiss 3T3 cells. *J. Biol. Chem.*, **265**, 11841–8.

Staddon, J. M., Herrenknecht, K., Smales, C. and Rubin, L. L. (1995a). Evidence that tyrosine phosphorylation may increase tight junction permeability. *J. Cell Sci.*, **108**, 609–19.

Staddon, J. M., Smales, C., Schulze, C. *et al.* (1995b). p120, a p120-related protein (p100) and the cadherin/catenin complex. *J. Cell Biol.*, **130**, 369–81.

Stewart, P. A. and Wiley, M. J. (1981). Developing nervous tissue induces formation of blood–brain barrier characteristics in invading endothelial cells: a study using quail-chick transplantation chimeras. *Dev. Biol.*, **84**, 183–92.

Tsukita, S., Oishi, K., Akiyama, T. *et al.* (1991). Specific proto-oncogenic tyrosine kinases of src family are enriched in cell-to-cell adherens junction where the level of tyrosine phosphorylation is elevated. *J. Cell Biol.*, **113**, 867–79.

Van der Geer, P. and Hunter, T. (1994).
Phosphopeptide mapping and
phosphoamino acid analysis by
electrophoresis and chromatography on
thin-layer cellulose plates. *Electrophoresis*,
15, 544–54.

Zhong, Y., Saitoh, T., Minase, T. *et al.*
(1993). Monoclonal antibody 7H6 reacts
with a novel tight-junction associated
protein distinct from ZO-1, cingulin and
ZO-2. *J. Cell Biol.*, **120**, 477–83.

32 Chemotherapy and chemosensitization

R. BÉLIVEAU, M. DEMEULE, E. BEAULIEU and L. JETTÉ

- Chemotherapy for brain tumors
- Multidrug resistance
- Chemosensitization
- New approaches

Chemotherapy for brain tumors

Brain tumors are the second and fourth leading causes of cancer mortality in children and in young adults between the age of 15 and 34 respectively. Clinical progress in the treatment of these malignancies has been slow. Surgery is difficult because tumor cells infiltrate into surrounding brain, making complete resection impossible. Physical localization of the tumor in deep cortex or in highly functional areas is also a problem. Radiotherapy is limited by low brain tolerance and by the infiltration of tumor cells into normal brain. Adjuvant chemotherapy is thus essential to the treatment of some types of brain tumors. Response to chemotherapy depends on the concentration of drugs reaching the tumor, blood flow inside the tumor, inherent or acquired drug resistance of the cancer and integrity of the blood–brain barrier (BBB).

The role of the BBB in resistance to chemotherapy of brain tumors remains unclear and controversial (Tomita, 1991; Lesser and Grossman, 1993; Stewart, 1994; Conrad *et al.*, 1995). The main argument in favor of an active role is the fact that most chemotherapeutic agents achieve only low concentrations in the brain and that lipophilic agents crossing the BBB are those producing an increase, although modest, in median survival of

patients. The main argument suggesting a lack of involvement of the BBB in the failure of chemotherapy is the disruption of the barrier in brain tumors. The level of disruption varies according to the tumor type; vessels in glial tumors are non-fenestrated, while non-glial and metastatic tumors are fenestrated (Shibata, 1989). The ambiguity becomes even stronger when the concept of the brain-adjacent tumor (BAT) is considered. These peripheral tumor cells invading the normal brain tissue have an intact BBB with a low permeability to anticancer drugs. The inefficiency of the treatment would then come from the survival of these cancer cells. Finally, brain tumor cells have been shown to have a low mitotic index, making them less susceptible to anticancer agents that kill actively dividing cells. The resistance to treatment would then be independent of the BBB, but inherent to the tumor cells.

Factors responsible for clinical drug resistance are either pharmacological or cellular. The pharmacological factors are those related to drug exposure. They depend on drug concentration, time of exposure, vascular access, blood flow and hypoxia, which reduces the action of certain drugs. Cellular factors include: (1) increased repair of DNA; (2) inactivation or reduced activation of the drugs; (3) reduction in the affinity of the target enzyme; (4) alteration of drug transport across the membrane. Biochemical properties of the drugs that affect their access to the brain compartment were identified: lipid solubility, low molecular size, weak ionization in plasma, poor protein binding and the presence or absence of a specific transport system (Brecher, 1994; Abbott and Romero, 1996).

Primary tumors

The nitrosoureas (BCNU, CCNU and methyl-CCNU), which are widely used against brain tumors, are cell-cycle-nonspecific alkylating agents and their main toxicity is due to cross-linking of DNA (Brecher, 1994). These lipid-soluble agents, which readily penetrate the CNS, were initially used to treat malignant gliomas. Results obtained in patients with these brain tumors treated with BCNU remain controversial (Conrad et al., 1995). A modest prolongation in median survival was observed in patients receiving BCNU after surgery and radiation (50 weeks) compared to patients receiving surgery and radiation (40 weeks). The use of antibiotic cell-cycle-specific agents that prevent DNA transcription and replication (adriamycin, daunomycin, bleomycin and actinomycin D) has been limited since these agents penetrate the CNS poorly (Brecher, 1994). The anti-mitotic agent vincristine in combination with other alkylating agents including lomustine (CCNU) and the water-soluble procarbazine (PCV regimen) had no effect on the median survival of patients with glioblastomas but increased that of patients with anaplastic astrocytomas (151 weeks) when compared with BCNU (81 weeks) (Levin et al., 1990). Oligodendrogliomas, uncommom glial tumors in young adults, also present some sensitivity to the PCV regimen. Other drugs such as methotrexate, the epipodophyllotoxins (VP-16 and VM-26), platinum derivatives (cisplastin or carboplatin) and the inhibitor of thymidylate synthetase, 5-fluorouracil, when administered alone or in combination, gave disappointing results (Mousseau, 1994) and are very little used. Treatment of low-grade astrocytomas and ependymomas usually consists of surgical resection followed sometimes by limited radiotherapy. Chemotherapy for these tumors has only a limited role in the treatment of patients with recurrent disease and may include different agents. Beneficial effects of adjuvant chemotherapy in

patients with medulloblastoma, the most common CNS malignancy in childhood, are not yet clear. No improvement in survival of patients with this disease treated with chemotherapy was observed in many studies. However, improved 5- and 10-year survivals were observed in patients treated with adjuvant vincristine and lomustine for 1 year following resection and radiation (Lesser and Grossman, 1993). Tumors of the pineal region, which include a heterogeneous group of tumors, showed modest sensitivity to a variety of agents. Recently, promising new drugs have entered clinical trials for malignant gliomas (Conrad et al., 1995). These drugs include: (1) temozolomide, with which partial responses (40–50%) were reported for patients with newly diagnosed and recurrent high-grade astrocytomas, (2) topotecan, a topoisomerase I inhibitor, and (3) taxol.

Metastatic tumors

Cancer cells forming brain metastases originate mostly from lung or breast cancers, colorectal carcinoma, melanoma and urinary organ tumors. These metastases, which often occur after primary chemotherapic treatment or radiotherapy, are more chemo-resistant. The fact that some of these primary solid tumors are very refractory to chemotherapy may explain why brain metastases of these tumors are insensitive to antitumor drugs. It was suggested that chemotherapy for brain metastases could be effective only if it was effective for systemic tumors, since brain metastases originating from small cell lung carcinomas and germ cells respond with similar rates to metastases at other sites (Buckner, 1991). However, in spite of the fact that an objective response of 45% was obtained for patients with brain metastases from small cell lung carcinomas treated with a combination of multidrug chemotherapy and radiotherapy, only a small gain in the median survival was observed with this therapy (Cumin et al., 1995). In addition, BCNU used in combination with teniposide (VM-26) against brain metastases was shown to be poorly effective, regardless of their origin, with a median survival time of 14.6 weeks for the whole group (Grau et al., 1994). Since patients with brain metastases from extracerebral origin usually die of systemic disease rather than from cerebral disease, it is still not clear to what extent the shutdown of the BBB may have a significant beneficial impact for these patients receiving chemotherapy.

Multidrug resistance

Mechanisms by which the cells become resistant to multiple anti-neoplastic agents include the multidrug resistance (MDR) phenotype, overexpression of glutathione-S-transferase and alteration of topoisomerase I or II activity. P-glycoprotein (P-gp) is associated with MDR and was previously shown to be highly expressed in normal brain capillaries (Beaulieu *et al.*, 1995; Jetté *et al.*, 1995). It could limit the efficiency of chemotherapy by two mechanisms. P-gp in the BBB may restrict the entry of drugs by pumping them out of the brain or by expulsing them out of the tumor cells, thus preventing them from reaching cytotoxic concentrations (Henson *et al.*, 1992). Neutralization of this mechanism of resistance in surrounding tumor-infiltrated brain and in disseminated tumor cells with normal BBB may be very helpful in increasing the exposure of primary brain tumors and metastases to chemotherapeutic agents.

Immunohistochemical studies suggested that P-gp is mainly localized on luminal membranes of the normal and tumoral vascular endothelium of the brain (Cordon-Cardo *et al.*, 1989; Tanaka *et al.*, 1994). The isolation of luminal membranes with

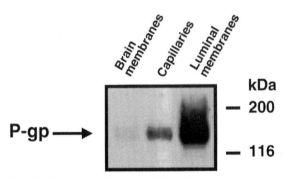

Fig. 32.1. Immunodetection of P-gp in brain membranes. After solubilization, proteins from whole brain membranes (30 µg), brain capillaries (3 µg) and luminal membranes isolated from the brain endothelium (3 µg) were separated by SDS-PAGE. Immunodetection of P-gp was performed by Western blotting with monoclonal antibody C219.

electron dense silica-polyanion (Jacobson *et al.*, 1992) confirmed that P-gp is localized at this site (Fig. 32.1). Western blot detection showed that P-gp is enriched 17-fold in the luminal membranes compared to isolated brain capillaries (Beaulieu *et al.*, 1997). The expression of P-gp on the luminal side of the BBB capillaries suggests that P-gp is responsible for the low penetration of some drugs like vinblastine and ivermectin through this barrier (Schinkel *et al.*, 1994).

Chemosensitization

Blocking P-gp function at the BBB could enhance the concentration of chemotherapeutic drugs into the cerebral compartment and increase the sensitivity of brain tumors to anticancer drugs (Fig. 32.2). Pharmacological agents that enhance the intracellular concentration of chemotherapeutic drugs and restore the sensitivity of cancer cells, whether they interact directly or not with P-gp, have been termed chemosensitizers or resistance modifying agents (RMA). They include calcium channel blockers (verapamil, diltiazem, nifedipine), calmodulin antagonists (trifluoperazine), cardiovascular drugs (dipyridamole, quinidine), steroidal agents (tamoxifen, progesterone, megestrol acetate), antibiotics (erythromycin), antimalarials (quinine, quinacrine), immunomodulators and their derivatives (cyclosporin A, FK-506, SDZ PSC-833), synthetic peptides (SDZ 280–446), retinoids, monoclonal antibodies (MRK-16, UIC-2), and many other compounds (Lum *et al.*, 1993). Recent studies tend to focus on the search for very potent chemosensitizers, which are less toxic and alter specifically and efficiently P-gp activity without affecting other physiological functions.

The interaction of some RMA with P-gp expressed at the BBB sites has been studied in cultured brain capillary endothelial cells (BCEC) and isolated brain capillaries. Agents such as verapamil, diltiazem, quinidine, testosterone, progesterone and cyclosporin A are able to enhance the uptake of vincristine or the accumulation of rhodamine-123 in BCEC (Hegmann *et al.*, 1992; Tsuji *et al.*, 1992). Furthermore, basal to apical transport of vincristine and some peptides could be blocked by verapamil (Tatsuta *et al.*, 1992;

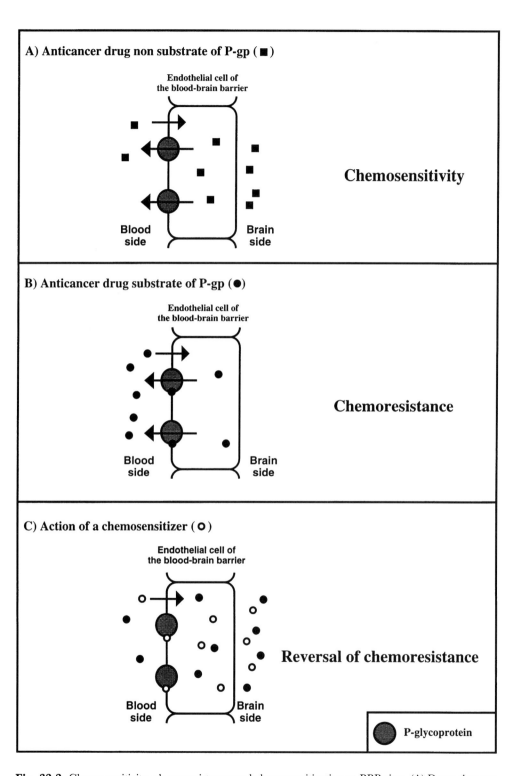

Fig. 32.2. Chemosensitivity, chemoresistance and chemosensitization at BBB sites. (A) Drugs that are not P-gp substrates can accumulate into the brain compartment. (B) Anticancer drugs that are P-gp substrates are actively extruded out of the endothelial cells and back into the blood compartment. (C) Pharmacological blockade of P-gp function by a chemosensitizer allows the penetration of chemotherapeutic drugs through the endothelial cells and their accumulation into the brain compartment.

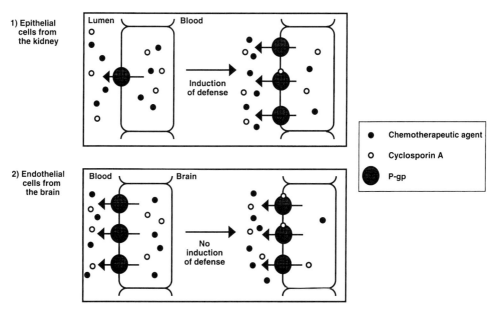

Fig. 32.3. Interaction of the chemosensitizer cyclosporin A with P-gp expressed in the kidney and at BBB sites. *In vivo* experiments have demonstrated that daily administration of cyclosporin A to rats results in an increased level of P-gp expression in normal tissues such as kidney and liver. However, P-gp expression in BBB is not increased by CsA administration. The high density of P-gp expressed in the luminal membrane of brain endothelial cells allows very few molecules of cyclosporin A or chemotherapeutic agents to accumulate into the brain compartment.

Chikhale *et al.*, 1995). P-gp expressed in BCEC also transports cyclosporin A and this uptake is modified by verapamil, quinidine and steroidal hormones (Tsuji *et al.*, 1993; Sakata *et al.*, 1994). Photoaffinity labeling studies performed with isolated brain capillaries have shown that P-gp can be labeled with $[^{125}I]$-arylazidoprazosin or a $[^3H]$-azido-cyclosporin derivative. This labeling is inhibited in the presence of reserpine, verapamil, quinidine, cyclosporin A and SDZ PSC-833 (Jetté *et al.*, 1995). In agreement with results obtained with cancer cell lines, SDZ PSC-833 was the most potent RMA among those tested (Gavériaux *et al.*, 1991).

In vivo experiments have demonstrated that daily administration of cyclosporin A to rats results in an increased level of P-gp expression in normal tissues such as kidney and liver, but not in brain capillaries (Fig. 32.3) (Jetté *et al.*, 1995, 1996). From these observations, it seems that P-gp could act as a mechanism of protection that is induced when the cells encounter cytotoxic compounds. The lack of induction in brain capillaries could be due to

the already high endogenous level of expression and the luminal localization of P-gp in this tissue (Beaulieu *et al.*, 1997). This hypothesis is supported by the fact that cyclosporin A, when co-administered, modifies doxorubicin distribution in many mouse tissues except brain (Colombo *et al.*, 1994). SDZ PSC-833, a non-immunosuppressive analog of cyclosporin which is already being tested in clinical trials as a RMA, presents a higher affinity than CsA for P-gp (Gavériaux *et al.*, 1991) and has a higher brain penetration compared to cyclosporin A (Lemaire *et al.*, 1996). P-gp conformation also appears to be modified following exposure of resistant cells to SDZ PSC-833, since the binding of a specific antibody to P-gp is altered (Jachez *et al.*, 1994). P-gp exists as a dimer in brain capillaries and RMA such as CsA or SDZ PSC-833 do not alter its oligomeric state (Jetté *et al.*, 1997).

Pre-administration of SDZ PSC-833 to rats increases the passage of cyclosporin A into the brain whereas the latter compound does not modify that of SDZ PSC-833 (Lemaire *et al.*, 1996). SDZ PSC-833 was first thought to be not transported by P-gp (Archinalmattheis *et al.*, 1995). However, a more recent study has proposed SDZ PSC-833 as a P-gp substrate at the BBB site (Lemaire *et al.*, 1996). Administration of SDZ PSC-833 also leads to hypersensitivity to cyclosporin A and ivermectin, and to alterations of CNS functions (Didier and Loor, 1995). Daily administration of SDZ PSC-833 to rats results in an increased level of P-gp in brain capillaries. However, the induced P-gp was not functional since it was unable to bind drugs (Jetté *et al.*, 1998). This is clearly distinct from the P-gp induction by CsA observed in other tissues, where P-gp remained functional. Thus, distinct RMA, even if they are structurally related, may affect P-gp function by different mechanisms, and their potency may vary in function of the targeted tissue or tumor. Distinct RMA, even if they are structurally related, may affect P-gp function by different mechanisms, and their potency may vary in function of the targeted tissue or tumor. It also re-emphasizes the need to study the interactions of new potential chemosensitizers with P-gp expressed at the BBB sites.

New approaches

Different approaches (Tomita, 1991; Inamura *et al.*, 1994; Lesser and Grossman, 1994; Conrad *et al.*, 1995) have been used to increase CNS penetration of drugs normally shut out by the BBB: (1) continous infusion of combined water-soluble and lipid-soluble chemotherapeutic agents with different toxicity profiles; (2) intra-arterial chemotherapy or high-dose intravenous chemotherapy followed by bone marrow transplantation, which showed similar survival rates as conventional chemotherapy; (3) intracavitary or interstitial chemotherapy using different approaches among which the release of highly concentrated agents impregnated on biodegradable polymers may be promising; (4) BBB disruption by osmotic agents in combination with chemotherapy. In this kind of approach, a new bradykinin analog (RMP-7) was shown to selectively increase permeability of tumor capillaries to methotrexate and leave normal capillaries intact in rats; (5) Chemo-biotherapy, which combines cytokines such as interferons and more traditional chemotherapeutic agents.

Conventional chemotherapeutic approaches, although useful in some cases to reduce radiotherapy doses for example, still give modest results in terms of response rate and median survival. The main causes of failure are related to drug delivery and drug resistance. In addition to what was described above, two other proteins, MRP (multidrug resistance associated protein) and LRP (lung resistance protein), have recently been reported to be expressed in different tissues and are involved in multidrug resistance (Flens *et al.*, 1996; Izquierdo *et al.*, 1996). These two proteins may also be important for chemo-resistance of brain metastases from solid tumors. MRP appears to be especially involved in gliomas, where its mRNA levels correlate with resistance to etoposide, adriamycin and vincristine (Abe *et al.*, 1994). It is only through the understanding of the molecular aspects of the phenomena involved in drug delivery and drug resistance that more efficient clinical treatments of brain tumors can be envisioned.

References

Abbott, N. J. and Romero, I. (1996). Transporting therapeutics across the blood–brain barrier. *Mol. Med. Today*, 106–13.

Abe, T., Hasegawa, S., Taniguchi, K., *et al.* (1994). Possible involvement of multidrug-resistance-associated protein (MRP) gene expression in spontaneous drug resistance to vincristine, etoposide and adriamycin in human glioma cells. *Int. J. Cancer*, **58**, 860–4.

Archinalmattheis, A., Rzepka, R. W., Watanabe, T. *et al.* (1995). Analysis of the interactions of SDZ PSC 833 ([3′-keto-bmt1]-val2]-cyclosporin), a multidrug resistance modulator, with P-glycoprotein. *Oncol. Res.*, **7**, 603–10.

Beaulieu, E., Demeule, M., Pouliot, J.-F. *et al.* (1995). P-glycoprotein of blood brain barrier: cross-reactivity of MAb C219 with a 190-kDa protein in bovine and rat isolated brain capillaries. *Biochim. Biophys. Acta*, **1233**, 27–32.

Beaulieu, É., Demeule, M., Ghitescu, L. and Béliveau, R. (1997). P-glycoprotein is strongly expressed in the luminal membranes of the endothelium of blood vessels in the brain. *Biochem. J.*, **326**, 301–7.

Brecher, M. S. (1994). Principles of chemotherapy. In *Brain Tumors in Children: Principles of Diagnosis and Treatment*, 2nd edn, ed. M. E. Cohen and P. K. Duffner, pp. 117–46. New York: Raven Press.

Buckner, J. C. (1991). The role of chemotherapy in the treatment of patients with brain metastases from solid tumors. *Cancer Metast. Rev.*, **10**, 335–41.

Chikhale, E. G., Burton, P. S. and Borchardt, R. T. (1995). The effect of verapamil on the transport of peptides across the blood–brain barrier in rats: kinetic evidence for an apically polarized efflux mechanism. *J. Pharmacol. Exp. Ther.*, **273**, 298–303.

Colombo, T., Zucchetti, M. and Dincalci, M. (1994). Cyclosporine-A markedly changes the distribution of doxorubicin in mice and rats. *J. Pharmacol. Exp. Ther.*, **269**, 22–7.

Conrad, C. A., Milosavljevic, V. P. and Yung, W. K. (1995). Advances in chemotherapy for brain tumors. *Neurol. Clin.*, **13**, 795–812.

Cordon-Cardo, C., O'Brien, J. P., Casals *et al.* (1989). Multidrug-resistance gene (P-glycoprotein) is expressed by endothelial cells at blood–brain barrier sites. *Proc. Natl. Acad. Sci. USA*, **86**, 695–8.

Cumin, I., Lacroix, H., Mahé, M. *et al.* (1995). Efficacy of combination multidrug chemotherapy (mitomycin, ifosfamide and cisplatin) and radiotherapy for treatment of brain metastases in non small cell lung. *Bull. Cancer*, **82**, 57–62.

Didier, A. D. and Loor, F. (1995). Decreased biotolerability for ivermectin and cyclosporin A in mice exposed to potent P-glycoprotein inhibitors. *Int. J. Cancer*, **63**, 263–7.

Flens, M. J., Zaman, G. J. R., van der Valk, P. *et al.* (1996). Tissue distribution of the multidrug resistance protein. *Am. J. Pathol.*, **148**, 1237–47.

Gavériaux, C., Boesch, D., Jachez, B. *et al.* (1991). SDZ PSC 833, a non-immunosuppressive cyclosporin analog, is a very potent multidrug-resistance modifier. *J. Cell. Pharmacol.*, **2**, 225–34.

Grau, J. J., Estapé, J., Daniels, M. and Mané, J. M. (1994). BCNU plus teniposide (VM26) as a first line chemotherapy for brain metastases regardless of the origin. *Int. J. Oncol.*, **4**, 961–4.

Hegmann, E. J., Bauer, H. C. and Kerbel, R. S. (1992). Expression and functional activity of P-glycoprotein in cultured cerebral capillary endothelial cells. *Cancer Res.*, **52**, 6969–75.

Henson, J. W., Cordon-Cardo, C. and Posner, J. B. (1992). P-glycoprotein expression in brain tumors. *J. Neuro-Oncol.*, **14**, 37–43.

Inamura, T., Nomura, T., Bartus, R. T. and Black, K. L. (1994). Intracarotid infusion of RMP-7, a bradykinin analog: a method for selective drug delivery to brain tumors. *J. Neurosurg.*, **81**, 752–8.

Izquierdo, M. A., Scheffer, G. L., Flens, M. J. *et al.* (1996). Broad distribution of the multidrug resistance-related vault lung resistance protein in normal human tissues and tumors. *Am. J. Pathol.*, **148**, 877–87.

Jachez, B., Cianfriglia, M. and Loor, F. (1994). Modulation of human P-glycoprotein epitope expression by temperature and/or resistance-modulating agents. *Anti-Cancer Drugs*, **5**, 655–65.

Jacobson, B. S., Schnitzer, J. E., McCaffery, M. and Palade, G. (1992). Isolation and partial characterization of the luminal plasmalemma of microvascular endothelium from rat lungs. *Eur. J. Cell Biol.*, **58**, 296–306.

Jetté, L., Murphy, G. F. and Béliveau, R. (1998). Drug binding to P-glycoprotein is inhibited in normal rat tissues following SDZ-PSC 833 treatment. *Int. J. Cancer*, in press.

Jetté, L., Murphy, G. F., Leclerc, J.-M. and Béliveau, R. (1995). Interaction of drugs with P-glycoprotein in brain capillaries. *Biochem. Pharmacol.*, **50**, 1701–9.

Jetté, L., Beaulieu, E., Leclerc, J.-M. and Béliveau, R. (1996). Cyclosporin A treatment induces overexpression of P-glycoprotein in the kidney and other tissues. *Am. J. Physiol.*, **270**, F756–65.

Jetté, L., Potier, M. and Béliveau, R. (1997). P-glycoprotein is a dimer in the kidney and brain capillary membranes: effect of cyclosporin A and SDZ-PSC 833. *Biochemistry*, **36**, 13929–37.

Lemaire, M., Bruelisauer, A., Guntz, P. and Sato, H. (1996). Dose-dependent brain penetration of SDZ PSC 833, a novel multidrug resistance-reversing cyclosporin, in rats. *Cancer Chemother. Pharmacol.*, **38**, 481–6.

Lesser, G. J. and Grossman, S. A. (1993). The chemotherapy of adult primary brain tumors. *Cancer Treat. Rev.*, **19**, 261–81.

Lesser, G. J. and Grossman, S. (1994). The chemotherapy of high-grade astrocytomas. *Sem. Oncol.*, **21**, 220–35.

Levin, V. A., Silver, P., Hannigan, J. *et al.* (1990). Superiority of post-radiotherapy adjuvant chemotherapy with CCNU, procarbazine, and vincristine (PCV) over BCNU for anaplastic gliomas: NCOG 6G61 final report. *Int. J. Rad. Oncol., Biol. Phys.*, **18**, 321–4.

Lum, B. L., Gosland, M. P., Kaubisch, S. and Sikic, B. I. (1993). Molecular targets in oncology: implications of the multidrug resistance gene. *Pharmacotherapy*, **13**, 88–109.

Mousseau, M. (1994). La chimiothérapie des tumeurs cérébrales: bases biologiques de son efficacité limitée. *Bull. Cancer*, **81**, 414–24.

Sakata, A., Tamai, I., Kawazu, K. *et al.* (1994). In vivo evidence for ATP-dependent and P-glycoprotein-mediated transport of cyclosporin A at the blood-brain barrier. *Biochem. Pharmacol.*, **48**, 1989–92.

Schinkel, A. H., Smit, J. J. M., van Tellingen, O. *et al.* (1994). Disruption of the mouse mdr1a P-glycoprotein gene leads to a deficiency in the blood–brain barrier and to increased sensitivity to drugs. *Cell*, **77**, 491–502.

Shibata, S. (1989). Ultrastructure of capillary walls in human brain tumors. *Acta Neuropathol.*, **78**, 561–71.

Stewart, D. J. (1994). A critique of the role of the blood-barrier in the chemotherapy of human brain tumors. *J. Neuro-Oncol.*, **20**, 121–39.

Tanaka, Y., Abe, Y., Tsugu, A., Takamiya, Y. *et al.* (1994). Ultrastructural localization of P-glycoprotein on capillary endothelial cells in human gliomas. *Virchows Archiv.*, **425**, 133–8.

Tatsuta, T., Naito, M., Oh-hara, T. *et al.* (1992). Functional involvement of P-glycoprotein in blood–brain barrier. *J. Biol. Chem.*, **267**, 20383–91.

Tomita, T. (1991). Interstitial chemotherapy for brain tumors: review. *J. Neuro-Oncol.*, **10**, 57–74.

Tsuji, A., Terasaki, T., Takabatake, Y. *et al.* (1992). P-glycoprotein as the drug efflux pump in primary cultured bovine brain capillary endothelial cells. *Life Sci.*, **51**, 1427–37.

Tsuji, A., Tamai, I., Sakata, A. *et al.* (1993). Restricted transport of cyclosporin A across the blood–brain barrier by a multidrug transporter, P-glycoprotein. *Biochem. Pharmacol.*, **46**, 1096–99.

33 Lipid composition of brain microvessels

JEAN-MARIE BOURRE

- Introduction
- Changes in fatty acids in relation to the diet, and alterations during development and aging
- Lipid synthesis and energy substrates
- Lipoprotein receptors and fatty acid transport
- Various lipid-related enzymatic activities
- Protection against peroxidation
- Fatty acid synthesizing systems
- Lipid metabolism in cultured cells

Introduction

Membrane lipids containing fatty acids are important as they play a direct role in the structure and function of cells, including brain endothelial cells. Moreover, these latter cells transfer fatty acids from the blood to the brain cells. Brain is the second organ in terms of lipid content, after adipose tissue; in brain, lipids do not provide any energy, but play a structural role: they participate in the structure of membranes, and thus mediate their functions. This transfer is obligatory for essential fatty acids of dietary origin, but it is not yet known whether the essential linoleic ($18:2(n\text{-}6)$) and alpha-linolenic ($18:3(n\text{-}3)$) acids are transferred, or whether it is the longer chains that are in fact transferred (mainly arachidonic acid, $20:4(n\text{-}6)$; and docosahexaenoic acid, $22:6(n\text{-}3)$, DHA).

Thus brain microvessel metabolism controls brain membrane polyunsaturated fatty acids. This is of special importance as, for instance, alterations in dietary ($n\text{-}3$) polyunsaturated fatty acids change the fatty acid profile of brain cell membranes (neurons, astrocytes and oligodendrocytes) and subcellular fractions (myelin and nerves endings) (Bourre et al., 1984), and thus alter brain structure and functions including learning performance. This has been documented in animal models (Bourre et al., 1989), and in human infants. In animals, during development, different structures within the brain may vary in their capacity to synthesize DHA, and this may be correlated with the regional growth rate (Pawlosky et al., 1996); in human infants fed formula milks the amount of DHA produced may not reach the DHA level observed in breast-fed newborn infants (Salem et al., 1996).

Consequently, it is very important to determine how polyunsaturated fatty acids are transferred from the blood to the brain, and whether dietary fatty acids are lengthened and desaturated at the level of the blood–brain barrier, since the two essential dietary precursors (linoleic and alpha-linolenic acids) are almost absent in brain membranes, and only their derived very long polyunsaturated chains are found. It is possible that microvessels play a role in the metabolism of essential fatty acids during their transfer from the circulation to the brain (metabolism and eicosanoid formation).

Changes in fatty acids in relation to the diet, and alterations during development and aging

A diet deficient in some polyunsaturated fatty acids induces alterations in fatty acids in brain capillaries (Matheson *et al.*, 1981; Homayoun *et al.*, 1988) and choroid plexus (Homayoun *et al.*, 1988), and recovery is extremely slow after substitution of a non-deficient diet (Homayoun *et al.*, 1988). During aging (Tayarani *et al.*, 1989), the percentage of total saturated fatty acids does not change. In contrast, monounsaturated fatty acids increase and polyunsaturated fatty acids decrease.

Changes in dietary fatty acids, such as alpha-linolenic acid deficiency, alter the fatty acid composition of the brain microvessels, and the efficiency of the blood–brain barrier (Ziylan *et al.*, 1992); a diet deficient in alpha-linolenic acid induces a greater transport of sucrose from blood to brain in some brain regions, but not of alpha-aminoisobutyric acid or L-phenylalanine.

Lipid synthesis and energy substrates

A number of metabolic activities and mechanisms related to lipids have been found in brain microvessels. These vessels use ketone bodies for energy production, and lipid synthesis is altered during development (Homayoun *et al.*, 1988). More precisely, the rate of CO_2 production (an index of oxidative metabolism) from glucose is slightly higher than from aceto-acetate, D-hydroxybutyrate, acetate and butyrate. Thus, ketone bodies can be used as a source of energy by brain capillaries. All the above substrates are also used for the synthesis of lipids, which *in vitro* is suppressed by the addition of albumin in the incubation medium. The incorporation of glucose into total lipids is ten times higher than that of other precursors. However, glucose is almost exclusively found in the glycerol backbone of phospholipids, especially in phosphatidylcholine.

Ketone bodies, as well as glucose, are incorporated mainly into phospholipids, whereas acetate and butyrate are mainly incorporated into neutral lipids. The rank order contribution of the various substrates to fatty acid synthesis is: butyrate > acetate > ketone bodies > glucose. All precursors, except glucose, are used for sterol synthesis.

Lipoprotein receptors and fatty acid transport

Lipoprotein receptors are present in these microvessels (Pitas *et al.*, 1987; Martin-Nizard *et al.*, 1989; Méresse *et al.*, 1989), but not albumin receptors (Pardridge *et al.*, 1985). It has been hypothesized that the entry of polyunsaturated fatty acids into the brain correlates with the high-density lipoprotein-induced methylation of phosphatidylethanolamine and phospholipase A2 (Magret *et al.*, 1996); it has been demonstrated that the conversion of phosphatidylethanolamine into phosphatidylcholine by a sequence of three methylation reactions is stimulated by the apolipoprotein E-free subclass of high density lipoprotein (HDL_3) in isolated bovine brain capillary membranes. Both methyl transferase and phospholipase A2 activity depend on HDL_3 concentration in the medium, and are strictly dependent on the binding (HDL_3 modified by tetranitromethane is no longer able to bind to specific receptors, and does not induce activation of these enzymatic activities).

This suggests that the phosphatidylcholine pool arising from phosphatidylethanolamine could be used as a pathway for the supply of polyunsaturated fatty acids to the brain.

Various lipid-related enzymatic activities

Lipoprotein-lipase (Brecher and Kuan, 1979; Shirai *et al.*, 1986) and diacylglycerol lipase and kinase (Hee-Cheong *et al.*, 1985) have been detected in rabbit and rat microvessels. HDL-lipoprotein-sphingomyelin is taken up and utilized (Homayoun *et al.*, 1989). Arachidonyl-CoA synthetase (Morand *et al.*, 1987) and non-specific acyl-CoA synthetase (Carré *et al.*, 1989) are present and play a role in fatty acid activation. The exact importance of phosphoinositide metabolism remains to be elucidated (Joo, 1992). Brain microvessels also produce HETE (Moore *et al.*, 1990).

Protection against peroxidation

Protection systems against peroxidation are altered in brain capillaries during development and aging. Between days 7 and 60 after birth, glutathione peroxidase is constant in microvessels, while glutathione reductase increases, a similar time course is observed in brain homogenate. In contrast, catalase in microvessels decreases, as it does in brain homogenate, but the activity is higher in microvessels than in brain (Buard et al., 1992).

During adulthood and aging (Tayarani et al., 1987, 1989), glutathione peroxidase and glutathione reductase levels do not change in brain capillaries, but increase in cerebrum and cerebellum. Catalase declines in brain capillaries, but is stable in cerebrum and cerebellum. The activities of the three enzymes are significantly higher in brain capillaries than in cerebrum and cerebellum. Superoxide dismutase increases in brain and in isolated capillaries.

Concentrations of trace elements related to protection against peroxidations are altered during aging. Copper content in capillaries increases during development and then levels off, whereas it continues to increase in cerebrum and cerebellum. Zinc increases in brain capillaries, but not in cerebrum and cerebellum. Manganese content remains stable in brain and capillaries.

Fatty acid synthesizing systems

It has not yet been determined how cerebral microvessels participate in the uptake of essential fatty acids by the brain. Precursors (linoleic and alpha-linolenic acid) are almost absent in the brain, thus they have to be desaturated either in the liver or at the level of the blood–brain barrier or the blood–CSF barrier, since enzymatic activities in the brain are nearly nil after early development (Bourre et al., 1990, 1992). In fact, the fatty acids present in cerebral membranes are not the precursors, but longer chain fatty acids, mainly arachidonic acid (20:4 (n-6)) and docosahexaenoic acid (22:6 (n-3)). The key enzyme that controls all transformations (chain lengthening and desaturation) is delta-6-desaturase, which transforms linoleic acid (18:2(n-6)) into gamma-linolenic acid (18:3 (n-6)) and alpha-linolenic acid (18:3 (n-3)) into stearidonic acid (18:4 (n-3)). Another protein, cytochrome b5 reductase, is involved in the desaturation of fatty acids.

Delta-6-desaturase was measured in rat brain microvessels and choroid plexus by incubation in the presence of radioactive linoleic acid (Bourre et al., 1997). In 21-day-old animals, delta-6 desaturase was not detected in brain microvessels. In contrast, it was present in choroid plexus (about 21 pmol/min/mg protein). In comparison, the activity in brain was much lower (about 1 pmol/min/mg protein) and higher in liver (about 55 pmol/min/mg protein). Interestingly, during development the activity in choroid plexus peaked at day 6 after birth and declined slightly thereafter. These results show that delta-6 desaturase was not detectable in brain microvessels but was present in choroid plexus.

Thus, brain microvessels do not contain measurable amounts of delta-6 desaturase (by direct measurement of the enzymatic activity), in contrast with endothelial cells in culture, as determined by synthesis of long polyunsaturated chains from precursors added to the culture medium (Moore et al., 1991). It can be speculated that differentiation of brain endothelial cells leads to disappearance of delta-6 desaturase. A similar hypothesis is also probably valid in skin, where delta-6 desaturase is also absent (Ziboh and Chapkin, 1988). It is known that endothelial cells in culture rapidly lose markers found in the microvessels, such as gamma-glutamyl-transpeptidase or alkaline phosphatase (Roux et al., 1994).

As microvessels contain measurable amounts of very long chain polyunsaturated fatty acids, such as arachidonic and docosahexaenoic acids, these fatty acids must be supplied by the blood. It has been recently demonstrated that docosahexaenoic acid is taken up by the microvessels from developing rat brain (Anderson et al., 1993). This acid synthesizes endothelial cell membrane lipids, but could be transferred to the other brain cells.

As delta-6 desaturase was not detected in brain microvessels during development, very long unsaturated chains found in nervous tissue are probably not synthesized in the microvessels; this is in agreement with the hypothesis that they are either synthesized by the liver or supplied directly by the diet (Bourre et al., 1989; Scott and Bazan, 1989).

Lipid metabolism in cultured cells

Lipid synthesis in primary cultures of microvascular endothelial cells from rat brain is very active. These cells are able to synthesize all their lipids (phospholipids and neutral lipids) from various water-soluble compounds such as glucose, acetate, aceto-acetate and beta-hydroxybutyrate; the ketone bodies being the preferred substrates for lipid synthesis. The metabolic pathway is different for glucose, which is preferentially incorporated into phospholipids. The existence of an inverse relationship between serum lipoprotein levels and lipid synthesis suggests that cultured endothelial cells are able to take up lipids (such as cholesterol) contained in lipoproteins. Consequently, lipids in endothelial cells could be supplied either by intracellular synthesis or by serum lipoproteins. Activity in cultured cells is at variance with that observed in isolated capillaries: it is regulated by serum lipoproteins (Roux *et al.*, 1989).

Cultured murine cerebro-microvascular endothelia are able to convert linoleic acid into arachidonic acid, and alpha-linolenic acid into EPA but not DHA; although the uptake of linoleic and alpha-linolenic acid is similar, alpha-linolenic acid is more extensively elongated and desaturated (Moore *et al.*, 1990). The blood–brain barrier can play an important role in the elongation and desaturation of essential fatty acids during transfer from the circulation into the brain. Primary rat cultures of neurons do not produce DHA, but primary cultures of astrocytes do (Moore *et al.*, 1991). However, it is not totally certain whether results concerning fatty acid metabolism, obtained with cultured cells, can provide information about the actual situation *in vivo*. In fact, age is an important parameter, as delta-6-desaturase levels are high in brain during development, but low thereafter (Bourre *et al.*, 1990, 1992). Moreover, delta-6 desaturase is extremely low in adult brain microvessels (Bourre *et al.*, 1997).

Co-culture with astrocytes changes the fatty acid composition of bovine brain capillary endothelial cells (Bénistant *et al.*, 1995). Co-culture increases arachidonic concentration, at the expense of linoleic acid, and DHA is increased at the expense of its precursors. Interestingly, the changes induced by co-culture are found only in phospholipids (especially phosphatidylcholine, phosphatidylethanolamine and phosphatidylserine), but not in phosphoinositides and other lipid classes. Only (n-3) fatty acids were altered in capillary endothelial cells from adrenal cortex co-cultured under the same conditions.

DHA is the major (n-3) polyunsaturated fatty acid in rat brain microvessels (Homayoun *et al.*, 1988) and in bovine retinal microvessels; its concentration is restored in bovine retinal endothelial cells in co-culture when the medium is enriched in this fatty acid (Lecomte *et al.*, 1996). The very high concentration of polyunsaturated fatty acids in retinal microvessels raises the question of the pathogenic processes leading to diabetic neuropathy through oxidation products derived from these fatty acids.

Table 33.1 shows distribution of radioactivity in the various main lipids in brain microvessels after incubation with radioactive linoleic acid. Radioactivity in sphingomyelin was low; as expected since sphingomyelin is known not to contain polyunsaturated fatty acids. The low radioactivity in cholesterol is probably due to degradation of the labelled linoleic acid to labelled acetate units, which are in turn utilized to synthesize cholesterol or saturated and monounsaturated fatty acids found in sphingomyelin. The high labelling of free fatty acids in capillaries could be because endothelial cells are low in fatty-acid-binding proteins, at least in heart, and this may result in accumulation of free fatty acids.

Interestingly, the role of choroid plexus remains to be determined. It could be proposed as an

Table 33.1. *Linoleic acid incorporation in isolated 21-day-old brain capillaries.*

	Capillaries
Cholesterol	3.0 ± 0.8
Cholesterol ester	4.2 ± 1.4
Free fatty acids	19.9 ± 4.8
Phosphatidylethanolamine	6.9 ± 0.4
Phosphatidylinositol + phosphatidic acid	1.5 ± 0.1
Phosphatidylserine	6.7 ± 1.0
Phosphatidylcholine	55.8 ± 2.7
Sphingomyelin	1.9 ± 0.5

alternative pathway for supplying brain tissue with very long unsaturated chains via the CSF lipoproteins. Thus, choroid plexus metabolism must be taken into account in the delivery of lipids to the brain, at least at the level of polyunsaturated fatty acids. It is not known whether the choroid plexus uses all the very long chain fatty acids it synthesizes or whether some are also transported to the brain. As monolayer cultures are now possible,

it would be interesting to measure their delta-6 desaturase activity.

Acknowledgments

The author is most grateful to INSERM for supporting this work, and to A. Strickland for reviewing this manuscript.

References

Anderson, G. J. , Hohimer, A. R. and Willeke, G. B. (1993). Uptake of docosahexaenoic acid by microvessels from developing rat brain. *Life Sci.*, **53**, 1089–98.

Bénistant, C., Dehouck, M. P., Fruchart, J. C. *et al.* (1995). Fatty acid composition of brain capillary endothelial cells: effect of the coculture with astrocytes. *J. Lipid Res.*, **36**, 2311–19.

Bourre, J. M. and Piciotti, M. (1992). Delta-6 desaturation of alpha-linolenic acid in brain and liver during development and aging in the mouse. *Neurosci. Lett.*, **141**, 65–8.

Bourre, J. M., Pascal, G., Durand, G. *et al.* (1984). Alterations in the fatty acid composition of rat brain cells (neurons, astrocytes and oligodendrocytes) and of subcellular fractions (myelin and synaptosomes) induced by a diet devoid of n-3 fatty acids. *J. Neurochem.*, **43**, 342–8.

Bourre, J. M., François, M., Youyou, A. *et al.* (1989). The effects of dietary α-linolenic acid on the composition of nerve membranes, enzymatic activity, amplitude of electrophysiological parameters, resistance to poisons and performances of learning tasks in rats. *J. Nutr.*, **119**, 1880–92.

Bourre, J. M., Piciotti, M. and Dumont, O. (1990). Delta-6 desaturase in brain and liver during development and aging. *Lipids*, **25**, 354–6.

Bourre, J. M., Dinh, L. Bolthias, C. *et al.* (1997). Possible rôle of the choroid plexus in the supply of brain tissue with polyunsaturated fatty acids. *Neurosci. Lett.*, **224**, 1–4.

Brecher, P. and Kuan, H. T. (1979). Lipoprotein lipase and acid lipase activity in rabbit brain microvessels. *J. Lipid Res.*, **20**, 464–71.

Buard, A., Clement, M. and Bourre, J. M. (1992). Developmental changes in enzymatic systems involved in protection against peroxidation in isolated rat brain microvessels. *Neurosci. Lett.*, **141**, 72–4.

Carré, J. B., Morand, O., Homayoun, P. *et al.* (1989). Purified rat brain microvessels exhibit both acid and neutral sphingomyelinase activities, *J. Neurochem.*, **52**, 1294–9.

Hee-Cheong, M., Fletcher, T., Kryski, S. K. and Severson, D. L. (1985). Diacylglycerol lipase and kinase activities in rat brain microvessels. *Biochim. Biophys. Acta*, **833**, 59–68.

Homayoun, P. and Bourre, J. M. (1987). Ketone body utilization for energy production and lipid synthesis in isolated rat brain capillaries. *Biochem. Biophys. Acta*, **922**, 345–50.

Homayoun, P., Durand, G., Pascal, G. and Bourre, J. M. (1988). Alteration in fatty acid composition of adult rat brain capillaries and choroid plexus induced by a diet deficient in n-3 fatty acids: slow recovery after substitution with a nondeficient diet. *J. Neurochem.*, **51**, 45–8.

Homayoun, P., Bentejac, M., Lecerf, J. and Bourre, J. M. (1989). Uptake and utilization of double-labeled high-density lipoprotein sphingomyelin in isolated brain capillaries of adult rats. *J. Neurochem.*, **53**, 1031–5.

Joo, F. (1992). The cerebral microvessels in culture, an update. *J. Neurochem.*, **58**, 1–17.

Lecomte, M., Paget, C., Ruggiero, D. *et al.* (1996). Docosahexaenoic acid is a major n-3 polyunsaturated fatty acid in bovine retinal microvessels. *J. Neurochem.*, **66**, 2160–7.

Magret, V., Elkhalil, L., Nazih-Sanderson, F. *et al.* (1996). Entry of polyunsaturated fatty acids into the brain: evidence that high-density lipoprotein-induced methylation of phosphatidylethanolamine and phospholipase A$_2$ are involved. *Biochem. J.*, **316**, 805–11.

Martin-Nizard, F., Meresse, S., Cecchelli, R. *et al.* (1989). Interactions of high-density lipoprotein 3 with brain capillary endothelial cells. *Biochim. Biophys. Acta*, **1005**, 201–8.

Matheson, D. F., Oei, R. and Roots, B. I. (1981). Effect of dietary lipid on the acyl group composition of glycerophospholipids of brain endothelial cells in the developing rat. *J. Neurochem.*, **36**, 2073–9.

Méresse, S., Delbart, C., Fruchart, J. C. and Cecchelli, R. (1989). Low-density lipoprotein receptor on endothelium of brain capillaries. *J. Neurochem.*, **53**, 340–5.

Moore, S. A., Yoder, E. and Spector, A. A. (1990). Role of the blood–brain barrier in the formation of long-chain n-3 and n-6 fatty acids from essential fatty acid precursors. *J. Neurochem.*, **55**, 391–402.

Moore, S. A., Yoder, E., Murphy, S. *et al.* (1991). Astrocytes, not neurons, produce docosahexaenoic acid (22:6 n-3) and arachidonic acid (20:4 n-6). *J. Neurochem.*, **56**, 518–24.

Morand, O., Carré, J. B., Homayoun, P. *et al.* (1987). Arachidonyl-coenzyme-A synthetase and nonspecific acyl-coenzyme-A synthetase activities in purified rat brain microvessels. *J. Neurochem.*, **48**, 1150–6.

Pardridge, W. M., Eisenberg, J. and Cefalu, W. T. (1985). Absence of albumin receptor on brain capillaries in vivo or in vitro. *Am. J. Physiol.*, **249**, E264–E267.

Pawlosky, R. J., Ward, G. and Salem, N. (1996). Essential fatty acid uptake and metabolism in the developing rodent brain. *Lipids*, **31**, 103–7.

Pitas, R. E., Boyles, J. K., Lee, S. H. *et al.* (1987). Lipoproteins and their receptors in the central nervous system, characterization of the lipoproteins in cerebrospinal fluid and identification of apolipoprotein B,E(LDL) receptors in the brain. *J. Biol. Chemistry*, **262**,14352–60.

Roux, F. S., Mokni, R., Hughes, C. C. *et al.* (1989). Lipid synthesis by rat brain microvessel endothelial cells in tissue culture, *J. Neuropathol. Exp. Neurol.*, **48**, 437–47.

Roux, F., Durieu-Trautman, O., Chaverot, N. *et al.* (1994). Regulation of gamma-glutamyl transpeptidase and alkaline phosphatase activities in immortalized rat brain microvessel endothelial cells. *J. Cell. Physiol.*, **159**, 101–13.

Salem, N., Wegher, B., Mena, P. and Uauy, R. (1996). Arachidonic and docosahexaenoic acids are biosynthesized from their 18-carbon precursors in human infants. *Proc. Natl. Acad. Sci. USA*, **93**, 49–54.

Scott, B. L. and Bazan, N. G. (1989). Membrane docosahexaenoate is supplied to the developing brain and retina by the liver. *Proc. Natl. Acad. Sci. USA*, **86**, 2903–7.

Shirai, K., Saito, Y., Yoshida, S. and Matsuoka, N. (1986). Existence of lipoprotein lipase in rat brain microvessels. *Tohoku J. Exp. Med.*, **149**, 449–50.

Tayarani, I., Chaudiere, J., Lefauconnier, J. M. and Bourre, J. M. (1987). Enzymatic protection against peroxidative damage in isolated brain capillaries. *J. Neurochem.*, **48**, 1399–402.

Tayarani, I., Cloez, I., Clément, M. and Bourre, J. M. (1989). Antioxidant enzymes and related trace elements in aging brain capillaries and choroid plexus. *J. Neurochem.*, **53**, 817–24.

Ziboh, V. A. and Chapkin, R. S. (1988). Metabolism and function of skin lipids. *Prog. Lipid Res.*, **27**, 81–105.

Ziylan, Z. Y., Bernard, G. C., Lefauconnier, J. M. *et al.* (1992). Effect of dietary n-3 fatty acid deficiency on blood-to-brain transfer of sucrose, -aminoisobutyric acid and phenylalanine in the rat. *Neurosci. Lett.*, **137**, 9–13.

34 Brain microvessel antigens

BÜRKHARD SCHLOSSHAUER

Introduction

Understanding the structure–function relationship of the BBB depends on the identification of the molecular components involved. One approach to address this topic is based on the generation of monospecific antibodies starting typically from heterogeneous immunogen fractions. The resulting antibodies are then used to identify the corresponding antigens and determine their function, therefore following a structure-to-function strategy. This chapter is focused on antigens of this experimental history, whereas antibodies for characterized vascular endothelial proteins such as glucose transporters, transferrin- and VEGF receptors, junction proteins etc. will be discussed elsewhere. Besides being helpful to reveal the molecular architecture of the BBB, antigens could be employed as diagnostic indexes to evaluate BBB integrity under pathological conditions *in vivo* or, for example, as differentiation markers in *in vitro* models.

HT7/Neurothelin

One of the most thoroughly studied antigens present on brain microvessels is HT7/neurothelin. In two independent approaches using as immunogens either tissue homogenates or purified cell membranes of the embryonic chicken retina, monoclonal antibodies (MAb) HT7 and 1W5 were generated. The corresponding antigens, which have subsequently been shown to be identical, have been termed HT7 (Risau *et al.*, 1986) and neurothelin (Schlosshauer and Herzog, 1990), respectively. As deduced from cDNA sequencing, the antigen has 246 amino acids with a predicted molecular weight of 26 893 daltons. The protein belongs to the immunoglobulin superfamily, being composed of a short intracellular tail, a transmembrane domain and an extracellular region (Seulberger *et al.*, 1990). The extracellular protein region is characterized by two C2-type immunoglobulin domains with the characteristic sandwich of ß-sheets. Immunoglobulin domains are stabilized by disulphide bonds based on the presence of four cysteine residues. The transmembrane region contains a leucine zipper-like motif with leucines every seventh amino acid residue. In the HT7/neurothelin sequence, there are three leucines and a phenylalanine surrounded by some hydrophobic amino acids at the fourth site. The leucine zipper and the charged amino acid glutamate within the transmembrane region could be of functional relevance by interacting with other membrane components.

Five potential glycosylation sites have been identified in the HT7/neurothelin sequence. Depending on the tissue and electrophoresis protocol used, major HT7/neurothelin bands appear as a smear in the range of 41–52 kDa. Additional bands at 58/69 kDa can be found depending on the developmental stage and tissue type analysed (Schlosshauer and Herzog, 1990). About 40% of the native protein mass is due to saccharide moieties, as shown by enzymatic deglycosylation of native HT7/neurothelin by endoglycosidase F/N-glycosidase F (Schlosshauer, 1991).

HT7/neurothelin homologous antigens have been identified in man (M6, EMMPRIN, human basigin BSG) (Kasinrerk *et al.*, 1992; Biswas *et al.*, 1995), rabbit (4D4 antigen) (Schuster *et al.*, 1996), rat (OX-47 antigen, CE9) (Fossum *et al.*, 1991; Nehme *et al.*, 1993), mouse (gp42, mouse basigin, mouse HT7) (Altruda *et al.*, 1989; Miyauchi *et al.*, 1990; Seulberger *et al.*, 1992) and chicken (5A11) (Fadool and Linser, 1993*b*). In the transmembrane domain a stretch of 29 amino acids is completely conserved in all species analysed. Between human and mouse homologues, 58% of the amino acids are identical and 80% of the changes are conservative (Miyauchi *et al.*, 1991). Between mouse and chicken homologues 70% identity is evident in the cytoplasmic domain and 40% in the extracellular domain. Three of the five potential N-glycosylation sites present in the sequence of the chicken antigen are preserved in the murine homologue (Seulberger *et al.*, 1992). Southern blots indicate that the HT7/neurothelin gene is unique in the chicken genome (Seulberger *et al.*, 1990). The murine basigin gene is located on chromosome 10, spans 7.5 kb and consists of seven exons and six introns. Whether a protein polymorphism exists, remains controversial (Miyauchi *et al.*, 1995). The human basigin gene has been mapped at chromosome 19 (Kaname *et al.*, 1993).

HT7/neurothelin is possibly associated with the cytoskeleton. Immunofluorescence data indicate the colocalization of ankyrin together with the antigen in the blood–eye barrier forming pigment epithelium *in situ*. In addition, the antigen can be biochemically copurified with spectrin (Rizzolo and Zhou, 1995). Furthermore, immunocytochemical double labeling of cultured pigment epithelial cells reveals coincidence of HT7/neurothelin and actin. Disruption of actin filaments by cytochalasin D causes disintegration of the ordered cell surface distribution of HT7/neurothelin, whereas depolymerization of microtubules using demecolcine does not affect antigen distribution (Schlosshauer *et al.*, 1995).

HT7/neurothelin is expressed on BBB-specific endothelial cells including the endothelium of the pecten oculi within the chicken vitreous (Gerhardt *et al.*, 1996). It is not expressed on vascular endothelial cells of the developing brain before the onset of BBB formation. Electron microscopic images of immunogold-labeled specimens suggest that HT7/neurothelin is specifically expressed by endothelial cells but not other perivascular cell types. Extraembryonic blood vessels of the chorioallantoic membrane of fertilized chicken eggs and systemic vessels reveal essentially no immunoreactivity (Risau *et al.*, 1986). In brain circumventricular organs such as pituitary, where endothelial cells do not form tight junctions and therefore lack BBB characteristics, HT7/neurothelin is absent in microvessels. In the choroid plexus the barrier is formed by epithelial cells facing the ventricle, whereas endothelial cells form fenestrated capillaries. Also in this area, HT7/neurothelin expression is correlated with barrier functions and found only on epithelial but not on endothelial cells (Albrecht *et al.*, 1990). The antigen is exposed on the luminal surface of vascular endothelial cells.

Although HT7/neurothelin expression allows one to distinguish BBB-specific endothelial cells from non-barrier forming vascular endothelial cells, it should be emphasized that other cells types synthesize the antigen, too. These include blood–eye barrier forming pigment epithelial cells, epithelial cells at transport interfaces such as in kidney tubules (Risau *et al.*, 1986), erythroblasts (Unger *et al.*, 1993) and, for example, radial Müller glial cells (Fadool and Linser, 1994). In other species homologous antigens have been identified in fibroblasts (Altruda *et al.*, 1989), peripheral granulocytes (Kasinrerk *et al.*, 1992), activated B and T lymphocytes (Fossum *et al.*, 1991), embryonal carcinoma cells (Miyauchi *et al.*, 1990), lung carcinoma cells (Biswas *et al.*, 1995), spermatozoa (Cesario *et al.*, 1995) and most pronounced in brown adipocytes (Nehme *et al.*, 1995). Most interestingly, the apparent molecular weights of HT7/neurothelin and homologues differ in different tissues and cells, suggesting cell type specific synthesis of different isoforms or specific post-translational modifications. Northern blot analysis revealed major transcripts of 2 kb and minor transcripts of 1.4 kb in brain, kidney and erythroblasts of chicken (Seulberger *et al.*, 1990). Different glycosylation patterns of HT7/neurothelin are evident in retina, kidney and liver of the chicken (Fadool and Linser, 1993*a*). In rats 40% of the extracellular domain of the antigen is endoproteolytically cleaved resulting in a redistribution of the antigen from the posterior to the anterior tail of spermatozoa (Cesario *et al.*, 1995). Therefore, distinct HT7/neurothelin forms are likely to be differentially distributed in various tissues, cell types, and cell compartments.

Within the nervous system of chicken, HT7/neurothelin expression is subject to stringent control mechanisms. During the early stages of development *in ovo* (first week of incubation), endothelial cells are devoid of HT7/neurothelin. Antigen expression in brain microvessels starts with the differentiation of astrocytes and the concomitant formation of the BBB. Glial cells are likely to induce endothelial antigen expression. This notion is based on the observation that HT7/neurothelin negative systemic blood vessels forced to invade brain tissue, become HT7/neurothelin positive in a similar way as when systemic vessels are exposed to glia-conditioned media (Risau *et al.*, 1986; Schlosshauer and Herzog, 1990; Lobrinus *et al.*, 1992).

Mechanisms of antigen induction and cell surface distribution have been investigated in several cell types of different species. Challenging human T-lymphocytes by addition of phytohemagglutin *in vitro*, results in elevated immunoreactivity for M6 (Kasinrerk *et al.*, 1992). Metabolic activation of rat adipose tissue that occurs upon exposure to the cold results in a 3-fold increase in the level of CE9

mRNA. The level of CE9 mRNA in hepatocytes is increased about 2-fold after administration of thyroid hormone or Concanavalin A (Nehme *et al.*, 1995).

The functions of HT7/neurothelin and homologous antigens have been addressed in various systems. In the course of studies focused on the mechanisms of tumor cell invasion, the human homologues, termed EMMPRIN and M6, located on the surface of distinct tumor cells, stimulate expression of metalloproteinases in fibroblasts. One of these enzymes, collagenase, could degrade extracellular matrix (ECM) proteins as an initial step in metastasis (Biswas *et al.*, 1995). That EMMPRIN/M6 has indirect impact on ECM integrity is further supported by the notion that M6 is expressed by granulocytes in patients with rheumatoid arthritis. This could indicate a role for M6 in protease induction and the consequent matrix degradation that occurs in arthritic joints (Kasinrerk *et al.*, 1992).

In summary, HT7/neurothelin represents a tightly regulated cell surface glycoprotein of the immunoglobulin superfamily expressed on BBB specific endothelial cells. It could serve receptor functions mediating different cell–cell interactions.

140 kDa protein/pAP N

For the generation of the monoclonal antibody 7–1C3, isolated rat brain microvessels were employed as immunogen (Krause *et al.*, 1988). Western blot analysis indicates that the corresponding antigen recognized by MAb 7–1C3 is a 140 kDa protein being glycosylated as suggested by binding of the two lectins Concanavalin A and *Ulex europeus* agglutinin. Microsequencing of the N-terminal end of the 140 kDa protein after Edman degradation revealed 18 amino acids that are identical to the N-terminus of aminopeptidase N (pAP N; EC 3.4.11.2). For technical reasons sequence analysis was performed on the 140 kDa protein isolated from kidney. Subsequent sequencing of a 372 bp cDNA fragment employing reverse transcriptase–polymerase chain reaction in conjunction with RNA from cerebral microvessels and kidney AP N deduced primers indicates a 100% identity of both including the terminal sequence of the 140 kDa protein. In conclusion, the 140 kDa protein/pAP N is most likely aminopetidase N (Kunz *et al.*, 1994).

Within the brain, MAb 7–1C3 labels arterioles, capillaries, and post-capillary segments, whereas larger blood vessels are not immunoreactive. Sinusoidal capillaries of the choroidal plexus and the area postrema are devoid of the antigen. In contrast to vascular endothelial cells, which do not reveal any immunolabeling either on the luminal or on the abluminal surface, exclusively perivascular pericytes express the antigen in the brain. Analysis of confocal microscopic images reveals that the antigen is confined to defined bands around the capillary wall. This coincides with the topography of pericytes, which ensheath cerebral microvessels in a discontinuous manner. That endothelial cells are 140 kDa protein/pAP N negative could be further substantiated by immuno double-labeling for 140 kDa protein/pAP N and factor VIII-related antigen; the latter being fairly homogeneously distributed on vascular endothelial cells. Cell culture experiments indicate that 140 kDa protein/pAP N is expressed on the cell surface. The antigen becomes internalized after 2 days *in vitro* leaving pericytes devoid of any immunoreactivity.

During development before the formation of the BBB no MAb 7–1C3 binding is found in the rat brain. Shortly before birth (embryonic day 21) the antigen becomes detectable and reaches adult levels at day 8 post-partum. Besides the peripheral nervous system immunoreactivity is also evident in non-nervous tissue such as liver, small intestine and kidney. These immunocytochemical data are corroborated by Northern blot analysis. In the kidney, antibody binding is strictly confined to the apical surface of proximal tubules, being terminated abruptly near the zonula occludens.

In the course of experimental autoimmune encephalomyelitis (EAE), microvascular 140 kDa protein/pAP N expression transiently declines. Acute EAE is induced *in vivo* by challenging rats with intravenously injected T cells, which had been stimulated with myelin basic protein. Therefore, perturbation of 140 kDa protein/pAP N expression reflects aspects of the inflammatory vascular response (Kunz *et al.*, 1995).

In summary, in the brain 140 kDa protein/

pAP N has been identified as aminopetidase N expressed at the BBB on microvascular pericytes, whose function could be the extracellular inactivation of peptides such as enkephalins.

Endothelial-barrier antigen (EBA)

The monoclonal antibody anti-EBA (renamed SMI 71) was produced from mice immunized with rat brain homogenates. On nitrocellulose blots of electrophoresed samples of enriched brain microvessels the antibody identifies three proteins with apparent molecular weights of 23 kDa, 25 kDa and 30 kDa (Sternberger and Sternberger, 1987). As revealed by sequencing, these proteins represent histones, which are likely to be unspecifically bound by the antibody, an IgM (L. Sternberger, personal communication). Some IgMs tend to display unspecific histone binding.

Designation of the antibody is based on the observation that anti-EBA reacts fairly specifically with brain endothelia that have a selective permeability barrier. In CNS regions lacking BBB characteristics such as the choroid plexus and area postrema, microvessels are weakly reactive or completely nonreactive. Pial and parenchymal vessels of the optic nerve are strongly immunopositive for EBA, whereas vessels of the dura and the sciatic nerve are essentially negative (Lawrenson *et al.*, 1995). Heart, adrenal, skeletal muscle, intestine and various other organs are devoid of immunoreactivity. In the spleen, a patchy staining pattern on some vessels is evident as well as on cells with small diameters (presumably Langerhans cells) in the epidermis of the skin. Transport epithelia do not express EBA. Immunogold labeling revealed that at the BBB, EBA is selectively expressed on the luminal surface of endothelial cells, but absent from neurons, pericytes, and glial cells.

In the developing rat brain the antigen is absent from endothelial cells at embryonic day 18, but present in low amounts as early as 3 days post-partum. Marked immunoreactivity, as in adulthood, is observed first at day 40 (Ibiwoye *et al.*, 1994). Therefore, EBA expression is somewhat delayed in comparison to the formation of the BBB as judged from the ability of brain capillaries to function as a barrier for serum proteins. Likewise, in fetal neocortex transplanted into the adult parietal cortex, EBA is not expressed for 2 weeks after transplantation. However, at later times, transplant vessels become anti-EBA positive (Rosenstein *et al.*, 1992). Aging does not influence EBA expression with the exception of the hippocampus, where in the 26-month-old rat the number of EBA-immunoreactive microvessels is significantly reduced. Streptozotocin-induced diabetes does not change the EBA expression (Mooradian *et al.*, 1993). Following stab wound injury with a concurrent loss of BBB properties, affected microvessels fail to demonstrate antibody binding. Subsequent regeneration of the BBB is accompanied by re-expression of EBA. Similarly, in rats inoculated with myelin basic protein, in order to induce experimental allergic encephalomyelitis, anti-EBA reactivity is abolished in inflammatory brain microvessels. Only after the lesion has resolved, does EBA immunoreactivity become re-established (Sternberger *et al.*, 1989).

EBA represent marker proteins predominantly expressed on the luminal surface of endothelial cells. Changes of EBA expression are largely correlated with the formation of the BBB or its experimentally induced breakdown. The function of EBA has not yet been elucidated.

Gp4A4

Immunization of mice with cultured bovine brain microvessel endothelial cells led to MAb 4A4 (Raub *et al.*, 1994). The antigen recognized by the antibody represents a heterogeneous group of cell surface glycoproteins with molecular weights of 50–65 kDa and 85 kDa called gp4A4. The antigen is sensitive to neuraminidase and N-glycase. Of the apparent molecular weight, 22% is due to N-linked oligosaccharides. Sulfation and phosphorylation of gp4A4 can be shown by metabolic radiolabeling and subsequent immunoprecipitation. Two-dimensional gel electrophoresis reveals a microheterogeneity with isoelectric variants with pIs of 3.8–4.8. The antigen resists carbonate extraction, but partitions into a detergent Triton TX-114 phase indicating that gp4A4 represents a group of integral membrane proteins. In monolayer cultures gp4A4 is turned over slowly, being constitutively recycled for >40 h. There are about 150 000 molecules per cell. The expression of gp4A4 is enhanced by a soluble factor secreted by C6 glial cells (Raub *et al.*, 1990).

Gp4A4 is expressed by endothelial cells of brain microvessels. However, it is not BBB-specific, but found on various endothelia with some exceptions such as the fenestrated endothelium of the choroid plexus. Gp4A4 is also found on transporting epithelia in choroid plexus, bile duct, and kidney tubules. Cerebral endothelial cells display a homogeneous surface distribution of gp4A4. The function of the antigen is still unknown.

EBM antigen

A rat brain fraction enriched with microvessels by Ficoll gradient centrifugation was employed to produce the hybridoma cell line, which secreted the monoclonal antibody anti-EBM (endothelium of brain microvessels) (Michalak *et al.*, 1986). The corresponding antigen has not yet been identified. In brain, the antibody reacts with endothelial cells of microvessels, but not with endothelia of arteries, veins and the choroid plexus. Endothelial cells of other organs such as liver, kidney and heart are also negative. However, in kidney the brush border of proximal tubuli and in liver the bile canaliculi are immunoreactive. Immuno-electron microscopic localization of EBM antigen indicates that it is present in significant amounts in granules dispersed throughout the cytoplasm as well as on the luminal surface of brain endothelial cells. The abluminal membrane is devoid of the antigen. The function of the EBM antigen remains to be elucidated.

Proteins recognized by polyclonal antisera

In order to produce polyclonal antisera, which display a distinct specificity for brain endothelial cells, enriched plasma membranes of bovine BBB microvessels were employed to immunize rabbits. After preabsorption of the antiserum with rat liver and kidney powder, one antiserum preferentially immunoprecipitates a 46 kDa protein (Pardridge *et al.*, 1986) present on capillaries in brain, but not heart, liver and kidney. However, the corresponding antigen is expressed in the epithelial lining of biliary ducts in liver. In the brain, endothelial cells are the only immunoreactive cell type. Immunocytochemistry of cultured endothelial cells reveals that the antiserum avidly binds to lateral membranes. The function and the molecular identity of the 46 kDa antigen has not yet been evaluated. Therefore, it is unknown whether the antigen represents, for example, a distinct isoform of HT7/neurothelin.

A second antiserum reacted with a protein triplet of 45 kDa, 53 kDa and 200 kDa (Pardridge *et al.*, 1990). The antiserum marks the luminal and antiluminal endothelial cell surface, in addition to the tight junctional area (Farrell and Pardridge, 1991). No structures in kidney, liver, heart, and urinary bladder are immunopositive. In the choroid plexus only the 200 kDa protein is present. Whether any relation exists between these antisera has not been reported. This immunological approach demonstrates that by virtue of immunogen purification and subsequent fractionation of polyspecific antisera, distinct BBB components can be identified.

PAL-E and MECA-32

PAL-E and MECA-32 might be considered *contra-BBB antigens*, because both components are expressed in endothelial cells only as long as these cells are not induced to express BBB characteristics. The monoclonal antibody PAL-E was obtained after a mouse had been challenged with cell suspensions of human lymph node metastases of melanoma (Schlingemann *et al.*, 1985). The antibody stains capillaries and small-sized veins, but not arterioles. Blood vessels of the normal brain are PAL-E negative. Most interestingly, brain microvessels become positive once the BBB breaks down under pathological conditions such as in glioblastoma, anaplastic astrocytoma and other brain tumors (Leenstra *et al.*, 1990). Similarly, brain vessels without BBB under normal conditions, such as the area postrema and choroid plexus, show PAL-E reactivity. In addition, at 6

weeks gestation age before the formation of the BBB, microvessels of the developing human brain do express the PAL-E antigen. PAL-E staining is located on the cell membrane of endothelial cells.

MAb MECA-32 recognizes protein bands of molecular weights 50–55 kDa under reducing conditions and 100–120 kDa bands under nonreducing conditions. Cloning of MECA-32 indicates that the protein although associated with the cell surface, has no signal sequence and no transmembrane domain (R. Hallmann, personal communication). It binds specifically to mouse endothelium and therefore to blood vessels in essentially all organs. In the brain, BBB microvessels are devoid of the antigen, whereas endothelial cells of the choroid plexus are immunoreactive. Before differentiation of the BBB, MECA-32 is expressed in brain microvessels. Around day 16 of gestation brain microvasculature becomes MECA-32 negative (Hallmann *et al.*, 1995).

These contra-BBB antigens provide a very helpful index for the integrity of the BBB under pathological conditions *in vivo* and experimental conditions *in vitro*. Both antigens could be components of gene programmes that switch from non-barrier to barrier functions during development and vice versa during the manifestation of distinct diseases.

Concluding remark

The different antigens described add to the list of more common BBB components such as γ-glutamyl-transpeptidase, alkaline phosphatase and others. It is likely that these antigens are not interrelated on a molecular level and represent novel proteins of the BBB. Further understanding of these antigens promises to facilitate future insights into BBB functioning.

Acknowledgment

I am grateful to H. Bauch, R. Dermietzel, P. Gordon-Weeks, R. Hallmann, W. M. Pardridge, L. Sternberger, and H. Wolburg for inspiring discussions and critical reading of the manuscript.

References

Albrecht, U., Seulberger, H., Schwarz, H. and Risau., W. (1990). Correlation of blood–brain barrier function and HT7 protein distribution in chick brain circumventricular organs. *Brain Res.*, **535**, 49–61.

Altruda, F., Ccrvella, P., Gaete, M. L. *et al.* (1989). Cloning of cDNA for a novel mouse membrane glycoprotein (gp42), shared identity to histocompatibility antigens, immunoglobulins and neural cell adhesion molecules. *Gene*, **85**, 445–52.

Biswas, C., Zhang, Y., Decastro, R. *et al.* (1995). Human tumor cell-derived collagenase stimulatory factor (renamed EMMPRIN) is a member of the immunoglobulin superfamily. *Cancer Res.*, **55**, 434–9.

Cesario, M. M., Ensrud, K., Hamilton, D. W. and Bartles, J. R. (1995). Biogenesis of the posterior-tail plasma membrane domain of the mammalian spermatozoon, targeting and lateral redistribution of the posterior-tail domain-specific transmembrane protein CE9 during spermiogenesis. *Dev. Biol.*, **169**, 473–86.

Fadool, J. M. and Linser, P. J. (1993a). Differential glycosylation of the 5A11/HT7 antigen by neural retina and epithelial tissues in the chicken. *J. Neurochem.*, **60**, 1354–64.

Fadool, J. M. and Linser, P. J. (1993b). 5A11 antigen is a cell recognition molecule which is involved in neuronal-glial interactions in avian neural retina. *Dev. Dynam.*, **196**, 252–62.

Fadool, J. M. and Linser, P. J. (1994). Spatial and temporal expression of the 5A11/HT7 antigen in the chick embryo – association with morphogenetic events and tissue maturation. *Roux. Arch. Devel. Biol.*, **203**, 328–39.

Farrell, C. L. and Pardridge, W. M. (1991). Ultrastructural localisation of blood–brain barrier-specific antibodies using immunogold-silver enhancement techniques. *J. Neurosci. Meths.*, **37**, 103–10.

Fossum, S., Mallett, S. and Barclay, A. N. (1991). The MRC OX-47 antigen is a member of the immunoglobulin superfamily with an unusual transmembrane sequence. *Eur. J. Immunol.*, **21**, 671–9.

Gerhardt, H., Liebner, S. and Wolburg, H. (1996). The pecten oculi of the chicken as a new in vivo model of the blood–brain barrier. *Cell Tissue Res.*, **285**, 91–100.

Hallmann, R., Mayer, D. N., Berg, E. L. *et al.* (1995). Novel mouse endothelial cell surface marker is suppressed during differentiation of the blood–brain barrier. *Dev. Dynam.*, **202**, 325–32.

Ibiwoye, M. O., Sibbons, P. D., Howard, C. V. and van Velzen, D. (1994). Immunocytochemical study of a vascular barrier antigen in the developing rat brain. *J. Comp. Pathol.*, **111**, 43–53.

Kaname, T., Miyauchi, T., Kuwano, A. *et al.* (1993). Mapping basigin (BSG), a mcmber of the immunoglobulin superfamily, to 19p13.3. *Cytogenet. Cell. Genet.*, **64**, 195–7.

Kasinrerk, W., Fiebiger, E., Stefanova, I. *et al.* (1992). Human leukocyte activation antigen M6, a member of the Ig superfamily, is the species homologue of rat OX-47, mouse basigin, and chicken HT7 molecule. *J. Immunol.*, **149**, 847–54.

Krause, D., Vatter, B. and Dermietzel, R. (1988). Immunochemical and immunocytochemical characterization of a novel monoclonal antibody recognizing a 140 kDa protein in cerebral pericytes of the rat. *Cell Tissue Res.*, **252**, 543–55.

Kunz, J., Krause, D., Kremer, M. and Dermietzel, R. (1994). The 140 kDa-protein of blood–brain barrier-associated pericytes is identical to aminopeptidase N. *J. Neurochem.*, **62**, 2375–86.

Kunz, J., Krause, D., Gehrmann, J. and Dermietzel, R. (1995). Changes in the expression pattern of blood–brain barrier-associated pericytic aminopepti-dase N (pAP N) in the course of acute experimental autoimmune encephalomyelitis. *J Neuroimmunol*, **59**, 41–55.

Lawrenson, J. G., Ghabriel, M. N., Reid, A. R. *et al.* (1995). Differential expression of an endothelial barrier antigen between the CNS and the PNS. *J. Anat.*, **186**, 217–21.

Leenstra, S., Das, P. K., Troost, D. *et al.* (1990). PAL-E, monoclonal antibody with immunoreactivity for endothelium specific to brain tumours. *The Lancet*, **335**, 671.

Lobrinus, J. A., Juillerat-Jeanneret, L., Darekar, P. *et al.* (1992). Induction of the blood–brain barrier specific HT7 and neurothelin epitopes in endothelial cells of the chick chorioallantoic vessels by a soluble factor derived from astrocytes. *Dev. Brain Res.*, **70**, 207–11.

Michalak, T., White, F. P., Gard, A. L. and Dutton, G. R. (1986). A monoclonal antibody to the endothelium of rat brain microvessels. *Brain Res*, **379**, 320–8.

Miyauchi, T., Kanekura, T., Yamaoka, A. *et al.* (1990). Basigin, a new, broadly distributed member of the immunoglob-ulin superfamily, has strong homology with both the immunoglobulin V domain and the beta-chain of major histocompatibility complex class II antigen. *J. Biochem.*, **107**, 316–23.

Miyauchi, T., Masuzawa, Y. and Muramatsu, T. (1991). The basigin group of the immunoglobulin superfamily: complete conservation of a segment in and around transmembrane domains of human and mouse basigin and chicken HT7 antigen. *J. Biochem.*, **110**, 770–4.

Miyauchi, T., Jimma, F., Igakura, T. *et al.* (1995). Structure of the mouse basigin gene, a unique member of the immunoglobulin superfamily. *J. Biochem. Tokyo.*, **118**, 717–24.

Mooradian, A. D., Grabau, G. and Uko-eninn, A. (1993). In situ quantitative estimates of the age-related and diabetes-related changes in cerebral endothelial barrier antigen. *Brain Res.*, **309**, 41–4.

Nehme, C. L., Cesario, M. M., Myles, D. G. *et al.* (1993). Breaching the diffusion barrier that compartmentalizes the transmembrane glycoprotein CE9 to the posterior-tail plasma membrane domain of the rat spermatozoon. *J. Cell. Biol.*, **120**, 687–94.

Nehme, C. L., Fayos, B. E. and Bartles, J. R. (1995). Distribution of the integral plasma membrane glycoprotein CE9 (MRC OX-47) among rat tissues and its induction by diverse stimuli of metabolic activation. *Biochem. J.*, **310**, 693–8.

Pardridge, W. M., Yang, J., Eisenberg, J. and Mietus, L. J. (1986). Antibodies to blood–brain barrier bind selectively to brain capillary endothelial lateral membranes and to a 46 kDa protein. *J. Cereb. Blood Flow Metab.*, **6**, 203–11.

Pardridge, W. M., Yang, J., Buciak, J. L. and Boado, R. J. (1990). Differential expression of 53- and 45-kDa brain capillary-specific proteins by brain capillary endothelium and choroid plexus in vivo and by brain capillary endothelium in tissue culture. *Mol. Cell. Neurosci.*, **1**, 20–8.

Raub, T. J., Kuentzel, S. L. and Sawada, G. A. (1990). Expression, characterization and recycling of a sulfated membrane glycoprotein on bovine brain microvessel endothelial in vivo and in culture. *J. Cell. Biol.*, **111**, 183a.

Raub, T. J., Sawada, G. A. and Kuentzel, S. L. (1994). Expression of a widely distributed, novel sulfated membrane glycoprotein by bovine endothelia and certain transporting epithelia. *J. Histochem. Cytochem.*, **42**, 1237–50.

Risau, W., Hallmann, R., Albrecht, U. and Henke-Fahle, S. (1986). Brain induces the expression of an early cell surface marker for blood–brain barrier-specific endothelium. *The EMBO J.*, **5**, 3179–83.

Rizzolo, L. J. and Zhou, S. M. (1995). The distribution of Na$^+$,K$^+$-ATPase and 5A11 antigen in apical microvilli of the retinal pigment epithelium is unrelated to alpha-spectrin. *J. Cell. Sci.*, **108**, 3623–33.

Rosenstein, J. M., Krum, J. M., Sternberger, L. A. *et al.* (1992). Immunocytochemical expression of the endothelial barrier antigen (EBA) during brain angiogenesis. *Dev. Brain Res.*, **66**, 47–54.

Schlingemann, R. O., Dingjan, G. M., Emeis, J. J. *et al.* (1985). Monoclonal antibody PAL-E specific for endothelium. *Lab. Invest.*, **52**, 71–6.

Schlosshauer, B. (1991). Neurothelin: molecular characteristics and developmental regulation in the chick CNS. *Development*, **113**, 129–40.

Schlosshauer, B. and Herzog, K.-H. (1990). Neurothelin, an inducible cell surface glycoprotein of blood–brain barrier-specific endothelial cells and distinct neurons. *J. Cell. Biol.*, **110**, 1261–74.

Schlosshauer, B., Bauch, H. and Frank, R. (1995). Neurothelin, amino acid sequence, cell surface dynamics and actin colocalization. *Eur. J. Cell Biol.*, **68**, 159–66.

Schuster, V. L., Lu, R., Kanai, N. *et al.* (1996). Cloning of the rabbit homologue of mouse 'basigin' and rat 'OX-47': kidney cell type-specific expression, and regulation in collecting duct cells. *Biochim. Biophys. Acta.*, **1311**, 13–19.

Seulberger, H., Lottspeich, F. and Risau, W. (1990). The inducible blood–brain barrier specific molecule HT7 is a novel immunoglobulin-like cell surface glycoprotein. *The EMBO J.*, **9**, 2151–8.

Seulberger, H., Unger, C. M. and Risau, W. (1992). HT7, neurothelin, basigin, gp42 and OX-47 – many names for one developmentally regulated immuno-globulin-like surface glycoprotein on blood–brain barrier endothelium, epithelial tissue barriers and neurons. *Neurosci. Lett.*, **140**, 93–7.

Sternberger, N. H. and Sternberger, L. A. (1987). Blood–brain barrier protein recognized by monoclonal antibody. *Proc. Natl. Acad. Sci. USA*, **84**, 8169–73.

Sternberger, N. H., Sternberger, L. A., Kies, M. W. and Shear, C. R. (1989). Cell surface endothelial proteins altered in experimental allergic encephalomyelitis. *J. Neurobiol.*, **21**, 241–8.

Unger, C. M., Seulberger, H., Breier, G. *et al.* (1993). Expression of the HT7 gene in blood–brain barrier. In *Frontiers in Cerebral Vascular Biology, Transport and its Regulation*, ed. L. R. Drewes and A. L. Betz, pp. 211–15. New York: Plenum Press.

321

35 Molecular dissection of tight junctions: occludin and ZO-1

SHOICHIRO TSUKITA, MIKIO FURUSE and MASAHIKO ITOH

- Barrier function of tight junctions
- ZO-1: a peripheral membrane protein localizing at tight and adherens junctions
- Identification of occludin: an integral membrane protein localizing at tight junctions
- Molecular architecture of tight junctions
- Occludin and ZO-1 at endothelial cells
- Perspective

Barrier function of tight junctions

The establishment of compositionally distinct fluid compartments by various types of cell sheets is crucial for the development and function of most organs in multicellular organisms. Since these cell sheets consist of two-dimensionally arranged cells, some mechanism is required to seal cells to create a primary barrier to the diffusion of solutes through the paracellular pathway. This mechanism is thus essential for morphogenesis of the multicellular system, and the tight junction, an element of epithelial and endothelial junctional complexes, is now believed to be directly involved in this mechanism (Schneeberger and Lynch, 1992; Gumbiner, 1987, 1993). The brain is an important compartment that is protected by a barrier of endothelial cell sheets bearing well-developed tight junctions. This is referred as the blood–brain barrier.

In thin-section electron microscopy, tight junctions appear as a series of discrete sites of apparent fusion, involving the outer leaflet of the plasma membrane of adjacent cells (Farquhar and Palade, 1963). In freeze-fracture electron microscopy, this junction appears as a set of continuous, anastomosing intramembrane strands or fibrils in the P-face (the outwardly facing cytoplasmic leaflet) with complementary grooves in the E-face (the inwardly facing extracytoplasmic leaflets) (Staehelin, 1974). It has remained controversial whether the strands are predominantly lipid in nature, that is, cylindrical lipid micelles, or represent linearly aggregated integral membrane proteins (Kachar and Reese, 1982; Pinto da Silva and Kachar, 1982). However, given the detergent stability of tight junction strands visualized by negative staining (Stevenson and Goodenough, 1984) and freeze fracture (Stevenson et al., 1988), it was thought to be unlikely that these elements are composed solely of lipids.

ZO-1: a peripheral membrane protein localizing at tight and adherens junctions

ZO-1 was defined as an antigen for monoclonal antibodies that recognize tight junctions in epithelial cells (Stevenson et al., 1986). It is a peripheral membrane protein with a molecular mass of 220 kDa underlying the cytoplasmic surface of plasma membranes. In epithelial cells, ZO-1 is exclusively localized at tight junctions, with the exception that it is highly concentrated at the undercoat of plasma membranes of the slit diaphragm in kidney glomeruli. In non-epithelial cells such as cardiac muscle cells and fibroblasts, ZO-1 is precisely colocalized with cadherins to form adherens junctions (Howarth *et al.*, 1992; Itoh *et al.*, 1991, 1993). The molecular mechanism of this peculiar behavior of ZO-1 remains elusive. In endothelial cells, this adherens junction versus tight junction problem of ZO-1 has not been analyzed or discussed in detail. ZO-1 has been used as a specific marker for tight junctions also in endothelial cells, but this should be reevaluated as described below.

The structure of ZO-1 has been analyzed by cDNA cloning and sequencing (Itoh *et al.*, 1993; Tsukita *et al.*, 1993; Willott *et al.*, 1993). The amino-terminal half of this molecule displays significant similarity to the product of the lethal(1)discs large1 (*dlg*) gene in *Drosophila*. The *dlg* gene product (and also the amino-terminal half of ZO-1) contains putative functional domains. From the amino-terminus, there are filamentous, SH3, and guanylate kinase domains. The amino-terminal filamentous domain contains three internal repeats, which are called PDZ repeats. Various proteins localizing just beneath plasma membranes are now found to contain PDZ repeats, indicating a gene family called MAGUK (membrane-associated guanylate kinase homologues) family.

In addition to ZO-1, other peripheral proteins have been identified to be localized at tight junctions. ZO-2, with a molecular mass of 160 kDa, was identified as a ZO-1-binding protein by immunoprecipitation (Gumbiner *et al.*, 1991). This molecule also shows sequence similarity to the *dlg* product, indicating that it is a member of the MAGUK family (Jesaitis and Goodenough, 1994). Furthermore, monoclonal antibodies identified two other tight junction-specific peripheral membrane proteins named cingulin and 7H6 antigen (Citi *et al.*, 1988; Zhong *et al.*, 1993). Despite intensive studies, the functions of these tight junction-associated peripheral membrane proteins totally remain elusive, although it is presumed that they are involved in the formation, maintenance, and regulation of tight junctions.

Identification of occludin: an integral membrane protein localizing at tight junctions

To clarify the structure and functions of tight junctions at the molecular level, an integral membrane protein working at tight junctions had to be identified. However, this integral membrane component remained elusive for quite some time. A procedure was established for isolating cadherin-based cell-to-cell adherens junctions from the rat liver (Tsukita and Tsukita, 1989). During the course of identification of novel proteins enriched in this fraction, ZO-1 was also found to be concentrated, indicating that not only adherens, but also tight junctions are enriched in this fraction (Itoh *et al.*, 1993). An attempt was then made to identify the putative integral membrane protein localizing at tight junctions using this isolated junctional fraction. To obtain a powerful antigen, we isolated the junctional fraction from chicken liver and injected it into rats to generate monoclonal antibodies.

Three mAbs that are specific for a ~65 kDa protein were obtained (Furuse *et al.*, 1993). This antigen was not extractable from plasma membranes without detergent, suggesting that it is an integral membrane protein. Immunofluorescence and immunoelectron microscopy with these mAbs showed that this ~65 kDa membrane protein is exclusively localized at tight junctions of both epithelial and endothelial cells. Labels were detected directly over the points of membrane contact in tight junctions by ultra-thin section electron microscopy, and directly over the intramembranous particle strands of tight junctions by immuno-freeze fracture electron microscopy (Fujimoto, 1995). It was therefore concluded that these mAbs recognize an integral membrane protein localizing at tight junctions. This antigen was then designated occludin from the Latin word *occludere*.

To further clarify the nature and structure of chick occludin, its cDNA was cloned and sequenced. It encoded a 504 amino acid polypeptide with a calculated molecular mass of 56 kDa. A search of the database identified no proteins with significant homology to occludin. A most striking feature of its primary structure was revealed by a

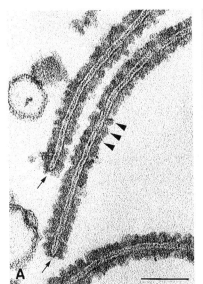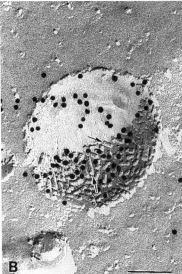

Fig. 35.1. Ultrastructure of the multilamellar structures enriched in Sf9 cells overexpressing chicken occludin. (A) Ultrathin electron microscopic images of isolated multilamellar structures fixed with 0.1% tannic acid. Each lamella has a membrane loop at both ends (arrows). In each lamella, the outer leaflets of opposing membranes are fused with no gaps like tight junctions, and their cytoplasmic surface is characterized by closely-arranged dense protrusions, which may be morphological counterparts of the long cytoplasmic domain of occludin (arrowheads). (B) Immunoelectron microscopic images of freeze-fracture replicas of occludin-enriched structures labeled with anti-chicken occludin mAb. Several particles occasionally align to form a short strand (arrows). Bar, 100 nm.

hydrophilicity plot (see Fig. 35.2). (1) In the amino-terminal half, occludin contains four transmembrane domains. (2) A carboxyl-terminal half consisting of ~250 amino acid residues resides in the cytoplasm. (3) Charged amino acids mostly locate in the cytoplasm. (4) The content of tyrosine and glycine residues is very high in the extracellular domains.

Compared with adhesion molecules working at other intercellular junctions such as adherens junctions and desmosomes, those at tight junctions should be structurally and functionally unique. They must tightly obliterate the intercellular space for the barrier function in epithelial and endothelial cell sheets, and form a continuous strand within the membrane to form a fence against membranous lipids and proteins. To determine whether or not occludin fulfills these criteria for tight junction adhesion molecules, chicken occludin was overexpressed in insect Sf9 cells by recombinant baculovirus infection (Furuse *et al.*, 1996). Most of the overexpressed occludin molecules did

not appear on the cell surface, but were concentrated in peculiar multilamellar structures in the cytoplasm. Thin-section electron microscopy revealed that each lamella was transformed from intracellular membranous cisternae in which the luminal space was completely collapsed. Furthermore, the outer leaflets of opposing membranes in each lamella appeared to be fused with no gaps, like tight junctions (Fig. 35.1). Short tight junction-like intramembranous particle strands were occasionally observed in freeze-fracture replicas of these multilamellar structures, which were specifically labeled by anti-occludin mAb. These findings favor the notion that occludin is one of the major cell adhesion molecules in tight junctions.

Considering that tight junctions play a key role as a barrier in endothelial cells (and also in epithelial cells), it would be important in cell biological as well as in medical research to analyze the expression and localization of occludin in various pathological states of human samples and to modulate the functions of occludin not only at the cell cul-

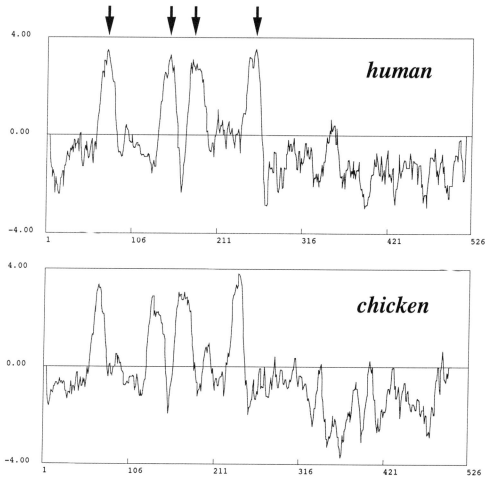

Fig. 35.2. Hydrophilicity plots for human and chicken occludin. Hydrophilic and hydrophobic residues are in the lower and upper part of the frames, respectively. The axis is numbered in amino acid residues. At the amino-terminal half of each occludin, there are four major hydrophobic, potentially membrane-spanning, regions (arrows).

ture but also at the whole body levels. As described above, occludin was identified in the chicken, and none of our mAbs and pAbs raised against chicken occludin cross-reacted with the murine and human homologues (Furuse *et al.*, 1993). Several investigators, including ourselves, have attempted to isolate cDNA encoding mammalian homologues, based upon the assumption that the occludin amino acid sequence is rather evolutionarily conserved due to its functional importance. However, these efforts have only recently been successful.

During attempts to identify the mammalian homologues of occludin, we learned from the Gen-Bank database, using the biological sequence search program Mpsrch, that a 675 nucleotide sequence showing similarity to part of the carboxyl terminal domain of chicken occludin had been found in close proximity to the human neuronal apoptosis inhibitory protein gene (Roy *et al.*, 1995). To determine whether or not this sequence really encodes part of the human homologue of occludin, PCR was performed with two oligonucleotides as primers, using an expression cDNA library of human cultured cells. A DNA fragment was obtained that allowed us to isolate a full length cDNA encoding human occludin (Ando-Akatsuka *et al.*, 1996). The cDNAs encoding murine and canine occludin homologues were also isolated and sequenced by

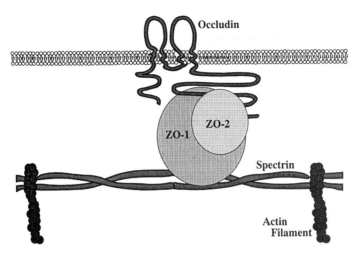

Fig. 35.3. Schematic drawing of the possible molecular architecture of tight junctions. Both ZO-1 and ZO-2 are directly associated with occludin.

the same procedure. The amino acid sequences of the three mammalian (human, murine, and canine) occludins are closely related (~90% identity), whereas they diverged considerably from those of chicken (~50% identity). However, the hydrophilicity profile of chicken occludin is highly conserved in human occludin (Fig. 35.2).

Molecular architecture of tight junctions

The identification of occludin allowed us to analyze the detailed molecular architecture of tight junctions, in terms of the interaction of occludin with tight-junction peripheral proteins at the molecular level. Based on distance from the plasma membrane, tight-junction peripheral proteins can be subclassified into two categories. The first class includes ZO-1 and ZO-2, which are localized in the immediate vicinity of plasma membranes. The second class includes cingulin and the 7H6 antigen, which are localized more than 40 nm from the plasma membranes. We showed that the GST-fusion protein of the carboxyl-terminal half cytoplasmic domain of occludin specifically associates with 220 and 160 kD bands among the various membrane peripheral proteins in the extract from the isolated junction fraction (Furuse et al., 1994). These two bands were identified as ZO-1 and ZO-2, respectively, by immunoblotting and the domain

responsible for this binding was narrowed down to the carboxyl-terminal ~150 amino acid sequence of occludin. Furthermore, using the various recombinant ZO-1 and ZO-2 proteins produced by recombinant baculovirus infection, we found that the amino-terminal halves of ZO-1 and ZO-2 directly and independently bound to the cytoplasmic domain of occludin (Itoh et al., in preparation). Spectrin tetramers are associated with ZO-1 at ~10–20 nm from their midpoint (Itoh et al., 1991), and spectrin was specifically trapped in a column containing the GST-occludin fusion protein (Furuse et al., 1994). Thus there may be a molecular linkage between occludin and actin filaments as shown in Fig. 35.3, since an intimate spatial relationship between tight junctions and actin-based cytoskeletons has been observed (Madara, 1988). It remains elusive where other tight junction peripheral proteins such as cingulin and the 7H6 antigen should be placed in this scheme, how the integrity of this molecular organization is regulated, and how this molecular organization is important for the functions of tight junctions.

Occludin and ZO-1 at endothelial cells

We produced various mAbs and pAbs that recognize mammalian occludin homologues by immunofluorescence microscopy and immunoblotting. One

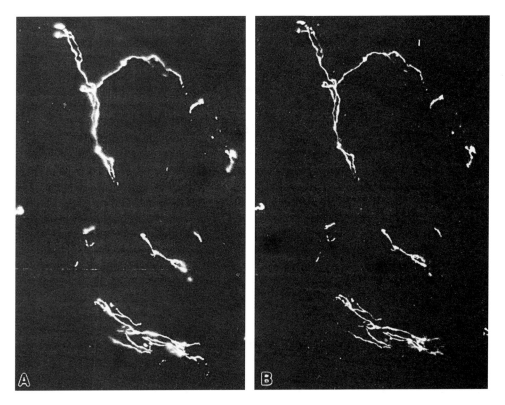

Fig. 35.4. Double immunofluorescence staining of a frozen section of guinea pig brain with a rat mAb against mouse occludin (A) and a mouse mAb against ZO-1 (B). Both occludin and ZO-1 are highly concentrated at the junctional complex region of endothelial cells of microvessels.

of these mAbs, named MOC37, recognized all mammalian occludins as far as examined (Saitou *et al.*, submitted). Using MOC37 and anti-ZO-1 mAb, the expression level and localization of occludin and ZO-1 in various epithelial and endothelial cells was compared by immunofluorescence microscopy. In epithelial cells, the intensity of the occludin signal from tight junctions appeared to correlate well with the number of tight junction strands, which have been so far determined by freeze-fracture. For example, in the kidney, the occludin signal was intense from the distal tubules, whereas it was very weak from the proximal tubules.

In the brain, spinal cord, and peripheral nerves, the endothelial cells bear well-developed tight junctions, which are thought to be a morphological counterpart for the blood–brain barrier. In these endothelial cells, the occludin signal was remarkably intense (Fig. 35.4). By contrast, most of the endothelial cells in non-neuronal tissue such as intestine, kidney and heart were stained only very weakly with anti-occludin mAb. Some blood vessels were rather intensely stained in these tissues, but the nature of these occludin-positive endothelial cells remains to be elucidated. The ZO-1 signal was very intense in endothelial cells not only from neuronal, but also from non-neuronal tissue. These findings indicate that in endothelial cells, the development of tight junctions correlates well with the intensity of the occludin signal, but not with that of ZO-1. It is possible that in endothelial cells, ZO-1 is not restricted to tight junctions, but also associated with the cadherin system as observed in fibroblasts and cardiac muscle cells.

Perspective

Now that the mammalian occludins have been identified, the organization and function of tight junctions can be structurally and functionally examined at the molecular level. Using various types of cultured human, murine and canine (MDCK) cells, the barrier function of tight junctions and the regulation mechanisms involved can be experimentally analyzed by modulating occludin gene expression or by blocking it with antisense probes or with antibodies. For example, it can now be determined whether upon the overexpression of occludin cDNA, the number of tight junction strands, as seen in freeze-fracture replicas, will increase, with concomitant upregulation of the barrier function. Through the production of various transgenic and occludin gene knock-out mice,

we will learn how tight junction formation is involved in the morphogenesis of various organs and whether or not tight junction dysfunction is related to various pathological states such as inflammation and tumor metastasis. The modulation of tight junction functions, especially its barrier function, is also interesting in relation to drug delivery, and it should be possible to modulate the blood–brain barrier through up- or down-regulating occludin synthesis and/or functions in brain endothelial cells.

References

Ando-Akatsuka, Y., Saitou, M., Hirase, T. *et al.* (1996). Iterspecies diversity of the occludin sequence: cDNA cloning of human, mouse, dog, and rat-kangaroo homologues. *J. Cell Biol.*, **133**, 43–7.

Citi, S., Sabanay, H., Jakes, R. *et al.* (1988). Cingulin, a new peripheral component of tight junctions. *Nature (Lond.)*, **33**, 272–6.

Farquhar, M. G. and Palade, G. E. (1963). Junctional complexes in various epithelia. *J. Cell Biol.*, **17**, 375–409.

Fujimoto, K. (1995). Freeze-fracture replica electron microscopy combined with SDS digestion for cytochemical labeling of integral membrane proteins. Application to the immunogold labeling of intercellular junctional complexes. *J. Cell Sci.*, **108**, 3443–9.

Furuse, M., Hirase, T., Itoh, M. *et al.* (1993). Occludin: a novel integral membrane protein localizing at tight junctions. *J. Cell Biol.*, **123**, 1777–88.

Furuse, M., Itoh, M., Hirase, T. *et al.* (1994). Direct association of occludin with ZO-1 and its possible involvement in the localization of occludin at tight junctions. *J. Cell Biol.*, **127**, 1617–26.

Furuse, M., Fujimoto, K., Sato, N. *et al.* (1996). Overexpression of occludin, a tight junction-associated integral membrane protein, induces the formation of intracellular multilamellar bodies bearing tight junction-like structures. *J. Cell Sci.*, **109**, 429–35.

Gumbiner, B. (1987). Structure, biochemistry, and assembly of epithelial tight junctions. *Am. J. Physiol.*, **253**, C749–C758.

Gumbiner, B. (1993). Breaking through the tight junction barrier. *J. Cell Biol.*, **123**, 1631–3.

Gumbiner, B., Lowenkopf, T. and Apatira, D. (1991). Identification of a 160 kDa polypeptide that binds to the tight junction protein ZO-1. *Proc. Natl. Acad. Sci. USA*, **88**, 3460–4.

Howarth, A. G., Hughes, M. R. and Stevenson, B. R. (1992). Detection of the tight junction-associated protein ZO-1 in astrocytes and other nonepithelial cell types. *Am. J. Physiol.*, **262**, C461–469.

Itoh, M., Yonemura, S., Nagafuchi, A. *et al.* (1991). A 220-kD undercoat-constitutive protein: its specific localization at cadherin-based cell-cell adhesion sites. *J. Cell Biol.*, **115**, 1449–62.

Itoh, M., Nagafuchi, A., Yonemura, S. *et al.* (1993). The 220-kD protein colocalizing with cadherins in non-epithelial cells is identical to ZO-1, a tight junction-associated protein in epithelial cells: cDNA cloning and immunoelectron microscopy. *J. Cell Biol.*, **121**, 491–502.

Jesaitis, L. A. and Goodenough, D. A. (1994). Molecular characterization and tissue distribution of ZO-2, a tight junction protein homologous to ZO-1 and the Drosophila discs-large tumor suppresser protein. *J. Cell Biol.*, **124**, 949–61.

Kachar, B. and Reese, T. S. (1982), Evidence for the lipidic nature of tight junction strands. *Nature (Lond.)*, **296**, 464–6.

Madara, J. L. (1988). Tight junction dynamics: is paracellular transport regulated ? *Cell*, **53**, 497–498.

Pinto da Silva, P. and Kachar, B. (1982). On tight junction structure. *Cell*, **28**, 441–50.

Roy, N., Mahadevan, M. S., McLean, M. *et al.* (1995). The gene for neuronal apoptosis inhibitory protein is partially deleted in individuals with spinal muscular atrophy. *Cell*, **80**, 167–78.

Schneeberger, E. E. and Lynch, R. D. (1992). Structure, function, and regulation of cellular tight junctions. *Am. J. Physiol.*, **262**, L647–L661.

Staehelin, L. A. (1974). Structure and function of intercellular junctions. *Int. Rev. Cytol.*, **39**, 191–282.

Stevenson, B. R. and D. Goodenough (1984). Zonula occludentes in junctional complex-enriched fractions from mouse liver: preliminary morphological and biochemical characterization. *J. Cell Biol.*, **98**, 1209- 21.

Stevenson, B. R., Siliciano, J. D., Mooseker, M. S. and Goodenough, D. A. (1986). Identification of ZO-1: a high molecular weight polypeptide associated with the tight junction (zonula occludens) in a variety of epithelia. *J. Cell Biol.*, **103**, 755–66.

Stevenson, B. R., Anderson, J. M. and Bullivant, S. (1988). The epithelial tight junction: Structure, function and preliminary biochemical characterization. *Mol. Cell. Biochem.*, **83**, 129–45.

Tsukita, Sh. and Tsukita, Sa. (1989). Isolation of cell-to-cell adherens junctions from rat liver. *J. Cell Biol.*, **108**, 31–41.

Tsukita, Sh., Itoh, M., Nagafuchi, A. *et al.* (1993). Submembranous junctional plaque proteins include potential tumor suppresser molecules. *J. Cell Biol.*, **123**, 1049–53.

Willott, E., Balda, M. S., Fanning, A. S. *et al.* (1993). The tight junction protein ZO-1 is homologous to the Drosophila discs-large tumor suppresser protein of septate junctions. *Proc. Natl. Acad. Sci. USA*, **90**, 7834–8.

Zhong, Y., Saitoh, T., Minase, T. *et al.* (1993). Monoclonal antibody 7H6 reacts with a novel tight junction-associated protein distinct from ZO-1, cingulin and ZO-2. *J. Cell Biol.*, **120**, 477-83.

36 Phosphatidylinositol pathways

R. E. CATALÁN

- General considerations concerning the phosphatidylinositol cycle
- Blood–brain barrier and the metabolism of phosphoinositides
- Modulation of the PI pathway by endothelin in the blood–brain barrier

General considerations concerning the phosphatidylinositol cycle

The discovery of the 'phosphoinositide effect' by Hokin and Hokin as early as in 1953 (Hokin and Hokin, 1953) demonstrating that acetylcholine could stimulate the incorporation of $^{32}P_i$ into phosphatidylinositol (PI) and phosphatidic acid (PA), revealed the association between hormone action and phospholipid turnover. Later, the agonist-induced phosphoinositide turnover and its relationship to Ca^{2+} signaling were described (Michell, 1975). The fact that the hydrolysis of phosphatidylinositol bisphosphate (PIP_2) by a phosphoinositide-specific phospholipase C yields two second messengers: 1,2-diacylglycerol (DAG), which activates protein kinase C and inositol 1,4,5-trisphosphate (IP_3) which mobilizes Ca^{2+} from intracellular stores, was demonstrated (Streb et al., 1983).

Although reported some years ago, this phosphoinositide field is currently one of the most interesting fields in biochemistry, which has witnessed during the past decade a tremendous increase in the knowledge of the PI pathway. To gain more insights into this field the following roles are studied: the nuclear metabolism of the PI cycle, the role of phosphatases and the role of higher phosphorylated forms as IP_4, IP_5 and IP_6 (Heslop et al., 1985; Malviya et al., 1990; Henzi and McDermott, 1992). In this regard, phosphoinositide-mediated signal transduction in the nervous system is no exception, and a general view of the PI pathway is now available (Fisher et al., 1992). Nevertheless, we must point out that the knowledge about the molecular mechanisms that regulate the PI pathway in the blood–brain barrier (BBB) is far from complete. Thus, there is little data obtained by cerebral microvascular endothelial cells and cerebral capillaries on the phosphoinositide metabolism. Besides, we must point out that the BBB involved in the maintenance of neuronal function is present in a complex cellular system, and that brain microvessels represent the major component of the BBB. These capillaries have three major functions: protection of the brain from milieu; selective transport; and metabolism or modification of blood/brain-borne substances. Although methods for the culture of brain microvessel endothelial cells have already been described (Audus and Borchardt, 1986), there are several lines of evidence suggesting that cultured brain microvessel endothelial cells rapidly lose their characteristics of differentiated barrier in culture (Risau and Walburg, 1990). In this regard, the use of isolated microvessels may provide a suitable approach for elucidating the biochemical functioning of the BBB (Catalán et al., 1989a,b; 1991; 1992, 1993a,b; 1995; 1996a,b,c).

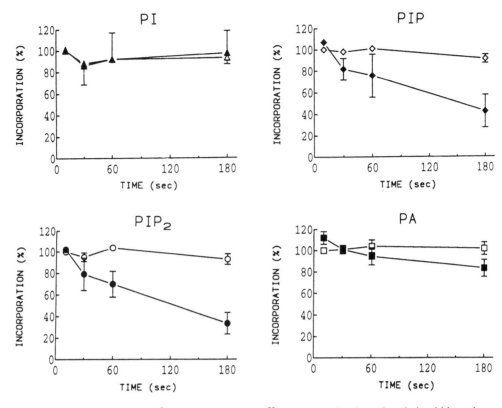

Fig. 36.1. Time-course for Ca^{2+}-ionophore effect on $^{32}P_i$ incorporation into phosphoinositide and PA. Brain microvessels, prelabeled for 90 min with 100 μCi/ml of [^{32}P]orthophosphate were stimulated with 5 μM ionophore A23187 for the time indicated. Data are expressed as percentage of incorporation with respect to the control value. Results represent the mean ± SE from three separate experiments performed in triplicate ($P<0.05$). From Catalán *et al.*, 1995, reprinted by permission of Elsevier Science Inc., 655 Ave. of the Americas, New York, NY 10010.

Blood–brain barrier and the metabolism of phosphoinositides

As stated earlier there is little data reported about the metabolism of phosphoinositides in the BBB. In this regard, the first data were reported by Zeleznikar *et al.* (1983) describing an alpha$_1$-adrenergic receptor-mediated PI effect in canine cerebral capillaries. The existence of the bradikinin receptor, in brain microvessels, that is coupled to phosphoinositide turnover via a pertussis toxin insensitive G protein was described later (Homayoun and Harik, 1991). The regulatory role for protein kinase C in phospholipid signaling pathways in rat brain microvessels was also described (Catalán *et al.*, 1992). In addition, it was found that ADP induces inositol phosphate-independent intracellular Ca^{2+}

mobilization in brain capillary endothelial cells (Frelin *et al.*, 1993) and that the induction of Ca^{2+} mobilization and phosphoinositide metabolism in cultured bovine cerebral microvascular endothelial cells is triggered by platelet activating factor (PAF) (Lin and Rui, 1994).

Most of the work on BBB has been carried out using cerebral microvessels. Thus, the experiments in steady-state conditions showed that increased intracellular Ca^{2+} concentration caused a rapid and marked loss of labeling of phosphatidylinositol monophosphate (PIP) and PIP$_2$, but not from PI and PA (Fig. 36.1). Interestingly, this was concommitantly accompanied by a different effect on inositol phosphates, a rise in labeling of inositol bisphosphate (IP$_2$) and inositol monophosphate (IP), but there was no significant production of IP$_3$

Table 36.1. *Production of inositol phosphates by Ca^{2+} ionophore A23187 in brain microvessels*

Treatment	IP	IP$_2$	IP$_3$
Control	5120±85	170±25	93±20
Ionophore	6383±120*	321+28*	97±12

Brain microvessels were prelabeled with 10 μCi/ml of myo-[2-^{3}H]inositol for 90 min and stimulated by 5 μM ionophore A23187. Inositol phosphates were isolated by HPLC. Data expressed in cpm represent the mean ± SE of two experiments performed in triplicate. Asterisks indicate significant differences from the control value. $P<0.05$. From Catalán *et al.* (1995), reprinted by permission of Elsevier Science Inc., 655 Ave of the Americas, New York, NY 10010.

(Table 36.1). These results suggest that both PIP and PIP$_2$ are hydrolyzed by a Ca^{2+}-activated phosphodiesterase and a Ca^{2+}-activated phosphomonoesterase, respectively. The possibility that PIP$_2$ is hydrolyzed by a phosphodiesterase to yield DAG and IP$_3$, which is rapidly hydrolyzed by a phosphatase (and therefore IP$_3$ cannot be detected) cannot be considered, taking into account that previous data from brain (Brammer and Weaver, 1989) suggest that this hypothesis is unlikely. The phenomenon of a net decrease in polyphosphoinositide levels instead of a complete replenishment may be explained by a partial inhibition of both PI and PIP kinases due to the increased levels of intracellular Ca^{2+}. In this regard, there is a considerable inhibition of endogenous phosphoinositide phosphorylation by Ca^{2+} in isolated membranes. Moreover, these findings agree well with data reported by some authors, where PI kinase (Kai *et al.*, 1966) and PIP kinase (Kai *et al.*, 1968) were shown to be more active in the absence of Ca^{2+}. Nevertheless, there is a partial resynthesis of polyphosphoinositides from PA and PI, as demonstrated by the fact that these phospholipids showed unchanged steady-state radioactivity levels. Studies in synthesis conditions, showing markedly increased labeling by Ca^{2+} ionophore, are compatible with a partial functioning of phosphoinositide cycle (Fig. 36.2). Furthermore, the fact that polyphosphoinositide labeling can be maintained without significant changes in synthesis under experimental conditions (where

ATP increases its specific activity with time) suggests that isolated microvessels display an ability to synthesize PIP and PIP$_2$ sufficient to withstand partially the great increase in the breakdown of these phospholipids by intracellular Ca^{2+}.

Due to the Ca^{2+} ionophore effects on phosphoinositide cycle, it is tempting to speculate that in the blood–brain barrier there may be a reciprocal control mechanism between polyphosphoinositide metabolism and mobilization of Ca^{2+}. Thus, whereas the intracellular levels remain increased after agonist-stimulated PIP$_2$ hydrolysis, both Ca^{2+}-mediated inhibition of PIP and PIP$_2$ resynthesis and activation of PIP phosphodiesterasic breakdown, but not of PIP$_2$, take place. Moreover, there is an increased conversion of PIP$_2$ into PIP. In this way, Ca^{2+} might regulate the responsiveness of the trisphosphoinositide signaling pathway, thus preventing a further increase of Ca^{2+} mobilization. It was suggested by Berridge (1987) that PIP hydrolysis releasing IP$_2$ and DAG provides a mechanism for activating protein kinase C without affecting intracellular Ca^{2+} stores. The return to the initial phosphoinositide levels might occur by a protein kinase C mediated activation of phosphoinositide kinases. Thus, TPA (a potent protein kinase C activator) induced activation of phosphoinositide kinases and staurosporine (an inhibitor of protein kinase C) reversed this effect (Catalán *et al.*, 1992). Thus, as a general statement, these results support a regulatory role for protein kinase C in the phospholipid signaling pathway in the BBB.

Apart from calcium and kinase activities, other components of the transduction cascade can interact with the PI cycle. This is the case with arachidonic acid and its role in modulating activities of signaling proteins. In this regard, cerebral microvessels respond to increased intracellular Ca^{2+} with an arachidonate production as previous steps for eicosanoid production, reported to be active in cerebral microvessels (Koide *et al.*, 1985).

In conclusion, the data available in this particular field indicate that, first, the PI pathway is active in brain microvessels and second, that the vessels are an appropriate substrate to study the components of the PI cycle and its specific relationships with other systems such as those mentioned earlier. It must be underlined that the knowledge of these aspects may have important implications in several

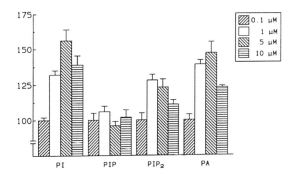

Fig. 36.2. Dose–response relationships for Ca^{2+}-ionophore A23187-induced changes on ^{32}P incorporation into phosphoinositides and PA. Brain microvessels were prelabeled for 30 min with 100 µCi/ml of [^{32}P]orthophosphate, then stimulated with different concentrations of ionophore A23187 for 5 min. Data are expressed as percentage of incorporation with respect to control value. Results represent the mean ± SE from three separate experiments performed in triplicate ($P < 0.05$). From Catalán *et al.*, 1995, reprinted by permission of Elsevier Science Inc., New York.

pathophysiological events, such as preventing the impairment of the BBB following the Ca^{2+} antagonists treatment of hypertension. Demonstration of functional interaction of the PI pathway with other mechanisms of the signal transduction cascade is an open question of potential importance for understanding the regulation of the BBB function.

Modulation of the PI pathway by endothelin in the blood–brain barrier

Taking into account the above facts, the role of some modulatory agents on the BBB–PI relationship needs special attention. One of these regulators is endothelin. Endothelin, the most potent vasoconstrictor substance found, was first described in the cardiovascular system (Yanagisawa *et al.*, 1988) and the presence of endothelin peptides in the brain was clearly demonstrated (Kohzuki *et al.*, 1991).

Cerebral endothelium microvessels possibly regulate the local blood flow within the brain through the production of endothelin (Yoshimoto *et al.*, 1990). It was also reported (Stanimirovic *et al.*, 1993) that endothelin induces an increase of cerebrovascular endothelium permeability, and the induction by endothelin of adhesion molecule expression in brain microvascular endothelial cells was also described (McCarron *et al.*, 1993). Moreover, endothelial cells from rat brain microvessels express receptor sites for endothelin. Some of these receptor sites are coupled to phospholipase C. Thus, as cited (Vigne *et al.*, 1990) endothelin-1 stimulates DNA synthesis involving PI hydrolysis, and increases intracellular Ca^{2+} mobilization in brain capillary endothelial cells (Vigne *et al.*, 1990, 1991). Moreover, endothelin inhibits cholera toxin stimulated adenylyl cyclase and increases phospholipase C activity (Ladoux and Frelin, 1991; Stanimirovic *et al.*, 1993; 1994; Purkiss *et al.*, 1994).

The studies on the effect of endothelins on the PI pathway in the BBB reveal several important points. The most significant is that endothelins are effective in inducing hydrolysis of PI and subsequent resynthesis in intact cerebral microvessels (Fig. 36.3). This hydrolysis is mediated by phospholipase C activation since there was a rapid production of inositol phosphates (Fig. 36.4) together with an increase of DAG mass (Fig. 36.5). However, it must be taken into consideration that other phospholipases (i.e. phospholipase D) and/or other phospholipids (i.e. phosphatidylcholine) might be involved in the overall PA production, as well as DAG generation (Catalán *et al.*, 1995).

As reported earlier, many endothelin responses are mediated by phospholipase C activation in other tissues and cells (Yanagisawa and Masaki, 1989). However, it should be pointed out that there are substantial differences in the mechanism of action of endothelin among different species and cells. In this regard, we must underline that the study and the elucidation of the signal transduction pathways involved in the endothelin actions are relevant in determining the significance of this peptide in the BBB. Intact cerebral microvessels constitute a tissue that has not been sufficiently elucidated in the previous studies on endothelin signal transduction. Studies done in isolated capillary endothelial cells show that both phospholipase C and A_2 are involved. As stated earlier, cerebral endothelial cells rapidly lose their characteristics of differentiated barrier in culture, and therefore, intact cerebral microvessels appear to be a better model for the study of the BBB functionality than

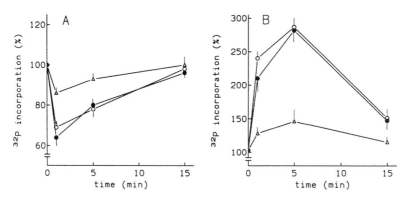

Fig. 36.3. Time-course of endothelin effects on ^{32}P incorporation into PIP$_2$ (A) and PA (B). After pre-labeling for 30 min with 100 μCi/ml [^{32}P]orthophosphate, microvessels were stimulated with 10^{-7} M of each endothelin isoform. Data are expressed as percentage of variation with respect to control values. Endothelin-1 (●), endothelin-2 (○), endothelin-3 (△). Results represent the mean ± SE from three separate experiments performed in triplicate ($P < 0.05$). From Catalán *et al.*, 1996c, reprinted by permission of Lippincott-Raven Publishers.

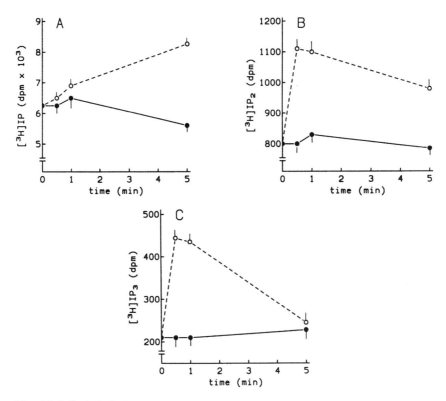

Fig. 36.4. Endothelin-induced inositol phosphates production. Cerebral microvessels were prelabeled with myo-(2-^{3}H)inositol (29 Ci/ml) for 120 min and then 10^{-7} M endothelin-1 was added for the time indicated. Results are expressed as dpm incorporated into each inositol phosphate. A is IP, B is IP$_2$, C is IP$_3$, ●, control; ○,endothelin-1. Results represent the mean ± SE from three separate experiments performed in triplicate ($P < 0.05$). From Catalán *et al.*, 1996c, reprinted by permission of Lippincott-Raven Publishers.

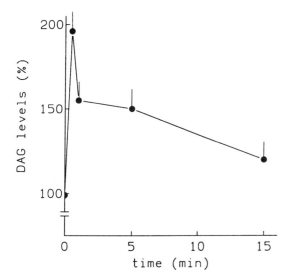

Fig. 36.5. Effect of endothelin-1 on diacylglycerol production. Microvessels were treated with 10^{-7} M endothelin-1 for the time indicated. DAG separated by thin layer chromatography and quantified. Data are expressed as percentage of variation with respect to the control value at zero time (100). Results represent the mean ± SE from three separate experiments performed in triplicate ($P<0.05$). From Catalán *et al.*, 1996*c*, reprinted by permission of Lippincott-Raven Publishers.

the cultured endothelial cells. In this particular case, there are controversial data about the ability of these cells in culture to secrete endothelin (Yoshimoto *et al.*, 1990; Vigne *et al.*, 1990) and about the kinetic characteristics of inositol phosphate production by stimulation with the peptide (Vigne *et al.*, 1990; Ladoux and Frelin, 1991; Stanimirovic *et al.*, 1993; 1994; Purkiss *et al.*, 1994). Moreover, it has been described that cultured endothelial cells could be a kind of injured cell since they produce more endothelin than the microvessel itself (Yoshimoto *et al.*, 1990).

Furthermore, the possibility of interactions of endothelin with other related transduction systems

is worth mentioning. Thus, an enhanced production of a PAF-like material by endothelin was identified by standard and biological probes in platelets, such as induction of aggregation, PA production, increase of endogenous protein phosphorylation and the reversal of these responses by a PAF antagonist. The effects evoked by endothelins on phosphoinositide metabolism and PAF production were to a certain extent dependent on the presence of extracellular Ca^{2+}. In addition, endothelin induced changes in Ca^{2+} dynamics, evoking an initial and rapid intracellular mobilization and influx of Ca^{2+} and later a maintained Ca^{2+} influx (Catalán *et al.*, 1996*c*).

The involvement of endothelin in the pathogenesis of vascular disorders such as strokes, hypertension and subarachnoid hemorrhage (Sakurai and Goto, 1993) and in the function of the BBB (Vigne *et al.*, 1991) were reported. Therefore, a precise knowledge of the molecular mechanism of endothelin action on the BBB is a requisite for the development of an effective therapy. For instance, the therapeutic use of both PAF and Ca^{2+} antagonists in BBB diseases where endothelin is involved has the potential for effectiveness. As a general conclusive statement, the role of endothelin in different intracellular signal transduction processes for controlling, among other functions, endothelial permeability is an open question that merits further study.

Acknowledgment

I would like to thank my collaborators who are listed as co-authors in the publications. Part of the data in this chapter is reproduced from recent publications with the permission of Elsevier Science Inc. and Raven Press. The work reviewed here was supported by grants from the Fundación Ramón Areces and DGICYT.

References

Audus, K. L. and Borchardt, R. T. (1986). Characterization of an in vitro blood–brain barrier model system for studying drug transport and metabolism. *Pharmaceut. Res.*, **3**, 81–7.

Berridge, M. J. (1987). Inositol trisphosphate and diacylglycerol: two interacting second messengers. *Ann. Rev. Biochem.*, **5**, 159–93.

Brammer, M. J. and Weaver, K. (1989). Kinetic analysis of A23187-mediated polyphosphoinositide breakdown in rat cortex arise primary by degradation of inositol trisphosphate. *J. Neurochem.*, **53**, 399–407.

Catalán, R. E., Martínez, A. M., Aragonés, M. D. and Díaz, G. (1989*a*). Evidence for a regulatory action of vanadate on protein phosphorylation in brain microvessels. *Biochem. Biophys. Res. Comm.*, **163**, 771–9.

Catalán, R. E., Martínez, A. M., Aragonés, M. D. and Fernández, I. (1989*b*). Substance P stimulates translocation of protein kinase C in brain microvessels. *Biochem. Biophys. Res. Comm.*, **164**, 595–600.

Catalán, R. E., Martínez, A. M., Aragonés, M. D., Miguel, B. G., Díaz, G. and Hernández, F. (1991). Pertussiss toxin-insensitive regulation of phosphatidyli-nositol hydrolysis by vanadate in brain microvessels. *Biochem. Int.*, **25**, 985–93.

Catalán, R. E., Martínez, A. M., Aragonés, M. D. *et al.* (1992). Phorbol esters stimulate phosphoinositide phosphoryla-tion and phosphatidylcholine metabo-lism in brain microvessels. *Biochem. Int.*, **27**, 231–42.

Catalán, R. E., Martínez, A. M., Aragonés, M. D. *et al.* (1993*a*). Platelet-activating factor stimulates protein kinase C translocation in cerebral microvessels. *Biochem. Biophys. Res. Comm.*, **192**, 446–51.

Catalán, R. E., Martínez, A. M., Aragonés, M. D. and Díaz, G. (1993*b*). Identification of GTP binding proteins in brain microvessels and their role in phosphoinositide turnover. *Biochem. Biophys. Res. Comm.*, **195**, 952–7.

Catalán, R. E., Martínez, A. M., Aragonés, M. D. *et al.* (1995). Involvement of calcium in phosphoinositide metabolism in the blood–brain barrier. *Cell. Signal.*, **7**, 261–7.

Catalán, R. E., Martínez, A. M., Aragonés, M. D. and Hernández, F. (1996*a*). Protein phosphorylation in the blood–brain barrier. Possible presence of MARCKS in brain microvessels. *Neurochem. Int.*, **28**, 59–65.

Catalán, R. E., Martínez, A. M., Aragonés, M. D. *et al.* (1996*b*). Endothelin stimulates protein phosphorylation in blood–brain barrier. *Biochem. Biophys. Res. Comm.*, **219**, 366–9.

Catalán, R. E., Martínez, A. M., Aragonés, M. D. *et al.* (1996*c*). Endothelin stimulates phosphoinositide hydrolysis and PAF synthesis in brain microvessels. *J. Cereb. Blood Flow Metab.*, **16**, 1325–34.

Fisher, S. K., Heacock, A. M. and Agranoff, B. N. (1992). Inositol lipids and signal transduction in the nervous system: an update. *J. Neurochem.*, **58**, 18–38.

Frelin, C., Breittmayer, J. R. and Vigne, P. (1993). ADP induces inositol phosphate-independent intracellular Ca²⁺ mobilization in brain capillary endothelial cells. *J. Biol. Chem.*, **268**, 8787–92.

Henzi, V. and MacDermott, A. B. (1992). Characteristic and function of Ca²⁺ and inositol 1,4,5-trisphosphate-releasable shares of Ca²⁺ in neurons. *Neuroscience*, **46**, 251–73.

Heslop, J. P., Irvine, R. F., Tashjaian, A. H. and Berridge, M. J. (1985). Inositol tetrakis- and pentakisphosphates in GH4 cells. *J. Exp. Biol.*, **119**, 394–401.

Hokin, M. R. and Hokin, L. E. (1953). Enzyme secretion and incorporation of ³²P into phospholipids of pancreas slices. *J. Biol. Chem.*, **203**, 967–77.

Homayoun, P. and Harik, S. I. (1991). Bradykinin receptors of cerebral microvessels stimulate phosphoinositide turnover. *J. Cereb. Blood Flow Metab.*, **11**, 557–66.

Kai, M., While, G. L. and Hathorne, J. N. (1966). The phosphatidylinositol kinase of rat brain. *Biochem. J.*, **101**, 328–37.

Kai, M., Salway, J. G. and Hathorne, J. N. (1968). The diphosphoinositide kinase of rat brain. *Biochem. J.*, **106**, 791–801.

Kohzuki, M., Chai, S. Y., Paxinos, G. *et al.* (1991). Localization and characterization of endothelin receptor binding sites in the rat brain visualized by in vitro autoradiography. *Neuroscience*, **42**, 245–60.

Koide, T., Gotoh, O., Asano, T. and Thorgeirsson, G. (1985). Alterations of the eicosanoid synthetic capacity of rat brain microvessels following ischemia: relevance to ischemic brain edema. *J. Neurochem.*, **44**, 85–93.

Ladoux, A. and Frelin, C. (1991). Endothelins inhibit adenylate cyclase in brain capillary endothelial cells. *Biochem. Biophys. Res. Comm.*, **180**, 169–73.

Lin, A.-Y and Rui, Y.-C (1994). Platelet activating factor induced calcium mobilization and phosphoinositide metabolism in cultured bovine cerebral microvascular endothelial cells. *Biochim. Biophys. Acta*, **1224**, 323–8.

Malviya, A. N., Roque, P. and Vincendon, G. (1990). Stereospecific inositol 1,4,5-³²P trisphosphate binding to isolated rat liver nuclei: evidence for inositol trisphosphate receptor-mediated calcium release from the nucleus. *Proc. Natl Acad. Sci. USA*, **87**, 9270–4.

McCarron, R. M., Wang, L., Stanimirovic, D. B. and Spatz, M. (1993). Endothelin induction of adhesion molecule expression on human brain microvascu-lar endothelial cells. *Neurosci. Lett.*, **156**, 31–4.

Michell, R. H. (1975). Inositol phospho-lipids and cell surface receptors function. *Biochim. Biophys. Acta*, **415**, 81–147.

Purkiss, J. R., West, D., Wilkes, L. C. *et al.* (1994). Stimulation of phospholipase C in cultured microvascular endothelial cells from human frontal lobe by histamine, endothelin and purinoceptor agonists. *Br. J. Pharmacol.*, **111**, 1163–9.

Risau, W. and Walburg, H. (1990). Development of the blood–brain barrier. *Trends Neurosci.*, **13**, 174–8.

Sakurai, T. and Goto, K. (1993). Endothelins. Vascular actions and clinical implications. *Drugs*, **46**, 795–804.

Stanimirovic, D. B., McCarron, R., Bertrand, N. and Spatz, M. (1993). Endothelins release ⁵¹Cr from cultured human cerebromicrovascular endothelium. *Biochem. Biophys. Res. Comm.*, **191**, 1–8.

Stanimirovic, D. B., Yamamoto, T., Uematsu, S. and Spatz, M. (1994). Endothelin-1 receptor binding and cellular signal transduction in cultured human brain endothelial cell. *J. Neurochem.*, **62**, 592–601.

Streb, H., Irvine, R. F., Berridge, M. J. and Schulz, I. (1983). Release of Ca²⁺ from a nonmitochondrial store in pancreatic cells by inositol-1,4,5-trisphosphate. *Nature*, **396**, 67–8.

Vigne, P., Marsault, R., Beittmayer, J. P. and Frelin, C. (1990). Endothelin stimulates phosphatidinositol hydrolysis and DNA synthesis in brain capillary endothelial cells. *Biochem. J.*, **266**, 415–20.

Vigne, P., Ladoux, C. and Frelin, C. (1991). Endothelins activate Na⁺/H⁺ exchange in brain capillary endothelial cells via a high affinity endothelin-3 receptor that is not coupled to phospholipase C. *J. Biol. Chem.*, **266**, 5925–8.

Yanagisawa, M. and Masaki, T. (1989). Endothelin, a novel endothelium-derived peptide. *Biochem. Pharmacol.*, **38**, 1877–83.

Yanagisawa, M., Kurihara, M., Kimura, S. *et al.* (1988). A novel potent vasoconstrictor peptide produced by vascular endothelial cells. *Nature*, **332**, 411–15.

Yoshimoto, S., Ishizaki, Y., Kurihara, H. *et al.* (1990). Cerebral microvessels endothelium is producing endothelin. *Brain Res.*, **508**, 283–5.

Zeleznikar, Jr., R. J., Quit, E. E. and Drewes, L. R. (1983). An alpha$_1$-adrenergic receptor mediated phosphatidylinositol effect in canine cerebral microvessels. *Mol. Pharmaco.*, **24**, 163–7.

37 Nitric oxide and endothelin at the blood–brain barrier

SYLVIE M. CAZAUBON and PIERRE OLIVIER COURAUD

- Introduction
- Nitric oxide
- Endothelin
- Conclusion

Introduction

Endothelial cells play a key role in the local control of vascular tone, by releasing a variety of relaxing and contracting factors. The very labile 'endo-thelium-derived relaxing factor' first described by Furchgott and coworkers (Furchgott and Zawadzki, 1980) was later identified as nitric oxide (NO), the biological activity of which is now known to extend far beyond vasorelaxation, to host defence and neuromodulation. Together with several cyclooxy-genase products (thromboxane A2, endoperoxides), endothelin largely contributes to endothelium-derived vasoconstricting activity. As with NO, it soon became obvious during the past decade that endothelin isopeptides (ET-1, -2, -3) are pleiotropic factors not only involved in vasoconstriction, but also in a number of physiological processes, such as cell proliferation or hormone secretion, and cardiovascular disorders, such as hypertension or stroke (Masaki and Yanagisawa, 1992). This chapter focuses on our current knowledge of the roles of NO and ETs in the control of cerebral circulation and cellular interactions at the level of the blood–brain barrier (BBB).

Nitric oxide

NO biosynthesis: cellular distribution and regulation

NO synthase isoforms NO is a small, relatively stable free-radical gas that diffuses through cell membranes and reacts with a number of cellular targets. It is synthesized by NO synthase (NOS) from L-arginine. At least three distinct NOS iso-forms (Table 37.1), more than 50% homologous, have been characterized at the molecular level (Dawson and Snyder, 1994; Gross and Wolin, 1995): two of them are constitutively expressed, one in endothelial cells (eNOS) and one in neurons (nNOS, also identified to NADPH-diaphorase); the third NOS isoform (iNOS), initially identified in macrophages, is inducible by cytokines and inflammatory agents, such as lipopolysaccharide, in many different cell types. The constitutive iso-forms eNOS and nNOS, positively regulated via calcium/calmodulin binding, generally produce low amouts of NO, in comparison with the large quantities synthesized by iNOS.

Cellular distribution of NOS isoforms in the brain

ENDOTHELIAL CELLS The presence of the con-stitutive eNOS has been described in the endothe-

Table 37.1. Cellular distribution and regulation of NOS isoforms

NOS	Cellular distribution	Regulation	Stimuli	Biological activities
nNOS	Neurons Astrocytes	Ca^{2+}/Calmodulin	NMDA	Neurotoxicity
eNOS	Endothelial cells	Ca^{2+}/Calmodulin	Substance P Acetylcholine ADP	CBF increase Inhibition of lymphocyte adhesion
iNOS	Endothelial cells Astrocytes Microglial cells	Cytokines LPS	TNF-α INF-γ	Cytotoxicity

lial layer of cerebral vessels (Faraci and Brian, 1994). A number of vasoactive agents such as acetylcholine, ADP, serotonin or substance P have been shown to stimulate eNOS and NO release through activation of their respective receptors on brain microvessel endothelial cells. In addition, in the same cells, combinations of cytokines (TNF-α, IFN-γ, IL-1ß), potentiated by catecholamines, induce iNOS expression (Kilbourn and Belloni, 1990; Durieu-Trautmann *et al.*, 1993), this effect being counteracted by NO itself (Borgerding and Murphy, 1995), glucocorticoids or IL-4.

GLIAL CELLS Astrocytes, in addition to their critical role in maintaining a balanced environment in the nervous system, are known to constitute, together with microglial cells, a major cerebral source of cytokines. The capacity of these glial cells to release NO has been documented more recently (Murphy *et al.*, 1993; Mollace and Nistico, 1995). There is evidence that a constitutive form of NOS, possibly nNOS, is expressed in astrocytes at a low level: interestingly, as shown by NADPH-diaphorase activity, the highest expression was observed in endfeet of perivascular astrocytes, in contact with the blood vessels (Murphy *et al.*, 1993). The activity of this constitutive isoform can be stimulated *in vitro* by several calcium-elevating agonists such as noradrenaline and quisqualate.

The inducible iNOS isoform was found to be expressed in cultures of murine microglial cells, astrocytes and human astrocytoma upon stimulation by inflammatory cytokines (IFN-γ, IL-1β, TNF-α) and/or LPS. As reported above for brain endothelial cells, the induction capacity of these immunological agents is potentiated by catecholamines (Murphy *et al.*, 1993; Mollace and Nistico, 1995).

NEURONS The constitutive nNOS isoform has been primarily localized to discrete populations of neurons (about 2% of all neurons), in distinct areas such as cerebral cortex, hippocampus, and cerebellum. This expression could not be correlated with neurotransmitter pattern. In the cerebral cortical and retinal blood vessels, nNOS was found in autonomic nerves in the outer, adventitial layers (Dawson and Snyder, 1994). Elevation of calcium levels by glutamate or neuropeptides is a key regulator of nNOS: the calcium-activated phosphatase calcineurin dephosphorylates and activates nNOS. However, phosphorylation by protein kinase C, cAMP- or cGMP-dependent protein kinase decreases nNOS catalytic activity. In addition, some neurons may express low levels of eNOS (Irikura *et al.*, 1995), especially in CA1 pyramidal cells of the hippocampus, where it might be implicated in long-term potentiation (Dawson and Snyder, 1994).

Biological activity of NO

NO and intracellular signaling pathways

ACTIVATION OF SOLUBLE GUANYLYL CYCLASE One of the main cellular targets of NO is certainly the soluble guanylyl cyclase, a hemoprotein whose enzymatic activity is stimulated by formation of an NO–heme complex (Gross and Wolin, 1995). Endothelium-released NO activates soluble guanylyl cyclase and increases cGMP levels in vascular smooth muscle cells: cGMP activates a Ser/Thr protein kinase and leads ultimately to dephosphorylation of myosin light chains, causing vasodilation. In astrocytes, NO also stimulates the cGMP/cGMP-dependent protein kinase pathway, which contributes to the regulation of calcium entry. Similarly, the cyclooxygenases (the constitutive COX-1 and cytokine-inducible COX-2 isoforms), which are also hemoproteins, are activated by NO through NO–heme formation, leading to up-regulation of prostaglandin release.

INHIBITION OF ACTIVITY OF THIOL-CONTAINING PROTEINS In addition to hemoproteins, the activity of a number of thiol-containing proteins can be regulated by NO through S-nitrosation. Glyceraldehyde-3-phosphate dehydrogenase activity is thus inhibited by S-nitrosation, with important consequences for energy metabolism in the cell, and possibly for leukocyte infiltration into the brain, as recently suggested by the observation that this enzyme directly associates with adhesion molecules in cerebral endothelial cells (Fédérici *et al.*, 1996). Interestingly, the *N*-methyl-D-aspartate (NMDA) receptor-channel, which is responsible for neuronal production of NO, is also inhibited by S-nitrosation (Lei *et al.*, 1992), suggesting that NO is involved in a negative-feedback loop in NO-producing neurons.

NO in the cerebral vasculature

VASODILATION AND CONTROL OF CEREBRAL BLOOD FLOW NO is a potent vasodilator in most vascular beds, including cerebral arteries and arterioles (Faraci and Brian, 1994). In normal conditions, local injection of NOS inhibitors has been reported to constrict cerebral vessels and to decrease cerebral blood flow (CBF): this suggests that the basal tone of brain vessels is controled by constitutive release of NO, probably from endothelial cells, but probably also from perivascular astrocytes and neurons.

Following CO_2 inhalation, the increase in regional CBF has been demonstrated to be mediated essentially by NO produced by nNOS, endothelium thus being not a major source of NO during hypercapnia (Irikura *et al.*, 1995; Wang *et al.*, 1995).

NEUROTOXICITY During strokes, the capacity of NO to maintain CBF may contribute to limit brain damage. However, upon reoxygenation, the reaction of NO with superoxide to generate peroxynitrite, a highly reactive compound, is implicated in neurotoxicity (Chan, 1996). Using selective inhibition of the nNOS, as well as targeted disruption of the nNOS gene, it has been established recently that the initial protective effect is mediated by endothelial NO production, while neuronal NO overproduction, resulting from the glutamatergic activation of NMDA receptors, appears to exacerbate ischemic brain injury (Huang *et al.*, 1994). During septic shock, neurotoxicity also appears as a consequence of massive release of NO following cytokine-induced expression of iNOS in cerebral endothelial cells, perivascular astrocytes and microglial cells.

REGULATION OF BBB PERMEABILITY Administration of NO-releasing compounds, as well as the iNOS-inducer lipopolysaccharide, increases the permeability of BBB to various tracer drugs (Shukla *et al.*, 1995). Furthermore, during phenylephrine-induced acute hypertension in rats, albumin permeability through cerebral venules was significantly blocked by topical application of NOS inhibitors (Mayhan, 1995). Altogether, these observations suggest that NO contributes to disruption of the BBB during bacterial infection or acute hypertension.

A tonic suppressive effect of NO has been demonstrated on the adhesion of leukocytes to brain endothelium and their infiltration through the BBB, which may have beneficial effects during ischemia by limiting inflammatory processes in the cerebral parenchyma (Nathan, 1992).

Endothelin

ET biosynthesis: cellular distribution and regulation

ET peptide family ET, originally isolated as a vasoconstrictor peptide secreted by endothelial cells (Yanagisawa and Masaki, 1989), is a peptide of 21 amino acid residues with two disulfide bridges (Fig. 37.1). The human genome encodes not only this peptide, now called ET-1, but also two isopeptides: ET-2 and ET-3 (Inoue *et al.*, 1989). ETs were found to be highly homologous to

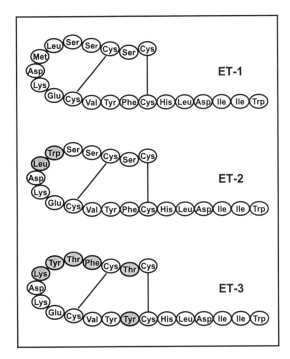

Fig. 37.1. Amino acid sequences of human peptides from the endothelin family. Filled circles indicate amino acid residues different from those of the ET-1 sequence.

a family of peptides, the snake venom sarafotoxins S6, both families of peptides activating the same receptors in brain.

Processing of precursors Gene sequences predict that all the ETs are derived from preproendothelin precursors of 160 to 238 amino acids, depending on isopeptides and species. Preproendothelins are first cleaved by furin at dibasic pairs of amino acids to yield proendothelins (commonly called 'big ETs') of 37 to 41 amino acids. Final processing to the 21 amino acid mature peptides is achieved via a specific endothelin converting enzyme (ECE). This latter enzyme has been cloned, expressed and characterized as a phosphoramidon-sensitive and thiorphan-insensitive metalloendopeptidase (Shimada *et al.*, 1994). A number of related ECEs displaying different tissue distributions and selectivities were subsequently identified.

Cellular distribution of ETs in the brain

ENDOTHELIAL CELLS Like macrovascular endothelial cells, primary or immortalized brain micro-

vascular endothelial cells have been shown to constitutively produce ET-1 (Durieu-Trautmann *et al.*, 1991, 1993). Polar secretion of ET-1 was observed in culture, the majority of synthesized peptide being released across the basal membrane (Yoshimoto *et al.*, 1991). Since ET-1 does not cross the BBB, this observation indicates that microvascular endothelial cells are responsible for local ET-1 production in brain. This response can be positively stimulated by thrombin, several neuropeptides and cytokines. Inhibition of ET-1 formation was found to be mediated by NO or by NO-releasing complexes produced by astrocytes *in vitro* (Fédérici *et al.*, 1995; Flowers *et al.*, 1995), suggesting that astrocytes may be involved in a regulatory loop of ET-1 production at the level of the BBB.

ASTROCYTES Whether astrocytes are capable of synthesizing ETs remains a matter of debate. Evidences for the expression of ET-1 mRNA as well as ET-3-like immunoreactivity in rat astrocytes have been presented (MacCumber *et al.*, 1990; Ehrenreich *et al.*, 1991), but other reports failed to demonstrate the presence of ETs in astrocytes (Hama *et al.*, 1992). Moreover, there is evidence showing that during ischemia, ETs are secreted in excess, not only by endothelial cells but also by astrocytes (Yamashita *et al.*, 1994).

Biological activity of ETs

ET receptor subtypes and intracellular signaling pathways ET biological activity is mediated by binding to specific cell surface receptors (ET_A-R, ET_B-R), which belong to the superfamily of receptors with seven transmembrane domains, coupled to heterotrimeric G proteins (Arai *et al.*, 1990; Sakurai *et al.*, 1990). Pharmacological studies have shown that ET_A-R preferentially binds ET-1, while ET_B-R binds all three ETs with similar affinities. Although a larger diversity of ET receptors has been proposed on the basis of physiological and pharmacological studies, no additional subtype receptor has been cloned yet.

Investigations of the intracellular signaling events following ET receptor stimulation indicate that phosphatidylinositol hydrolysis and calcium mobilization are crucial in many short-term responses mediated by either ET_A-R or ET_B-R. Both receptors, however, exhibit opposite effects on the cAMP cascade: ET_A-R mediates activation of adenylyl cyclase/cAMP-dependent protein kinase, whereas ET_B-R displays an inhibitory action on this pathway (Aramori and Nakanishi, 1992).

Cellular distribution of ET receptors

ENDOTHELIAL CELLS Most of the data concerning the expression of ET receptors by endothelial cells were collected from studies using peripheral macrovascular endothelial cells and indicate the presence of ET_B-R on these cells (ET_{B2}-R), pharmacologically distinct from those expressed in smooth muscle cells (ET_{B1}-R). Whether brain microvascular endothelial cells also express ET_{B2}-R, or ET_A-R remains to be elucidated.

ASTROCYTES Perivascular astrocytes have been identified as ET targets. The pharmacological and functional characterization of ET receptor subtypes expressed in primary cultures of rat astrocytes, reveal the preferential expression of ET_B-R (Lazarini et al., 1996). It has been observed that ET_B-R expression in astrocytes is up-regulated during differentiation (Hama et al., 1992), and that C6 glioma express ET_A-R (Ambar and Sokolovsky, 1993). Altogether, these data suggest that ET_B-R expression may be associated with astrocytic differentiation.

ETs in the central nervous system

CBF REGULATION AND BBB INTEGRITY ET-1, as a prominent vasoactive agent, plays a significant role in the CBF regulation. Intrathecal infusion of ET-1 causes a sustained reduction of the spinal cord blood flow and results in a prolonged breakdown of the blood–spinal cord barrier (Westmark et al., 1995). Enhanced ET-1 secretion along the axis of the spinal cord, correlating with barrier breakdown, has been observed after injury (McKenzie et al., 1995). It has also been reported that patients with acute nonhemorrhagic cerebral infarction present a marked elevation in plasma ET-1 level, which may induce severe and prolonged constriction of collateral vessels (Ziv et al., 1992). The availability of ET-receptor antagonists crossing the BBB, has recently allowed confirmation of the involvement of endogenous ETs in a variety of pathologies including cerebral focal ischemia and subarachnoid hemorrhage.

NEUROTOXIC/NEUROTROPHIC FACTOR SECRETION Activation of endothelial cells by several vasoactive hormones, neurotransmitters and cytokines increases the production of ET-1, which in turn, by an autocrine loop, induces the release of NO. Since ET-1 stimulates the secretion of NGF by astrocytes in vitro (Ladenheim et al., 1993), the balance between ET-1 and NO may be of key importance in the local modulation of neuronal function and/or survival.

ASTROCYTE PROLIFERATION ET-1 acts as a growth factor for astrocytes, potentiating DNA synthesis and proliferation (MacCumber et al., 1990; Couraud et al., 1991). In primary cultures of astrocytes, these responses are mediated by ET_B-R, which was found to be functionally coupled to the mitogen-activated protein kinase pathway (Cazaubon et al., 1993, 1994). Another important consequence of ET response is the inhibition of gap junction permeability of astrocytes (Giaume et al., 1992), which could contribute to the mitogenic action of ETs on these cells. ETs could therefore play a significant role in glial proliferation during brain development, and reactive gliosis associated with brain injury or inflammation.

BRAIN DEVELOPMENT Dramatic advances have been made in ET research with the breeding of ET-1, ET_A-R and ET_B-R knockout mice, which exhibit dramatic deficiencies in the development of neural crest-derived tissues (Baynash et al., 1994; Kurihara et al., 1994).

Conclusion

The multiple roles of NO at the level of the cerebral vasculature illustrate the dual bioactivity of this compound in the brain. ETs also display beneficial as well as detrimental effects. The multiplicity of production sites and cellular targets in cerebral vessels and perivascular brain tissue, for both NO and ETs, constitutes the basis of a complex network of interactions (Fig. 37.2), involving endothelial cells, smooth muscle cells/pericytes, astrocytes, microglial cells and neurons. This concept of cross-talks between the two systems is supported by the observations of the balance between NO-

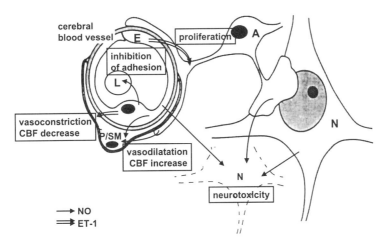

Fig. 37.2. Schematic representation of biological activities of NO (single arrows) and ET-1 (double arrows) at the level of the BBB and perivascular cells. E: endothelial cell, L: lymphocyte, P/SM: pericyte/smooth muscle cell, A: astrocyte, N: neuron.

mediated vasodilatation and ET-1-mediated vaso-constriction, the prevention by NO of ET-1 formation, the neurotoxicity of NO contrasting with the capacity of ET-1 to promote neurotrophin release.

It is likely that discovery of new selective inhibitors of NO overproduction and ET action, with high biological stability and BBB permeability index, will condition further developments to clinical applications.

Acknowledgments

We are grateful to Prof. A.D. Strosberg for constant support, Dr. S. Timsit and C. Fédérici for helpful discussions.

References

Ambar, I. and Sokolovsky, M. (1993). Endothelin receptors stimulate both phospholipase C and phospholipase D activities in different cell lines. *Eur. J. Pharmacol.*, **245**, 31–41.

Arai, H., Hori, S., Aramori, I. *et al.* (1990). Cloning and expression of a cDNA encoding an endothelin receptor. *Nature*, **348**, 730–5.

Aramori, I. and Nakanishi, S. (1992). Coupling of two endothelin receptor subtypes to differing signal transduction in transfected chinese hamster ovary cells. *J. Biol. Chem.*, **267**, 12468–74.

Baynash, A. G., Hosoda, K., Giaid, A. *et al.* (1994). Interaction of endothelin-3 with endothelin B receptor is essential for development of epidermal melanocytes and enteric neurons. *Cell*, **79**, 1277–85.

Borgerding, R. A. and Murphy, S. (1995). Expression of inducible Nitric oxide synthase in cerebral endothelial cells is regulated by cytokine-activated astrocytes. *J. Neurochem.*, **65**, 1342–7.

Cazaubon, S., Parker, P. J., Strosberg, A. D. and Couraud, P. O. (1993). Endothelins stimulate phosphorylation and activity of p42/mitogen-activated protein kinase in astrocytes. *Biochem. J.*, **293**, 381–6.

Cazaubon, S. M., Ramos-Morales, F., Fischer, S. *et al.* (1994). Endothelin induces tyrosine phosphorylation and GRB2 association of SHC in astrocytes. *J. Biol. Chem.*, **269**, 24805–9.

Chan, P. H. (1996). Role of oxidants in ischemic brain damage. *Stroke*, **27**, 1124–9.

Couraud, P. O., Durieu-Trautmann, O., Le Nguyen, P. *et al.* (1991). Functional endothelin-1 receptors in rat astrocytoma C6. *Eur. J. Pharmacol.*, **206**, 191–8.

Dawson, T. M. and Snyder, S. H. (1994). Gases as biological messengers: nitric oxide and carbon monoxide in the brain. *J. Neurosci.*, **14**, 5147–59.

Durieu-Trautmann, O., Foignant-Chaverot, N., Perdomo, J. *et al.* (1991). Immortalization of brain capillary endothelial cells with maintenance of structural characteristics of the blood–brain barrier endothelium. *In vitro Cell. Dev. Biol.*, **27A**, 771–8.

Durieu-Trautmann, O., Fédérici, C., Créminon, C. *et al.* (1993). Nitric oxide and endothelin secretion by microvessel endothelial cells: regulation by cyclic nucleotides. *J. Cell. Physiol.*, **155,** 104–11.

Ehrenreich, H., Kehrl, J. H., Anderson, R. W. *et al.* (1991). A vasoactive peptide, endothelin-3, is produced by and specifically binds to primary astrocytes. *Brain Res.*, **538**, 54–8.

Faraci, F. M. and Brian, J. E. (1994). Nitric oxide and the cerebral circulation. *Stroke*, **25**, 692–703.

Fédérici, C., Camoin, L., Creminon, C. *et al.* (1995). Cultured astrocytes release a factor that decreases endothelin-1 secretion by brain microvessel endothelial cells. *J. Neurochem.*, **64**, 1008–15.

Fédérici, C., Camoin, L., Hattab, M. *et al.* (1996). Association of the cytoplasmic domain of intercellular-adhesion molecule-1 with glutaraldehyde-3-phosphate dehydrogenase and ß-tubulin. *Eur. J. Biochem.*, **238**, 173–80.

Flowers, M. A., Wang, Y., Stewart, R. J. *et al.* (1995). Reciprocal regulation of endothelin-1 and endothelial constitutive NOS in proliferating endothelial cells. *Am. J. Physiol.*, **269**, H1988–1997.

Furchgott, R. and Zawadzki, J. (1980). The obligatory role of endothelial cells in the relaxation of arterial smooth muscle by acetylcholine. *Nature*, **288**, 373–6.

Giaume, C., Cordier, J. and Glowinski, J. (1992). Endothelins inhibit junctional permeability in cultured rat astrocytes. *Eur. J. Neurosci.*, **4**, 877–81.

Gross, S. S. and Wolin, M. S. (1995). Nitric oxide: pathophysiological mechanisms. *Annu. Rev. Physiol.*, **57**, 737–69.

Hama, H., Sakurai, T., Kasuya, Y. *et al.* (1992). Action of endothelin-1 on rat astrocytes through the ETB receptor. *Biochem. Biophys. Res. Comm.*, **186**, 355–62.

Huang, Z., Huang, P. L., Panahian, N. *et al.* (1994). Effects of cerebral ischemia in mice deficient in neuronal oxide synthase. *Science*, **265**, 1883–5.

Inoue, A., Yanagisawa, M., Kimura, S. *et al.* (1989). The human endothelin family: three structurally and pharmacologically distinct isopeptides predicted by three separate genes. *Proc. Natl. Acad. Sci. USA*, **86**, 2863–7.

Irikura, K., Huang, P. L., Ma, J. *et al.* (1995). Cerebrovascular alterations in mice lacking neuronal nitric oxide synthase expression. *Proc. Natl. Acad. Sci. USA*, **92**, 6823–7.

Kilbourn, R. G. and Belloni, P. (1990). Endothelial cell production of nitrogen oxides in reponse to interferon γ in combination with tumor necrosis factor, interleukin-1, or endotoxin. *J. Intl. Cancer Inst.*, **82**, 772–5.

Kurihara, Y., Kurihara, H., Suzuki, H. *et al.* (1994). Elevated blood pressure on craniofacial abnormalities in mice deficient in endothelin-1. *Nature*, **368**, 703–10.

Ladenheim, R., Lacroix, I., Foignant-Chaverot, N. *et al.* (1993). Endothelins stimulate c-*fos* and nerve growth factor expression in astrocytes and astrocytoma. *J. Neurochem.*, **60**, 260–6.

Lazarini, F., Strosberg, A. D., Couraud, P. O. and Cazaubon, S. M. (1996). Coupling of ET$_B$ endothelin receptor to mitogen-activated protein kinase stimulation and DNA synthesis in primary cultures of rat astrocytes. *J. Neurochem.*, **66**, 459–65.

Lei, S. Z., Pan, Z. H., Aggarwal, S. K. *et al.* (1992). Effect of nitric oxide production on the redox modulatory site of the NMDA receptor-channel complex. *Neuron*, **8**, 1087–99.

MacCumber, M. W., Ross, C. A. and Snyder, S. H. (1990). Endothelin in brain: receptors, mitogenesis and biosynthesis in glial cells. *Proc. Natl. Acad. Sci. USA*, **87**, 2359–63.

Masaki, T. and Yanagisawa, M. (1992). Physiology and pharmacology of endothelins. *Med. Res. Rev.*, **12**, 391–421.

Mayhan, W. G. (1995). Role of nitric oxide in disruption of the blood–brain barrier during acute hypertension. *Brain Res.*, **686**, 99–103.

McKenzie, A. L., Hall, J. J., Aihara, N. *et al.* (1995). Immunolocalization of endothelin in the traumatized cord: relationship to blood–spinal cord barrier breakdown. *J. Neurotrauma.*, **12**, 257–68.

Mollace, V. and Nistico, G. (1995). Release of nitric oxide from astroglial cells: a key mechanism in neuroimmune disorders. *Adv. Neuroimmunol.*, **5**, 421–30.

Murphy, S., Simmons, M. L., Agullo, L. *et al.* (1993). Synthesis of nitric oxide in CNS glial cells. *Trends Neuron. Sci.*, **16**, 323–8.

Nathan, C. (1992). Nitric oxide as a secretory product of mammalian cells. *FASEB J.*, **6**, 3051–64.

Sakurai, T., Yanagisawa, M., Takuwa, Y. *et al.* (1990). Cloning of a cDNA encoding a non-isopeptide-selective subtype of the endothelin receptor. *Nature*, **348**, 732–5.

Shimada, K., Takahashi, M. and Tanzawa, K. (1994). Cloning and functional expression of endothelin-converting enzyme from rat endothelial cells. *J. Biol. Chem.*, **269**, 18275–8.

Shukla, A., Dikshit, M. and Srimal, R. C. (1995). Nitric oxide modulates blood–brain barrier permeability during infections with an inactivated bacterium. *Neuroreport*, **6**, 1629–32.

Wang, Q., Pelligrino, D. A., Baughman, V. L. *et al.* (1995). The role of neuronal nitric oxide synthase in regulation of cerebral blood flow in normocapnia and hypercapnia in rats. *J. Cereb. Blood Flow Metab.*, **15**, 774–8.

Westmark, R., Noble, L. J., Fukuda, K. *et al.* (1995). Intrathecal administration of endothelin-1 in the rat: impact on spinal cord blood flow and the blood–spinal cord barrier. *Neurosci. Lett.*, **192**, 173–6.

Yamashita, K., Niwa, M., Kataoka, Y. *et al.* (1994). Microglia with an endothelin ET$_B$ receptor aggregate in rat hippocampus CA1 subfields following transient forebrain ischemia. *J. Neurochem.*, **63**, 1042–51.

Yanagisawa, M. and Masaki, T. (1989). Endothelin, a novel endothelium-derived peptide. *Biochem. Pharmacol.*, **38**, 1877–83.

Yoshimoto, S., Ishizaki, Y., Sasaki, T. and Murota, S. (1991). Effect of carbon dioxide and oxygen on endothelin production by cultured porcine cerebral endothelial cells. *Stroke*, **22**, 378–83.

Ziv, I., Fleminger, G., Djaldetti, R. *et al.* (1992). Increased plasma endothelin-1 in acute ischemic stroke. *Stroke*, **23**, 1014–16.

38 Role of intracellular calcium in regulation of brain endothelial permeability

N. JOAN ABBOTT

Introduction

Calcium is an important trigger and regulator of endothelial cell physiology. Historically, most information has come from the study of endothelial cells in culture, chiefly cells from large vessel endothelia such as aorta and umbilical vein. More recently, cultured microvascular endothelial cells have been investigated, and some studies have been done on endothelial cells in intact and split-open vessels, or covering the surface of cardiac valves. Studies on brain microvascular endothelium have begun more recently. This chapter reviews studies on the mechanisms governing changes in intracellular calcium involved in the normal physiology of systemic endothelium, evidence that calcium contributes to the control of endothelial permeability in both non-brain and brain endothelium, and cellular mechanisms demonstrated in brain microvascular endothelial cells.

Mechanisms controlling elevation of intracellular calcium in mammalian cells

Cytoplasmic free calcium controls a large number of cellular functions, from the activation of enzymes, to secretory processes and contraction. In mammalian cells, elevation of intracellular calcium occurs from two sources: Ca^{2+} release from intracellular stores, and Ca^{2+} influx across the plasma membrane. Two major classes of tetrameric calcium channels control intracellular calcium release, the ryanodine receptor (RR), and the inositol trisphosphate receptor (InsP$_3$R) (Berridge, 1993). In skeletal muscle, the RR is directly coupled to dihydropyridine receptors in the T-tubular plasmalemma, so that membrane depolarization during an action potential leads to intracellular calcium release. In cardiac muscle and some neurons, the coupling between the plasmalemma and the RR is indirect, depolarization causing a small amount of calcium entry through voltage-dependent ion channels, which in turn triggers intracellular calcium release. A range of agonists acting on G-protein linked receptors is able to release calcium from intracellular stores by activating membrane phospholipase C and generation of $InsP_3$, which acts on $InsP_3R$ to release calcium. Diacylglyerol produced in parallel with $InsP_3$ can activate protein kinase C (PKC) and exert control over further cellular processes. It is not clear whether the RR- and $InsP_3R$-controlled calcium stores correspond to a single organelle compartment, or whether they are separate, or interconnected.

For individual cell types, it is possible to determine the relative contribution of the different intracellular release mechanisms, since $InsP_3$-sensitive calcium release is blocked by heparin and caffeine, while the RR is blocked by Ruthenium Red and ryanodine, and activated by caffeine and heparin. Both mechanisms can be modulated by intracellular calcium and ATP (Ehrlich et al., 1994). Calcium release from $InsP_3$-sensitive stores can control processes throughout the cell, due to the high 'space constant' of $InsP_3$ (Kasai and Petersen, 1994), while calcium influx through the cell membrane tends to control local events such as exocytosis and calcium-induced calcium release (CICR).

Calcium influx through voltage operated channels is found in relatively few cell types, chiefly excitable cells such as nerve and muscle. Non-excitable cells have other routes for calcium entry, including nonselective cation channels, second messenger activated channels, and stretch-activated channels (Fasolato et al., 1994; Otun et al., 1996). It has recently become apparent that depletion of intracellular stores, e.g. via receptor activated $InsP_3$ generation, leads to calcium entry through activation of plasmalemmal ion channels. This process has been called capacitative Ca^{2+} influx, store-dependent Ca^{2+} influx or store-operated Ca^{2+} influx, and the associated current called 'calcium release activated current' or I_{CRAC}. Recently a consensus term 'store operated calcium influx' has been agreed, with I_{SOC} the term for the underlying ionic current (Favre et al., 1996).

Calcium elevation in endothelial cells

Calcium elevation in endothelial cells follows the basic plan outlined above. The activation of plasmalemmal receptors by vasoactive agents including bradykinin, acetylcholine and ATP in aortic endothelial cells causes a biphasic elevation of intracellular $[Ca^{2+}]$, an initial release of calcium from intracellular stores, and a subsequent prolonged influx of calcium across the plasma membrane (reviewed in Adams et al., 1993; Himmel et al., 1993). The calcium rise activates Ca^{2+}-dependent K^+ channels, whose activity can thus be used to monitor the $[Ca^{2+}]_i$ elevation. The biphasic rise in calcium is accompanied by a biphasic increase both in the open probability of unitary currents and the amplitude of I_{SOC} (Sauvé et al., 1988; Rusko et al., 1992).

There is evidence for the co-existence of $InsP_3$-sensitive and caffeine-sensitive (RR) stores in cultured bovine aortic endothelial cells (Thuringer and Sauvé 1992; Zieglestein et al., 1994a; Rusko et al., 1995). Since calcium can modulate both systems, with increased activity at low $[Ca^{2+}]_i$ and reduced activity at high $[Ca^{2+}]_i$, both positive and negative feedback interactions between the two systems are observed (Ehrlich et al., 1994; Otun et al., 1996). The balance between the $InsP_3R$- and RR-controlled calcium release systems appears to be different between cultured and freshly-dissociated aortic endothelial cells, with caffeine reported to release a smaller fraction of intracellular calcium in cultured than in freshly dissociated cells (Buchan and Martin, 1991; Rusko et al., 1995). The intracellular calcium pools are rapidly depleted when ATP levels are reduced (Ziegelstein et al., 1994b).

Role of calcium in regulating endothelial permeability

A well-documented role for changes in intracellular calcium is the control of endothelial permeability by regulating the tightness of the paracellular pathway. In endothelia, as in epithelia, the cleft between adjacent cells is bridged by a junctional complex including tight junctions (zonula occludens), gap junctions, and adherens junctions (zonula adherens) (Gumbiner, 1993; Dejana and Del Maschio, 1995; Dejana et al., 1995). The complexity of the tight junctions varies along the length of the vascular tree, from the most complete and complex junctions in arterioles, to poorly organized junctions with frequent open pathways in post-capillary venules (Simionescu *et al.*, 1975). The tightness of microvascular junctions also varies between different tissues, from relatively leaky in mesenteric vessels (transendothelial electrical resistance or TEER ~ 3 Ω cm^2, Crone and Christensen, 1981) to extremely tight in brain endothelium (TEER 1–3000 Ω cm^2, Crone and Olesen, 1982; Butt *et al.*, 1990). There is a general inverse correspondence between TEER and the interendothelial membrane separation within the tight junction, as revealed by tilting the thin sections in the electron microscope, with the tightest microvessels having no measurable gap between apposed membranes (Ward *et al.*, 1988; Schulze and Firth, 1992).

The transmembrane protein occludin acts as the link between adjacent membranes (Furuse *et al.*, 1993; McCarthy *et al.*, 1996), while associated cytoplasmic molecules include ZO-1, cingulin, ZO-2, and a newly detected small GTP-binding protein rab13 (Furuse *et al.*, 1994; Dejana *et al.* 1995). These associated molecules may contribute to anchorage of the tight junction to the actin microfilaments of the cytoskeleton, and/or may mediate signal transduction (Dejana *et al.*, 1995), both from cell:cell contacts to intracellular processes, and from intracellular signals to regulation of the tight junction.

Gap junctions between endothelial cells are seen in large vessels but are rare or absent in microvessels (Simionescu *et al.*, 1975); they are likely to be important in coordinating function along the length of the endothelial lining. Possible electrical coupling via gap junctions between endothelial cells and surrounding smooth muscle, pericytes or macrophages is more controversial (Davies *et al.*, 1988; Beny, 1990; Dejana *et al.*, 1995).

Adherens junctions between endothelial cells contain cadherins (transmembrane glycoproteins) that mediate the cell:cell attachment, stabilized by extracellular Ca^{2+}, and a submembranous zone of cytoplasmic proteins and actin microfilaments (Dejana *et al.*, 1995). Adherens junctions are a prerequisite for assembly of both tight and gap junctions.

An important function of all endothelia is to regulate exchange between the blood and the tissue interstitium. Most exchange of small solutes occurs in the capillary and post-capillary segments of the vasculature. The post-capillary venules are also the site of the most conspicuous modulation of permeability by vasoactive agents (Olesen, 1989). Agents like histamine and thrombin induce a rapid and short-lived (minutes) increase in vascular permeability, while cytokines and hypoxia induce a delayed and sustained response that develops in hours to days (Dejana *et al.*, 1995).

Vasoactive agents shown to increase endothelial permeability *in vivo* include thrombin, histamine, bradykinin, LPS, LTB4, PAF, cytokines (TNF-α, IL-1, γ-IFN), VEGF, and ANF, while adenosine, β-adrenergic agonists, PGE$_1$, PGE$_2$ and PGI$_2$ cause a decreased permeability (Allen and Coleman, 1995; Dejana *et al.*, 1995). The pattern observed in cultured endothelial cells is similar, although histamine, ANF and adenosine have been reported respectively to increase and to decrease permeability in different preparations (Dejana *et al.*, 1995).

The mechanisms linking receptor activation to change in paracellular permeability are of major interest. In general, agents increasing intracellular $[Ca^{2+}]$ and stimulating PLC cause increased permeability, while raising cAMP decreases permeability, but there are some exceptions (Dejana *et al.*, 1995). Where the cytoskeleton has been examined, stabilization of the actin cytoskeleton reduces endothelial permeability, while inhibition of microfilament assembly increases permeability.

In studies on individual mesenteric microvessels loaded with calcium-sensitive dye, Curry and coworkers have shown parallel changes in endothelial $[Ca^{2+}]_i$ and hydraulic conductivity (representing permeability of the paracellular pathway) in response to vasoactive agents (Curry, 1992). The permeability increase was dependent on calcium influx controlled by the electrochemical gradient across the membrane (He and Curry, 1994). However, elevation of cAMP reduced the permeability increase caused by ATP but without changing the biphasic calcium elevation (He and Curry, 1993). This suggested that cAMP acts on some downstream element linking elevation of calcium to tight junction regulation, e.g. via a calmodulin dependent actin–myosin cascade.

Histamine causes endothelial cells to retract from each other, and has been shown to increase the phosphorylation of myosin light chain kinase (MLC_{20}) in human umbilical vein endothelial cells (Moy *et al.*, 1993). Elevation of cAMP prevented cell retraction in response to histamine. These studies show that modulation of myosin light chain kinase activity may be an important step in the control of endothelial barrier function.

Modulation of blood–brain barrier permeability *in situ*

As indicted above, the brain endothelium forming the blood–brain barrier is ~50–100 times tighter than that of systemic endothelium, as seen by the much higher TEER (1–3000 Ω cm^2). Most studies of BBB modulation have been done on pial microvessels of the frog or rat, which retain BBB properties (Bundgaard, 1982; Butt *et al.*, 1990). Although the brain microvasculature is generally more resistant to modulation by inflammatory mediators than the systemic vasculature (Greenwood, 1992), modulation of pial vessel permeability has been demonstrated in both the frog (Olesen, 1989) and in mammals (Abbott and Revest, 1991; Greenwood 1992). Table 38.1 lists vasoactive agents that have been shown to increase BBB permeability, as seen by a drop in TEER, or extravasation of dyes and other tracers. All these agents are capable of being released in the vicinity of the cerebral microvasculature, in normal physiology or in pathology. For many of the agents, there is evidence that the effects are mediated by specific receptors. Thus in rat pial vessels, histamine and bradykinin (but not serotonin) caused a dose-

Table 38.1. *Vasoactive agents reported to increase blood–brain barrier permeability*

Histamine, serotonin (5-HT), bradykinin
Purine nucleotides : ATP, ADP, AMP
Phospholipase A_2, Platelet activating factor, PAF
Arachidonic acid, prostaglandins, leukotrienes
Interleukins : IL-1α, IL-1β, IL-2
Macrophage inflammatory proteins MIP-1, MIP-2
Complement-derived polypeptide C3a-desArg
Free oxygen radicals.

From information in Olesen, 1989; Greenwood, 1992.

dependent drop in TEER (Butt, 1995), and the increased permeability caused by histamine could be blocked by the H_2 antagonist cimetidine (Fig. 38.1, Butt and Jones, 1992). The fact that the calcium ionophore A23187 caused a reversible drop in TEER of frog pial vessels with a time course similar to that of many of the inflammatory mediators, suggested that increased permeability was linked to elevation of $[Ca^{2+}]_i$ (Olesen, 1989).

Activation of phospholipase C in isolated brain microvessels and cultured brain endothelial cells

In order to investigate the receptor pharmacology and signal transduction mechanisms at the BBB, early studies used isolated microvessels in binding and biochemical assays (Joó, 1985). More recently, primary cultures of brain endothelial cells and immortalized cell lines that preserve aspects of a BBB phenotype have been used (Joó, 1992; Abbott *et al.*, 1992, 1995). Where studies have been done on clonal cell lines of passaged cells, more variability is reported (Frelin and Vigne, 1993), suggesting the results may be affected by a phenotypic drift away from the receptor profile expressed in situ.

Table 38.2 summarizes studies in which addition of vasoactive agents has been shown to cause either hydrolysis of inositol phosphates, or elevation of intracellular calcium, compatible with activation of PLC.

In primary cultured human brain endothelial cells used up to passage 10, the action of histamine to increase inositol phosphate hydrolysis was blocked by mepyramine, suggesting action via an H_1 receptor (Purkiss *et al.*, 1994). This is in contrast to the *in situ* studies, which showed increased permeability via H_2 receptor activation (Butt and Jones, 1992; Sarker and Fraser, 1994).

In studies with purinceptor agonists on primary rat brain endothelial cells, using fura-2 to monitor elevation of $[Ca^{2+}]_i$, the order of potency of ATP>ADP>AMP, and the progressive desensitization to ATP, were consistent with presence of a P_2 receptor (Revest *et al.*, 1991). Using a flow cytometric method to measure intracellular calcium, and measurements of inositol phosphate production in a clonal population of bovine brain endothelial

Table 38.2. *Vasoactive agents activating phospholipase C in cultured brain endothelium, measured as elevation of $[Ca^{2+}]_i$ or inositol phosphate hydrolysis*

Agonist	Brain endothelial preparation	Reference
Elevation of $[Ca^{2+}]_i$		
Histamine, bradykinin ATP, ADP, AMP	Rat, primary culture	Revest *et al.*, 1991
ATP/UTP, ADP	Bovine, passaged clone	Frelin *et al.*, 1993
Histamine, ATP, UTP	Rat, primary culture RBE4, immortalized	Nobles *et al.*, 1995
Endothelin	Rat, passaged clone	Frelin and Vigne, 1993
Bradykinin	Bovine, passaged clone	Frelin and Vigne, 1993
Phosphoinositide hydrolysis		
α_2-adrenergic, bradykinin, arginine vasopressin, endothelin B, angiotensin II	Microvessels	Drewes, 1993
ATP/UTP, ADP	Bovine, passaged clone	Vigne *et al.*, 1994
Histamine, endothelin, ATP, UTP	Human, up to passage 10	Purkiss *et al.*, 1994
Endothelin	Human, passaged	Stanimirovic *et al.*, 1994

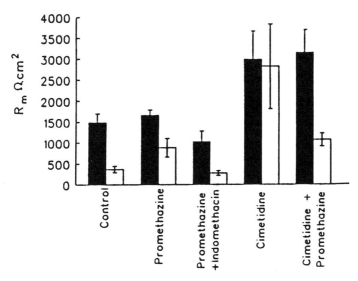

Fig. 38.1. H_2 histamine receptor mediates BBB opening in the rat. Effect of presurgical treatment with histamine receptor antagonists and cyclo-oxygenase inhibitor on basal resistance (R_m = TEER) (filled bars) and the histamine-mediated decrease in resistance (open bars). Neither promethazine alone nor promethazine plus indomethacin affected basal resistance. The decrease in resistance during histamine was partly blocked by promethazine alone but not by promethazine plus indomethacin. The H_2 receptor antagonist cimetidine caused a 100% increase in the basal resistance and completely blocked the histamine-mediated decrease in resistance. An equivalent increase in basal resistance was observed with the combined treatment of cimetidine plus promethazine, but the effect of histamine was ony partially blocked. From Butt and Jones, 1992, with permission.

A.

B.

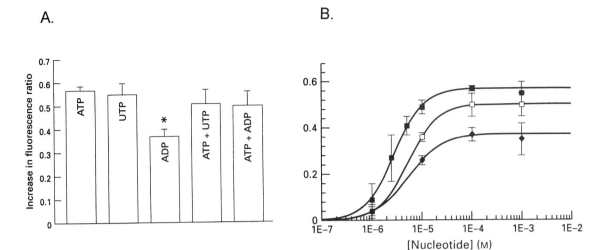

Fig. 38.2. Evidence that ATP, UTP and ADP act at the same receptor on immortalized rat brain endothelial cells RBE4. Change in fluorescence ratio from fura-2 loaded cells is a measure of change in $[Ca^{2+}]_i$.
(A) Comparison of effects of ATP, UTP and ADP, and combinations of agonists (mean $\pm$ SEM, $n = 7-14$ cells). All agents were applied at 100 μM for 20 s. The combinations ATP + UTP, and ATP + ADP gave responses no greater than for ATP alone (*$P < 0.05$).
(B) Evidence from dose–response curves that ATP and ADP act at the same receptor; nucleotides were applied at the concentrations shown (mean $\pm$ SEM, $n =$ at least four experiments per point). Curves were fitted with the Hill equation, with no parameters fixed. The p[A_{50}] values were 2.79 μM for ATP (■), 5.23 μM for ADP (□) and 5.33 μM for ATP + ADP(◆). The depression of the response to ATP in the presence of ADP is consistent with competition for the same receptor. From Nobles *et al.*, 1995, with permission.

cells, Frelin *et al.* (1993) distinguished a receptor for ATP/UTP coupled to PLC, and a separate ADP receptor capable of mobilizing intracellular calcium but without activation of PLC. They subsequently reported additional evidence for an atypical P$_{2Y}$ purinoceptor coupled to PLC (Vigne *et al.*, 1994b). On cultured human brain endothelial cells used up to passage 10, ATP and UTP, but not 2-methylthioATP (2MeSATP, P$_{2Y}$ agonist) or β,γ-methylene ATP (P$_{2X}$ agonist) gave measurable changes in inositol phosphate hydrolysis (Purkiss *et al.*, 1994), suggesting the main type of receptor present was activated by ATP and UTP. Studies on intracellular calcium using fura-2 in primary and immortalized (RBE4) rat brain endothelial cells reached a similar conclusion, and while ADP was effective on the ATP/UTP (P$_{2U}$) receptor, there was no evidence for a separate ADP receptor (Fig. 38.2., Nobles *et al.*, 1995). Taken together, these studies show some variability in expression of

purine/pyrimidine receptors in cultured brain endothelial cells, that may reflect the differences in species, passage number and phenotype of the cells.

The reported effects of bradykinin are also somewhat variable. A bradykinin receptor causing elevation of intracellular calcium was found in primary cultured rat brain endothelial cells (Revest *et al.*, 1991), and in a proportion of RBE4 cells (Abbott *et al.*, 1995). However, while Frelin and Vigne (1993) detected a bradykinin-induced elevation of intracellular calcium in a clonal population of bovine brain endothelial cells, they found no response in cloned rat brain capillary endothelial cells. The bradykinin B$_2$ analogue RMP7, in clinical trials for therapeutic blood–brain barrier opening for drug delivery to the brain, caused elevation of $[Ca^{2+}]_i$ in primary rat brain microvascular endothelial cells (Doctrow *et al.*, 1994).

Taken together these results show that there is

greater consistency among primary cultured brain endothelial cells and cell lines immortalized from early passage primary cells (e.g. RBE4), than among clonal populations of unspecified passage number.

Endothelins and arginine vasopressin cause hydrolysis of inositol phosphates and elevation of $[Ca^{2+}]_i$ in brain endothelium (Drewes, 1993; Frelin and Vigne, 1993; Stanimirovic *et al.*, 1994; Spatz *et al.*, 1995), but do not cause detectable increase in BBB permeability to small solutes *in situ* (Faraci, 1989). This highlights the interesting question as to how agonists that activate the same intracellular second messenger systems nevertheless can exert different effects on cell physiology. The reported 'cross-talk' among cAMP, cGMP and Ca^{2+}-dependent intracellular signalling mechanisms in brain capillary endothelial cells (Vigne *et al.*, 1994a; Nobles and Abbott, 1996) may be one way in which more subtle differentiation of effector actions can occur.

Intracarotid injection of hypertonic solutions *in vivo* is known to cause reversible BBB opening, and the mechanism has been assumed to involve endothelial shrinkage and pulling apart of tight junctions (Rapoport and Robinson, 1986). However, exposure to hypertonic mannitol increased monolayer permeability and elevated $[Ca^{2+}]_i$ in primary cultured rat brain endothelial cells (Nagashima *et al.*, 1994), suggesting a role for this second messenger in the osmotic opening of the BBB.

Conclusions and future directions

This review has shown that a number of the inflammatory mediators reported to increase the permeability of the blood–brain barrier also cause activation of PLC and elevation of intracellular $[Ca^{2+}]$, consistent with a Ca^{2+}-dependent contractile mechanism for opening brain endothelial tight junctions. Direct evidence from experiments in

which $[Ca^{2+}]_i$, endothelial contraction and tight junctional permeability are monitored simultaneously is now required. Although an InsP$_3$-sensitive calcium pool that can be mobilized by agonists acting on G-protein coupled receptors has been identified in brain endothelium, it is not known whether CICR and RR receptors are also involved, and whether mechanisms exist for amplification and attenuation of the response via this route. Although cross-talk has been detected between several second messenger systems, interactions with further systems such as the arachidonic acid pathway (Easton and Fraser, 1994), and the physiological implications, remain to be explored. Full understanding of the mechanisms for BBB modulation will offer opportunities not only for deliberate BBB opening for drug delivery, but also for therapeutic intervention to reduce BBB permeability occurring in pathologies such as stroke and multiple sclerosis.

While this review has concentrated on the role of calcium in regulating brain endothelial tight junctions, other roles for calcium in controlling endothelial secretion (NO, prostacyclin), and vascular tone are likely to prove equally important. Finally, it will be necessary not only to consider the ways in which the endothelium coordinates its activities along the length of the vessel, but also how endothelial function is integrated with that of the other cell types surrounding the endothelium, many of which (astrocytes, smooth muscle, neurons, microglia) are also capable of releasing and receiving chemical signals.

Acknowledgement

Our work on modulation of intracellular calcium in brain endothelial cells was supported by the MRC and the Wellcome Trust.

References

Abbott, N. J. and Revest, P. A. (1991). Control of brain endothelial permeability. *Cereb. Brain Metab. Rev.*, **3**, 39–72.

Abbott, N. J., Hughes, C. C. W., Revest, P. A. and Greenwood, J. (1992). Development and characterization of a rat brain capillary endothelial culture: towards an in vitro blood–brain barrier. *J. Cell Sci.*, **103**, 23–38.

Abbott, N. J., Roux, F., Couraud, P.-O. and Begley, D. J. (1995). Studies on an immortalized brain endothelial cell line: differentiation, permeability and transport. In *New Concepts of a Blood–Brain Barrier*, ed. J. Greenwood, D. J. Begley and M. B. Segal, pp. 239–49. New York: Plenum Press.

Adams, D. J., Rusko, J. and Van Slooten, G. (1993). Calcium signalling in vascular endothelial cells: Ca^{2+} entry and release. In *Ion Flux in Pulmonary Vascular Control*, ed. E. K. Weir, J. R. Hume and J. T. Reeves, NATO ASI Series, vol 251, pp. 259–75. New York: Plenum Press.

Allen, M. J. and Coleman, R. A. (1995). β$_2$-Adrenoceptors mediate a reduction in endothelial permeability in vitro. *Eur. J. Pharmacol.*, **274**, 7–15.

Beny, J.-L. (1990). Endothelial and smooth muscle cells hyperpolarized by bradykinin are not dye coupled. *Am. J. Physiol.* **258**, H836–41.

Berridge, M. J. (1993). Inositol trisphosphate and calcium signalling. *Nature*, **361**, 315–25.

Buchan, K. W. and Martin, W. (1991). Bradykinin induces elevations of cytosolic calcium through mobilization of intracellular and extracellular pools in bovine aortic endothelial cells. *Br. J. Pharmacol.*, **102**, 35–40.

Bundgaard, M. (1982). Ultrastructure of frog cerebral and pial microvessels and their impermeability to lanthanum ions. *Brain Res.*, **241**, 57–65.

Butt, A. M. (1995). Effect of inflammatory agents on electrical resistance across the blood–brain barrier in pial microvessels of anaesthetized rats. *Brain Res.*, **696**, 145–50.

Butt, A. M. and Jones, H. C. (1992). Effect of histamine and antagonists on electrical resistance across the blood–brain barrier in rat brain-surface microvessels. *Brain Res.*, **569**, 100–105.

Butt, A. M., Jones, H. C. and Abbott, N. J. (1990). Electrical resistance across the blood–brain barrier in anaesthetized rats: a developmental study. *J. Physiol.*, **429**, 47–62.

Crone, C. and Christensen, O. (1981). Electrical resistance of a capillary endothelium. *J. Gen. Physiol.*, **77**, 349–71.

Crone, C. and Olesen, S.-P. (1982). Electrical resistance of brain microvascular endothelium. *Brain Res.*, **241**, 49–55.

Curry, F. E. (1992). Modulation of venular microvessel permeability by calcium influx into endothelial cells. *FASEB J.*, **6**, 2456–66.

Davies, P. F., Olesen, S.-P., Clapham, D. E. *et al.* (1988). Endothelial communication. *Hypertension*, **11**, 563–72.

Dejana, E. and Del Maschio, A. (1995). Molecular organization and functional regulaton of cell to cell junctions in the endothelium. *Thromb. Haemostas.*, **74**, 309–12.

Dejana, E., Corada, M. and Lampugnani, M. G. (1995). Endothelial cell-to-cell junctions. *FASEB J.*, **9**, 910–18.

Doctrow, S. R., Abelleira, S. M., Curry, L. A. *et al.* (1994). The bradykinin analog RMP-7 increases intracellular free calcium levels in rat brain microvascular endothelial cells. *J. Pharmacol. Exp. Ther.*, **271**, 229–37.

Drewes, L. (1993). Phosphoinositide turnover in the brain microvasculature. In *The Blood–Brain Barrier*, ed. W. M. Pardridge, pp. 289–302. New York: Raven Press.

Easton, A. S. and Fraser, P. A. (1994). Evidence that arachidonic acid disruption of the blood–brain barrier is mediated by free radicals in the anaesthetized rat. *J. Physiol.*, **475**, 71P.

Ehrlich, B. E., Kaftan, E, Bezprozvannaya, S. and Bezprozvanny, I. (1994). The pharmacology of intracellular Ca^{2+}-release channels. *Trends Pharmacol. Sci.*, **15**, 145–9.

Faraci, F. M. (1989). Effects of endothelin and vasopressin on cerebral blood vessels. *Am. J. Physiol.*, **26**, H799–803.

Fasolato, C., Innocenti, B. and Pozzan, T. (1994). Receptor-activated Ca^{2+} influx: how many mechanisms for how many channels. *Trends Pharmacol. Sci.*, **15**, 77–83.

Favre, C. J., Nüsse, O., Lew, D. P. and Krause, K.-H. (1996). Store-operated Ca^{2+} influx: what is the message from the stores to the membrane? *J. Clin. Med.*, **128**, 19–26.

Frelin, C. and Vigne, P. (1993). Brain microvascular vasoactive agents: receptors and mechanisms of action. In *The Blood–Brain Barrier*, ed. W. M. Pardridge, pp. 249–65. New York: Raven Press.

Frelin, C., Breittmayer, J. P. and Vigne, P. (1993). ADP induces inositol phosphate-independent intracellular Ca^{2+} mobilization in brain capillary endothelial cells. *J. Biol. Chem.*, **268**, 8787–692.

Furuse, M., Hirase, T., Itoh, M. *et al.* (1993). Occludin: A novel integral membrane protein localizing at tight junctions. *J. Cell Biol.*, **123**, 1777–88.

Furuse, M., Itoh, M, Hirase, T. *et al.* (1994). Direct association of occludin with ZO-1 and its possible involvement in the localization of occludin at tight junctions. *J. Cell Biol.*, **127**, 1617–26.

Greenwood, J. (1992). Experimental manipulations of the blood–brain and blood–retinal barriers. In *Physiology and Pharmacology of the Blood–Brain Barrier*, ed. M. W. B. Bradbury, pp. 460–486. Berlin: Springer Verlag.

Gumbiner, B. M. (1993). Breaking through the tight junction barrier. *J. Cell Biol.*, **123**, 1631–3.

He, P. and Curry, F. E. (1993). Differential actions of cAMP on endothelial [Ca^{2+}]i and permeability in microvessels exposed to ATP. *Am. J. Physiol.* 265, H1019–23.

He, P. and Curry, F. E. (1994). Endothelial hyperpolarization increases [Ca^{2+}]i and venular microvessel permeability. *J. Appl. Physiol.*, **76**, 2288–97.

Himmel, H. M., Whorton, R. and Strauss, H. C. (1993). Intracellular calcium, currents, and stimulus-response coupling in endothelial cells. *Hypertension*, **21**, 112–27.

Joó, F. (1985). The blood–brain barrier in vitro: Ten years of research on microvessels isolated from the brain. *Neurochemi. Int.*, **7**, 1–25.

Joó, F. (1992). The cerebral microvessels in culture, an update. *J. Neurochem.* **58**, 1–17.

Kasai, H. and Petersen, O. H. (1994). Spatial dynamics of second messengers: IP$_3$ and cAMP as long-range and associative messengers. *Trends Neurosci.*, **17**, 96–101.

McCarthy, K. M., Skare, I. B., Stankewich, M. C. *et al.* (1996). Occludin is a functional component of the tight junction. *J. Cell Sci.*, **109**, 2287–98.

Moy, A. B., Shasby, S. S., Scott, B. D. and Shasby, D. M. (1993). The effect of histamine and cyclic adenosine monophosphate on myosin light chain phosphorylation in human umbilical vein endothelial cells. *J. Clin. Invest.*, **92**, 1198–206.

Nagashima, T., Shijing, W., Mizoguchi, A. and Tamaki, N. (1994). A possible role of calcium ion in osmotic opening of blood–brain barrier. *J. Auton. Nerv. Syst.*, **49**, S145–149.

Nobles, M. and Abbott, N. J. (1996). Effects of cyclic nucleotides on the increase in [Ca^{2+}]i caused by external ATP in the brain endothelial cell line, RBE4. *J. Physiol.*, **491**, 38P.

Nobles, M., Revest, P. A., Couraud, P.-O and Abbott, N. J. (1995). Characteristics of nucleotide receptors that cause elevation of cytoplasmic calcium in immortalized rat brain endothelial cells (RBE4) and in primary cultures. *Br. J. Pharmacol.*, **115**, 1245–52.

Olesen, S.-P. (1989). An electrophysiological study of microvascular permeabilty and its modulation by chemical mediators. *Acta Physiol. Scand.*, **136**, Suppl 579, 1–28.

Otun, H., Aidulis, D M., Yang, J. M. and Gillespie, J. I. (1996). Interactions between inositol trisphosphate and Ca^{2+} dependent Ca^{2+} release mechanisms on the endoplasmic reticulum of perme-abilised bovine aortic endothelial cells. *Cell Calcium*, **19**, 315–25.

Purkiss, J. R., West, D., Wilkes, L. C. *et al.* (1994). Stimulation of phospholipase C in cultured microvascular endothelial cells from human frontal lobe by histamine, endothelin and purinoceptor agonists. *Br. J. Pharmacol.*, **111**, 1041–6.

Rapoport, S. I. and Robinson, P. J. (1986). Tight junctional modification as the basis of osmotic opening of the blood–brain barrier. *Ann. NY Acad. Sci.*, **481**, 250–66.

Revest, P. A., Abbott, N. J. and Gillespie, J. I. (1991). Receptor-mediated changes in intracellular [Ca^{2+}] in cultured rat brain capillary endothelial cells. *Brain Res.*, **549**, 159–61.

Rusko, J., Tanzi, F., van Breemen, C. and Adams, D. J. (1992). Calcium-activated potassium channels in native endothelial cells from rabbit aorta: conductance, Ca^{2+} sensitivity and block. *J. Physiol.*, **455**, 601–21.

Rusko, J., Van Slooten, G. and Adams, D. J. (1995). Caffeine-evoked, calcium-sensitive membrane currents in rabbit aortic endothelial cells. *Br. J. Pharmacol.*, **115**, 133–41.

Sarker, M. H. and Fraser, P. A. (1994). Histamine receptor activation and the regulation of cerebro-microvascular permeability in the anaesthetized rat. *J. Physiol.*, **475**, 60–61P.

Sauvé, R., Parent, L., Simoneau, C and Roy, G. (1988). External ATP triggers a biphasic activation process of a calcium-dependent K$^+$ channel in cultured bovine aortic endothelial cells. *Pflügers Archiv.*, **412**, 469–81.

Schulze, C. and Firth, J. A. (1992). Interendothelial junctions during blood–brain barrier development in the rat: morphological changes at the level of individual tight junctional contacts. *Dev. Brain Res.*, **69**, 85–95.

Simionescu, M., Simionescu, N. and Palade, G. E. (1975). Segmental differentiation of cell junctions in the vascular endothelium. *J. Cell Biol.*, **67**, 863–85.

Spatz, M., Stanimirovic, D. and McCarron, R. M. (1995). Endothelin as a mediator of blood–brain barrier function. In *New Concepts of a Blood–Brain Barrier*, ed. J. Greenwood, D. J. Begley and M. B. Segal, pp. 47–61. New York: Plenum Press.

Stanimirovic, D. B., Yamamoto, T., Uematsu, S. and Spatz, M. (1994). Endothelin-1 receptor binding and cellular signal transduction in cultured human brain endothelial cells. *J. Neurochem.*, **62**, 592–601.

Thuringer, D. and Sauvé, R. (1992). A patch clamp study of the Ca^{2+} mobilization from internal stores in bovine aortic endothelial cells. I. Effects of caffeine on intracellular Ca^{2+} stores. *J. Memb. Biol.*, **130**, 125–37.

Vigne, P., Lund, L. and Frelin, C. (1994a). Cross talk among cyclic AMP, cyclic GMP, and Ca^{2+}-dependent intracellular signalling mechanisms in brain capillary endothelial cells. *J. Neurochem.*, **62**, 2269–74.

Vigne, P., Feolde, E., Breittmayer, J. P and Frelin, C. (1994b). Characterization of the effects of 2-methylthio-ATP and 2-chloro-ATP on brain capillary endothelial cells: similarities to ADP and differences from ATP. *Br. J. Pharmacol.*, **112**, 775–80.

Ward, B. J., Bauman, K. F. and Firth, J. A. (1988). Interendothelial junctions of cardiac capillaries in rats: their structure and permeability properties. *Cell Tiss. Res.*, **252**, 57–66.

Ziegelstein, R. C., Spurgeon, H. A., Pili, R. *et al.* (1994a). A functional ryanodine-sensitive intracellular Ca^{2+} store is present in vascular endothelial cells. *Circ. Res.*, **74**, 151–6.

Ziegelstein, R. C., Cheng, L., Aversano, T. *et al.* (1994b). Increase in rat aortic endothelial free calcium mediated by metabolically sensitive calcium release from endoplasmic reticulum. *Cardiovasc. Res.*, **28**, 1433–9.

39 Cytokines and the blood–brain barrier

ROUMEN BALABANOV and PAULA DORE-DUFFY

- Introduction
- Vascular cells as producers of cytokines
- EC as the target of locally released cytokines
- Cytokines, the BBB and pathophysiology of CNS diseases
- Cytokines and BBB permeability
- Mechanism of action
- Concluding remarks

Introduction

The blood–brain barrier (BBB), by virtue of its strategic position, is an important regulatory organ involved in complex communication mechanisms that regulate homeostasis. Soluble biological response modifiers (BRMs), identified as early as 1926, were shown to be capable of mediating this bi-directional regulatory system (Zinssern and Tamiya, 1926). The BBB is not only a constant target of BRMs, but synthesizes its own unique repertoire, which includes eicosanoids, growth factors, chemokines and cytokines. In this chapter discussion is restricted to the classic cytokines and the role of the BBB as both the target and producer of these biologically potent molecules.

Cytokines are a heterogeneous group of paracrine and autocrine regulatory glycoproteins. They form a complex network of signals that coordinate diverse pathophysiological events such as BBB development and differentiation (Woodroofe, 1995), response to injury (Beneviste, 1992), and involvement in many acute and chronic neurological diseases (Morgani-Kossmann *et al.*, 1992). The cytokines are capable of inducing long-term responses characterized by phenotypic changes, alteration of cell–cell contacts, and functional reprogramming (Paul and Seder, 1994). A better understanding of cytokine regulatory pathways functioning at the BBB is important to our overall understanding of this complex structure and its role in CNS disease.

Vascular cells as producers of cytokines

Because homogeneous populations of CNS endothelial cells (EC) are difficult to obtain, much of our knowledge of the EC as a producer of cytokines comes from studies performed on EC of non-CNS origin such as the human umbilical vein endothelial cell (HUVEC). EC release a variety of cytokines depending on the culture conditions and their physiology (Pober and Cortan, 1990). Quiescent CNS EC from murine origin have been reported to produce interleukin-1 (IL-1), interleukin-6 (IL-6), and granulocyte–macrophage-colony stimulating factor (GM-CSF) when analyzed for protein and/or cytokine specific messenger RNA (mRNA) (Table 39.1). Permanent CNS lines from the SJL/j mouse produce IL-6, but not IL-1 (Fabry *et al.*, 1993). In another study spontaneous

Table 39.1. *Cytokine production by the BBB cells**

Cell	Stimulus	Cytokine	Ref.
1. EC	Culture	IL-α, IL-1β, IL-6, GM-CSF	(1), (2)
	LPS IL-1	IL-α, IL-1β, IL-6, GM-CSF	(1), (2)
	HTLV	IL-6	(2)
	RSV	TGF-β	(3)
	HIV	IL-1, IL-6 IFN-γ, TNF-α	(4), (5)
2. PC-EC	Co-culture	TGF-β	(6), (7)
3. SMC/PC	Culture IL-1, LPS	IL-1β, IL-6 GM-CSF	(1)

*Table includes data obtained from CNS EC and PC. References: (1) Fabry *et al.*, 1993; (2) Rott *et al.*, 1993; (3) Moordian and Diglio, 1991; (4) Moses and Nelson, 1994; (5) Tyor *et al.*, 1992; (6) Antonelli-Oldrige *et al.*, 1989; (7) Shepro and Morel, 1993.

IL-6 secretion could be diminished by employing serum-free culture media (Rott *et al.*, 1993).

The cytokine repertoire is altered upon exposure to exogenous stimuli known to activate EC (Table 39.1). These agents are diverse and include cytokines, coagulation factors, bacterial products, and viral particles (Antonelli-Oldrige *et al.*, 1989; Moordian and Diglio, 1991; Tyor *et al.*, 1992; Fabry *et al.*, 1993; Rott *et al.*, 1993; Moses and Nelson, 1994). Transfection of murine BALB/c EC with a human T-cell leukemia virus-1 (HTLV-1) *tax* gene-containing plasmid upregulated IL-6 mRNA expression (Rott *et al.*, 1993). Rous sarcoma virus (RSV) transformed rat cerebral EC were found to secrete the active form of TGF-β (Moordian and Diglio, 1991). However similar findings were reported in co-cultures of EC and pericytes (PC) (Antonelli-Oldrige *et al.*, 1989). Human CNS EC secrete significantly higher levels of IL-6 following infection with the human immunodeficiency virus (HIV) (Moses and Nelson, 1994). Similarly, in brain tissue from patients with acquired immunodeficiency syndrome (AIDS), EC stained positively for IL-6, IL-1, and less frequently for IFN-γ and TNF-α (Tyor *et al.*, 1992).

CNS pericytes (PC) are another important cytokine-producing cellular constituent of the microvascular wall, physically located near the EC and completely surrounded by basement membrane. CNS PC have been implicated in many normal and pathological conditions, but their function is still not well understood (Shepro and Morel, 1993). Fabry and colleagues (1993) reported that smooth muscle/pericytes produce IL-1β, IL-6 and GM-CSF. Expression is augmented by lipopolysaccharide (LPS). In another co-culture system containing EC and PC from retina, Antonelli-Oldrige and colleagues (1989) reported the production of the active form of TGF-β1. In our laboratory, conditioned media from 4-day-old and primary rat CNS PC were found to contain little to no TGF-β1, no IL-1β and TNF-α . However, this repertoire is substantially altered upon exposure to an activating or stress signal where TGF-β is augmented (P. Dore-Duffy, unpublished observations). TGF-β1 also downregulates cytokine-mediated EC activation (Dore-Duffy *et al.*, 1994) as well as inhibiting EC proliferation (Antonelli-Oldrige *et al.*, 1989). It is possible that EC and PC use TGF-β1 in endogenous regulation of endothelial activation.

EC as the target of locally released cytokines

Evidence has accumulated that cytokines as well as other biologically active components can induce a functional and phenotypic change in the endothelium (Mantouani *et al.*, 1992; Augustin *et al.*, 1994). The quiescent endothelium is nonadhesive, antithrombotic and fibrinolytic. Upon exposure to cytokines summarized in Table 39.2 the endothelium becomes dysfunctional or 'activated'. The activated endothelium becomes hyperadhesive, prothrombotic and proinflammatory (Pober, 1988; Pober and Cortan, 1990). While the mechanisms governing EC activation are unclear, evidence points to a major role for locally released cytokines (Beneviste, 1992). The source of these cytokines may be the vascular cells, nearby non-vascular cells, or leukocytes, drawn to sites of infection or injury.

Uncommitted or naive T lymphocytes produce

Table 39.2. *CNS endothelial cell response to cytokines*

Cytokine	Effect	Ref.
IFN-γ	↑MHC class I	(1), (2)
	class II Ag	(3), (4)
	↑ICAM-1	(5), (6)
	↑TNF-Rs	(7)
IFN-β	↓IFN-γ effects	(8)
TNF-α	↑VCAM-1	(3), (9)
	↑ELAM-1	(10), (11), (12)
IL-1	↑ICAM-1, TNF-R	(1), (13)
	↑IL-α, IL-1β	(4), (11)
	IL-6, GM-CSF	(12)
TGF-β	↓IL-1, TNF-α	(14), (15)
	IFN-γ effects	(6)

↑↓ – increase of decrease respectively.
References: (1) Fabry *et al.*, 1992; (2) Wong and Dorovini-Zis, 1992; (3) Dore-Duffy *et al.*, 1994*b*; (4) Bebo and Linuthicum, 1995; (5) McCarron *et al.*, 1985; (6) Dore- Duffy *et al.*, 1996; (7) Huynh and Dorovini-Zis, 1993; (8) Huynh *et al.*, 1995; (9) Fabry *et al.*, 1993; (10) Kim *et al.*, 1992; (11) Claudio *et al.*, 1994; (12) Vires *et al.*, 1993; (13) Rott *et al.*, 1993; (14) Dore-Duffy *et al.*, 1994*a*; (15) Fabry *et al.*, 1995.

IL-2 (Weinberg and English, 1990). Once they become effector cells they produce cytokines considered to be of the TO pattern – (IL-2, IL-3, IL-4, IL-5, IL-6, IL-10, GM-CSF, IFN-γ, lymphotoxin (LT) and TNF-α (Mossmann and Coffran, 1989). T cells can be induced to polarize to either a T1 pattern (IFN-γ , TNFα , LT, IL-3, GM-CSF, +/-, IL-2), or a T2 pattern of cytokine release (IL-4, IL-5, IL-6, IL-10 and IL-13). Polarization to one pattern or another appears to be related to factors such as pathogen, specific antigen chemokines and/or macrophage-directed factors (Swain, 1995). Other cytokines such as TGF-β1 have also been implicated in regulation of cytokine producing phenotype (Paul and Seder, 1994). Thus, endothelial exposure to cytokine in the *in vivo* setting is complicated. Results from experiments in which endothelial cell lines are exposed to a single cytokine may inappropriately simplify a complex *in vivo* condition.

Proinflammatory cytokines (T1 pattern) control the expression of several groups of adhesion molecules including intercellular adhesion molecule-1 (ICAM-1), vascular cell adhesion molecule-1 (VCAM-1) and endothelial leukocyte adhesion molecule-1 (ELAM-1, E-selectin). Cytokines such as IL-1, TNF-α and IFN-γ upregulate the expression of ICAM-1 on rat, mouse and human CNS EC cultures (Fabry *et al.*, 1992; Wong and Dorovini-Zis, 1992; Dore-Duffy *et al.*, 1994*b*). TNF-α and IL-1 increase the expression of E-selectin on CNS microvessels and primary cultures (Dore-Duffy *et al.*, 1994*b*). VCAM-1 is upregulated by exposure to TNF-α, IL-1, but not IFN-γ . IFN-β and TGF-β1 have no effect on quiescent EC, but do inhibit cytokine-mediated activation of EC or preactivated EC (Dore-Duffy *et al.*, 1994*a*). It is possible that TGF-β1 (Antonelli-Oldrige *et al.*, 1989; Dore-Duffy *et al.*, 1994*a*; Huynh *et al.*, 1995) may be involved in regulation of activation. A loss of this regulatory ability may result in perpetuation of activation and/or chronic inflammatory activity.

In combination, cytokines may induce fundamentally different results. Exposure of CNS EC to both IL-1β and TNF-α or IFN-γ, and TNF-α can result in synergistic induction of E-selectin, and ICAM-1 and MHC class II molecules respectively (Pober and Cortan, 1990) as both IL-1 and IFN-γ increase TNF receptors (Bebo and Linuthicum, 1995). Hydrogen peroxide and possibly other by-products of oxidative metabolism, which on their own activate the endothelium, when combined with T1 cytokines inhibit activation (Bradley *et al.*, 1993).

It is unclear whether patterns of cytokine induction and EC activation analyzed in non-CNS EC parallel those of CNS EC. Organ specific differences in EC are not well characterized. Human CNS EC express a higher basal level of ICAM-1 than non-CNS EC. CNS EC are more sensitive to cytokine induction of ICAM-1, express ICAM-1 earlier and maintain elevated expression for a longer period of time following cytokine removal (Wong and Dorovini-Zis, 1992). E-selectin, originally thought to be a transiently expressed endothelial activation antigen when analyzed *in vitro*, is now thought to persist *in vivo*. In CNS microvessels exposed to TNF-α, E-selectin persisted for up to 48 hours (Dore-Duffy *et al.*, 1994*b*). In primary culture, TNF-α-stimulated CNS EC transiently expressed E-selectin.

Cytokines, the BBB and pathophysiology of CNS diseases

The local release of cytokines by cells of the immune system has considerable pathological significance. Expression of EC surface proteins has been shown to characterize CNS microvascular tissue at sites of infection (Moses and Nelson, 1994), vascular injury (Wakefield *et al.*, 1994), stroke (Kim *et al.*, 1995), traumatic brain injury (Kochanek and Hallenbek, 1992; Matsuo *et al.*, 1994) and inflammatory disease (Raine *et al.*, 1990; Washington *et al.*, 1994). The etiological mechanisms that result in induction of these molecules may be fundamentally different, but the role played by activated endothelium in CNS disease shares basic tenets. These include: augmented leukocyte adhesion and migration, enhanced expression of immunologically relevant antigens and alteration in BBB function and integrity resulting in permeability and/or edema. Specific aspects of the role played by the BBB in CNS disease are covered elsewhere in this book.

EC expression of adhesion molecules and their interaction with appropriate ligands on the surface of leukocytes promotes leukocyte sequestration or tethering to the microvascular wall (Male *et al.*, 1990; Bevilacqua, 1993; McCarron *et al.*, 1993). Activation augments both the migration of naive and committed leukocytes as well as enhancing the chances of tethering by upregulation on translocation of appropriate adhesion proteins to the luminal surface (Bevilacqua, 1993; McCarron *et al.*, 1993). With the development of molecular techniques that allow targeting of specific genes, leukocyte–EC tethering and migration is now known to involve multiple adhesion molecules (Ley, 1995). While one adhesion molecule may have a primary role in leukocyte tethering in normal mice, in the absence of this molecule in knockout mice another protein is often able to substitute functionally (Sligh *et al.*, 1993). In CNS, EC pretreatment of cultured monolayers with IFN-γ, IL-1, or TNF-α significantly increased T-cell adhesion in a dose and time dependent manner (Bevilacqua, 1993; McCarron *et al.*, 1993), and in one study independently of antigen specificity (Male *et al.*, 1990). Fabry and colleagues reported that TGF-β2 inhibits basal and cytokine-induced leukocyte adhesion, and inhibits IL-1-, TNF-α-, and IFN-γ-induced leukocyte migration (Fabry *et al.*, 1995).

IFN-γ, in addition to its ability to induce adhesion proteins, controls the expression of a specific set of molecules, important to immune function (McCarron *et al.*, 1985). The major histocompatability complex (MHC) class I and class II molecules are involved in antigen processing and presentation as well as specific interactions with T and B lymphocytes (McCarron *et al.*, 1985, 1993; Male *et al.*, 1990). The MHC Class II molecule, which must be induced, and the MHC Class I molecule, which is constitutively produced in low levels on quiescent CNS EC, are not always co-expressed on activated EC. In multiple sclerosis (MS), a chronic neurological disease of the CNS characterized by perivascular leukocyte infiltration, isolated microvessels taken from periplaque areas had lower percentages of microvessel fragments expressing MHC class II molecules than vessels isolated from uninvolved brain tissue from the same patient (Washington *et al.*, 1994). The reverse was true for expression of adhesion molecules E-selectin and VCAM-1. This suggests that MHC class II-dependent leukocyte EC interactions may precede a generalized endothelial activation. Upregulation of the numerous adhesion molecules seen in MS microvessels may be a result of cytokine release by nonspecifically recruited naive leukocytes, which make up the majority of the migrating cells (Raine and Scheinberg, 1988). In rats immunized with myelin basic protein (MBP), adhesion molecules are sequentially upregulated following immunization (Dore-Duffy *et al.*, 1996). The expression of MHC class II molecules, ICAM-1 and VCAM-1 precedes the development of clinical symptoms. Upregulation of constitutively expressed MHC class I molecules occurs only at 12–14 days post-immunization, concurrent with expression of clinical evidence of neurological disease. This may suggest that during this stage CD8+ T-lymphocytes involved in cytolytic MHC class I-dependent mechanisms are most pronounced. A T1 pattern of cytokine release would be compatible with these activities. MS is discussed in greater detail in a previous chapter of this book.

Cytokines and BBB permeability

From both *in vivo* and *in vitro* studies it is clear that cytokines have a profound effect on the structural integrity and/or barrier function of the CNS endothelium. Cytokine-induced changes may involve gross breakdown of the BBB with massive extravasation of blood-borne elements to a more subtle change in regulation of transport mechanisms (Kim *et al.*, 1992; Claudio *et al.*, 1994; Saija *et al.*, 1995). Much of our understanding of the role played by cytokines in barrier disruption comes from morphological studies in pathological tissue, *in vivo* toxicology studies, and from *in vitro* studies using cell models of the BBB.

Development of *in vitro* models of the blood–brain barrier have been attempted by a number of laboratories (Huynh and Dorovini-Zis, 1993; Vires *et al.*, 1993; Fabry *et al.*, 1995; Gillies and Su, 1995; Huynh *et al.*, 1995). Confluent EC monolayers dedifferentiate and lose many barrier characteristics, as well as the multicelluar nature of CNS endothelium. Despite these shortcomings such systems can provide useful clues to the role of cytokines in barrier permeability. TNF-α, IL-1 and IL-6 have been shown to increase permeability as measured by changes in transendothelial resistance (TEER) (Vires *et al.*, 1993). Decreased TEER (over 50%) was observed within 60 min of cytokine addition. It is unlikely that such rapid changes in permeability could be due to induction of new proteins, but may be associated with translocation and/or altered matrix protein–adhesion molecule interactions. In a similar system, IFN-γ increased the permeability of EC monolayers (Huynh and Dorovini-Zis, 1993). Exposure of EC to IFN-γ for 72–96 hours resulted in pronounced morphological changes, which included loss of organized cytoskeletal alignment and contact inhibition. Cells exhibited loose swirls and areas of cellular overlap (Huynh and Dorovini-Zis, 1993). These authors suggested that such ultra-structural changes result in increased vascular permeability. The mechanisms of action are

unknown. In a subsequent study the same authors found that IFN-β antagonized IFN-γ mediated changes in permeability (Huynh *et al.*, 1995). Further, IFN-α2b has been shown to augment barrier characteristics (Gillies and Su, 1995). It is unclear whether other cytokines such as TGF-β1, known to downregulate endothelial activation, also restore normal vascular permeability. However, a direct correlation between EC activation and vascular permeability has not thus far been shown. Thus, expression of adhesion protein on vascular tissue can not be used as an indicator of barrier damage. Rather, it simply represents endothelial activation.

Mechanism of action

The cytokines elicit cellular responses through surface receptor coupling mechanisms (Roit *et al.*, 1993). Cytokine receptors based on their intrinsic protein kinase (PTK) activity are classified into two groups (Miyajima *et al.*, 1992): (1) *Cytokine receptor type I*, which has intrinsic PTK activity. These receptors are engaged by the interleukins (IL-2, IL-3, IL-4, IL-5, IL-6, IL-7, IL-8, IL-9, IL-11, IL-12, IL-13, IL-14, IL-15), colony-stimulating factors GM-CSF, G-CSF), erythropoetin (EPO) and growth hormone (GH) (Miyajima *et al.*, 1993). They activate the Ras/MAP kinase signaling pathway, which is involved downstream in the transcriptional control of the target genes via NF-IL6 (C/ERBb) and AP-1 (jun/fos related proteins) transcription factors. (2) *Cytokine receptor type II* lacks its own PTK activity, but transduces the cytokine signals by interactive PTK (Darnell *et al.*, 1994). JAK (Just Another or JAnus Kinase) kinases are physically associated with the intercellular receptor domain either constitutively or in response to ligand binding. They transduce signals by phosphorylating STAT (Signal Transducers and Activators of Transcription) proteins. This recently described JAK/STAT signal pathway mediates the cytokine effects of interferons (IFNs) and IL-10 (Darnell *et al.*, 1994; Schindler and Darnell, 1995). Once activated, STAT proteins interact with each other and form homo- and heterodimers, that translocate into the nucleus. There are two classes of STAT responsive regulatory sequences differentiating the interferon responses: GAS

(Gamma Activating Sequences) controlling IFN-γ inducible genes, and ISRE (Interferon-Stimulated Responses Element), mediating mainly IFN-α/β responses. Other cytokines (EGF, PDGF, IL-6, CSFs) may also utilize them in their signal pathways. GAS elements are recognized by a homodimer of STAT 1, as well as the other closely related proteins STAT 3, STAT 5 and STAT 6 (Schindler and Darnell, 1995). ISRE is recognized by a complex containing STAT 1, STAT 2 and p48, referred to also as ISGF3. It mediates IFN-β inhibition of MHC class II molecule expression by reducing the functional competence of the IFN-γ-inducible and JAK-activated CIITA (Class II TransActivator), an essential factor for this expression (Lu *et al.*, 1995). The knowledge for JAK and STAT families continues to expand as well as the evidence showing that some other cytokines (EGF, PDGF, IL-6, CSFs) use them in their signal pathways.

TNF-α and IL-1 induced-signal events include phospholipid hydrolysis, protein tyrosine phosphorylation, and elevation of cAMP (Ray *et al.*, 1992; Scholtze *et al.*, 1994). Stimulus-sensitive sphingomyelinase generates ceramide-activated protein kinases. Activated PTK transduces the ligand signal to either Ras/MAP kinase or inositol-phospholipid pathways (Scholtze *et al.*, 1994). The activated protein kinases further involve transcription factors such as NF-κB, NF-IL6, AP-1 and CREB controlling *cis*-activating sequences of the TNF-α, and IL-1 inducible target genes (Miyajima *et al.*, 1992). NF-κB plays an important role in regulating cytokine induced activation (Collins *et al.*, 1995). In resting EC, NF-κB binding proteins are in an inactive cystolic form due to complex formation with inhibitory protein IκB-α (Baldwin, 1996; Sun *et al.*, 1993). Upon EC activation IκB-α is phosphorylated and subsequently degraded by proteosomes, a nonlysomal proteolytic pathway, allowing NF-κB translocation into the nucleus (Liou and Baltimore, 1993). Although NF-κB transcription factor system is critical, it is not sufficient for cytokine-induced expression of adhesion molecules. The process also requires other cytokine-activated transcription factors such as NF-IL6, AP-1, ATF/CREB and STAT 1. This may account for the synergism seen with multiple cytokines (Collins *et al.*, 1995).

Concluding remarks

The BBB has become the focus of intensive research over the last decade. Interest has developed in the BBB as a multicellular regulatory organ whose fine-tuned homeostatic mechanisms involve complex crosstalk between the cellular constituents of the BBB, and between the BBB and nonvascular cells such as microglial cells, astrocytes and cells of the immune system. Deciphering the language of these crosstalk mechanisms, which involve not only cytokines but a host of biologically active components, will require the use of experimental systems that accurately duplicate the multicellular nature of the BBB, coupled with molecular approaches that involve gene targeting. This knowledge is likely to yield important new insights leading to the development of therapeutic strategies aimed at modulation of BBB function and EC and PC differentiation. The BBB is not passive. Rather, it is an active participant in maintenance of homeostasis and in neuroimmune networks centered at the microvasculature.

References

Antonelli-Oldrige, A., Saunders, K., Smith, S. and D'Amore, P. (1989). An activated form of transforming growth factor is produced by cocultures of endothelial cells and pericytes. *Proc. Natl. Acad. Sci. USA*, **86**, 4544–88.

Augustin, H., Kozian, D. and Johnson, R. (1994). Differentiation of endothelial cell: analysis of the constitutive and activated endothelial cell phenotypes. *Bio-Essays*, **16**(12), 901–6.

Baldwin, A. (1996). The NF-κB and IκB proteins: new discoveries and insights. *Annu. Rev. Immunol.*, **14**, 649–81.

Bebo and Linuthicum, D. (1995). Expression of mRNA for 55 kDa and 75 kDa tumor necrosis factor receptors in mouse cerebrovascular endothelium of interleukin-1β, interferon-γ and TNF-α on cultured cells. *J. Neuroimmunol.*, **62**, 116–67.

Beneviste, E. (1992). Inflammatory cytokines within the central nervous system: sources, function and mechanism of action. *Am. J. Physiol.*, **263**, C1–16.

Bevilacqua, M. P. (1993). Endothelial-leukocyte adhesion molecules. *Annu. Rev. Immunol.*, **11**, 767–804.

Bradley, J. R., Johnson, D. R. and Pober, J. S. (1993). Endothelial activation by hydrogen peroxide. Selective increases of intercellular adhesion molecule-1 and major histocompatibility complex class I. *Am. J. Pathol.*, **142**(5), 1598–609.

Claudio, L., Martiney, J. and Brosman, C. (1994). Ultrastructural studies of the blood–retinal barrier after exposure to interleukin-1 or tumor necrosis factor-α in rat. *Lab. Invest.*, **70**(6), 850–61.

Collins, T., Read, M., Neish, A. *et al.* (1995). Transcriptional control of endothelial cell adhesion molecules: NF-kB and cytokine-inducible enhancers. *FASEB J.*, **9**, 899–909.

Darnell, J., Kerr, L. and Stark, G. (1994). JAK-STAT pathways and transcriptional activation in response to IFNs, and other extracellular signaling proteins. *Science*, **264**, 1415–20.

Dore-Duffy, P., Balabanov, R., Washington, R. and Swanborg, R. (1994*a*). Transforming growth factor-β1 inhibits cytokine-induced CNS endothelial cell activation. *Mol. Chem. Neuropathol.*, **22**, 161–17.

Dore-Duffy, P., Washington, R. and Balabanov, R. (1994*b*). Cytokine-mediated activation of CNS microvessels: A system for examining antigenic modulation of CNS endothelial cells, and evidence for long-term expression of the adhesion protein E-selectin. *J. Cereb. Blood Flow Metab.*, **14**, 837–44.

Dore-Duffy, P., Balabanov, R., Rafols, J. and Swanborg, R. (1996). Recovery phase of acute experimental autoimmune encephalomyelitis in rats corresponds to development of endothelial cell unresponsiveness to interferon gamma activation. *J. Neurosci. Res.*, **44**, 223–34.

Fabry, Z., Waldschmidt, M., Hendrickson, D. *et al.* (1992). Adhesion molecules on murine brain microvascular endothelial cells: expression and regulation of ICAM-1 and Lgp 55. *J. Neuroimmunol.*, **36**, 1–11.

Fabry, Z., Fitzimmons, K., Herlein, J. *et al.* (1993). Production of cytokines interleukin 1 and 6 by murine brain microvessel endothelium and smooth muscle pericytes. *J. Neuroimmunol.*, **43**, 23–34.

Fabry, Z., Taphan, D., Fee, D. *et al.* (1995). TGF-β2 decreases migration of lymphocytes in vitro and homing of cells into the central nervous system in vivo. *J. Immunol.*, **155**, 325–32.

Gillies, M. and Su, T. (1995). Interfon-α2b enhances barrier function of bovine retinal microvascular endothelium in vitro. *Microvasc. Res.*, **49**, 277–88.

Huynh, H. and Dorovini-Zis, K. (1993). Effects of interferon-gamma on primary cultures of human brain microvessel endothelial cells. *Am. J. Pathol.*, **142**, 1265–78.

Huynh, H., Oger, J. and Dorovini-Zis, K. (1995). Interferon-β downregulates interferon-γ-induced class II MHC molecule expression and morphological changes in primary cultures of human brain microvessel endothelial cells. *J. Neuroimmunol.*, **60**, 63–73.

Kim, J. S., Chopp, M., Chen, H. *et al.* (1995). Adhesive glycoproteins CD11a and CD18 are upregulated in the leukocytes from patients with ischemic stroke and transient ischemic attacks. *J. Neurol. Sci.*, **128**, 45–50.

Kim, K., Wass, C., Cross, A. and Opal, S. (1992). Modulation of blood–brain barrier permeability by tumor necrosis factor and antibody to tumor necrosis factor in rat. *Lymphokine Cytokine Res.*, **11**(6), 293–8.

Kochanek, P. M. and Hallenbek, J. M. (1992). Polymorphonuclear leukocytes and monocytes/macrophages in the pathogenesis of cerebral ischemia and stroke. *Stroke*, **23**, 45–50.

Ley, K. (1995). Gene-targeted mice in leukocyte adhesion research. *Microcirculation*, **2**(2), 141–50.

Liou, H. and Baltimore, D. (1993). Regulation of the NF-kB/Rel transcription factor and IkB inhibitor system. *Curr. Opin. Cell Biol.*, **5**, 477–87.

Lu, H., Riley, J., Babcock, G. *et al.* (1995). Interferon (IFN) beta acts downstream of IFN-gamma-induced class II transactivator messenger RNA accumulation to block major histocompatibility complex class II gene expression and requires the 48-kD DNA-binding protein, ISGF3-gamma. *J. Exp. Med.*, **182**(5), 1517–25.

Male, D., Pryce, G., Hughes, C. and Lantos, P. (1990). Lymphocyte migration into brain in vitro: control by lymphocyte activation, cytokines, and antigen. *Cell. Immunol.*, **127**, 1–11.

Matsuo, Y., Onedera, H., Shiga, Y. *et al.* (1994). Role of cell adhesion molecules in brain injury after transient middle cerebral artery occlusion in the rat. *Brain Res.*, **656**, 344–52.

McCarron, R., Kempski, O., Spatz, M. and McFarlin, D. (1985). Presentation of myelin basic protein by murine cerebral vascular endothelial cells. *J. Immunol.*, **134**(5), 3100–3.

McCarron, R., Wang, L., Racke, M. *et al.* (1993). Cytokine-regulated adhesion between encephalitogenic T lymphocytes and cerebrovascular endothelial cells. *J. Neuroimmunol.*, **434**, 23–30.

Miyajima, A., Kitamura, T., Harada, N. *et al.* (1992). Cytokine receptors and signal transduction. *Annu. Rev. Immunol.*, **10**, 295–331.

Miyajima, A., Mui, A., Ogoroshi, T. and Sakamaki, K. (1993). Receptors for granulocyte-macrophage colony-stimulating factor, interleukin-3 and interleukin-5. *Blood*, **82**, 1960–4.

Montovani, A., Bussolino, F. and Dejana, E. (1992). Cytokine regulation of endothelial cell function. *FASEB J.*, **6**, 2591–6.

Moordian, D. and Diglio, C. (1991). Production of a transforming growth factor-beta-like growth factor by RSV-transformed rat cerebral microvascular endothelial cells. *Tumor Biol.*, **12**, 171–83.

Morgani-Kossmann, M., Kossmann, T. and Wahl, S. (1992). Cytokines and neuropathology. *TIPS*, **13**, 286–91.

Moses, A., and Nelson, J. (1994). HIV infection of human brain capillary endothelial cells – implication for AIDS dementia. *Adv. Neuroimmunol.*, **4**, 239–47.

Mossmann, T. R. and Coffran, R. L. (1989). Th1 and Th2 cell: different patterns of lymphokine secretion lead to different functional properties. *Annu. Rev. Immunol.*, **7**, 145–73.

Paul, W. E. and Seder, R. A. (1994). Lymphocyte responses and cytokines. *Cell*, **72**, 241–51.

Pober, R. (1988). Cytokine-mediated activation of vascular endothelium. Physiology and pathology. *Am. J. pathol.*, **133**, 426–32.

Pober, J. and Cortan, R. (1990). Cytokines and endothelial cell biology. *Physiol. Rev.*, **70**, 427–51.

Raine, C. and Scheinberg, L. (1988). On immunopathology of plaque development and repair in multiple sclerosis. *J. Neuroimmunol.*, **120**, 189–201.

Raine, C., Lee, S., Sheinberg, L. C. *et al.* (1990). Adhesion molecules on endothelial cells in the central nervous system: an emerging area in the neuroimmunology of multiple sclerosis. *Clin. Immunol. Immunopathol.*, **57**, 173–87.

Ray, K., Thompson, N., Kennard, N. *et al.* (1992). Investigation of guanine-nucleotide binding protein involvement and regulation of cyclic AMP metabolism in interleukin 1 transduction. *Biochem. J.*, **282**, 743–53.

Roit, I., Brostoff, J. and Male, D. (1993). *Immunology*, 3rd edn. London: Mosby.

Rott, O., Tontsch, U., Fleticher, B. and Cash, E. (1993). Interleukin-6 production in 'normal' and HTLV-1 tax-expressing brain-specific endothelial cells. *Eur. J. Immunol.*, **23**, 1987–91.

Saija, A., Princi, P., Lanza, M. *et al.* (1995). Systemic cytokine administration can affect blood–brain barrier permeability in the rat. *Life Sci.*, **56**(10), 775–84.

Schindler, C. and Darnell, J. (1995). Transcriptional responses to polypeptide ligands: the JAK-STAT pathway. *Annu. Rev. Biochem.*, **64**, 621–51.

Scholtze, S., Machleidt, T. and Kronke, M. (1994). The role of diacyglycerol and ceramide in tumor necrosis factor and interleukin-1 signal transduction. *J. Leuk. Biol.*, **56**, 533–9.

Shepro, D. and Morel, N. (1993). Pericyte physiology. *FASEB J.*, **7**, 1031–8.

Sligh, J. E., Ballantyne, C. M., Rich, S. S. *et al.* (1993). Inflammatory and immune responses are impaired in mice deficient in intracellular adhesion molecule 1. *Proc. Natl. Acad. Sci. USA*, **90**, 8529–33.

Sun, S., Ganchi, P., Ballard, D. and Green, W. (1993). NF-kB controls expression of inhibitor IkBa: evidence for an inducible autoregulatory pathway. *Science*, **259**, 1912–15.

Swain, S. (1995). Who does the polarizing? *Curr. Biol.*, **59**(8), 849–51.

Tyor, W., Glass, J., Griffin, J. *et al.* (1992). Cytokine expression in the brain during acquired immunodeficiency syndrome. *Ann. Neurol.*, **31**, 349–60.

Vires, H., Brom-Rossemalen, M., van Oosten, M. *et al.* (1993). The influence of cytokines on the integrity of the blood–brain barrier in vitro. *J. Neuroimmunol.*, **64**, 37–43.

Wakefield, A. J., More, L. J., Difford, J. and McLaughlin, J. E. (1994). Immunohistochemical study of vascular injury in acute multiple sclerosis. *J. Clin. Pathol.*, **47**, 129–33.

Washington, R., Burton, J., Todd, R. F. III *et al.* (1994). Expression of immunologically relevant endothelial cell activation antigens on isolated central nervous system microvessels from patients with multiple sclerosis. *Ann. Neurol.*, **35**, 89–97.

Weinberg, A. D. and English, M. (1990). CD4+ Tcell subsets: lymphokine secretion of memory cells and of effector cells that develop from precursors. *J. Immunol.*, **144**, 1788–99.

Wong, D. and Dorovini-Zis, K. (1992). Upregulation intercellular adhesion molecule-1(ICAM-1) expression in primary cultures of human brain microvessel endothelial cells by cytokines and lipopolysaccharide. *J. Neuroimmunol.*, **39**, 11–22.

Woodroofe, M. (1995). Cytokine production in the central nervous system. *Neurology*, **45** (suppl), S6–10.

Zinssern, H. and Tamiya, T. (1926). An experimental analysis of bacterial allergy. *J. Exp. Med.*, **44**, 753–76.

40 Blood–brain barrier and monoamines, revisited

MARIA SPATZ and RICHARD M. McCARRON

Introduction

At the present time, it is generally accepted that the blood–brain barrier (BBB) represents a conglomeration of regulatory systems concerned with maintaining a homeostatic biochemical environment for the brain parenchyma. The concept of a barrier between the blood and brain originated almost a century ago with Ehrlich's studies demonstrating that injection of certain aniline dyes stained peripheral organs and tissues but not the brain (Ehrlich, 1902). This notion was expanded by Goldman (1909) who showed that directly injecting vital dyes into the cerebrospinal fluid (CSF) stained the entire brain without affecting peripheral organs and tissues. Notably, Goldman was the first to suggest that intraparenchymatous cerebral capillaries play a role in restricting the passage of the dyes between the blood and the brain or vice versa.

The morphological confirmation for existence of the BBB at the level of brain capillaries was demonstrated by electron microscopy (Reese and Karnovsky, 1967). It has been shown that the endothelial cells, which comprise the brain capillaries

and microvessels but not those in the peripheral vasculature, are connected by continuous belts of tight junctions, devoid of fenestrae and containing a few vesicles. Interestingly, the microvascular endothelium of the choroid plexus and circumventricular organs lack these properties; the blood–CSF barrier of the choroid plexus is formed by tight junctions between epithelial cells (Lindvall et al., 1980; Rapoport, 1976). The morphological barrier functions by presenting a continuous membrane that tightly regulates passage of substances between the blood and the brain. In addition, the cytoplasmic subcellular structural and metabolic composition of endothelium also provides, in many instances, a barrier to agents originating from the blood or the brain. Nevertheless, three distinct mechanisms may permit the entry of substances into the brain: (1) some residual leakiness of the BBB as demonstrated by the entry of a low concentration of albumin into the central nervous system (CNS); (2) diffusion across the BBB as determined by the lipid solubility of the particular compound; and (3) various selective uni- or bi-directional transport systems (Gillis, 1976; Bradbury, 1979).

Monoamines are among many substances from

the peripheral circulation shown to have a limited access to the brain. These observations not only led to investigations of the mechanisms responsible for this phenomenon but also provided an impetus for discovering their biosynthesis in the brain. Since their detection, numerous wide-ranging studies of monoamines have been concerned with their role as vasoactive substances and neurotransmitters under physiological and pathological conditions. Although this subject has been previously described in various forms, the focus of this chapter is related to the function of monoamines at the BBB (Hardebo and Owman, 1980*a*; Head *et al.*, 1980; Hardebo *et al.*, 1981; Spatz and Mrsulja, 1982; Owman, 1983; Kobayashi *et al.*, 1985; Spatz, 1986; Kalaria and Harik, 1987; Palmer *et al.*, 1989; Owman and Hardebo, 1990; Joo, 1993). This review encompasses the past and present state of knowledge about monoamine uptake, metabolic pathways, receptors, and BBB permeability under physiological and pathological conditions.

General aspects of monoamines

The monoamines, known also as biogenic amines, which possess a 3,4-dihydroxyphenyl (catechol) nucleus and an amino group, are derivatives of 3,4-dihydroxyphenylamine and are referred to as catecholamines (i.e. dopamine (DA), norepinephrine (NE), and epinephrine (E)). 5-Hydroxytryptamine (5-HT), commonly known as serotonin, also belongs to the family of monoamines. Unlike their precursors, an insignificant amount of the catecholamines and 5-HT were shown to cross the BBB (Weil-Malherbe *et al.*, 1961; Oldendorf, 1971; Pardridge and Oldendorf, 1977).

Uptake and metabolic pathway of monoamine precursors

Tyrosine, phenylalanine and 3,4-dihydroxyphenylalanine (L-DOPA) (the catecholamine precursors) and tryptophan (serotonin precursor) share an uptake site at the BBB for large neutral amino acids (e.g. methionine, isoleucine, leucine, threonine, L-DOPA). These amino acids are transported at the blood–brain interface through a

sodium-dependent facilitated carrier-mediated 'L system' (Oldendorf, 1971; Wade and Katzman, 1975*a,b*; Pardridge and Oldendorf, 1977). The circulating phenylalanine or tyrosine is more likely than L-DOPA to serve as catecholamine precursors in the brain, since L-DOPA is not detectable in peripheral blood. The uptake of these amino acids as well as tryptophan is stereoselective, but the passage of a given substance through the BBB is more complex, depending on the concentration of the circulating amino acids competing for the same site of the BBB transporter (Nagatsu, 1973; Pardridge and Oldendorf, 1977). It should be noted that there is no evidence of phenylalanine hydroxylase (the enzyme which converts phenylalanine into tyrosine) in the cellular constituents of the BBB. On the other hand, tyrosine hydroxylase (TH), an enzyme catalyzing the conversion of L-tyrosine into L-DOPA, was detected in isolated brain microvessels, pial vessels, and parenchymal arterioles (Lai *et al.*, 1975; Hardebo *et al.*, 1979*b*; Head *et al.*, 1980; Lindvall *et al.*, 1980; Hervonen *et al.*, 1981). Regardless, there is no direct proof that the microvascular elements can synthesize L-DOPA from tyrosine. It was suggested that the detected activity of this enzyme in isolated microvessels reflects TH activity in the contaminant nerve endings (Lai and Spector, 1978). Interestingly, we have also found TH activity in some endothelial cell (EC) cultures derived from brain microvessels of 2 to 3-day-old rats (unpublished observation). However, its exact localization and significance are not presently established even though the purity of the EC culture was greater than 95%.

In contrast to the neuronal localization of TH, aromatic L-amino acid decarboxylase (AADC) (E.C. 4.1.1.28), which catalyzes the conversion of L-DOPA to DA and that of 5-hydroxytryptophan (5-HTP) to 5-HT, is distributed both intra- and extraneuronally (Nagatsu, 1973). Bertler *et al.* and subsequently others have proven that cerebral but not peripheral vessels possess an enzymatic barrier for L-DOPA and DA by demonstrating capillary accumulation of L-DOPA after DOPA-decarboxylase and monoamine oxidase (MAO) inhibition (Bertler *et al.*, 1964, 1966; Hardebo *et al.*, 1977*b*). Others who have shown the presence of the aromatic acid decarboxylase, DOPA-decarboxylase, in the cerebral capillary endothelium, also found an increased uptake of L-DOPA and 5-HTP from blood into the brain following inhibition of this enzyme (Bertler *et al.*, 1964; Hardebo and Owman, 1980a). They suggested that this enzyme may also be engaged in the enzymatic barrier mechanism of other circulating amino acids.

Exogenous L-DOPA or 5-HTP was repeatedly shown to raise the brain concentrations of DA or 5-HT, respectively, after either intravenous or intra-peritoneal injection (for review, see Oldendorf, 1971; Wade and Katzman, 1975b; Hardebo and Owman, 1980a). These studies demonstrated that the regional uptake of L-DOPA operated at about the same rate in various brain areas in spite of marked regional variation in catecholamine concentration. The decarboxylation of L-DOPA also occurred at a similar rate in all regions. Based on these observations it was concluded that the rate of L-DOPA entry into the brain appears to be controlled by the neutral amino acid transport system and not by the decarboxylase-trapping mechanism (Wade and Katzman, 1975b). Each of these substances was demonstrated in the EC of the intraparenchymal capillaries and pericytes by a histofluorescent technique (Owman and Rosengren, 1967; Lai *et al.*, 1975; Hardebo *et al.*, 1979a). The specificity of the detected reaction was confirmed by inhibitors of AADC, which decreased the fluorescence in these cells.

AADC activity was also demonstrated in isolated brain microvessels, which showed a higher concentration of this enzyme than was seen in either brain filtrate or mesenteric artery preparations (Lai *et al.*, 1975). The demonstrated 5-HT formation from L-tryptophan in cerebromicrovascular EC cultures indicated the presence of AADC activity and provided, for the first time, evidence for extraneuronal synthesis of 5-HT in these cells (Maruki *et al.*, 1984). Moreover, the presence of L-DOPA decarboxylase in the brain is not limited to intraparenchymatous capillary EC since it was also seen in the EC of the pia arachnoid and epithelial cells of the choroid plexus (Hardebo *et al.*, 1979b; Lindvall *et al.*, 1980; Hervonen *et al.*, 1981).

Dopamine-β-hydroxylase (DBH), which catalyzes the conversion of DA to NE, is also capable of converting various phenylethylalamine derivatives. DBH is not considered the rate-limiting enzyme in the conversion of DA to NE. This enzyme was also thought to be localized in the neurons but its activity has been found extraneuronally in brain microvessels and EC cultures (Baranczyk-Kuzma, *et al.*, 1986; Hardebo and Owman, 1980a; Lai *et al.*, 1975; Nagatsu, 1973).

Phenylethanolamine-*N*-methyltransferase (PNMT), the enzyme that forms epinephrine (E) from NE, was originally detected in the adrenal medulla. Subsequently, small levels of PNMT and E were also detected in the heart and CNS (Nagatsu, 1973). Biochemical and immunohistochemical investigations more than a decade ago detected the existence of PNMT not only in the cerebromicrovascular fraction but also in the cultured endothelium (Spatz *et al.*, 1982). The presence of this capillary enzyme was not species-specific since it was demonstrated in rats and gerbils. The enzymatic activity was specific for phenylethanolamine and could not be substituted by β-phenylethylamine or tryptamine in a substrate using S-adenyl (methyl-^{14}C) methionine as a methyl donor in the reaction mixture (Nagatsu, 1973). The level of the capillary PNMT was 7- and 11-fold higher than in the brain parenchyma. Similar enrichment has been found in the vessels separated from the brains of adult gerbils. PNMT activity in the second to fourth generations of EC cultures was lower (40%) than that in the microvessels. Strong immunofluorescence specific for PNMT was also seen in the microvessels obtained from adult and 2-day-old rat brains (Spatz *et al.*, 1982). Vascular PNMT immunofluorescence showed a diffuse and net-like pattern that was more prominent in the precapillaries than in the capillaries. A slight-to-marked diffuse immunofluorescence specific for PNMT was also found in several generations of EC cultures. Thus, these findings indicated the presence of PNMT in both perimicrovascular nerve fibers and EC.

Uptake and metabolic pathway of monoamines

Normally, a low concentration of monoamines is detectable in the systemic circulation. As mentioned above, under physiological conditions, the passage of exogenously delivered monoamines is limited. The behavior of the amines has been attributed to their polar structure (Bradbury, 1979). On the other hand, as early as 1965, Hamberger and Masuoka suggested that the cerebral capillaries may also play an active role in removing and inactivating NE (Hamberger and Masuoka, 1965). The authors demonstrated NE uptake in pericytes and the capillary wall by a histofluorescence technique utilizing brain slices pretreated with a MAO inhibitor.

The evidently limited BBB passage and rapid metabolism of the monoamines prevented characterization of their *in vivo* uptake. A clearer understanding of the cerebromicrovascular involvement in the interactions between the BBB and monoamines was aided by *in vitro* studies of brain slices and especially isolated microvessels. It was shown that L-DA, L-NE, DL-metaraminol (M, the nonmetabolizable NE analog) and 5-HT were taken up by the microvessels by a temperature-, oxygen-, glucose-, sodium- and potassium-dependent as well as ouabain-sensitive process (Abe *et al.*, 1980*b*; Hardebo and Owman, 1980*b*; Spatz *et al.*, 1981*a,b*). This process was shared by other amines, since the uptake of [³H]-NE or [³H]-5-HT was cross-inhibited in the presence of other amines (DL-M, NE, E, or 5-HT) but not by their metabolites.

The ineffectiveness of synthetic amino acids characteristic of A- or L-transport systems or monoamine metabolites to affect the microvascular monoamine uptake provided evidence for distinct transport systems for these substances (Abe *et al.*, 1980*b*). In general, the properties of the microvascular uptake of the amines were unlike those described for other extraneuronal sites in peripheral organs in that they displayed sensitivity to M but not to normetanephrine and metanephrine. The monoamine uptake also showed features of neuronal uptake since a decrease of NE fluorophore accumulation was detected in the microvascular wall of brain tissue and a reduction in the uptake of amines (NE, M and 5-HT) into isolated microvessels was observed in the presence of inhibitors of neuronal uptake. The demonstrated inhibition of NE and M uptake by α- and β-adrenergic receptor antagonists suggested a receptor-mediated uptake of these amines (Abe *et al.*, 1980*b*; Hardebo and Owman, 1980*b*). In addition, both isolated brain microvessels and EC cultures were shown not only to take up the monoamines, but also to metabolize them (see below). Thus, considering all these observations together, there is no doubt that brain microvessels and cultured endothelium displayed features of neuronal and extraneuronal monoamine uptake somewhat similar to that described for pulmonary microvessels (Gillis, 1976).

The exact localization of the monoamines' uptake in the cerebral microvessels cannot be ascertained from these studies. The dependence of the amines' uptake on Na⁺-, K⁺-ATPase and the reported presence of this enzyme in the capillary basement membrane (even though a lesser activity of this enzyme was also localized in the luminal membrane) suggests an abluminal vascular uptake of the amines (Betz *et al.*, 1980). On the other hand, the observed good correlation between the increased NE and 5-HT passaged from blood-to-brain and the change in the cerebromicrovascular function (increased capillary NE and 5-HT uptake with attenuated activity of their degrading enzymes) in gerbils recovering from cerebral ischemia strongly suggest that the capillaries may also take up NE and 5-HT from the luminal side (see below).

Three different techniques were used to assess and/or detect monoamine metabolism: (1) histochemistry and immunohistochemistry; (2) biochemical measurements of the metabolites; and (3) detection of monoamine-metabolizing enzymes. The results of many of these procedures were aided and/or confirmed by the addition of specific inhibitors of the tested monoamines in brain capillaries. As we mentioned above, a MAO inhibitor was originally used to enhance the detection and localization of monoamines in brain tissue.

The methylated substances were the main metabolites formed by NE in brain microvessels after incubation in the presence of Ca^{2+} or Mn^{2+} ions (Spatz *et al.*, 1981*a*; Spatz and Mrsulja, 1982). In the absence of Ca^{2+}, NE was mainly converted to E; the deamination of NE was negligible in the presence or absence of bivalent ions. The metabolic rate of NE was oxygen-dependent and lower in cerebral microvessels obtained from 2-day-old rat brains than those separated from adult brains.

These studies suggested the existence of catechol-*O*-methyltransferase (COMT) and PNMT in the microvessels. Originally these findings prompted the biochemical and immunohistochemical detection of PNMT in microvessels described above. The lower metabolic rate of NE in early postnatal life also suggested that the COMT, which is responsible for NE demethylation, is not fully developed in the microvessels at this time. These findings are consistent with the functional immaturity of the cerebral microvessels and the reported greater penetration of the monoamines into the brain of newborns as compared to adults (Glowinski *et al.*, 1964).

Brain microvessels as well as EC derived from these structures converted 5-HT to 5-hydroxyindoleacetic acid (5-HIAA), which was dependent on the level of oxygen and MAO activity (Maruki *et al.*, 1984). MAO is mainly a mitochondrial enzyme, which is widely distributed in human and animal tissues and exists in two forms: MAO-A and MAO-B (Nagatsu, 1973). MAO-A preferentially catalyzes the deamination of 5-HT, DA, NE, metanephrine, normetanephrine and β-hydroxylated phenylethylamine (e.g. octopamine). MAO-B deaminates benzylamine, tryptamine, 5-*O*-methyltryptamine and phenylethylamine (Nagatsu, 1973; Baranczyk-Kuzma *et al.*, 1986). Both MAO-A and MAO-B are present in brain tissue, choroid plexus, capillaries, microvessels and EC derived from these vessels, in humans and various animal species (Abe *et al.*, 1980a; Lai *et al.*, 1975; Lindvall *et al.*, 1980; Lindvall and Owman, 1980; Spatz and Mrsulja, 1982). The level of MAO activity varied among the tested mammalian tissue. For example, the highest MAO activity was found in rat microvessels compared with other species (Kalaria and Harik, 1987). In gerbils, brain MAO-A activity is higher than that of MAO-B in capillaries. However, in brain parenchyma, enrichment of capillary MAO-A was found to be lower than that of MAO-B as compared to the respective enzyme activities (Spatz and Mrsulja, 1982). It is important to mention that the greater activity of MAO in the cerebral microvessels of rats compared with other species including humans, provided a partial explanation for the observed lower 1-methyl-4-phenyl-1,2,3,6-tetrahydropyridine (MPTP) brain toxicity (Kalaria and Harik, 1987).

COMT, in addition to MAO, is involved in catecholamine metabolism but through *O*-methylation. This enzyme is also present in various tissues; its activity was detected in the brain, isolated microvessels, cultured endothelium and smooth muscle derived from these vessels by both immunohistochemical and biochemical methods (Kaplan *et al.*, 1979; Lai and Spector, 1978; Spatz *et al.*, 1986a). Pretreatment of brain with 6-hydroxydopamine (6-OHDA), which causes neuronal degeneration had no effect on the content of MAO or COMT in the microvessels, indicating that these enzymes are extraneuronal (Lai and Spector, 1978).

Thus, demonstration of the enzymes involved in the metabolism of monoamines and their precursors as well as detection of their metabolites in brain microvessels, especially after denervation, indicates the presence of a biosynthetic and metabolic pathway for catecholamines and 5-HT in the microvascular compartment. In addition, the same or similar results obtained in studies of the monoamine metabolic pathway in the endothelium derived from capillaries and/or microvessels indicate that the main enzymatic barrier for the monoamines resides in the endothelium.

In conclusion, it should be reiterated that all of the investigated models concerned with the BBB and monoamines indicate that the enzymatic BBB is localized in the cerebral microvessels and their cellular elements. The lower NE and 5-HT metabolism in microvessels found in newborn compared to that found in adult rats (Spatz *et al.*, 1982) is consistent with the functional immaturity of cerebral microvessels and the reported greater penetration of the monoamines into the newborn than into adult animals (Glowinski *et al.*, 1964). Thus, the cerebral microvessels are most likely responsible for regulating the cerebral inflow and outflow of the amines in order to protect the proper brain environment.

At this point, the question arises whether the microvascular monoamine uptake and metabolic systems act solely as a 'guardian' of the brain or have a wider role at the level of BBB that includes maintaining microvascular tone and blood flow. Although this subject is still debatable and the relationship of monoamines to the BBB and cerebromicrovascular bed is not yet fully explored, there is sufficient information available concerning monoaminergic involvement in general microvascular function including BBB permeability (Raichle *et al.*, 1975; MacKenzie *et al.*, 1976; Grubb *et al.*,

1978; Domer *et al.*, 1980; Hardebo and Owman, 1980*b*; Harik *et al.*, 1980; Hartman *et al.*, 1980; Preskorn *et al.*, 1980, 1982; Hardebo *et al.*, 1981; Edvinsson, 1982; Spatz and Mrsulja, 1982; Harik and McGunigal, 1984; Kobayashi *et al.*, 1985; Harik, 1986; Kalaria and Harik, 1989).

Cerebromicrovascular monoaminergic innervation, receptors and function

First, we would like to draw attention to several lines of reported evidence regarding the cerebral capillary and/or microvascular adrenergic innervation, monoaminergic receptors, and their response to monoamines. The close association of both sympathetic (originating from cervical ganglia) and non-sympathetic catecholaminergic fibers originating from the locus ceruleus (LC) with cerebral intraparenchymal and pial small vessels and capillaries as demonstrated by histo- and immunofluorescence or electron microscopy provided the basis for peripheral and central innervation of the microvascular bed in the brain (Edvinsson, 1982; Edvinsson *et al.*, 1983; Hartman *et al.*, 1972; Kalaria and Harik, 1989; Nelson and Rennels, 1970; Owman and Hardebo, 1990; Rennels and Nelson, 1975; Swanson *et al.*, 1977). In addition, the detected electron-dense bodies containing lucent vesicles resembling synaptic bodies adhering to the membranes of isolated cerebral microvessels indicated a direct contact between the 'synapses' and the microvessels. Thus, these observations emphasized the possibility of an interaction between the microvessels and neurotransmitters (Suddith *et al.*, 1980). Both concepts were strengthened by a variety of investigations conducted both *in vitro* and *in vivo*.

The functional relationship between monoamines and cerebral capillaries was advanced through interruption of NE fibers in the LC, and by identification of monoaminergic receptors by specific binding studies or activation of signal transduction mechanisms.

The detection of NE depletion (90%) and increased density of β_2-adrenergic receptor binding sites in the cortex ipsilateral to the LC innervation supports the implied noradrenergic microvascular innervation and response to decreased endogenous input of NE (Kalaria and Harik, 1989). The 'denervation supersensitivity' of the brain microvessels following LC lesions resembled that observed after chronic reserpine treatment. Since reserpine is known to deplete both peripheral and central NE, the finding suggested that β_2-adrenergic receptors on the brain microvessels in the rat respond mainly to NE from LC terminals. In addition, this type of injury modulated ouabain binding in isolated microvessels suggesting that Na$^+$-, K$^+$-ATPase activity in the microvessels is controlled by the intrinsic adrenergic neurons in the LC (Harik, 1986). It also suggested that 'denervation of the LC' could affect the Na$^+$/K$^+$ exchange as well as electrolyte homeostasis in the brain. Furthermore, a reduction of β-adrenergic receptors on microvessels derived from the brain of spontaneously and experimental hypertensive rats, and rats and gerbils subjected to unilateral brain ischemia, suggested an altered control of an adrenergic regulatory mechanism of cerebral microvessels (Kalaria and Harik, 1989; Magnoni *et al.*, 1983, 1985).

It is still debatable whether DA nerve endings are present in close proximity to microvessels except in the striatum (Braun *et al.*, 1980). On the other hand, intraparenchymal microvessels, choroid plexus and pial vessels were shown to receive serotonergic innervation from the raphe nuclei (Edvinsson *et al.*, 1983; Reinhard *et al.*, 1979; see review in Spatz, 1986). Recent studies using tryptophan hydroxylase immunochemistry reevaluated the relationship of serotonergic terminals with intraparenchymal capillaries and microvessels. The results showed that the tryptophan hydroxylase terminals were identical to the previously described serotonin-containing varicosities (Cohen *et al.*, 1995*b*). These terminals were found intimately associated with microvessels in the frontoparietal cortex but not in the hippocampus. In addition, 5-HT was also in sympathetic nerves and released together with NE from these nerves. In view of these observations, 5-HT has been implicated to play a role in the neurogenic control of cerebral blood flow (CBF).

Cerebral (including pia arachnoid) capillaries, microvessels and EC derived from these structures contain β_2- and α_2-adrenergic receptors (Herbst *et al.*, 1979; Nathanson and Glaser, 1979; Friedman and Davis, 1980; Harik *et al.*, 1980; Nathanson, 1980; Palmer, 1980; Kobayashi *et al.*, 1981; Karnushina *et al.*, 1982, 1983; Spatz, 1986; Kalaria and Harik, 1989; Palmer *et al.*, 1989; Spatz *et al.*, 1993). The existence of both subtypes of β_1- and β_2-adrenergic receptors in cerebral microvessels was debatable since they were not demonstrable in all animal species. In addition, the coexistence of β_1- and α_1-adrenergic receptors with β_2-and α_2-adrenergic receptors was only recently detected in EC originating from capillaries and/or microvessels of human brain (Bacic *et al.*, 1992). In these cells, the response of cAMP to various monoaminergic agents in the presence or absence of respective selective receptor antagonists was used to characterize the type of receptors. The maximal stimulation of cAMP formation was 2–7-fold over that of basal (unstimulated) activity after exposure to NE, E, or isoproterenol. The sensitivity of the adenylate cyclase (AC) system of these EC to some adrenergic agonists varied depending on the origin of the EC (e.g. the AC levels of EC derived from large, rather than small microvessels or capillaries was greater than the levels of 6-fluoronorepinephrine (6-FL) and isoproterenol). The stimulation of cAMP induced by NE, E, phenylephrine (PhE) or 6-FL was prevented in EC treated with cholera toxin (which causes ADP-ribosylation of the stimulatory guanine nucleotide-binding protein (G_S)). However, ADP-ribosylation of the inhibitory guanine nucleotide-binding protein (G_i) by pertussis toxin had no effect on PhE- or 6-FL-induced formation of cAMP. These data indicate that activation of α_1-adrenergic receptors is mediated by signal transduction mechanisms associated with G_s protein. The findings also confirmed the presence of both types of β- and both α-adrenergic receptors coupled to AC in these cells. It remains to be clarified if any adrenergic receptor subtypes are also associated with phosphoinositol metabolism since reportedly α_1- or a subtype of α-receptors have been coupled to phosphoinositol hydrolysis and Ca^{2+} release in some tissues (Bacic *et al.*, 1992).

The reported responsiveness of cerebromicrovascular AC activity to DA has been scrutinized for some time since DA caused only a slight stimulation of cAMP over basal levels in the microvessels of animals (Palmer *et al.*, 1989). In addition, a substantial enhancement of endothelial cell AC activity was only seen at a nonphysiological concentration of DA in cultured EC derived from rat brain microvessels. However, in human cultured EC there was a marked stimulation of cAMP either with DA or the D_1 receptor agonist inhibitable by selective D_1-receptor antagonists (Bacic *et al.*, 1991). The sensitivity of the D_1-receptor linked to AC activity similar to the adrenergic receptor coupled to AC activity was greater in EC derived from large rather than small microvessels. The results of ADP-ribosylation using either cholera or pertussis toxins indicated the presence of D_1 (stimulatory) and D_2 (inhibitory) receptors on these cells (Bacic *et al.*, 1991). In addition, it was shown that the dopaminergic receptors can interact with either α_1-adrenergic or 5-HT receptors on the human EC at the AC level (Bacic *et al.*, 1991).

The characterization of 5-HT receptors on cerebromicrovascular endothelium has evolved only during the last several years (Cohen *et al.*, 1995*a*; Cohen and Hamel, 1996). Originally, the studies to detect these receptors on bovine microvessels were unsuccessful since only a few binding sites for 5-HT were found (Peroutka *et al.*, 1980). In addition, little or no effect of 5-HT on cAMP production was detected in either isolated microvessels or cultured EC derived from rat brain. Studies of human brain capillary and/or microvascular endothelium revealed that both cAMP and IP_3 formation were stimulated by 5-HT and inhibited by $5-HT_1$ receptor antagonists (Spatz *et al.*, 1993). However, a more extensive characterization of the human brain microvessels has demonstrated the expression of mRNA for $5-HT_{1D\alpha}$, $5-HT_{1D\beta}$ receptors (mainly on smooth muscle), $5-HT_{2\beta}$ and $5-HT_7$ receptors (EC, smooth muscle and fetal brain astrocytes) but not $5-HT_{2\alpha}$ receptors (Cohen *et al.*, 1995*a*; Cohen and Hamel, 1996). The authors suggested that $5-HT_{1D\beta}$ receptors may mediate intracerebral vasoconstriction, while activation of $5-HT_{2\beta}$ and $5-HT_7$ receptors may be involved in vasodilation and/or changes in permeability.

Other studies, using either isolated microvessels or cultured EC have clearly shown that the individual catecholamines (e.g. DA, NE, E) or 5-HT stimulate various vasoactive substances secreted by the microvascular cellular elements (for review, see Spatz, 1986; Spatz *et al.*, 1993). For example, each of these amines altered production of known vasodilatory and/or vasoconstrictive agents such as prostanoids, nitric oxide (NO), and endothelin. In addition, the β-adrenergic agonist isoproterenol was demonstrated to potentiate the production of NO induced by interferon-γ and tumor necrosis factor-α (Durieu-Trautmann *et al.*, 1993). All of these agents may affect not only permeability but also microvascular tone and blood flow in the brain. NE was also shown to enhance degradation of glycogen in cultured EC and muscle cells derived from capillaries and microvessels of rat brain (Spatz *et al.*, 1986*b*). In contrast, 5-HT stimulated glycogen synthesis. These studies suggested that these two amines may play opposing roles controlling the microvascular energy metabolism since glycogen degradation results from increased requirements for energy.

In conclusion, the demonstrated existence of most monoaminergic and serotonergic nerve endings in the vicinity of cerebral intraparenchymal microvessels and the presence of their respective functional receptors detected in the isolated microvessels, EC, or muscle cells emphasize not only the possibility but the high probability of a capillary and microvascular interaction with monoamines released either from the brain or blood. In addition, the above-mentioned capability of the microvascular cellular elements to take up, utilize, and degrade the individual amines strongly suggests that the interplay between the constituents of the BBB and monoamines is complex and affects both the microvessels and the amines. It can also be surmised that prior to their degradation, the circulating and released monoamines from either blood or brain may influence the reactivity of the brain microvessels.

Monoamines, BBB permeability, and cerebral blood flow (CBF)

Implications of monoamines participating in altering BBB permeability have been long-standing even though the existence of an enzymatic barrier toward monoamines was already recognized at the level of the BBB. Many of these studies have been

contradictory, either supporting or negating this concept (Raichle *et al.*, 1975; Grubb *et al.*, 1978; Domer *et al.*, 1980; Hartman *et al.*, 1980; Johansson and Martinsson, 1980; Preskorn *et al.*, 1980, 1982; Hardebo *et al.*, 1981; Gulati *et al.*, 1984; Kobayashi *et al.*, 1985; Sarmento *et al.*, 1991). This discrepancy was most likely related to the route of administration and concentration of the amines as well as being dependent on the animal species. Nevertheless, in the mid-1970s, the first convincing studies demonstrated that stimulation of the LC with carbachol (cholinergic agonist), increased brain vascular permeability and reduced the CBF (Raichle *et al.*, 1975). These events were abolished by the α-adrenergic blocker phentolamine, thus supporting the hypothesis that central adrenergic receptors regulated both the BBB and CBF. Subsequent reports showed that adrenergic agents that stimulate α-adrenergic receptors in the LC not only increased BBB permeability to radiolabelled H_2O (Preskorn *et al.*, 1982) but also to albumin (Sarmento *et al.*, 1990). The latter event was accompanied by increased pinocytosis.

Recently it has also been shown that electrical stimulation (ES) of the LC increased BBB permeability to Na^+-fluorescein (NaF), which was augmented by pretreatment with β-adrenergic antagonists (Sarmento *et al.*, 1994). On the other hand, the ES-stimulated BBB permeability to NaF was reduced by α-adrenergic receptor antagonists. Similar studies *in vitro* conducted on bovine cerebromicrovascular endothelium (BCEC) used two model systems simulating the *in vivo* transport of monoamines (i) from blood-to-brain, and (ii) from brain-to-blood (apical or basal side of BCEC exposed to adrenergic substances, respectively) (Borges *et al.*, 1994). The data indicated that α-adrenergic agonist clenbuterol dose-dependently induced changes in BCEC permeability to NaF, which was prevented by prazosin, the α-adrenergic receptor antagonist. In addition a β₂-adrenergic agonist-reduced BCEC permeability was also observed in the presence or absence of NE. Both α- and β-adrenergic receptor-mediated alterations in EC permeability were inhibited with vincristine (inhibitor of fluid-phase pinocytosis) or by eliminating glucose in the incubating medium. BCEC exposed from the basal side to α- or β-adrenergic agonists showed a reduced passage of NaF (brain-to-blood). These findings support the supposition of α-adrenergic receptor-mediated increased passage of substances (most likely by pinocytosis) across the brain endothelium (blood-to-brain). However, the effect of β-adrenergic receptors is still unclear since the β-adrenergic receptor agonist decreased both the EC permeability in models simulating the transport from both blood-to-brain and from brain-to-blood. This contradiction between the *in vivo* and *in vitro* studies is not surprising since the *in vivo* results most likely represent an integrated response of endothelial and other cells, which together might contribute to alteration of the BBB.

The 5-HT induction of BBB permeability to macromolecules has been controversial since many investigators could not confirm the original observation of Westergaard (1975). He had demonstrated an enhanced vesicular passage of horseradish peroxidase from blood–brain after 5-HT administration in mice (Westergaard, 1975). However, neither intraventricularly nor intravenously injected 5-HT in rats or monkeys influenced BBB permeability to radiolabelled insulin or to Evans' Blue (Hardebo *et al.*, 1981; Gulati *et al.*, 1984). In recent years, Sharma *et al.* demonstrated that the intravenously administered 5-HT increase in BBB permeability to macromolecules, ^{131}Na, but not to lanthenium, is a transient phenomenon mediated by 5-HT$_2$ receptors in rats and mice (Sharma *et al.*, 1995). On the other hand, intravascular but not extravascular application of 5-HT, which reduced the electrical resistance, was reversed by either ketanserin (5-HT$_2$ receptor antagonist) or verapamil (Ca^{2+} entry blocker) in frog pial vessels (Olesen, 1985). This study suggested that 5-HT receptor-mediated influx of Ca^{2+} causes endothelial contraction and opening of tight junctions permitting an influx of small ions rather than large molecules (e.g. NaF). As mentioned before, the contradictory reports regarding the effect of 5-HT on BBB permeability may be dose-, route-, or species-dependent. With regard to CBF, it has been shown that intravascular 5-HT does not change the CBF unless given with inhibitors of 5-HT degradation or as a synthetic diffusible 5-HT. In these instances and after osmotic opening of the BBB, 5-HT induces a reduction in cerebral O$_2$ and glucose consumption as well as a decrease in CBF.

Attenuated BBB permeability to monoamines and CBF

The BBB has been shown to be compromised in many diseases of the brain (e.g. hypertension, sepsis, experimental allergic encephalomyelitis (EAE), stress, and ischemia). Experimental hypertension or hyperosmolar insult, which morphologically opens the BBB, were shown to increase markedly the intravenously injected E uptake into the brain as well as to raise the CBF (Hardebo *et al.*, 1977*a*; Westergaard *et al.*, 1977; Edvinsson *et al.*, 1978; Johansson and Martinsson, 1980; Owman and Hardebo, 1990). Such an event caused an accumulation of monoamines in the cerebromicrovascular wall (Hardebo *et al.*, 1979*a*). The mechanism responsible for the CBF response, which is coupled to the cerebral metabolic rate of oxygen (CMRO$_2$), was attributed to entry of E into the brain and activation of NE-sensitive neurons. This conclusion was supported by the observed inhibition of the increased CBF with propranolol (PPL), the β-adrenergic receptor antagonist.

Other studies involving experimental endotoxemia have demonstrated that intravenous injection of endotoxic *E. coli* lipopolysaccharide (LPS) disrupts the BBB, increases CMRO$_2$, decreases CBF, and raises the level of NE and E in the blood and CSF (Westerlind *et al.*, 1991). In addition, a variable uptake of these monoamines was observed in the brain. PPL pretreatment decreased the CMRO$_2$ but did not affect the CBF, suggesting that the former but not the latter effect was β-adrenergic in origin. The observed diverse responses of CMRO$_2$ and CBF to LPS could not be entirely explained by the effect of the increased passage of the NE and/or E. Therefore, it was suggested that a simultaneous release of other vasoactive substances such as prostaglandins or 5-HT could also have been involved in this process.

It has also been known that sepsis may be associated with metabolic acidosis and/or arterial hypoxia (Westerlind *et al.*, 1995*a,b*). Normally, the intact BBB protects the brain against changes in blood pH. However, endotoxemia with metabolic acidosis not only increases the CMRO$_2$ but also increases the CBF, both of which are preventable by pretreatment with PPL, indicating β-adrenergic mediation. It is therefore possible that the penetration of hydrogen ions in addition to the monoamines may alter the response of the CBF to LPS. Arterial hypoxia, which by itself has no effect on $CMRO_2$ but increases the CBF, also alters the CBF response to LPS. In addition, a release of NE from the brain to the blood was detected in hypoxia, whereas the uptake and release of monoamines was variable in hypoxia/endotoxemia. However, while the BBB function appears to be disturbed in each case, it is not clear whether the altered catecholamines are entirely responsible for the effect on CBF.

It has been observed that systemic catecholamine concentrations, vasoactive amines and cerebral levels of monoamines are all affected during the development of EAE and may be involved in the modulation of clinical signs of disease (Linthicum and Frelinger, 1982; Waxman *et al.*, 1984; Brosnan *et al.*, 1985; Krenger *et al.*, 1986; Weselmann *et al.*, 1987). Since previous experiments demonstrated BBB permeability changes in EAE, as well as multiple sclerosis (Kristensson and Wisniewski, 1977; Lossinsky *et al.*, 1989; McDonald and Barnes, 1989; Simmons *et al.*, 1987), the mechanism by which some of the above factors may influence EAE may involve their effects on vascular permeability.

In addition to affecting BBB permeability, these factors may modulate pathogenesis by other mechanisms. Alterations in BBB permeability seen during EAE correlated with changes in the expression of surface antigens by EC (Sternberger *et al.*, 1989). Furthermore, NE can modulate the expression of Ia antigen (an important factor in the pathogenic mechanism of EAE) by astrocytes (Frohman *et al.*, 1988). Studies regarding Ia expression on cerebral vascular endothelial cells clearly indicate the potential involvement of monoamines in the modulation of Ia antigen expression (Spatz *et al.*, 1990). This study demonstrated that isoproterenol (β-adrenergic agonist) and forskolin significantly inhibited the level of Ia antigen expression induced by interferon-γ. Treatment with the $β_1/β_2$ antagonist PPL or the $α_2$-adrenergic antagonist yohimbine, but not the $β_1$-antagonist atenolol, partially blocked the ability of isoproterenol to inhibit Ia antigen expression. Concomitant experiments utilizing these factors to assess their effects on the levels of cAMP revealed a possible correlation between cAMP levels and Ia expression. The precise nature of this correlation may involve additional second messengers, such as activation of cAMP-dependent protein kinase A modulation of protein kinase C through α-adrenergic receptors. These findings suggest a role for adrenergic receptors in the regulation of blood–brain interactions and imply that disturbances in monoamines may also be involved in immune-mediated diseases such as EAE.

It is also noteworthy that the opening of the BBB to macromolecules (e.g. Evans' Blue) and brain edema induced by either heat or immobilization stress is associated with a 4- to 6-fold increase of 5-HT in the plasma and brain (Sharma and Dey, 1986*a,b*; Sharma *et al.*, 1994). Since these changes were prevented by pretreatment with a 5-HT synthesis inhibitor (*p*-chlorophenylalanine), a 5-HT receptor antagonist (cyproheptadone) or indomethacin (an inhibitor of prostaglandin synthesis), it was concluded that 5-HT and possibly prostaglandins were instrumental in altering BBB permeability induced by stress.

Cerebral ischemia induced either by unilateral (1 h) or bilateral (15 min) occlusion of the common carotid artery in gerbils resulted in increased BBB permeability to monoamines (Abe *et al.*, 1980*a*; Hervonen *et al.*, 1980). However, a selective change in the passage of the amines from blood-to-brain was only seen following bilateral carotid occlusion and reperfusion. The observed enhanced BBB permeability of exogenous 5-HT occurred prior to that of NE (24 and 72 h after reperfusion, respectively). The greatest number of animals showing an altered BBB permeability to NE was found after 7 days of re-established CBF when the BBB permeability was also increased for dextran (molecular weight 60 000) (Hervonen *et al.*, 1980). To elucidate the mechanisms of these events, experiments were designed to investigate the uptake and metabolism of the amines as well as the level of their degrading enzymes in cerebral microvessels obtained from ischemic gerbils at times coinciding with the absence and presence of increased BBB permeability to 5-HT and NE (Abe *et al.*, 1980*a*).

These studies have shown that neither the uptake of 5-HT, NE, and M nor the deamination of 5-HT and NE was affected after ischemia without reperfusion, even though MAO activity was reduced in the cerebral microvessels isolated from these animals. On the other hand, increased specific 5-HT capillary uptake (40% above normal) with a significantly decreased metabolism as well as the lowest MAO-A activity were first found 24 h after postischemic reperfusion of blood. The enhanced NE and metanephrine uptake into the microvessels was not observed until 72 h following the release of arterial occlusion, but the activity of COMT and NE methylation was enhanced during ischemia and reperfusion when compared with respective sham controls (Abe *et al.*, 1980a; Spatz *et al.*, 1981a). Thus, the observed periods of increased capillary uptake of 5-HT and NE and the reduced MAO activity as well as deamination of 5-HT, but not the elevated levels of COMT and methylated NE, corresponded well with the increased BBB permeability of the amines demonstrable in parallel *in vivo* studies. However, neither the *in vivo* nor the *in vitro* studies explored whether the enhanced time-dependent selective uptake of monoamines was mediated by their respective receptors.

Comments

This summarized review represents a historical survey of studies concerned with the BBB and monoamines. It is quite apparent that the major contribution to understanding this barrier system to monoamines took place between the mid-1960s and 1980s. In the last decade, relatively few investigators have addressed the subject, particularly studies regarding further definition of cerebral capillary and/or microvascular transport of the monoamines, their localization, and regulation. It is a challenging task since it requires both the chemical and biochemical characterization of the luminal and basement membranes, whose acquisi-

tion in sufficient amounts is rather difficult. Nevertheless, recent advances in molecular biology should be helpful in achieving this goal in the future.

There is no doubt that *in vitro* models have been useful for studying cerebral capillary microvascular or endothelial function and the mechanisms related to the role of monoamines at the level of the BBB. Notwithstanding, characterization of the BBB and the monoamines cannot be completely clarified unless an *in vitro* model is developed which will have greater similarity to the morphological, biochemical, and physiological paradigms existing *in vivo*. Such a model will have to address the interaction between the individual cellular elements of the BBB (endothelium, pericytes, glia, or smooth muscle cells and their neurogenic inputs) as well as delineating their individual properties. Future *in vitro* models will not only be of great use to studies concerning the monoamine system, but they will also be applicable to the investigation of other systems that potentially may have clinical ramifications. Finally, it should be reiterated that the *in vitro* system cannot be equated with *in vivo* function. There is still a necessity for developing and utilizing animal models to study physiological and pathological phenomena such as the interaction between monoamines and the BBB. Thus, the presently accessible techniques combining molecular biology and immunochemistry provide a great impetus to facilitate investigations *in vitro* and *in vivo* in what has been only recently a relatively neglected field.

Acknowledgment

The authors appreciate the skillful editing of Devera G. Schoenberg, M.Sc.

References

Abe, T., Abe, K., Micic, D. *et al.* (1980a). Studies on the blood–brain barrier (BBB) to monoamines. In *Circulatory and Developmental Aspects of Brain Metabolism*, ed. M. Spatz, B. B. Mrsulja, Lj. Rakic and W. D. Lust, pp. 215–23. New York: Plenum Publishing Corporation.

Abe, T., Abe, K., Rausch, W. D. *et al.* (1980b). Characteristics of some monoamine uptake systems in isolated cerebral capillaries. In *The Cerebral Microvasculature*, ed. H. M. Eisenberg and R. L. Suddith, pp. 45–55. New York: Plenum Publishing Corporation.

Bacic, F., Uematsu, S., McCarron, R. M. and Spatz, M. (1991). Dopaminergic receptors linked to adenylate cyclase in human cerebromicrovascular endothelium. *J. Neurochem.*, **57**,1774–9.

Bacic, F., McCarron, R. M., Uematsu, S. and Spatz, M. (1992). Adrenergic receptors coupled to adenylate cyclase in human cerebromicrovascular endothelium. *Metab. Brain Dis.*, **7**, 125–37.

Baranczyk-Kuzma, A., Audus, K. L. and Borchardt, R. T. (1986). Catecholamine-metabolizing enzymes of bovine brain microvessel endothelial cell monolayers. *J. Neurochem.*, **46**, 1956–60.

Bertler, A., Falck, B., Owman, C. and Rosengrenn, E. (1966). The localization of monoaminergic blood–brain barrier mechanisms. *Pharmacol. Rev.*, **18**, 369–85.

Bertler, A., Falck, B. and Rosengrenn, E. (1964). The direct demonstration of a barrier mechanism in the brain capillaries. *Acta Pharmacol. Toxicol.*, **20**, 317–21.

Betz, A. L., Firth, J. A. and Goldstein, G. W. (1980). Polarity of the blood–brain barrier: distribution of enzymes between the luminal and antiluminal membranes of the brain capillary endothelial cell. *Brain Res.*, **192**, 17–28.

Borges, N., Shi, F., Azevedo I. and Audus, K. L. (1994). Changes in brain microvessel endothelial cell monolayer permeability induced by adrenergic drugs. *Eur. J. Pharmacol.*, **269**, 243–8.

Bradbury, M. (1979). *The Concept of a Blood-Brain Barrier.* New York: John Wiley and Sons.

Braun, U., Braun, G. and Sargent T., III. (1980). Changes in blood–brain permeability resulting from d-amphetamine, 6-hydroxydopamine and pimozide measured by a new technique. *Experientia*, **36**, 207–9.

Brosnan, C. F., Goldmuntz, E. A., Cammer, W. *et al.* (1985). Prazosin, an alpha adrenergic receptor antagonist suppresses experimental allergic encephalomyelitis in the Lewis rat. *Proc. Natl. Acad. Sci. USA*, **82**, 5915–9.

Cohen, Z., Bouchelet, I., Yong, W. V. *et al.* (1995a). Differential expression of serotonin receptors 5-HT$_{1DI}$ and 5-HT$_{2A}$ mRNA in human brain vessels, vascular cells and astrocytes in culture. *Abst., Soc. Neurosci.*, **21**, 1853.

Cohen, Z., Ehret, M., Maitre, M. and Hamel, E. (1995b). Ultrastructural analysis of tryptophan hydroxylase immunoreactive nerve terminals in the rat cerebral cortex and hippocampus: their associations with local blood vessels. *Neuroscience*, **66**, 555–69.

Cohen, Z. and Hamel, E. (1996). Expression of 5-HT$_{1DJ}$, 5-HT$_{1F}$, 5-HT$_{2B}$, 5-HT$_{2C}$ and 5-HT$_7$ receptor mRNAs in human intraparenchymal microvessels and related cells in culture. *Abst., Soc. Neurosci.*, **22**, 1782.

Domer, F. R., Sankar, R., Cole, S. and Wellmeyer, D. (1980). Dose-dependent, amphetamine-induced changes in permeability of the blood–brain barrier of normotensive and spontaneously hypertensive rats. *Exp. Neurol.*, **70**, 576–85.

Durieu-Trautmann, O., Fédérici, C. *et al.* (1993). Nitric oxide and endothelin secretion by brain microvessel endothelial cells: regulation by cyclic nucleotides. *J. Cell. Physiol.*, **155**, 104–11.

Edvinsson, L. (1982). Sympathetic control of cerebral circulation. *Trends Neurosci.*, **5**, 425–9.

Edvinsson, L., Degeururce, A., Duverger, D. *et al.* (1983). Central serotonergic nerves project to the pial vessels of the brain. *Nature*, **306**, 55–7.

Edvinsson, L., Hardebo, J. E., MacKenzie, E. T. and Owman, C. (1978). Effect of exogenous noradrenaline on local cerebral blood flow after osmotic opening of the blood–brain barrier in the rat. *J. Physiol.*, *(Lond.)* **274**, 149–56.

Ehrlich, P. (1902). Uber die Beziehungen von Chemischer Constitution, Vertheilung, und pharmakologischer Wirkung (reprinted and translated in *Collected Studies in Immunity*, pp. 567–95. New York: Wiley, 1906).

Friedman, A. H. and Davis, J. N. (1980). Identification and characterization of adrenergic receptors and catecholamine-stimulated adenylate cyclase in hog pial membranes. *Brain Res.*, **183**, 89–102.

Frohman, E. M., Vayuvegula, B., van den Noort, S. and Gupta, S. (1988). Norepinephrine inhibits gamma-interferon induced major histocompatibility class II (Ia) antigen expression on cultured brain astrocytes via beta-2 adrenergic signal transduction mechanisms. *Proc. Natl. Acad. Sci. USA*, **85**, 1292–6.

Gillis, C. N. (1976). Extraneuronal transport of noradrenaline in the lung. In *The Mechanism of Neuronal and Extraneuronal Transport of Catecholamines*, ed. D. M. Paton, pp. 281–97. New York: Raven Press.

Glowinski, J., Axelrod, J., Kopin, I. J. and Wurtman, R. J. (1964). Physiological disposition of ^{3}H-norepinephrine in the developing rat. *J. Pharmaco.*, **146**, 48–53.

Goldman, E. E. (1909). Die äussere und innere Sekretion des gesunden und kranken Organismus im Lichte der 'vitale Farbung'. *Beit. Klin. Chirurg.*, **64**, 192–265.

Grubb, R. L., Jr Raichle, M. E. and Eichling, J. E. (1978). Peripheral sympathetic regulation of brain water permeability. *Brain Res.*, **144**, 204–7.

Gulati, A., Agarwal, S. K., Shukla, R. *et al.* (1984). Evidence for the lack of serotonergic mechanisms in the regulation of the blood–brain barrier. *Pharmacol. Res. Comm.*, **16**, 181–8.

Hamberger, B. and Masuoka, D. (1965). Localization of catecholamine uptake in rat brain slices. *Acta Pharmacol. Toxicol.*, **22**, 363–8.

Hardebo, J. E. and Owman, C. (1980a). Barrier mechanisms for neurotransmitter monoamines and their precursors at the blood–brain interface. *Ann. Neurol.*, **8**, 1–11.

Hardebo, J. E. and Owman, C. (1980b). Characterization of the *in vitro* uptake of monoamines into brain microvessels. *Acta Physiol. Scand.*, **108**, 223–9.

Hardebo, J. E., Edvinsson, L., MacKenzie, E. T. and Owman, C. (1977a). Regional brain uptake of noradrenaline following mechanical or osmotic opening of the blood–brain barrier. *Acta Physiol. Scand.*, **101**, 342–50.

Hardebo, J. E., Edvinsson, L., Owman, C. and Rosengren, E. (1977b). Quantitative evaluation of the blood–brain barrier capacity to form dopamine from circulating L-DOPA. *Acta Physiol. Scand.*, **99**, 377–84.

Hardebo, J. E., Edvinsson, L., MacKenzie, E. T. and Owman, C. (1979a). Histo-fluorescence study on monoamine entry into the brain before and after opening of the blood–brain barrier by various mechanisms. *Acta Neuropathol. (Berl.)*, **47**, 145–50.

Hardebo, J. E., Falck, B. and Owman, C. (1979*b*). A comparative study on the uptake and subsequent decarboxylation of monoamine precursors in cerebral microvessels. *Acta Physiol. Scand.*, **107**, 161–7.

Hardebo, J. E., Owman, C. and Wicklund, L. (1981). Influence of neuro-transmitter monoamines and neurotoxic analogues on morphologic blood–brain barrier function. In *Cerebral Microcirculation and Metabolism*, ed. J. Cervos-Navarro and E. Fritschka, pp. 177–80. New York: Raven Press.

Harik, S. I. (1986). Blood–brain barrier sodium/potassium pump: Modulation by central noradrenergic innervation. *Proc. Natl. Acad. Sci. USA*, **83**, 4067–70.

Harik, S. I. and McGunigal, T., Jr. (1984). The protective influence of the locus ceruleus on the blood–brain barrier. *Ann. Neurol.*, **15**, 568–74.

Harik, S. I., Sharma, V. K., Wetherbee, J. R., Warren, R. H. and Banerjee, S. P. (1980). Adrenergic receptors of cerebral microvessels. *Eur. J. Pharmacol.*, **61**, 207–8.

Hartman, B. K., Zide, D. and Udenfriend, S. (1972). The use of dopamine beta-hydroxylase as a marker for the central noradrenergic nervous system in rat brain. *Proc. Natl. Acad. Sci. USA*, **69**, 2722–6.

Hartman, B. K., Swanson, L. W., Raichle, M. E. *et al.* (1980). Central adrenergic regulation of cerebral microvascular permeability and physiologic evidence. *Adv. Exp. Med. Biol.*, **131**, 113–26.

Head, R. J., Hjelle, J. T., Jarrott, B. *et al.* (1980). Isolated brain microvessels: Preparation, morphology, histamine and catecholamine contents. *Blood Vessels*, **17**, 173–86.

Herbst, T. J., Raichle, M. E. and Ferrendelli, J. A. (1979). β-adrenergic regulation of adenosine 3′, 5′-monophosphate concentration in brain microvessels. *Science*, **204**, 330–4.

Hervonen, H., Spatz, M., Bembry, J. and Murray, M. R. (1981). Studies related to the blood–brain barrier to monoamines and protein in pia-arachnoid cultures. *Brain Res.*, **210**, 449–54.

Hervonen, H., Steinwall, O., Spatz, M. and Klatzo, I. (1980). Behaviour of the blood–brain barrier toward biogenic amines in experimental cerebral ischemia. In *The Cerebral Microvasculature*, ed. H. M. Eizenberg and R. L. Suddith, pp. 295–305. New York: Plenum.

Johansson, B. B. and Martinsson, L. (1980). β-Adrenoceptor antagonists and the dysfunction of the blood–brain barrier induced by adrenaline. *Brain Res.*, **181**, 219–22.

Joo, F. (1993). The blood–brain barrier *in vitro*: the second decade. *Neurochem. Int.*, **23**, 499–521.

Kalaria, R. N. and Harik, S. I. (1987). Blood–brain monoamine oxidase: Enzyme characterization in cerebral microvessels and other tissues from six mammalian species, including human. *J. Neurochem.*, **49**, 856–64.

Kalaria, R. N. and Harik, S. I. (1989). Evidence for innervation of cerebral microvessels by locus ceruleus noradrenergic neurons. In *Neurotransmission and Cerebrovascular Function*, vol. 1, ed. J. Seylaz and E. T. MacKenzie, pp. 191–4. Amsterdam: Elsevier.

Kaplan, G. P., Hartman, H. K. and Creveling, C. R. (1979). Immunohisto-chemical demonstration of catechol-O-methyl-transferase in mammalian brain. *Brain Res.*, **167**, 241–50.

Karnushina, I. L., Spatz, M. and Bembry, J. (1982). Cerebral endothelial cell culture. I. The presence of β$_2$ and α$_2$-adrenergic receptors linked to adenylate cyclase activity. *Life Sci.*, **30**, 849–58.

Karnushina, I. L., Spatz, M. and Bembry, J. (1983). Cerebral endothelial cell culture. II. Adenylate cyclase response to prostaglandins and their interaction with the adrenergic system. *Life Sci.*, **32**, 1427–35.

Kobayashi, H., Magnoni, M. S., Govoni, S. *et al.* (1985). Neuronal control of brain microvessel function. *Experientia*, **41**, 427–558.

Kobayashi, H., Memo, M., Spano, P. F. and Trabucchi, M. (1981). Identification of beta-adrenergic receptor binding sites in rat brain microvessels, using [^{125}I] iodo-hydroxybenzylpindolol. *J. Neurochem.*, **36**, 1383–8.

Krenger, W., Honegger, C. G., Feurer, C. and Cammisuli, S. (1986). Changes of neurotransmitter systems of chronic relapsing experimental allergic encephalomyelitis in the rat brain and spinal cord. *J. Neurochem.*, **47**, 1247–54.

Kristensson, K. and Wisniewski, H. M. (1977). Chronic relapsing experimental allergic encephalomyelitis: studies in vascular permeability changes. *Acta Neuropathol. (Berl.)*, **39**, 189–94.

Lai, F. M. and Spector, S. (1978). Studies on the monoamine oxidase and catechol-O-methyltransferase of the rat cerebral microvessels. *Archiv. In. Pharmacodyn.*, **233**, 227–34.

Lai, F. M., Udenfriend, S. and Spector, S. (1975). Presence of norepinephrine and related enzymes in isolated brain microvessels. *Proc. Natl. Acad. Sci. USA*, **72**, 4622–5.

Lindvall, M. and Owman C. (1980). Evidence for the presence of two types of monoamine oxidase in rabbit choroid plexus and their role in breakdown of amines influencing cerebrospinal fluid formation. *J. Neurochem.*, **34**, 518–22.

Lindvall, M., Hardebo, J. E. and Owman, C. (1980). Barrier mechanisms for neurotransmitter monoamines in the choroid plexus. *Acta Physiol. Scand.*, **108**, 215–21.

Linthicum, D. S. and Frelinger, J. A. (1982). Acute autoimmune encephalitis in mice. II. Susceptibility is controlled by the combination of H-2 and histamine sensitization genes. *J. Exp. Med.*, **155**, 31–8.

Lossinsky, A. S., Badmajew, V., Robson, J. A. *et al.* (1989). Sites of egress of inflammatory cells and horseradish peroxidase transport across the blood–brain barrier in a murine model of chronic relapsing experimental allergic encephalomyelitis. *Acta Neuropathol.*, **78**, 359–71.

MacKenzie, E. T., McCulloch, J. and O'Keane, M. (1976). Influence of endogenous norepinephrine on cerebral blood flow and metabolism. *Am. J. Physiol.*, **231**, 489–95.

Magnoni, M. S., Kobayashi, H., Cazzaniga, A. *et al.* (1983). Hypertension reduces the number of beta-adrenergic receptors in rat brain microvessels. *Circulation*, **67**, 610–3.

Magnoni, M. S., Kobayashi, H., Frattola, L. *et al.* (1985). Effect of common carotid occlusion on beta-adrenergic receptor function in cerebral microvessels. *Stroke*, **16**, 505–9.

Maruki, C., Spatz, M., Ueki, Y. *et al.* (1984). Cerebro-vascular endothelial cell culture: Metabolism and synthesis of 5-hydroxytryptamine. *J. Neurochem.*, **43**, 316–9.

McDonald, W. I. and Barnes, D. (1989). Lessons from magnetic resonance imaging in multiple sclerosis. *Trends Neurosci.*, **12**, 376–9.

Nagatsu, T. (1973). *Biochemistry of Catecholamines: Biochemical Methods.* Tokyo: University of Tokyo Press.

Nathanson, J. A. (1980). Cerebral microvessels contain a β_2-adrenergic receptor. *Life Sci.*, **26**, 1793–9.

Nathanson, J. A. and Glaser, G. H. (1979). Identification of β-adrenergic-sensitive adenylate cyclase in intracranial blood vessels. *Nature*, **278**, 567–9.

Nelson, E. and Rennels, M. (1970). Innervation of intracranial arteries. *Brain*, **93**, 475–90.

Oldendorf, W. H. (1971). Brain uptake of radiolabelled amino acids, amines and hexoses after arterial injection. *Am. J. Physiol.*, **221**, 1629–38.

Olesen, S. P. (1985). A calcium-dependent reversible increase in microvessels in frog brain induced by serotonin. *J. Physiol., (Lond.).* **361**, 103–13.

Owman, C. (1983). Autonomic innervation of blood vessels with special emphasis on human cerebrovascular nerves and corresponding amine receptors. *Gen. Pharmaco.*, **14**, 17–20.

Owman, Ch. and Hardebo, J. E. (1990). Experimental opening of the blood–brain barrier affects cerebral blood flow and alters flow response to circulating transmitter amines and peptides. In *Pathophysiology of the Blood–Brain Barrier*, ed. B. B. Johansson, Ch. Owman and H. Widner, pp. 113–30. Amsterdam: Elsevier Science Publishers.

Owman, C. and Rosengren, E. (1967). Dopamine formation on brain capillaries – an enzymatic blood–brain barrier mechanism. *J. Neurochem.*, **14**, 547–50.

Palmer, G. C. (1980). Beta-adrenergic receptors mediate adenylate cyclase responses in rat cerebral capillaries. *Neuropharmacology*, **19**, 17–23.

Palmer, G. C., McCreedy, S. A. and Freedman, L. R. (1989). Neurotransmitter coupled responses in the microvasculature of the brain under normal and pathological conditions. In *Regulatory Mechanisms of Neuron to Vessel Communication in the Brain*, ed. F. Battaini *et al.*, pp. 113–41. Berlin-Heidelberg: Springer Verlag.

Pardridge, W. M. and Oldendorf, W. H. (1977). Transport of metabolic substrates through the blood–brain barrier. *J. Neurochem.*, **28**, 5–12.

Peroutka, S. J., Moskowitz, M. A., Reinhard, J. F., Jr. and Snyder, S. H. (1980). Neurotransmitter receptor binding in bovine cerebral microvessels. *Science*, **208**, 610–2.

Preskorn, S. H., Hartman, B. K., Irwin, G. H. and Hughes, C. W. (1982). Role of the central adrenergic system in mediating amitriptyline induced alterations in the mammalian blood–brain barrier *in vivo*. *J. Pharmacol. Exp. Ther.*, **223**, 388–95.

Preskorn, S. H., Hartman, B. K., Raichle, M. E., Swanson L. W. and Clark, H. B. (1980). Central adrenergic regulation of cerebral microvascular permeability and blood flow: Pharmacologic evidence. *Adv. Exp. Med. Biol.*, **131**, 127–38.

Raichle, M. E., Hartman, B. K., Eichling J. O. and Sharpe, L. G. (1975). Central noradrenergic regulation of cerebral blood flow and vascular permeability. *Proc. Natl. Acad. Sci. USA*, **72**, 3726–30.

Rapoport, R. L. (1976). *Blood–Brain Barrier in Physiology and Medicine.* New York: Raven Press.

Reese, T. S. and Karnovsky, M. J. (1967). Fine structural localization of a blood-brain barrier to exogenous peroxidase. *J. Cell Biology*, **34**, 207–17.

Reinhard, J. F., Jr., Liebmann, J. E., Schlosberg, A. J. and Moskovitz, M. A. (1979). Serotonin neurons project to small blood vessels in the brain. *Science*, **106**, 85–7.

Rennels, M. and Nelson, E. (1975). Capillary innervation in the mammalian central nervous system. An electron microscopic demonstration. *Am. J. Anat.*, **144**, 233–41.

Sarmento, A., Albino-Teixeira, A. and Azevedo, I. (1990). Amitriptyline induced morphologic alterations of the blood–brain barrier. *Eur. J. Pharmacol.*, **176**, 69–74.

Sarmento, A., Borges, N. and Azevedo, I. (1991). Adrenergic influences on the control of blood–brain barrier permeability. *Naunyn-Schmiedberg Arch. Pharmacol.*, **343**, 633–7.

Sarmento, A., Borges, N. and Lima, D. (1994). Influence of electrical stimulation of locus coeruleus on the rat blood–brain barrier permeability to sodium fluorescein. *Acta Neurochirurg.*, **127**, 215–9.

Sharma, H. S., Olsson, Y. and Dey, P. K. (1995). Serotonin as a mediator of increased microvascular permeability of the brain and spinal cord: experimental observations in anaesthetised rats and mice. In *New Concepts of a Blood-Brain Barrier*, ed. D. J. Greenwood, J. Begley and M. B. Segal, pp. 75–80. New York: Plenum Press.

Sharma, H. S. and Dey, P. K. (1986*a*). Probable involvement of 5-hydroxytryptamine in increased permeability of blood–brain barrier under heat stress in young rats. *Neuropharmacology*, **25**, 161–7.

Sharma, H. S. and Dey, P. K. (1986*b*). Influence of long-term immobilization stress on regional blood–brain permeability, cerebral blood flow and 5-HT level in conscious normotensive young rats. *J. Neurol. Sci.*, **72**, 61–76.

Sharma, H. S., Westman, J., Nyberg, F. *et al.* (1994). Role of serotonin and prostaglandins in brain edema induced by heat stress. An experimental study in the young rat. *Acta Neurochirurg.* [suppl.], **60**, 65–70.

Simmons, R. D., Buzbee, T. M., Linthicum, D. C. *et al.* (1987). Simultaneous visualization of vascular permeability change and leukocyte egress in the central nervous system during autoimmune encephalomyelitis. *Acta Neuropathol. (Berl.)*, **74**, 191–3.

Spatz, M. (1986). Recent advances in the study of cerebrovascular receptors. In *Mechanisms of Secondary Brain Damage*, ed. A. Baethmann, K. G. Go and A. Unterberg, pp. 283–94. New York: Plenum Publishing.

Spatz, M. and Mrsulja, B. B. (1982). Progress in cerebral microvascular studies related to the function of the blood–brain barrier. In *Advances in Cellular Neurobiology* , vol. 3, ed. S. Federoff and H. Hertz, pp. 311–37. New York: Academic Press.

Spatz, M., Abe, T., Rausch, W. D. *et al.* (1981*a*). Studies on the nature and function of cerebral microvessel involvement in the blood–brain barrier for monoamines. In *Cerebral Microcirculation and Metabolism*, ed. J. Cervos-Navarro and E. Fritschka, pp. 23–8. New York: Raven Press.

Spatz, M., Maruki, C., Abe, T. *et al.* (1981*b*). The uptake and fate of the radiolabeled 5-hydroxytryptamine in isolated cerebral microvessels. *Brain Res.*, **220**, 214–9.

Spatz, M., Nagatsu, I., Maruki, C. *et al.* (1982). The presence of phenylethanolamine-*N*-methyltransferase in cerebral microvessels and endothelial cultures. *Brain Res.*, **240**, 191–4.

Spatz, M., Kaneda, N., Sumi, C. *et al.* (1986*a*). The presence of catechol-*o*-methyltransferase activity in separately cultured cerebromicrovascular endothelial and smooth muscle cells. *Brain Res.*, **381**, 363–7.

Spatz, M., Mrsulja, B. B., Wroblewska, B. *et al.* (1986*b*). Modulation of glycogen metabolism in cerebromicrovascular smooth muscle and endothelial cultures. *Biochemical and Biophysical Research Communication*, **134**, 484–91.

Spatz, M., Merkel, N., Wang, L. *et al.* (1990). Modulation of Ia expression on murine cerebral vascular endothelial cells. In *Pathophysiology of the Blood-Brain Barrier*, ed. B. B. Johansson, Ch. Owman and H. Widner, pp. 485–99. Amsterdam: Elsevier.

Spatz, M., Bacic, F., Merkel, N. *et al.* (1993). The regulatory functions of cerebromicrovascular endothelium. In *CNS Barriers and Modern CSF Diagnostics*, ed. K. Felgenhauer, M. Holzgraefe and H. W. Prange, pp. 41–59. Weinheim, New York: VCH Publishing.

Sternberger, N., Sternberger, L., Lies, M. and Shear, C. (1989). Cell surface endothelial proteins altered in experimental allergic encephalomyelitis. *J. Neuroimmunol.*, **1**, 241–8.

Suddith, R. L., Savage, K. E and Eisenberg, H. M. (1980). Ultrastructural and histochemical studies of cerebral capillary synapse. In *The Cerebral Microvasculature*, ed. H. M. Eisenberg and R. L. Suddith, pp. 139–45. New York: Plenum.

Swanson, L. W., Connelly, M. A. and Hartman, B. K. (1977). Ultrastructural evidence for central monoaminergic innervation of blood vessels in the paraventricular nucleus of the hypothalamus. *Brain Res.*, **136**, 166-73.

Wade, L. A. and Katzman, R. (1975*a*). Synthetic amino acids and the nature of L-DOPA transport at the blood–brain barrier. *J. Neurochem.*, **25**, 837–42.

Wade, L. A. and Katzman, R. (1975*b*). Rat brain regional uptake and decarboxylation of L-DOPA following carotid injection. *Am. J. Physiol.*, **228**, 352–9.

Waxman, F. J., Taquiam, J. M. and Whitacre, C. C. (1984). Cellular modification of clinical and histopathological expression of experimental allergic encephalomyelitis by the vasoactive amine antagonist cyproheptadine. *Cell. Immunol.*, **85**, 82–93.

Weil-Malherbe, H., Whitby, L. G. and Axelrod, J. (1961). The blood–brain barrier for catecholamines in different regions of the brain. In *Regional Neurochemistry*, ed. S. Kety and L. Eldes, pp. 284–91. Oxford: Pergamon.

Weselmann, U., Konkol, R. J., Leo, G. L. *et al.* (1987). Altered splenic catecholamine concentrations during experimental allergic encephalomyelitis. *Pharmacol., Biochem. Behav.*, **26**, 851–4.

Westergaard, E. (1975). Enhanced vesicular transport of exogenous peroxidase across cerebral vessels, induced by serotonin. *Acta Neuropathol. (Berl.)*, **32**, 42–97.

Westergaard, E. V., Deurs, B. and Bronsted, H. E. (1977). Increased vesicular transfer of horseradish peroxidase across cerebral endothelium evoked by active hypertension. *Acta Neuropathol. (Berl.)*, **37**, 141–52.

Westerlind, A., Larsson, L. E., Häggendal, J. and Ekström-Jodal, B. (1991). Prevention of endotoxin-induced increase of cerebral oxygen consumption in dogs by propranolol pretreatment. *Acta Anaesthesiol. Scand.*, **35**, 745–9.

Westerlind, A., Larsson, L. E., Häggendal, J. and Ekström-Jodal, B. (1995*a*). Effects of propranolol pretreatment on cerebral blood flow, oxygen uptake and catecholamines during metabolic acidosis following *E. coli* endotoxin in dogs. *Acta Anaesthesiol. Scand.*, **39**, 467–71.

Westerlind, A., Larsson, L. E., Häggendal, J. and Ekström-Jodal, B. (1995*b*). Effects of arterial hypoxia and β-adrenoceptor blockade on cerebral blood flow and oxygen uptake following *E. coli* endotoxin in dogs. *Acta Anaesthesiol. Scand.*, **39**, 472–8.

PART V

Pathophysiology in disease states

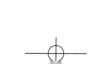

41 Cerebral amyloid angiopathy

HARRY V. VINTERS

- Introduction
- CAA associated with AD/SDAT/DS and 'aging'
- HCHWA-I/HCCAA
- HCHWA-D

Introduction

The term cerebral amyloid angiopathy (CAA) (synonymous with cerebral congophilic angiopathy and cerebrovascular amyloidosis) describes and defines a pathologic condition whereby the media of small arteries (arterioles), veins (venules) and adventitial component of capillaries is replaced by one of several fibrillar proteins that have a beta-pleated sheet configuration (Vinters, 1987). Whereas the older literature differentiates between primarily capillary and arteriolar amyloid deposition, modern conceptualization of CAA defines the microangiopathy based upon the biochemical composition of the primary molecule that constitutes the fibrillar amyloid deposits (Coria and Rubio, 1996). Thus, several forms of CAA are recognized:

1. CAA associated with Alzheimer disease/ senile dementia of Alzheimer type (AD/ SDAT), Down's syndrome (DS) and brain aging – biochemically composed of beta/A4 protein – is by far the most common form of CAA worldwide.
2. CAA in Icelandic patients who suffer from a hereditary form of cerebral hemorrhage – best described by the terms hereditary cerebral hemorrhage with amyloidosis, Icelandic (HCHWA-I); or, since the amyloid protein is a variant of gamma-trace/cystatin C,

hereditary cystatin C amyloid angiopathy (HCCAA) (Ólafsson et al., 1996).
3. CAA in Dutch patients who also experience frequent brain hemorrhage on a hereditary basis – by analogy to the Icelandic condition, referred to as HCHWA-D (Bornebroek et al., 1996; Maat-Schieman et al., 1996).
4. CAA associated with prion diseases – a group of rare, sometimes genetically determined neurodegenerative conditions that usually have a component of spongiform encephalopathy – in which prion protein (PrP) is deposited in vessel walls; hence the descriptive term PrP-CAA (Ghetti et al., 1996).
5. A very recently described and rare familial form of meningocerebrovascular amyloid (initially identified in a Hungarian kindred) associated with a mis-sense mutation in the gene encoding transthyretin (Vidal et al., 1996).

The emphasis in this chapter will be on CAA associated with AD/SDAT and DS, HCHWA-D and HCHWA-I. Whereas amyloid deposition occurs almost exclusively in microvessel walls – hence their inherent interest for anyone who studies the BBB or diseases that might affect it – in the entities described as (2) and (3) above, the other conditions show CAA as one manifestation of a more complex CNS amyloidosis (Glenner, 1983;

379

Kosik, 1992; Sekloe, 1994). Indeed, severe CAA as a component of AD/DS may represent one extreme of a phenotypic spectrum of brain amyloid deposition (Blumenthal and Premachandra, 1990; Vinters, 1992*a*), the other extreme of which is purely parenchymal beta/A4. For PrP-CAA, except in rare instances (for review see Ghetti *et al.*, 1996) microvascular amyloid deposition is minimal compared to brain parenchymal localization of PrP.

All forms of CAA are associated with one or both of two important groups of clinicopathologic conditions, i.e. (a) stroke, and (b) neurodegenerative conditions, especially with a major component of dementia. Stroke usually takes the form of cerebral hemorrhage (rarely ischemic infarct) (Vinters, 1992*b*), whereas dementia is almost certainly multifactorial and in many cases may not be causally related to the presence of amyloid within vessel walls. Some unique features of the various 'CAA syndromes', together with a consideration of their pathophysiologic features, merit consideration.

CAA associated with AD/SDAT/DS and 'aging'

CAA and brain parenchymal amyloid deposition were recognized as major brain parenchymal markers of 'neurodegeneration' almost from the time AD/SDAT was recognized shortly after the turn of the century. Elegant descriptions of the morphologic patterns of CAA that could be appreciated using classical histochemical methods appeared from the 1920s to the 1970s (for brief review, see Vinters *et al.*, 1996). While an association between CAA and dementing illnesses was suspected, the close association between CAA and AD/SDAT or brain aging was 'rediscovered' in the early 1980s by (among others) Glenner (1983, 1985). Even at the time the widely used 'Khachaturian criteria' (for the neuropathologic diagnosis of AD) were formulated, CAA was implicitly considered a less important diagnostic marker for the disease than an abundance of senile plaques and neurofibrillary tangles within brain (cortical) parenchyma. The isolation of a unique 4.2 kilodalton peptide (subsequently known as beta/A4) from meningeal arterioles of AD and DS patients (Glenner and Wong, 1984) – a finding that was later replicated in cortical parenchymal microvessels (Pardridge *et al.*, 1987) – refocused attention on cerebral microvascular amyloid as an important component of the neuropathologic spectrum of AD. In a simple autopsy survey of brains from elderly patients (including some with stroke and/or AD/SDAT), CAA was found to increase in severity with advancing age and to be widely distributed within cerebral cortex (Vinters and Gilbert, 1983). By the late 1980s and early 1990s, most biochemical/molecular work was aimed at understanding the mechanism of how beta/A4 comes to be deposited in excess in the brain substance and cerebral microvessel walls of AD patients, with emphasis on the former (for reviews see Kosik, 1992; Selkoe, 1994; Price *et al.*, 1995).

(a) Clinicopathologic consequences

CAA is known for producing non-traumatic intracerebral/intraparenchymal hemorrhage (Vinters, 1992*b*; Yong *et al.*, 1992). This occurs with CAA associated with AD/SDAT and HCHWA-I (HCCAA) as well as HCHWA-D, though it is not well documented with PrP-CAA. CAA-associated cerebral bleeds are almost always 'lobar' hemorrhages within the cerebral hemispheres, rarely cerebellar, almost never within the basal ganglia/thalamus or brainstem – common sites for hypertensive hemorrhages. Given the large 'universe' of patients who suffer from AD/SDAT, only a relatively tiny proportion develop brain parenchymal hematomas. Why CAA, which is found to some extent in virtually all brains of patients with AD/SDAT, should produce bleeds in so few of them has been a puzzling feature of AD/SDAT-associated CAA. Part of the explanation almost certainly lies in the finding that only a subset of patients with severe CAA develop CAA-associated (secondary) microvasculopathies, including fibrosis, microaneurysm formation and fibrinoid necrosis, which would be expected to lead to weakening of arteriolar walls with resultant hemorrhage (Mandybur, 1986; Vonsattel *et al.*, 1991). Precisely why this should occur in only a few AD/SDAT patients is unknown.

CAA of AD/SDAT is noted with other clinical presentations, including angiitis (usually granulomatous or giant cell arteritis), as a 'mass lesion' or with subarachnoid hemorrhage, all of which are extremely rare, even by comparison with cerebral hemorrhage (Vinters *et al.*, 1996). The contribution of CAA to brain ischemic lesions is controversial. Isolated examples of AD/SDAT patients with overwhelming CAA and cerebral macro- and/or microinfarcts are well described (Anders *et al.*, 1993), though larger studies (Vonsattel *et al.*, 1991) find no statistically significant association between occurrence/severity of CAA and brain ischemic lesions. Correlative clinicopathologic studies based on autopsy material in very elderly patients are complicated by the array of large and small vessel disease that is common in this age group. It would be valuable to know, for instance, whether CAA might contribute in a unique fashion to the development of dementia independent of its association with classical 'stroke' syndromes, e.g. through the mechanism of producing petechial hemorrhages, microinfarcts and demyelination (Greenberg *et al.*, 1993).

(b) Cellular/molecular pathogenesis

CAA is easily detectable in routine (H & E-stained) sections of brain by the finding within cortical arterioles of enacement of their media, and its replacement by a hyaline eosinophilic material which can conclusively be shown to represent amyloid using Congo Red or thioflavin stains with (respectively) polarization and fluorescent microscopy (Fig. 41.1). However, a more accurate method for demonstrating AD/CAA (and parenchymal/senile plaque amyloid) is to use anti-beta/A4 immunohistochemistry (Fig. 41.2), which highlights the major (though by no means only) protein within the vascular media. Beta/A4 is a unique 4.2 kDa protein representing the near-C-terminus portion cleaved from a much larger protein (amyloid precursor protein, APP) encoded by a gene on chromosome 21. Beta/A4 is a soluble product of physiologic cellular processing of APP. Pertinent to the pathogenesis of AD-associated CAA, anti-beta/A4 immunohistochemistry shows primarily extracellular amyloid deposits within arteriolar walls, whereas anti-APP antibodies tend to decorate smooth muscle (sm) cells themselves (Kawai *et al.*, 1993) though others (Frackowiak *et al.*, 1994) find sm to be immunolabelled with anti-

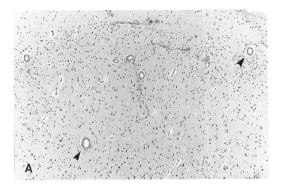
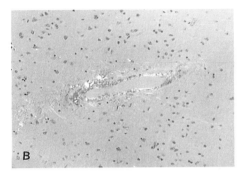
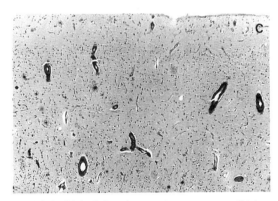

Fig 41.1. CAA, light microscopic appearance. CAA can be easily demonstrated using Congo Red, which shows thickened cortical arterioles (e.g. arrowhead) even without polarization microscopy (A). (B) demonstrates a comparable preparation (though at higher magnification) viewed *with* polarization – the 'birefringence' noted in the arterial wall was characteristically 'yellow/green' in color. (C) CAA can also be highlighted using the periodic acid–Schiff stain, as in this section. (Magnifications A ×80, B ×200, C ×80.)

beta/A4 in addition to APP, which coincides with our own experience. Vascular amyloid fibrils may first be formed within arteriolar abluminal basement membrane (bm) elements (Yamaguchi *et al.*,

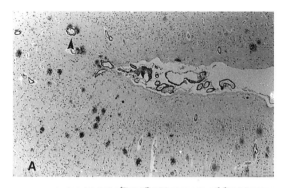

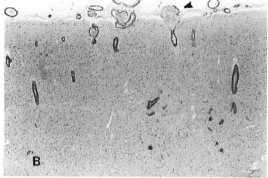

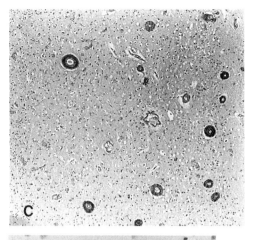

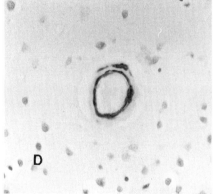

Fig. 41.2. CAA, immunohistochemistry. (A)–(C) are from sections immunostained with antibodies to beta/A4 or synthetic peptide representing a portion of beta/A4. (A) shows abundant immunoreactive cortical senile plaques as well as parenchymal and leptomeningeal arterial walls. Arrowhead indicates a beta/A4 immunoreactive artery with surrounding immunoreactive parenchymal material. (B) Section of cortex from a patient in whom beta/A4 immunoreactive material was almost exclusively arteriolar, i.e. there is a negligible parenchymal/SP component. (C) Severe CAA, immunoreactive arterioles viewed primarily in cross-section. (D) Severe CAA in cortex; section immunostained with anti-smooth muscle actin. Note that vessel wall shows preserved intimal/subintimal smooth muscle (sm) cells and occasional adventitial sm, though amyloid has replaced much of the media. (Magnifications A×55, B×50, C×80, D×515.)

1992); the bm may sequester beta/A4-containing APP segments, which are then cleaved further to produce amyloidogenic fragments. Beta/A4 can occur in various lengths (39–43 amino acids) and the 1–42/43 form is the most abundant in CAA (Roher *et al.*, 1993; Shinkai *et al.*, 1995). *In vitro* models examining APP metabolism in blood vessel-derived cultured cells are likely to assist in clarifying the cellular pathogenesis of CAA (Frackowiak *et al.*, 1995). Physiologic studies also

indicate that beta/A4 may have vasoactive properties and mediate endothelial damage (Thomas *et al.*, 1996).

Arteriolar CAA is clearly associated, based upon both ultrastructural and immunohistochemical studies, with smooth muscle (sm) cell degeneration (Fig. 41.3) (Vinters *et al.*, 1994; Wisniewski *et al.*, 1994). Of interest, however, is the observation that structural endothelial/BBB abnormalities within AD brain biopsy material are relatively slight and (in one patient studied) not especially accentuated with CAA; they include diminished mitochondrial density, increased capillary profiles containing pericytes (a possible 'second line of defence' for the BBB), and features that suggest 'leakiness' of inter-endothelial junctions (Stewart *et al.*, 1992).

ApoE and CAA Although the ε4 allele of apolipoprotien E (ApoE) is associated with beta/A4 deposition in AD cortex as senile plaques, the association between ApoE and CAA is less clear. Some groups have found ApoE ε4 to be an independent risk factor for CAA-related brain hemorrhage

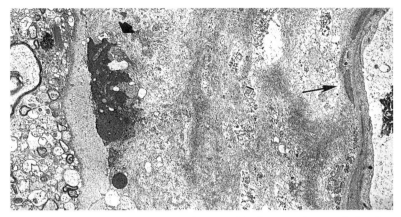

Fig. 41.3. Ultrastructural features of CAA. In this electron micrograph showing an affected arteriolar wall, lumen is at right of the figure, brain parenchyma (identifiable by presence of myelinated/unmyelinated fibers and astrocyte processes), at left. Whereas a thin layer of intact sm cells is identified immediately beneath the endothelium (arrow), for the most part these cells have been replaced by skeins of fibrillar material consistent in dimension with amyloid; the vessel wall was also prominently immunoreactive with ant-beta/A4. Arrowhead indicates electron-dense cytoplasmic debris (separated from brain parenchyma by basement membrane material), which may represent remnants of sm cells. For details, See Vinters *et al.* (1994).

(Greenberg *et al.*, 1995); others find an overrepresentation of the ApoE e2 allele in patients with autopsy/biopsy-proven CAA-related bleeding (Nicoll *et al.*, 1996), especially in patients with CAA lacking full CERAD criteria for AD/SDAT.

HCHWA-I/HCCAA

This tragic condition produces cerebral parenchymal hemorrhage in young Icelandic patients, typically within the third to fifth decades of life (Ólafsson *et al.*, 1996). Inherited as an autosomal dominant condition found in southwestern Iceland, apparently originating from a single 'founder' individual, it results from a point mutation in the gene encoding the cysteine protease inhibitor cystatin C (gamma-trace protein). This causes substitution of a single nucleotide (A for T) in codon 68, leading to replacement of leucine by glutamine in the protein. The resultant 'mutant' protein has an increased tendency to aggregate. It is deposited in cerebral cortical and meningeal arterial walls in a pattern reminiscent of AD/CAA; it can be demonstrated immunohistochemically using anti-cystatin C antibodies (Fig. 41.4); by light microscopy, HCHWA-I is virtually indistinguishable from AD/CAA. Extra-CNS deposits of amyloid are found in skin, salivary

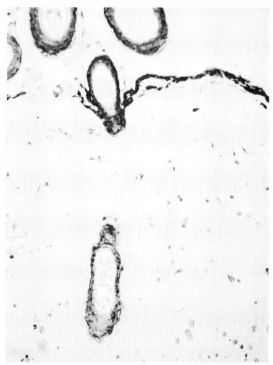

Fig. 41.4. HCHWA-I/HCCAA. Section from brain of an affected Icelandic patient immunostained with antibodies to synthetic peptide represesenting a portion of the gamma-trace molecule. Note staining of parenchymal and leptomeningeal arterial walls, as well as pial deposits of the protein. For details, see Vinters *et al.* (1990).

glands, lymphoid tissues and testes. Gamma-trace/cystatin C can also be demonstrated in non-Icelandic patients with the beta/A4 type of CAA, especially when associated with 'stroke' (Vinters *et al.*, 1990).

HCHWA-D

This condition shares features with both HCHWA-I and AD/CAA. Clinically, it shows an autosomal dominant pattern of inheritance; the causal abnormality is a point mutation at codon 693 of APP, resulting in an amino acid substitution at amino acid 22 of beta/A4. It presents as a 'recurrent stroke' syndrome resulting from cerebral hemorrhages, hemorrhagic and 'bland' infarcts (Bornebroek *et al.*, 1996) in patients with a mean age of approximately 50 years. Dementia often onsets after the initial 'stroke' and is probably multi-factorial,

resulting in part from encephalomalacic lesions but in part from unknown factors possibly related to beta/A4 deposition. The primary pathologic change is arteriolar beta/A4 deposition causing CAA – the light microscopic and even immunohistochemical appearances are similar to those of AD/CAA. Parenchymal ('plaque-like') deposition of beta/A4 occurs within cerebral cortex, but neurofibrillary tangles (characteristic of AD neuropathologic change) are inconspicuous (Maat-Shieman *et al.*, 1996).

Acknowledgments

Work in the author's laboratory supported in part by PHS grants P30 AG 10123 and P01 AG 12435. Carol Appleton assisted with preparation of photomicrographs.

References

Anders, K. H., Secor, D. L. and Vinters, H. V. (1993). Cerebral amyloid angiopathy (CAA) associated with ischemic necrosis. *J. Neuropathol. Exp. Neurol.*, **52**, 275.

Blumenthal, H. T. and Premachandra, B. N. (1990). The aging–disease dichotomy. Cerebral amyloid angiopathy – an independent entity associated with dementia. *J. Am. Geriat. Soc.*, **38**, 475–82.

Bornebroek, M., Haan, J., Maat-Schieman, M. L. C. *et al.* (1996). Hereditary cerebral hemorrhage with amyloidosis–Dutch type (HCHWA-D): I A review of clinical, radiologic and genetic aspects. *Brain Pathol.*, **6**, 111–14.

Coria, F. and Rubio, I. (1996). Cerebral amyloid angiopathies. *Neuropathol. and Appl. Neurobiol.*, **22**, 216–27.

Frackowiak, J., Zoltowska, A. and Wisniewski, H. M. (1994). Non-fibrillar beta-amyloid protein is associated with smooth muscle cells of vessel walls in Alzheimer disease. *J. Neuropathol. Exp. Neurol.*, **53**, 637–45.

Frackowiak, J., Mazur-Kolecka, B., Wisniewski, H. M. *et al.* (1995). Secretion and accumulation of Alzheimer's beta-protein by cultured vascular smooth muscle cells from old and young dogs. *Brain Res.*, **675**, 225–30.

Ghetti, B., Piccardo, P., Frangione, B. *et al.* (1996). Prion protein amyloidosis. *Brain Pathol.*, **6**, 127–45.

Glenner, G. G. (1983). Alzheimer's disease. The commonest form of amyloidosis. *Archiv. Pathol. and Lab. Med.*, **107**, 281–2.

Glenner, G. G. (1985). On causative theories in Alzheimer's disease. *Human Pathol.*, **16**, 433–5.

Glenner, G. G. and Wong, C. W. (1984). Alzheimer's disease and Down's syndrome: sharing of a unique cerebrovascular amyloid fibril protein. *Biochem. and Biophys. Res. Comm.*, **122**, 1131–5.

Greenberg, S. M., Vonsattel, J. P. G., Stakes, J. W. *et al.* (1993). The clinical spectrum of cerebral amyloid angiopathy: presentations without lobar hemorrhage. *Neurology*, **43**, 2073–9.

Greenberg, S. M., Rebeck, G. W., Vonsattel, J. P. G. *et al.* (1995). Apolipoprotein E e4 and cerebral hemorrhage associated with amyloid angiopathy. *Ann. Neurol.*, **38**, 254–9.

Kawai, M., Kalaria, R. N., Cras, P. *et al.* (1993). Degeneration of vascular smooth muscle cells in cerebral amyloid angiopathy of Alzheimer disease. *Brain Res.*, **623**, 142–6.

Kosik, K. S. (1992). Alzheimer's disease: a cell biological perspective. *Science*, **256**, 780–3.

Maat-Schieman, M. L. C., van Duinen, S. G., Bornebroek, M. *et al.* (1996). Hereditary cerebral hemorrhage with amyloidosis – Dutch type (HCHWA-D): II A Review of histopathological aspects. *Brain Pathol.*, **6**, 115–20.

Mandybur, T. I. (1986). Cerebral amyloid angiopathy: the vascular pathology and complications. *J. Neuropathol. and Exp. Neurol.*, **45**, 79–90.

Nicoll, J. A. R., Burnett, C., Love, S. *et al.* (1996). High frequency of apolipoprotein E e2 in patients with cerebral hemorrhage due to cerebral amyloid angiopathy. *Ann. Neurol.*, **39**, 682.

Ólafsson, I., Thorsteinsson, L. and Jensson, Ó. (1996). The molecular pathology of hereditary cystatin C amyloid angiopathy causing brain hemorrhage. *Brain Pathol.*, **6**, 121–6.

Pardridge, W. M., Vinters, H. V., Yang, J. *et al.* (1987). Amyloid angiopathy of Alzheimer's disease: amino acid composition and partial sequence of a 4200 Dalton peptide isolated from cortical microvessels. *J. Neurochem.*, **49**, 1394–401.

Price, D. L., Sisodia, S. S. and Gandy, S. E. (1995). Amyloid beta amyloidosis in Alzheimer's disease. *Curr. Opin. Neurol.*, **8**, 268–74.

Roher, A. E., Lowenson, J. D., Clarke, S. *et al.* (1993). Beta-amyloid-(1-42) is a major component of cerebrovascular amyloid deposits: implications for the pathology of Alzheimer disease. *Proc. Natl. Acad. Sci. USA*, **90**, 10836–40.

Selkoe, D. J. (1994). Alzheimer's disease: a central role for amyloid. *J. Neuropathol. and Exp. Neurol.*, **53**, 438–47.

Shinkai, Y., Yoshimura, M., Ito, Y. *et al.* (1995). Amyloid beta-proteins 1–40 and 1–42 (43) in the soluble fraction of extra- and intracranial blood vessels. *Ann. Neurol.*, **38**, 421–8.

Stewart, P. A., Hayakawa, K., Akers, M.-A. and Vinters, H. V. (1992). A morphometric study of the blood–brain barrier in Alzheimer's disease. *Lab. Invest.*, **67**, 734–42.

Thomas, T., Thomas, G., McLendon, C. *et al.* (1996). Beta-amyloid-mediated vasoactivity and vascular endothelial damage. *Nature*, **380**, 168–71.

Vidal, R., Garzuly, F., Budka, H. *et al.* (1996). Meningocerebrovascular amyloidosis associated with a novel transthyretin mis-sense mutation at codon 18 (TTRD18G). *Am. J. Pathol.*, **148**, 361–6.

Vinters, H. V. (1987). Cerebral amyloid angiopathy – a critical review. *Stroke*, **18**, 311–324.

Vinters, H. V. (1992a). Cerebral amyloid angiopathy and Alzheimer's disease: two entities or one? *J. Neurol. Sci.*, **112**, 1–3.

Vinters, H. V. (1992b). Cerebral amyloid angiopathy. In *Stroke. Pathophysiology, Diagnosis, and Management*, 2nd edn, ed. H. J. M. Barnett, J. P. Mohr, B. M. Stein and F. M. Yatsu, pp. 821–58. New York: Churchill Livingstone.

Vinters, H. V. and Gilbert, J. J. (1983). Cerebral amyloid angiopathy: incidence and complications in the aging brain. II. The distribution of amyloid vascular changes. *Stroke*, **14**, 924–8.

Vinters, H. V., Nishimura, G. S., Secor, D. L. and Pardridge, W. M. (1990). Immunoreactive A4 and gamma-trace peptide colocalization in amyloidotic arteriolar lesions in brains of patients with Alzheimer's disease. *Am. J. Pathol.*, **137**, 233–40.

Vinters, H. V., Secor, D. L., Read, S. L. *et al.* (1994). Microvasculature in brain biopsy specimens from patients with Alzheimer's disease: an immunohisto-chemical and ultrastructural study. *Ultrastruct. Pathol.*, **18**, 333–48.

Vinters, H. V., Wang, Z. Z. and Secor, D. L. (1996). Brain parenchymal and microvascular amyloid in Alzheimer's disease. *Brain Pathol.*, **6**, 179–95.

Vonsattel, J. P. G., Myers, R. H., Hedley-Whyte, E. T. *et al.* (1991). Cerebral amyloid angiopathy without and with cerebral hemorrhages: a comparative histological study. *Ann. Neurol.*, **30**, 637–49.

Wisniewski, H. M., Frąckowiak, J., Zóltowska, A. and Kim, K. S. (1994). Vascular beta-amyloid in Alzheimer's disease angiopathy is produced by proliferating and degenerating smooth muscle cells. *Amyloid: International Journal of Experimental Clinical Investigation*, **1**, 8–16.

Yamaguchi, H., Yamazaki, T., Lemere, C. A. *et al.* (1992). Beta amyloid is focally deposited within the outer basement membrane in the amyloid angiopathy of Alzheimer's disease. *Am. J. Pathol.*, **141**, 249–59.

Yong, W. H., Robert, M. E., Secor, D. L. *et al.* (1992). Cerebral hemorrhage with biopsy-proved amyloid angiopathy. *Arch. Neurol.*, **49**, 51–8.

42 Brain microvasculature in multiple sclerosis

CELIA F. BROSNAN and LUZ CLAUDIO

- Introduction
- Recognition of antigens within the CNS
- Proinflammatory cytokines and chemokines
- Response of the BBB to inflammatory mediators
- Regulation of inflammatory events in the CNS
- Cytokines and adhesion molecules in MS
- Edema formation in the CNS
- Astrogliosis
- Conclusions

Introduction

Multiple sclerosis (MS) is a chronic inflammatory demyelinating disorder of the central nervous system (CNS) that is the most common cause of acquired neurological dysfunction in young adults. The clinical manifestations and progression of MS vary widely amongst patients but are characterized by focal involvement of the optic nerves, spinal cord and brain that remit to a varying extent and recur over a period of years. Although the etiology remains unknown, there is strong circumstantial evidence to support the conclusion that it is mediated by an autoimmune attack directed against CNS myelin (Hafler and Weiner, 1995). A substantial genetic component to the disease process has been implicated by the observations that the risk for first degree relatives is increased over the general population, but environmental factors have also been shown to play a role (Ebers, *et al.*, 1995). Active lesions are characterized by perivascular cuffs of lymphocytes and macrophages centered on post-capillary venules, particularly in the periventricular white matter, the optic nerve and tract, the corpus callosum and brainstem. Older lesions are immunologically silent in terms of inflammation and comprise large astroglial scars and demyelinated axons (Raine, 1990). Lesions are rarely noted beyond the root entry zones of the cranial and spinal nerves. Despite intense efforts, no cure is currently available although a number of drugs have shown some remedial efficacy.

Damage to the blood–brain barrier (BBB) represents the earliest sign of lesion formation (Fig. 42.1), but pathological evidence of BBB damage is present to a varying degree in all MS lesions, including inactive demyelinated plaques (Kwon and Prineas, 1994; Claudio *et al.*, 1995). Gadolinium-enhanced magnetic resonance imaging (MRI) has demonstrated that alterations in BBB function precede the onset of clinical signs and, most probably, demyelination (Davie *et al.*, 1994). They also show that new lesions do not always impose upon old lesions, and that alterations in vascular permeability may persist for several weeks. The use of MRI

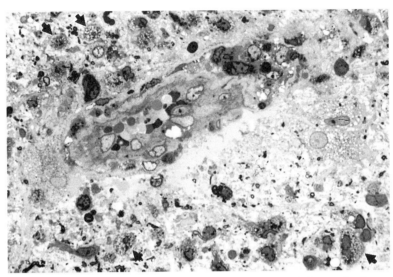

Fig. 42.1. Light micrograph showing extensive perivascular inflammation in an acute MS lesion. Note the presence of many lipid-laden macrophages (arrows) in the surrounding parenchyma, and the extensive edema and myelin degradation products. One micron section, ×300.

to study various aspects of the MS lesion are reviewed more extensively in Chapter 16. In this chapter, we discuss current concepts of the pathogenesis of lesion formation, particularly as it relates to the inflammatory process, and address the pathological evidence for BBB dysfunction in patients with MS.

In MS, the disruption of the BBB is thought to be due to the interaction of activated immunocompetent cells with CNS endothelial cells. Under normal conditions the BBB restricts the access of components of the immune system to the CNS compartment. Transport of immunoglobulins is controlled and the net negative charge of endothelial cells repels leukocytes. The absence, or low-level expression, of most adhesion molecules involved in the transmigration of inflammatory cells and the structure of the extracellular matrix reduces the traffic of leukocytes across the endothelial cell and their retention within the CNS parenchyma (reviewed by Brosnan *et al.*, 1992). During immune-mediated and inflammatory events, however, BBB function is lost, leukocytes invade the CNS and vasogenic edema develops (Figs. 42.1 and 42.2). Many of these initial events are difficult to monitor in tissue taken at autopsy because the state of tissue preservation is critical for the patho-

logical assessment of many aspects of vascular damage. However, they can be studied in a variety of animal models but most particularly in experimental allergic (autoimmune) encephalomyelitis (EAE), which is neuropathologically and clinically similar to MS. EAE is induced in susceptible species by sensitization with antigens associated with CNS myelin, and the release of proinflammatory cytokines by CD4[+] lymphocytes of the Th1 subset has been shown to be critical for disease expression (Miller and Karpus, 1994; Steinman, 1996). Studies in EAE indicate that changes in the permeability of the BBB are an early and significant component of lesion formation, and that clinical expression of disease correlates closely with the extent of edema in the CNS.

Studies that have focused on events occurring at the BBB in the primary demyelinating diseases have addressed four major questions: How do lymphocytes recognize and initiate an immune response directed against antigens located within the CNS compartment? What are the mechanisms involved in leukocyte trafficking into the CNS? Is there evidence that the specialized endothelial cells of the CNS respond differently to inflammatory mediators? How is damage to the BBB controlled and repaired?

387

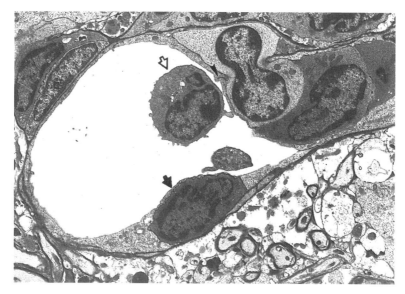

Fig. 42.2. Inflammatory cells at various stages of attachment and migration through a cerebral venule in a rat with EAE. Prior to sacrifice the animal was injected with the tracer horseradish peroxidase to assess compromised areas of the BBB. Note that the tracer permeates the area surrounding the migrating inflammatory cells that include macrophages (filled arrow) and lymphocytes (open arrow), the junctional complex (arrow head), as well as the perivascular space. ×9000 (reprinted with permission from Claudio *et al.*, (1990). *Am. J. Pathol.*, **137**, 1033–45).

Recognition of antigens within the CNS

The CNS has traditionally been considered to be an immunologically privileged site since allografts survive there longer than in most other tissues. The BBB is thought to contribute to this status by the low-level constitutive expression of MHC class I and class II molecules required for the activation and progression of an immune response, as well as by restricting lymphocyte trafficking into the CNS. However, although resting lymphocytes do not readily cross the BBB, small numbers of recently activated lymphocytes rapidly gain access to the CNS compartment in a non-antigen-specific manner (Hickey *et al.*, 1991). If they do not come in contact with the antigen then they leave, but if antigen is encountered then they become activated and initiate an immune response. Interestingly, studies in EAE have shown that remarkably few myelin-reactive lymphocytes are required to initiate the inflammatory cascade. They have also shown that these lymphocytes remain predominantly in a perivascular location, suggesting that

they control the inflammatory events occurring at the BBB (Cross, 1992; Steinman, 1996).

For immune reactions mediated by CD4+ lymphocytes, expression of MHC class II molecules is required for T cell activation to proceed. In the normal CNS, class II MHC molecules are present only at low levels on perivascular macrophages and parenchymal microglial cells. A primary role for the perivascular macrophage as the initial antigen presenting cell in EAE has been shown using a rat bone marrow chimera model by Hickey and colleagues (Hickey and Kimura, 1988; Williams *et al.*, 1994). Perivascular macrophages differ from the parenchymal microglia by their more rapid rates of turnover from peripheral bone-marrow-derived cells and by their greater constitutive expression of MHC class II. They can also be activated by proinflammatory cytokines such as IL-1 to express increased levels of MHC class II and to move away from the vessel wall (Cuff *et al.*, 1996*b*), suggesting that they may transport antigen to the draining lymph nodes, as has been shown for dendritic cells in the skin. Although studies *in vitro* have indicated that many different cell types can be induced by proinflammatory cytokines to express MHC class II, studies of the MS lesion have shown that increased expression is found principally in association with microglia, both within lesions and in the surrounding normal appearing white matter (Ulvestad *et al.*, 1994). Expression of MHC class II on astrocytes and endothelial cells in the MS lesion remains controversial at the present time and it is unlikely, given the experimental evidence, that endothelial cells play a direct role in antigen presentation and activation.

Proinflammatory cytokines and chemokines

Following activation in the CNS, antigen-presenting cells and Th1-type lymphocytes release a variety of soluble factors that lead to the influx of a large number of inflammatory cells to sites of antigen recognition. The chief mediators of this process appear to be the proinflammatory cytokines that include tumor necrosis factors (TNF)-α/β, interleukin-1 (IL-1)-α/β and interferon (IFN)-γ, as well as chemokines. These cytokines acting alone, or in concert, exert profound changes in endothelial cells that lead to increases in vascular permeability, blood flow and increased adhesiveness for circulating leukocytes (Pober *et al.*, 1986; see also Chapter 39). The nature of the inflammatory stimulus determines whether lymphocytes, monocytes or polymorphonuclear cells will predominate in the inflammatory exudate. Multiple steps are involved, each of which is mediated by a different set of released or induced factors, thus permitting considerable diversity in signaling by different combinations of the factors involved (reviewed by Springer, 1994).

The initial step in leukocyte recruitment involves the tethering and rolling of leukocytes along the surface of the activated endothelial cell. This process is mediated by cell-surface expression of the selectin family of adhesion molecules. Certain members of this family (P-selectin) are rapidly expressed on the cell surface following exposure to mediators of acute inflammation (such as thrombin or histamine) whereas others (E-selectin) are expressed following induction by cytokines such as IL-1 and TNF. The ligands for these receptors are

carbohydrates linked to specific mucin-like molecules. Firm adhesion to the endothelial cell is then effected by activation of the integrin family of adhesion molecules such as lymphocyte function associated antigen (LFA-1) and Mac-1, that interact with ligands of the immunoglobulin superfamily such as intercellular adhesion molecule-1 (ICAM-1) or ICAM-2. Activated lymphocytes may also express very late activation antigen-4 (VLA-4) that interacts with vascular cell adhesion molecule-1 (VCAM-1) on the endothelial cell. It has been proposed that ICAM-2 mediates lymphocyte trafficking through uninflamed tissues whereas induction of ICAM-1 mediates trafficking into inflamed tissues. The final step in this pathway is the migration of leukocytes across the endothelial cell wall (reviewed by Springer, 1994; Weller *et al.*, 1996). In the systemic vasculature diapedesis occurs predominantly via the junctional complex, however this is probably not the case for endothelial cells that express tight junctions (see below). Integrins are important for this final step in the extravasation of leukocytes and chemoattractants such as the chemokines or products of the activated complement cascade such as C5a impose directionality on this process.

A pivotal role for proinflammatory cytokines and adhesion molecule expression in disease development has been clearly demonstrated in EAE. T cells that can transfer EAE have been shown to express high levels of TNF and treatment of animals primed to develop EAE with neutralizing antibodies to TNFα and β, or with drugs known to block their release, has been shown to inhibit disease expression (Ruddle *et al.*, 1990; Selmaj, Raine and Cross, 1991). Interestingly, this effect correlates most closely with reduced inflammation in the CNS and with down-regulation of VCAM-1 expression on the CNS vasculature, supporting an important role for these cytokines as mediators of inflammation (Barten and Ruddle, 1994). Transgenic animals overexpressing TNFα in the CNS show spontaneous inflammatory demyelinating lesions that are accompanied by severe clinical deficits, eventually leading to death of the animal (Probert *et al.*, 1995).

IL-1 is thought to contribute to immune-mediated tissue injury by initiating inflammation, by activating other leukocytes (or glia) to produce cytokines, and by acting synergistically with cyto-kines such as TNFα and IFNγ. Injection of IL-1 into the CNS results in the induction of an inflam-matory response, reflecting in part the upregula-tion of various adhesion molecules on activated endothelial cells, as well as the induction of chemokines by perivascular cells including astro-cytes (reviewed by Brosnan *et al.*, 1992). In tissue culture studies, IL-1 has been shown to be a key cytokine involved in astrocyte activation, inducing the expression of various proinflammatory cyto-kines such as TNFα and IL-6, as well reactive nitrogen species (Lee *et al.*, 1995). In animals sensi-tized to develop EAE, injection of IL-1 has been shown to exacerbate disease whereas administra-tion of the soluble IL-1 receptor antagonist ame-liorated disease (Mannie *et al.*, 1987).

Chemokines are low molecular weight secreted proteins, that frequently possess structural motifs indicating that they bind to the extracellular matrix (Glabinski *et al.*, 1995). They have gener-ated much interest because of their ability to attract and activate specific subsets of leukocytes. So, for example, it has been shown that monocyte chemoattractant peptide-1 (MCP-1) specifically attracts monocytes and not neutrophils, and the closely related proteins macrophage inflammatory proteins 1α and1β have been shown to attract CD4 or CD8 expressing T cells depending on the memory phenotype of the cells involved, the rela-tive concentrations of these chemokines within the inflammatory milieu, and the presence of other proinflammatory cytokines. The receptors for chemokines, which are characterized by the pres-ence of seven transmembrane spanning domains, have been shown to be restricted on T cells to the activated or memory phenotype and to be upregu-lated on these cells by cytokines such as IL-2 (MacKay, 1996). Studies in EAE have shown that a tight temporal correlation exists between the lev-els of MCP-1 and clinical evidence of disease. In mice the primary site of expression appears to be in reactive astrocytes (Ransohoff *et al.*, 1993), whereas in rats, endothelial cells and perivascular macrophages have been found to be the initial sites of protein expression (Berman *et al.*, 1996). These factors can be rapidly induced in numerous cell types following exposure to the proinflamma-tory cytokines, particularly IFNγ, IL-1β and TNFα.

The fact that chemokines may represent a promis-ing target for therapeutic intervention has been supported by the observation that in the mouse model of EAE, antibodies against macrophage inflammatory protein-1α have been found to sig-nificantly protect animals against disease (Karpus *et al.*, 1995).

EAE has also been used to test whether anti-bodies directed at various adhesion molecules have the potential to be used as an effective therapeutic tool. At the height of clinical disease increased expression of ICAM-1, VCAM-1 and the high endothelial cell marker MECA-325 has been clearly documented on involved vessels, and their ligands LFA-1 and VLA-4 have been noted on inflammatory cells in the lesion, with kinetics that correlate well with clinical expression of disease (Cannella *et al.*, 1990; O'Neill *et al.*, 1991). How-ever, although antibodies to VLA-4 and to ICAM-1 and/or LFA-1 have proved effective in inhibit-ing disease in some studies, others have found that treatment with anti-ICAM-1 may lead to exacer-bation of disease (Yednock *et al.*, 1992; Canella *et al.*, 1993, reviewed by Brosnan *et al.*, 1997). Although the reasons for these discrepancies remain unclear at the present time, it is likely that they reflect differences in the dosage of antibody used. Taken together the results support a pivotal role for VLA-4 expression on T cells in order to gain access to the CNS. However, additional stud-ies have shown that the signal used to elicit T cell activation may significantly affect which adhesion-ligand pathway is used in the extravasation step.

Response of the BBB to inflammatory mediators

To address the question of whether the CNS vas-culature is altered in its response to proinflamma-tory cytokines, several laboratories have studied the effect of injecting cytokines such as TNFα, IL-1β or IFNγ into the CNS. The results strongly sup-port the conclusion that the nature of the inflam-matory response that ensues is dependent upon the specific areas of the CNS examined. If the injection sites include the meninges, ventricles or retina then the nature of the inflammatory res-ponse resembles that found in the systemic vasculature (reviewed by Brosnan *et al.*, 1992). If, however, the injection is made into the cerebral gray matter (hippocampus), then the response is altered both in its kinetics (proceeding more slowly in the CNS parenchyma) and in the nature of the cellular profile involved (consisting almost exclusively of mononuclear cells with few if any neutrophils) (Perry *et al.*, 1995). Although the mechanisms involved are not known at the present time, it is intriguing to note that astrocytic investment of blood vessels is more complete within the CNS parenchyma than it is at the other sites, suggesting that these cells may regulate inflammatory events occurring at the BBB (see also below). Of note here, however, in the context of MS is the observation that early lesions most frequently involve periventricular sites and the optic nerve head, supporting the conclusion that specific vascular beds within the CNS are particularly vulnerable to inflammation.

Further evidence for the specific vulnerability of different vascular beds within the CNS to inflammation has come from EAE. In the various animal models that have been studied, lesion distribution shows both an antigen- and species-specific variability. In the classic EAE models induced by sensitization to myelin antigens, lesions are predominantly found in the lumbar and cervical regions of the spinal cord, the optic nerve and brainstem, but the actual distribution of the lesions within the cord parenchyma differs depending on the species used. For example, in the Lewis rat the lesions frequently occur at the gray–white matter border whereas in the mouse inflammation is almost exclusively submeningeal in distribution. Factors that may be critical in determining the vulnerability of a particular vascular bed to inflammation include the distribution of vasoactive amines, sources of chemokines and/or lymphatic drainage pathways (Weller *et al.*, 1996). Interestingly, the susceptibility of a vascular bed to inflammation can be altered by trauma, even if the trauma does not occur in the immediate vicinity of the vessels affected but involves the neuronal tracts that terminate at those sites. Activation of microglia within the affected tissues is thought to contribute to this response (Williams *et al.*, 1994).

Another relevant area that has been addressed is whether there are adhesion molecules that are specific for the CNS. In the systemic circulation it has been shown that lymphocyte homing to peripheral lymphoid organs is mediated by tissue-specific 'addressins' present on high endothelial venules. It has also been suggested that during immune surveillance memory T cells may become 'imprinted' in such a way that they return to the tissues in which they first encountered antigen (Mackay, 1991). However, no evidence for brain-specific addressins has so far been detected in any of the studies that have investigated this question.

Regulation of inflammatory events in the CNS

In addition to cytokines that promote inflammation, it is now well recognized that there are other cytokines that down-regulate inflammation. These include transforming growth factor (TGF)-β, IL-10 and IL-4 as well as members of the type 1 IFNs, especially IFNβ. A principal mechanism involved in the anti-inflammatory properties of at least some of these cytokines is their down-regulatory effects on the activation of endothelial cells and macrophages (reviewed by Miller and Karpus, 1994).

TGFβ belongs to a large family of proteins with pleiotropic effects. Many of these are inhibitory to an immune response and include inhibition of lymphocyte activation and proliferation, down-regulation of macrophage activation, down-regulation of leukocyte adhesion to activated endothelial cells, and a decrease in the generation of cytotoxic lymphocytes. Because of its immunosuppressive activities, several groups have tested the effect of this cytokine in several autoimmune models. In EAE, TGFβ has been shown to be an effective inhibitor of disease expression, decreasing both the incidence and severity of the disease and inhibiting clinical relapses in animals with established disease (reviewed by Brosnan *et al.*, 1997). This regulatory activity has not been found to be specific for the CNS since TGFβ also effectively inhibits development of various forms of experimental arthritis, but the constitutive presence of TGFβ within the CNS has been implicated in the immunologically privileged status of the CNS environment (see also below). However, its role in inflammation remains controversial since both immunosuppressive and proinflammatory effects have been noted. In experiments that have specifically addressed the effect of TGFβ on inflammation in the CNS, it has been found to be an effective inhibitor of cellular inflammation, whereas effects on vascular permeability were found to be more complex. When administered into the systemic circulation TGFβ inhibited increases in vascular permeability (Pfister *et al.*, 1992). However, if given into the CNS (Cuff *et al.*, 1996*b*), or produced there by transgenic technology (Wyss-Coray *et al.*, 1995), then increases in vascular permeability have been noted. Leukocyte infiltration and increased vascular permeability are thought to be closely linked and studies that reduce leukocyte infiltration usually lead to decreases in vascular permeability. However, inflammation and vascular permeability were also found to be dissociated in a study of contact hypersensitivity in a P-selectin deficient mouse (Subramanian *et al.*, 1995). In EAE endogenous TGFβ secretion has been implicated in the recovery process and in disease suppression mediated by various tolerizing protocols (see Hafler and Weiner, 1995). TGFβ has been shown to be secreted by peripheral blood lymphocytes isolated from MS patients when either in remission or while symptoms were resolving (Beck *et al.*, 1991). Ongoing clinical trials are examining whether TGFβ may have immunosuppressive properties in patients with MS.

IL-4 and IL-10 have also been found to downregulate disease activity in animals sensitized to develop EAE, and increased levels of these cytokines have generally been found to correlate with later stages of the disease, as animals enter the recovery phase. IL-4 is primarily released by CD4$^+$ lymphocytes belonging to the Th2 subset and has been shown to downregulate the release of IL-12, a cytokine that is critical for the induction of a Th1-response. Since Th1 and Th2 lymphocytes appear to cross-regulate one another, this has led to the suggestion that increased expression of Th2-type cytokines may correlate with lesion regression and repair (see Brosnan *et al.* 1997). IL-10 has also been shown to be a potent inhibitor of activated macrophages, counteracting the effects of IFNγ. The extent to which these cytokines affect events occurring at the BBB has not been well defined, although treatment with IL-4 has been shown to lead to significant reduction in inflammation in the CNS, and IL-10 has been localized to astrocytic foot-processes in the normal CNS (Cannella and Raine, 1995). However, the effects of both of these cytokines are complex and inhibitory and stimulatory responses have been noted.

Inflammatory events have also been shown to be inhibited by soluble forms of both adhesion molecules and cytokine receptors that are either shed from activated cells or produced by alternative splicing of the mRNA (Burger and Dayer, 1995). These soluble factors are able to interact with their respective ligands and thus compete with membrane receptors. The efficiency with which this is achieved appears to reflect the relative affinities of the molecules involved for their specific ligands. In EAE, the IL-1 receptor antagonist and the soluble type I TNF receptor have been shown to be particularly effective inhibitors (Selmaj and Raine, 1995). It has also been suggested that the release of untethered chemokines into the circulation may serve to down-regulate the inflammatory response by interfering with the blood to tissue concentration gradient required for translocation across the vascular wall.

IFNβ is another cytokine that appears to directly affect events occurring at the BBB. In MS patients, MRI studies have shown that treatment with IFNβ leads to a rapid and dramatic reduction in enhancing lesions, suggesting that IFNβ, at least temporarily, inhibits the opening of the BBB (Stone *et al.*, 1995). Experiments *in vitro* also support a role for this cytokine in blocking endothelial cell activation mediated by proinflammatory cytokines (Huynh *et al.*, 1995). Currently, IFNβ is one of the few accepted modes of therapy for MS and has shown clinical efficacy particularly in the early phases of the disease process.

Cytokines and adhesion molecules in MS

To study the expression of cytokines, chemokines and adhesion molecule expression in MS and possible relationships to disease progression, two general approaches have been used. In one, peripheral blood and CSF samples have been studied for evidence of cytokines and soluble adhesion molecules at different stages of the disease process. In the other, immunohistochemistry and *in situ* hybridization procedures have been used to characterize the cell types expressing cytokines in the lesion at varying time in the disease process, and to correlate cytokine expression with adhesion molecules known to be involved in leukocyte trafficking.

As discussed above, following activation with proinflammatory cytokines, endothelial cells upregulate a wide range of adhesion molecules on their luminal surface. These adhesion molecules are equally rapidly shed, thus their presence within the circulation can be used as markers of recent, or ongoing, activation. Several groups have now reported increased levels of ICAM-1 in MS patients during exacerbation of the disease, which are associated with enhancing lesions by MRI (Rieckman *et al.*, 1994). Reductions were noted during remission or following high dose corticosteroid treatment (Tsukada *et al.*, 1993). Similarly, circulating VCAM-1 and L-selectin levels have also been found to be elevated during active disease, again correlating well with increased permeability of the BBB, as determined by gadolinium-enhanced MRI. These data support a role for increased adhesion molecule expression in disease progression (reviewed by Hartung *et al.*, 1995). Although many different cell types have been shown to express these markers, their presence within the circulation most probably reflects an endothelial cell source.

With respect to cytokines, several studies have now shown increased levels of interleukin-2, TNFα and IFNγ production from mitogen-stimulated peripheral blood mononuclear cells in patients with MS that correlate with attacks (Sharief and Hentges, 1991). Elevated levels of TNFα have also been detected in the CSF and peripheral blood of MS patients, with increasing levels correlating with lesion activity as determined by MRI, and increasing levels of IL-10 correlating with disease remission (see Miller and Karpus, 1994).

In tissues taken at autopsy, immunoreactivity for TNFα has been found at high levels in macrophages in the lesion center and on microglia outside of the lesion, and a few hypertrophic astrocytes, in acute active lesions. In adjacent normal appearing white matter, focal immunoreactivity for TNFα was frequently seen around blood vessels. Semi-quantitative analysis of cytokine expression in lesions of different ages, however, has suggested that TNFα levels may actually be higher in chronic-active lesions, correlating with high-level expression of the adhesion molecules VCAM-1 and VLA-4 (Hofmann *et al.*, 1989; Cannella and Raine, 1995). In lesions characterized by both inflammation and demyelination, *in situ* hybridization studies have shown that TNFα and IL-6 are the most widely and intensely expressed cytokines (Woodroofe and Cuzner, 1993). Taken together, these studies strongly support an important role for TNF as a mediator of the inflammatory process in MS.

Another cytokine that is expressed at high levels by invading inflammatory cells in the MS lesion is IL-6. This cytokine is a potent inducer of the acute phase response, constituting a rapid and general reaction against injury. IL-6, therefore, can also be found in the CNS of a number of disorders associated with traumatic incidents of varying kinds and antibodies to this cytokine have been shown to protect animals against EAE. In MS lesions in which both inflammation and demyelination were widespread, IL-6 was present at high levels in virtually all perivascular leukocytes, suggesting an important role for this cytokine in endothelial cell activation (Woodroofe and Cuzner, 1993).

In MS lesions, IL-1 is prominently expressed by macrophages in the lesion center as well as on microglia at the lesion edge. Levels of immunoreactivity were generally highest in acute lesions, remained high in chronic-active lesions, but were considerably lower in chronic silent lesions. IL-1 could also be detected in macrophages and microglia in autopsy tissues from other neurological diseases with prominent inflammatory infiltrates, but was essentially absent in non-inflamed areas of the brain, as well as in normal control tissues (Cannella and Raine, 1995).

Analysis of immunoreactivity for IL-4 in different types of MS lesions has shown high levels of reactivity in both acute and chronic active lesions. Expression was found predominantly at the edge of the lesion in association with small lymphocytes, microglial cells and foamy macrophages. Levels were generally lower in non-inflammatory lesions, but immunoreactivity for IL-4 could be found in all control tissues. High levels of

TGFβ were also found in acute MS lesions, particularly in association with the extracellular matrix around blood vessels. At these same locations, immunoreactivity for IL-10 was found exclusively on astrocytes with the astrocytic endfoot processes being particularly heavily stained. Interestingly, in CNS tissues taken at autopsy from non-neurological conditions, where evidence for proinflammatory cytokines was rare, reactivity for TGFβ and IL-10 was readily discernible in association with blood vessels, supporting the notion that these cytokines are involved in regulating immune responses occurring at the blood–brain barrier (Cannella and Raine, 1995).

To examine potential correlation between cytokine expression in the lesion and leukocyte trafficking to the CNS, several studies have examined MS lesions for expression of various families of adhesion molecules and their respective ligands. In normal brain tissue, these molecules were rarely detected or expressed constitutively at very low levels. However, in autopsy tissues, widespread expression of ICAM-1 on endothelial cells, and to a lesser extent on astrocytes, has been noted in the lesion, as well as in the immediate vicinity of the lesioned areas of the brain. In these same areas, immunoreactivity for LFA-1, the ligand for ICAM-1, has been found on most infiltrating leukocytes, as well as on a few microglia. Interestingly, as noted previously, expression of VCAM-1 on endothelial cells, and its ligand VLA-4 on leukocytes, was detected at higher levels in more chronic lesions, coincident with higher expression of TNFα (Brosnan et al., 1995; Cannella and Raine, 1995). As noted earlier, an important role for the VCAM-1/VLA-4 pathway was reported by Barten and Ruddle (1994) in their studies on the effect of antibodies against LT/TNF in the mouse model of EAE.

As might be expected, these adhesion molecule patterns have not been found to be specific for MS, and other inflammatory diseases, as well as to some extent non-inflammatory conditions, may also express quite significant levels of these adhesion molecules, particularly VCAM-1, on CNS elements. However, while VLA-4 expression was generally restricted to inflammatory cells in MS and other inflammatory conditions, in more chronic silent lesions, as well as in non-inflammatory CNS

disorders in which VCAM-1 was expressed, increased expression of VLA-4 was predominantly found on microglia. These results indicate, therefore, that endothelial cell activation is likely to be an important mechanism in disease expression in MS.

Edema formation in the CNS

One of the most serious consequences of inflammation in the CNS is the formation of edema and associated alterations in blood flow. Studies in EAE with various tracers, as well as ultrastructural morphometric studies, have demonstrated that leakage of serum proteins into the CNS parenchyma may occur by several different routes that include altered permeability of tight junctions, increased transcytotic transport and contraction of endothelial cells. In the venular bed these changes are closely associated with the perivascular transit of inflammatory cells, which migrate into the CNS via a transendothelial route as well as via a paracellular route (Figs. 42.1 and 42.2). Several studies have shown that attachment and migration of inflammatory cells occurs most frequently in the immediate vicinity of the junctional complex of veins and venules (Faustmann and Dermietzel, 1985; Lossinsky et al., 1989). Interestingly, studies in EAE have suggested that different subsets of inflammatory cells may follow different migratory pathways. Polymorphonuclear cells appear to migrate principally via the junctional complex whereas lymphocytes appear to induce the formation of channels or pores across the junctional complex. Macrophages have been frequently noted to migrate using a process resembling emperipolesis (Fig. 42.2). In these inflamed areas, the junctional complex has been found to be permeable to tracers which, using goniometer stage electron microscopy, can be seen to permeate throughout the junctional cleft. Thus, it seems that factors released by inflammatory cells can damage the junctional arrays making them more permeable to vascular solutes. In culture, this has been observed in endothelial cells exposed to TNFα and IFNγ (Rival et al., 1996).

Occasionally, interendothelial junctional arrays may be split apart by the direct action of inflam-

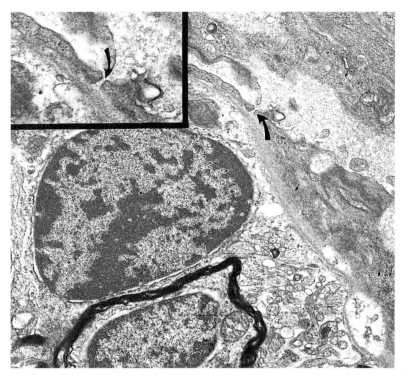

Fig. 42.3. Electron micrograph of an inflamed venule from a patient with acute MS. The curved arrow points to an interendothelial cell junction that has been split apart by the inflammatory process. Note also the large number of transcytotic vesicles present in the endothelial cells (small arrows). ×13 000, inset ×30 000.

matory cells. In these cases, the interendothelial space is widened forming a gap through which cells and blood solutes can penetrate into the CNS parenchyma. This has been observed both in EAE and MS (see Fig. 42.3), and is thought to be one of the mechanisms by which non-activated leukocytes gain access to the CNS compartment. Studies with other tight epithelia indicate that inflammatory cells can alter the permeability of the tight junctions by the release of proteolytic enzymes, factors that lead to alterations in Ca^{2+} flux, changes in the level of cAMP, and through reorganization of the cytoskeleton (reviewed by Brosnan *et al.*, 1992). An important role for proteases in mediating alterations in vascular permeability in the CNS has been demonstrated with intracerebral injection, particularly with enzymes that degrade the extracellular matrix (Rosenberg *et al.*, 1996) and by the ability of inhibitors of both metallo- and neutral proteases to reduce the severity of EAE in the Lewis rat (reviewed by Brosnan *et al.*, 1997).

In addition to these changes noted in inflamed veins, ultrastructural studies have detected changes in the normal morphological attributes of brain capillaries (characterized as having a diameter of 7 to 10 μm). In addition to the presence of tight junctions, endothelial cells of the BBB are characterized by a low level of endocytotic vesicles and a high content of mitochondria (Fig. 42.4). It has been suggested that these mitochondria provide the energy required to maintain the energy-dependent transport mechanisms that are also characteristic of the BBB. Studies in EAE, and to some extent in MS, have shown that as clinical disease progresses the mitochondrial content of the endothelial cells falls and the vesicular content rises such that at the height of disease the brain capillaries acquire the morphological attributes of those found in the systemic circulation (Fig. 42.4). As the animals recover, normal values for CNS capillaries are restored (Claudio *et al.*, 1989; Hawkins *et al.*, 1991). These data suggest, therefore, that during

A. Rat

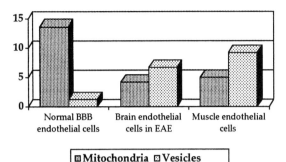

☒ **Mitochondria** ☐ **Vesicles**

B. Human

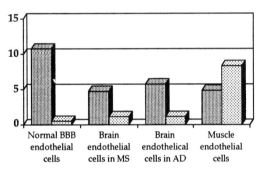

Fig. 42.4. Blood brain barrier endothelial cells lose their high mitochondrial content and acquire increased levels of vesicles during inflammation in rats with EAE, and in humans with MS and Alzheimer dementia. The values obtained for these parameters resemble those found in muscle endothelial cells which do not have a BBB. The data are expressed as the percentage of endothelial cell area occupied by the respective organelles. (A) Data obtained from rat tissues; (B) data obtained from human biopsy tissues. EAE, experimental autoimmune encephalomyelitis; MS, multiple sclerosis, AD, Alzheimer's disease.

EAE the brain capillaries transiently acquire the permeability properties of the systemic vasculature.

Although these plasmalemmal vesicles, or caveoli, were first identified as participants in an endocytotic process involved in transcytosis, more recent studies have shown that these sites are also actively involved in the concentration and internalization of small molecules, a process referred to as potocytosis. In addition, a variety of molecules known to function in signal transduction pathways have been found to be concentrated in caveolae

(Anderson, 1993). How these pathways are affected by proinflammatory cytokines remains to be determined; however, in the context of changes in vascular permeability it is of interest to note that second messenger systems associated with the response to nitric oxide (NO) have been localized to these sites.

In contrast to changes observed in inflamed veins and venules, these changes in the capillary network are not directly associated with inflammatory cells, but likely reflect the direct effect of inflammatory mediators, or their products, on endothelial cells and/or on vascular blood flow. Additional studies in EAE have suggested that the mitochondrial changes occur first. Although the mechanisms involved in this response remain unclear at the present time, it is known that several inflammatory mediators affect the normal function of mitochondria, perhaps through the generation of free radicals such as NO or reactive oxygen intermediates. In both EAE and MS, lesioned areas of the brain have been shown to contain significant levels of type II NOS, particularly in perivascular locations (reviewed by Brosnan *et al.*, 1995). NO is known to possess potent vasodilatory activity that could contribute to the formation of edema.

Changes in mitochondrial content in BBB endothelium have been described in various conditions. Quantitation of mitochondrial profiles in the aging monkey have shown a marked decrease, suggesting a loss of BBB function in aging (Mooradian, 1988). In epilepsy, it has been found that an increase in capillary mitochondria characterizes brain regions affected with seizures in humans (reviewed by Brosnan *et al.*, 1992). In mice with cerebral malaria, decreases in brain mitochondrial enzyme activity in cerebrovascular endothelium suggest a functional alteration of the BBB, which precedes histochemically detectable lesions (see Chapter 49). The diverse studies mentioned above suggest that BBB, mitochondrial content and enzymatic activity may fluctuate in pathological conditions. In this regard it is interesting to note that defects in mitochondrial function have been associated with MS-like illnesses (Harding, 1991). However, recent genetic analyses of patients with MS have failed to find evidence of a link with known mitochondrial mutations.

Ultrastructural changes related to the disruption of the BBB in MS can also be observed to extend beyond the endothelial cells (Claudio *et al.*, 1995). Perivascular fibrin and collagen deposits have been observed, which are also indicative of an increase in vascular permeability and reorganization of the extracellular matrix. It has also been suggested that the early deposition of fibrin may progress to an occlusive venous thrombosis (reviewed by Williams *et al.*, 1994). Pericytes may also show degenerative changes in MS. These cells have been shown to accumulate serum proteins in EAE and may serve as a secondary cellular barrier when the endothelial cells have been damaged. A similar role for astrocytes has been proposed and swollen astrocytic foot processes are frequently noted around blood vessels in active MS lesions.

Astrogliosis

Any discussion of alterations in BBB function in MS would be remiss without a discussion of the potential contribution of astrocytes to the observed changes. In addition to the loss of myelin, the other most characteristic feature of the MS plaque is the presence of a reactive gliosis. Reactive astrocytes in acute lesions or at the edge of chronic-active lesions display hypertrophy of the cell body (hypertrophic astrocytes), while those at the center of chronic-silent lesions display hypertrophy of their processes (fibrillary astrogliosis). Immunohistochemistry and *in situ* hybridization studies have shown that hypertrophic astrocytes can be a significant source of proinflammatory cytokines such as TNFα and IL-6, as well as potentially down-regulatory cytokines such as TGFβ and IL-10. In addition, growing evidence suggests that reactive astrocytes are a major source of reactive nitrogen intermediates in the lesion (Bo *et al.*, 1994). Because astrocytes *in vitro* can be readily activated by IFNγ to express class II MHC, it has also been suggested that they may perform this function *in vivo*. However, to date it has been difficult to show convincing class II MHC expression on astrocytes in either the normal or the inflamed CNS. Another important role for astrocytes in lesion development may be the production of chemokines such as MCP-1 and IP-10. Astrocytes are also a major

source of components of the clotting cascades, in particular tissue factor, a protease that is the major cellular initiator of the coagulation protease cascade resulting in the activation of thrombin (Eddleston *et al.*, 1993). Thus activation of these factors in reactive astrocytes may protect the brain against cerebral hemorrhage by increased expression of tissue factor, and subsequent induction of thrombin may lead to remodeling of the extracellular matrix.

Many inflammatory lesions release factors that promote angiogenesis and it is likely that new vessel growth is present in MS lesions. Since astrocytes are thought to participate in the induction of BBB function in endothelial cells, it is possible that the presence of a reactive gliosis may hinder this process. One might speculate, therefore, that either gliotic areas of the brain fail to maintain BBB function in CNS endothelial cells, or that new vessel growth into lesioned areas of the brain fails to establish normal BBB function. Although no data are currently available that specifically address this issue, experiments that have addressed the role of astrocytes in the repair of induced demyelinating lesions in the rat have shown that if progenitor-derived astrocytes that possess a phenotype more characteristic of type II astrocytes are transplanted along with oligodendrocytes, then disruption of blood vessels occurs resulting in areas of necrosis. However, if the cell mixture contains type I astrocytes, then lesion repair is enhanced (Franklin and Blakemore, 1995). These aspects of astrocyte–endothelial cell interactions will be important areas to study once the ability to select different populations of astrocytes becomes more feasible.

Conclusions

In conclusion, the data obtained from patients with MS, as well as that gleaned from the various model systems that have been used, strongly support the conclusion that alterations in BBB function are important correlates of disease activity. Strong circumstantial evidence also supports the conclusion that proinflammatory cytokines are the major mediators of endothelial cell activation. The extent to which this injury represents a direct attack on endothelial cells by components of the immune system, however, remains unclear. Deposits of terminal complexes of the complement cascade have been noted around vessels in MS lesions and the development of T cells that are cytotoxic for endothelial cells has been observed *in vitro* (Sedgwick *et al.*, 1990), but morphological evidence for endothelial cell loss or denudation remains rare both in MS and EAE. As noted earlier, however, it is difficult to assess endothelial cell changes in the very early stages of lesion formation. Finally, it should be noted that whilst the most striking alterations in BBB function are found in acute and chronic-active lesions, two recent studies have shown that even in chronic-silent lesions there is evidence for increased permeability of the BBB (Kwon and Prineas, 1994; Claudio *et al.*, 1995), suggesting that there is a low level persistent increase in vascular permeability even in the absence of ongoing inflammation that is not detectable by *in vivo* imaging techniques.

Taken together, the results indicate that therapies that target events occurring at the BBB are likely to significantly ameliorate or halt progression of disease and as such provide a major strategy for ongoing research and treatment in MS.

Acknowledgments

The authors would like to thank their colleagues for their continued support and interest. Supported in part by USPHS grants NS 11920, NS 31919 and NMSS grant 1089.

References

Anderson, R. G. (1993). Caveolae: where incoming and outgoing messengers meet. (Review). *Proc. Natl. Acad. Sci. (USA)*, **90**, 10909–13.

Barten, D. M. and Ruddle, N. H. (1994). Vascular cell adhesion molecule-1 modulation by tumor necrosis factor in experimental allergic encephalomyelitis. *J. Neuroimmunol.*, **51**, 123–134.

Beck, J., Rondot, P., Jullien, P. *et al.*, (1991). TGFβ-like activity produced during regression of exacerbations of multiple sclerosis. *Acta Neurol. Scand.*, **84**, 452–5.

Berman, J. W., Guida, M. P., Warren, J. *et al.* (1996). Localization of monocyte chemoattractant peptide-1 expression in the central nervous system in experimental autoimmune encephalomyelitis and trauma in the rat. *J. Immunol.*, **156**, 3017–23.

Bo, L., Dawson, T. M., Wesselingh, S. *et al.* (1994). Induction of nitric oxide synthase in demyelinating regions of multiple sclerosis brains. *Ann. Neurol.*, **36**, 778–6.

Brosnan, C. F., Cannella, B., Battistini, L. and Raine, C. S. (1995). Cytokine localization in multiple sclerosis lesions: correlation with adhesion molecule expression and reactive nitrogen species. *Neurology*, **45**, S16–21.

Brosnan, C. F., Claudio, L. and Martiney J. A. (1992). The blood–brain barrier during immune responses. *Semin. Neurosci.*, **4**, 193–200.

Brosnan, C. F., Racke, M. K. and Selmaj, K. (1997). An investigational approach to disease therapy in multiple sclerosis. In *Multiple Sclerosis: Clinical and Pathogenetic Basis.*, ed. C. S. Raine, H. F. MacFarland and W. W. Tourtellotte, pp. 325–340. London: Chapman and Hall.

Burger, D. and Dayer, J.-M. (1995). Inhibitory cytokines and cytokine inhibitors. *Neurology*, **45**, S39–S43.

Cannella, B. and Raine, C. S. (1995). The adhesion molecule profile and cytokine profile of multiple sclerosis lesions. *Ann. Neurol.*, **37**, 424–35.

Cannella, B., Cross, A. H. and Raine, C. S. (1990). Upregulation and coexpression of adhesion molecules correlate with relapsing autoimmune demyelination in the central nervous system. *J. Exp. Med*, **172**, 1521–4.

Cannella, B., Cross, A. H. and Raine, C. S. (1993). Anti-adhesion molecule therapy in experimental autoimmune encephalomyelitis. *J. Neuroimmunol.*, **46**, 43–55.

Claudio, L., Kress, Y., Norton, W. T. and Brosnan, C. F. (1989). Increased vesicular transport and decreased mitochondrial content in blood–brain barrier endothelial cells during experimental autoimmune encephalomyelitis. *Am. J. Pathol.*, **135**, 446–63.

Claudio, L., Raine, C. S. and Brosnan C. F. (1995). Evidence of persistent blood–brain barrier abnormalities in chronic-progressive multiple sclerosis. *Acta Neuropathol.*, **90**, 228–238.

Cross, A. (1992). Immune cell traffic control and the central nervous system. *Semin Neurosci.*, **4**, 213–219.

Cuff, C., Berman, J. W. and Brosnan, C. F. (1996a). The ordered array of perivascular macrophages is disrupted by IL-1-induced inflammation in the rabbit retina. *Glia*, **17**, 307–16.

Cuff, C. A., Martiney, J. A., Berman, J. W. and Brosnan, C. F. (1996b). Differential effects of transforming growth factor-β1 on IL-1-induced cellular inflammation and vascular permeability in the rabbit retina. *J. Neuroimmunol.*, **70**, 21–8.

Davie, C. A., Hawkins, C. P., Barker, G. J. *et al.* (1994). Serial proton magnetic resonance spectroscopy in acute multiple sclerosis. *Brain*, **117**, 49–58.

Ebers, G. C., Sadovnick, A. D. and Risch, N. J. (1995). A genetic basis for familial aggregation in multiple sclerosis. *Nature*, **377**, 150–1.

Eddelston, M., de la Torre, J. C., Oldstone, M. B. *et al.* (1993). Astrocytes are the primary source of tissue factor in murine central nervous system. *J. Clin. Invest.*, **92**, 349–58.

Faustmann, P. M. and Dermietzel, R. (1985). Extravasation of polymorphonuclear leukocytes from the cerebral microvasculature. Inflammatory response induced by alpha-bungarotoxin. *Cell Tissue Res.*, **242**, 399–407.

Franklin, R. J. M. and Blakemore, W. F. (1995). Glial cell transplantation and plasticity in the O-2A lineage - implications for CNS repair. *Trends Neurosci.*, **18**, 151–6.

Glabinski, A. R., Tani, M., Aras, S. *et al.* (1995). Regulation and function of central nervous system chemokines. [Review] *Int. J. Dev. Sci.*, **13**, 153–65.

Hafler, D. A. and Weiner, H. L. (1995). Immunological mechanisms and therapy in multiple sclerosis (Review). *Immunol. Rev.*, **144**, 75–107.

Harding, A. E. (1991). Neurological disease and mitochondrial genes. *Trends Neurosci.*, **14**, 132–8.

Harding, A. E., Riordan-Eva, P. and Govan, C. C. (1995). Mitochondrial DNA diseases: genotype and phenotype in Leber's hereditary optic neuropathy. *Muscle & Nerve*, **3**, S82–4.

Hartung, H-P, Archelos, J. J., Zielasek, J. *et al.* (1995). Circulating adhesion molecules and inflammatory mediators in demyelination: a review. *Neurology*, **45**, S22–S32.

Hawkins, C. P., MacKenzie, F., Tofts, P. *et al.* (1991). Patterns of blood–brain barrier breakdown in inflammatory demyelination. *Brain*, **114**, 801–10.

Hickey, W. F. and Kimura, H. (1988). Perivascular microglial cells of the central nervous system are bone marrow-derived and present antigen *in vivo*. *Science*, **239**, 290–2.

Hickey, W. F., Hsu, B. L. and Kimura, H. (1991). T-lymphocyte entry into the central nervous system. *J. Neurosci. Res.*, **28**, 254–60.

Hofman, F. M., Hinton, D. R., Johnson, K. and Merrill, J. E. (1989). Tumor necrosis factor identified in multiple sclerosis brain. *J. Exp. Med.*, **170**, 607–12.

Huynh, H. K., Oger, J. and Dorovini-Zis, K. (1995). Interferon-β downregulates interferon-induced class II MHC molecule expression and morphological changes in primary cultures of human brain microvessel endothelial cells. *J. Neuroimmunol.*, **60**, 63–73.

Karpus, W. J., Lukacs, N. W., McRae, B. L. *et al.* (1995). An important role for the chemokines macrophage inflammatory protein-1α in the pathogenesis of the T cell-mediated autoimmune disease, experimental autoimmune encephalomyelitis. *J. Immunol.*, **155**, 5003–10.

Kwon, E. E. and Prineas, J. W. (1994). Blood–brain barrier abnormalities in long-standing multiple sclerosis lesions. An immunohistochemical study. *J. Neuropath. Exp. Neurol.*, **53**, 625–36.

Lee, S. C., Dickson, D. W. and Brosnan, C. F. (1995). Interleukin-1, nitric oxide and reactive astrocytes. *Brain, Behav. Immun.*, **9**, 345–54.

Lossinsky, L. S, Badmajew, V., Robson, J. A. *et al.* (1989). Sites of egress of inflammatory cells and horseradish peroxidase transport across the blood–brain barrier in a murine model of chronic relapsing experimental allergic encephalomyelitis. *Acta Neuropathol. (Berl.)*, **78**, 359–71.

Mackay, C. R. (1991). T-cell memory: the connection between function, phenotype and migration pathways. *Immunol. Today*, **12**, 189–92.

Mackay, C. R. (1996). Chemokine receptors and T cell chemotaxis. *J. Exp. Med.*, **184**, 799–802.

Mannie, M. D., Dinarello, C. A. and Paterson, P. Y. (1987). Interleukin and myelin basic protein synergistically augment adoptive transfer activity of lymphocytes mediating experimental autoimmune encephalomyelitis in Lewis rats. *J. Immunol.*, **138**, 4229–35.

Miller, S. D. and Karpus W. J. (1994). The immunopathogenesis and regulation of T-cell-mediated demyelinating diseases. *Immunol. Today*, **15**, 356–61.

Mooradian, A. D. (1988). Effect of aging on the blood–brain barrier, [Review] *Neurobiol. Aging*, **9**, 31–9.

O'Neill, J. K., Butter, C. and Baker, D. (1991). Expression of vascular addressins and ICAM-1 by endothelial cells in the spinal cord during chronic-relapsing experimental allergic encephalomyelitis in the Biozzi AB/H mouse. *Immunology*, **72**, 520–5.

Perry, V. H., Bell, M. D., Brown, H. C. and Matyszak, M. K. (1995). Inflammation in the nervous system [Review] *Curr. Opin. Neurobiol.*, **5**, 636–41.

Pfister, H.-W., Frei, K., Ottnad, B. *et al.* (1992). Transforming growth factor β inhibits cerebrovascular changes and brain edema formation in the tumor necrosis factor-independent early phase of experimental pneumococcal meningitis. *J. Exp. Med.*, **176**, 265–8.

Pober, J. S., Gimbrone, M. A., Lapierre, L. A. *et al.*, (1986). Overlapping patterns of activation of human endothelial cells by interleukin-1, tumor necrosis factor and immun interferon. *J. Immunol.*, **137**, 1893–6.

Probert, L., Akassoglou, K., Parparakis, M. *et al.* (1995). Spontaneous inflammatory demyelinating disease in transgenic mice showing central nervous system-specific expression of tumor necrosis factor α. *Proc. Natl. Acad. Sci. (USA)*, **92**, 11294–8.

Raine, C. S. (1990). Demyelinating diseases. In *Textbook of Neuropathology*, 2nd edn, ed. Davis and Robertson, pp. 535–620. Baltimore: Williams and Wilkins.

Ransohoff, R. M., Hamilton, T. A., Tani, M. *et al.* (1993). Astrocyte expression of mRNA encoding cytokines IP-10 and JE/MCP-1 in experimental autoimmune encephalomyelitis. *FASEB J.*, **7**, 592–600.

Rieckman, P., Weichselbraun, I., Albrecht, M. *et al.* (1994). Serial analysis of circulating ICAM-1 in serum and cerebrospinal fluid of patients with active multiple sclerosis. Correlation with TNFα and blood–brain barrier damage. *Neurology*, **44**, 1523–6.

Rival, Y., Del Maschio, A., Rabiet, M. J. *et al.* (1996). Inhibition of platelet endothelial cell adhesion molecule-1 synthesis and leukocyte transmigration in endothelial cells by the combined action of TNF-alpha and IFN-gamma. *J. Immunol.*, **157**, 1233–41.

Rosenberg, G. A., Dencoff, J. E., Correa, N. Jr et al. (1996). Effect of steroids on CSF matrix metalloproteinases in multiple sclerosis: relation to blood–brain barrier injury. *Neurology*, **46**, 1626–32.

Ruddle, N. H., Bergman, C. M., McGrath, M. L., et al., (1990). An antibody to lymphotoxin and tumor necrosis factor prevents transfer of experimental allergic encephalomyelitis. *J. Exp. Med.*, **172**, 1193–1200.

Sedgwick, J. D., Hughes, C. C., Male, D. K., et al. (1990). Antigen-specific damage to brain vascular endothelial cells mediated by encephalitogenic and non-encephalitogenic CD4+ T cell lines in vitro. *J Immunol.*, **145**, 2474–81.

Selmaj, K. and Raine, C. S. (1995). Experimental autoimmune encephalomyelitis: immunotherapy with anti-tumor necrosis factor antibodies and soluble tumor necrosis factor antibodies. *Neurology*, **45**: S44–9.

Selmaj, K., Raine, C. S. and Cross, A. H. (1991). Anti-tumor necrosis factor therapy abrogates autoimmune demyelination. *Ann. Neurol.*, **30**, 694–700.

Sharief, M. K. and Hentges, R. (1991). Association between tumor necorsis factor-α and disease progression in patients with multiple sclerosis. *N. Engl. J. Med.*, **325**, 467–472.

Springer, T. A. (1994). Traffic signals for lymphocyte recirculation and leukocyte emigration: the multistep paradigm. *Cell*, **76**, 301–314.

Steinman, L. (1996). A few autoreactive cells in an autoimmune infiltrate control a vast population of non-specific cells: a tale of smart bombs and infantry [Review]. *Proc. Soc. Acad. Sci. (USA)*, **93**, 2253–6.

Stone, L. A., Frank, J. A., Albert, P. S. et al. (1995). The effect of interferon-β on blood–brain barrier disruptions demonstrated by contrast-enhanced magnetic resonance imaging in relapsing-remitting multiple sclerosis. *Ann. Neurol.*, **37**, 611–9.

Subramaniam, M., Saffaripour, S., Watson, S. R. et al. (1995). Reduced recruitment of inflammatory cells in a contact hypersensitivity response in P-selectin-deficient mice. *J. Exp. Med.*, **181**, 2277–82.

Tsukada, N., Miyaagi, K., Matsuda, M. et al., (1993). Increased levels of circulating ICAM-1 in multiple sclerosis and human T-lymphotropic virus type 1-associated myelopathy. *Ann. Neurol.*, **33**, 591–6.

Ulvestad, E., Williams, K., Bo, L. et al. (1994). HLA class II molecules (HLA-DR, DP, DQ) on cells in the human CNS studied in situ and in vitro. *Immunology*, **82**, 535–41.

Weller, R. O., Engelhardt, B. and Phillips, M. J. (1996). Lymphocyte targeting of the central nervous system: a review of afferent and efferent CNS-immune pathways. *Brain Pathol.*, **6**, 275–88.

Williams, K. C., Ulvestad, E., Hickey, W. F. (1994). Immunology of multiple sclerosis. *Clin. Neurosci.*, **2**, 229–45.

Woodroofe, M. N. and Cuzner, M. L. (1993). Cytokine mRNA expression in inflammatory multiple sclerosis lesions: detection by non-radioactive in situ hybridization. *Cytokine*, **5**, 583–88.

Wyss-Coray, T., Feng, L., Masliah, E. et al. (1995). Increased central nervous system production of extracellular matrix components and development of hydrocephalus in transgenic mice over expressing transforming growth factor β1. *Am. J. Path.*, **147**, 53–7.

Yednock, T. A., Cannon, C., Fritz, L. C. et al. (1992). Prevention of experimental autoimmune encephalomyelitis by antibodies against α4 β1 integrin. *Nature*, **356**, 63–6.

43 Hemostasis and the blood–brain barrier

MARK FISHER

- Introduction
- Tissue factor and the CNS
- Fibrinolysis and the CNS
- The antithrombotic system and the CNS
- Conclusions

Introduction

Hemostasis and the blood–brain barrier (BBB) is a subject of growing interest. This increased emphasis is largely due to the appreciation of the importance of the endothelial cell as a mediator of hemostasis pathways. The unique milieu of brain capillary endothelial cells suggests a potentially important role of the BBB as a regulator of hemostasis. This chapter will provide a brief review of hemostasis pathways, and discuss the current state of knowledge of hemostasis factors and the BBB.

The traditional mode of analysis of the coagulation cascade focuses on distinct 'intrinsic' and 'extrinsic' pathways that lead toward clot formation. That view has gradually shifted to an understanding that is, paradoxically, at once increasingly simple and yet more complex. A current view of the coagulation cascade is shown in Fig. 43.1. Note that there is no distinction between 'intrinsic' and 'extrinsic' pathways; that paradigm is useful for the laboratory analysis of coagulation disorders, but has only limited *in vivo* relevance (Furie and Furie, 1992). Also note that the entire cascade is driven by tissue factor. Finally, it is important to appreciate that this coagulation cascade represents only part of the process regulating clot formation.

The coagulation cascade is initiated by tissue factor, an integral membrane protein expressed by nonvascular cells. The extracellular domain of tissue factor serves as a receptor for Factor VII, and the tissue factor–VIIa complex then activates Factors IX and X (Furie and Furie, 1992). Ultimately, activated factors V and X will, on the membrane surface of activated platelets, convert prothrombin to thrombin (Tracy and Mann, 1986). Thrombin, in turn, generates fibrin monomer (from fibrinogen), which polymerizes to become a cross-linked fibrin clot (Furie and Furie, 1992).

The coagulation cascade is critically regulated by endothelial-dependent anti-thrombotic and fibrinolytic systems. Elements of these systems are represented in the central nervous system. Tissue factor, the primary instigator of the coagulation cascade, is also expressed by the CNS.

Tissue factor and the CNS

Initial studies of tissue factor in brain showed diffuse immunostaining throughout brain parenchyma (Drake *et al.*, 1989; Fleck *et al.*, 1990). The cellular source of brain tissue factor was not identified until Eddleston *et al.* (1993) reported their findings in murine brain. *In situ* hybridization using a tissue

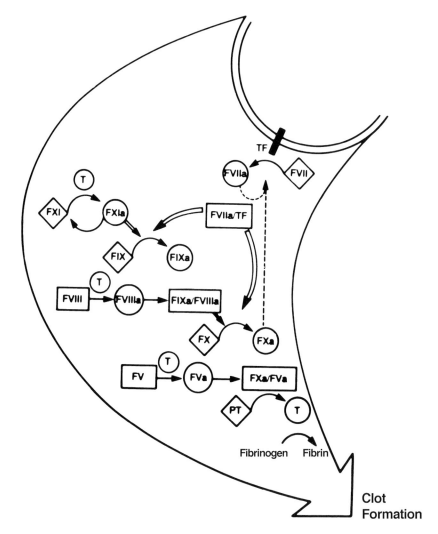

Fig. 43.1. Pathways of blood coagulation. Tissue factor (TF) initiates blood coagulation on the cell surface. Factor VII (FVII) binds to this receptor when plasma comes into contact with tissue factor. The tissue factor-activated factor VII complex activates factors IX (FIX) and X (FX). Feedback mechanisms, such as the conversion of prothrombin (PT) to thrombin (T) or other enzymes (dashed arrows), substantially accelerates blood clotting by proteolytic activation of factor VII to VIIa, factor XI (FXI) to XIa (FXIa), factor VIII (FVIII) to VIIIa (FVIIIa), and factor V (FV) to Va (FVa). This process generates fibrin, which polymerizes to form fibrin clot. Open arrows indicate enzymatic action on substrates; narrow solid arrows indicate conversion of protein from one functional state to another after peptide bond cleavage. (From Furie and Furie (1992), reprinted by permission of *The New England Journal of Medicine*, Massachusetts Medical Society).

factor probe showed hybridization that co-localized with the astrocyte marker glial fibrillary acidic protein (GFAP). Astrocytes of gray matter, including astrocyte endfeet surrounding the vasculature, were the primary source of brain tissue factor along with arachnoid cells; tissue factor was not definitely seen in microglia, neurons, oligodendrocytes, or endothelial cells. Moreover, both human and murine astrocyte cell lines expressed functional tissue factor protein (Eddleston *et al.*, 1993).

The significance of these findings can best be understood by reference to the 'hemostatic envelope' theory of tissue factor expression. Drake *et al.* (1989) demonstrated tissue factor in adventitia (rather than endothelia) of blood vessels and in fibrous capsules surrounding organs. This distribution suggests a 'barrier' function for tissue factor, in which organs are surrounded by a protective wall of tissue factor in order to prevent catastrophic hemorrhage.

Tissue factor localization to astrocytes, particularly astrocyte foot processes surrounding brain microvessels, suggests that tissue factor in the brain also functions as a 'hemostatic envelope'. It has been suggested that endothelia, of brain and other organs, may also have this function; *in vitro* studies show endothelial expression of tissue factor following stimulation by endotoxin and inflammatory cytokines interleukin-1 and tumor necrosis factor (Drake *et al*, 1993). These findings have not been duplicated *in vivo*. Thus, the hemostatic barrier within the brain appears to be largely dependent on astrocytes at the blood–brain barrier.

Some implications of this CNS localization of tissue factor have been described in a primate stroke model (Okada *et al.*, 1994). Following transient middle cerebral artery occlusion, intravascular fibrin deposition occurs in regions of extensive ischemic injury. Treatment with an anti-tissue factor monoclonal antibody demonstrated that this fibrin deposition is substantially mediated by tissue factor. Immunohistochemistry demonstrated perivascular tissue factor, probably expressed by astrocytes. It is likely that under ischemic conditions, endothelial injury exposes the hemostatic envelope, with tissue factor at the blood–brain barrier generating fibrin. Post-ischemia microvascular obstructions thus appear to be due in part to tissue factor at the blood–brain barrier.

Fibrinolysis and the CNS

Endothelial cells regulate thrombus formation in part by production of plasminogen activators. Plasminogen activators are serine proteases that have an important role in the dissolution of fibrin clot (i.e., fibrinolysis). Plasminogen activators convert the zymogen plasminogen into plasmin, the active protease that degrades fibrin. Two types of plasminogen activators have been described: tissue-

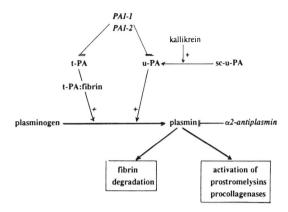

Fig. 43.2. The plasminogen activation system. Inhibitors are in italics. PA: plasminogen activator; t-PA: tissue-type PA; u-PA: urokinase-type PA; sc-u-PA: single-chain u-PA; PAI: PA inhibitor. + is activation; − is inhibition. (From Maragoudakis *et al.* (1994), p. 172, with permission).

type plasminogen activator (t-PA) and urokinase-type plasminogen activator (u-PA) (Fig. 43.2) (van Hinsbergh *et al.*, 1996).

In the absence of fibrin, t-PA is a poor enzyme. Both t-PA and plasminogen adsorb to fibrin, forming a ternary complex; in the presence of fibrin, the catalytic activity of t-PA is markedly enhanced (Lijnen and Collen, 1995). u-PA is synthesized as a single chain molecule (scu-PA), and is proteolytically cleaved to two chain u-PA (tcu-PA). tcu-PA is at least 20 times more effective as a plasminogen activator than scu-PA; the latter, however has fibrin specificity while tcu-PA does not (Lijnen and Collen, 1995).

The functional activity of t-PA and u-PA is determined by the interaction between the plasminogen activators and plasminogen activator inhibitors, as well as cellular receptors and matrix proteins. Plasminogen activator inhibitor-1 (PAI-1) and, to a lesser extent, plasminogen activator inhibitor-2 (PAI-2), both members of the serpin (serine protease inhibitor) superfamily, are the most important inhibitors of t-PA and u-PA. Endothelial cells have high-affinity binding sites for t-PA, u-PA, and plasminogen; of these, the u-PA receptor is the best characterized (van Hinsbergh *et al.*, 1996).

It is generally accepted that clot lysis *in vivo* is, in the systemic circulation, primarily dependent on t-PA; u-PA appears to be more important for peri-cellular proteolytic processes, including tissue remodeling and tumor invasion (Bachman, 1987). *In vitro* data using human umbilical vein endothelial cells demonstrate that induced release of u-PA is polar, with secretion primarily at the basolateral side. In contrast, induced release of t-PA shows no such polarity (van Hinsbergh *et al.*, 1990). Moreover, endothelium-derived urokinase has an important role in CNS angiogenesis (Rao *et al.*, 1996). These findings support the concept that u-PA function is directed toward tissue modeling.

Several lines of evidence suggest that fibrinolysis in the CNS microcirculation has distinctive features. Shatos and colleagues studied t-PA and u-PA expression in early-passage human brain-microvascular endothelial cells. In response to alpha-thrombin, brain endothelial cells showed extensive upregulation of u-PA mRNA and protein while exhibiting no significant change in t-PA expression. In contrast, systemic large and small vessel endothelial cells showed enhanced t-PA expression but little change in u-PA (Shatos *et al.*, 1995). A study of the distribution of t-PA *in vivo* showed complete absence of t-PA in large-vessel endothelia of non-human primates (Levin and del Zoppo, 1994); t-PA was found in adventitial vaso vasorum. A survey of brain vessels showed limited immunoreactivity for t-PA; only 3% of vessels were reactive for t-PA. Moreover, 90% of brain vessels exhibiting t-PA reactivity were arterioles and venules; only 3% of the t-PA reactive vessels were capillaries, despite capillaries representing nearly 40% of vessels sampled. Taken together, these *in vitro* and *in vivo* data suggest that brain capillaries have restricted expression of t-PA.

PAI-1, a rapid inhibitor of both t-PA and u-PA, is perhaps the primary regulator of plasminogen activation *in vivo* (Loskutoff *et al.*, 1993). PAI-1 is expressed by endothelial cells *in vitro* and *in vivo*, and is exclusively responsible for plasminogen activator inhibition in plasma (Loskutoff *et al.*, 1993; van Hinsbergh *et al.*, 1996). PAI-2, in contrast, is primarily expressed intracellulary (Bachman, 1995). Another inhibitor of urokinase (as well as plasmin and thrombin) is protease nexin-1; in the CNS, protease nexin-1 is found in astrocyte foot processes and is believed to be an important regulator of injury-related processes (Cunningham *et al.*, 1993).

Most studies of PAI-1 in brain have focused on its increased expression in neoplasms; PAI-1 mRNA has virtually no expression in normal human brain (Yamamoto *et al.*, 1994). Cell culture studies have shown (a) expression of PAI-1 by astrocytes (Kalderon *et al.*, 1990), and (b) downregulation of PAI-1 mRNA and, to a lesser extent, protein, produced by elevated glucose (Kollros *et al.*, 1994); neither of these findings have been confirmed *in vivo*. PAI-2 expression by human microglia has been demonstrated using immunocytochemistry (Akiyama *et al.*, 1993).

Zlokovic and colleagues have begun to delineate the relationship between brain t-PA and stroke. Because exogenous t-PA improves outcome in patients with acute stroke (National Institute of Neurological Disorders and Stroke, 1995), this issue is important. In rat brain, t-PA mRNA and protein are localized to microvascular endothelium (Zlokovic *et al.*, 1995). In the presence of either of two important stroke risk factors, diabetes or nicotine treatment (mimicking the effects of smoking), t-PA is substantially downregulated. In a streptozotocin-induced diabetes model, both t-PA and mRNA and protein are reduced; the latter was found to be completely depleted (Kittaka *et al.*, 1996). Subcutaneous ingestion of nicotine for two weeks completely depleted t-PA protein (Wang *et al.*, 1997). The importance of these findings was shown following transient (one hour) middle cerebral artery occlusion; infarct size increased by 36–41%. These findings thus demonstrate an association between expression of t-PA at the blood–brain barrier and neurological outcome in a large-vessel stroke model.

The antithrombotic system and the CNS

The major components of the antithrombotic (clot prevention) system are antithrombin-III, thrombomodulin, and the tissue factor pathway inhibitor. Antithrombin-III is a protease scavenger and an important inhibitor of thrombin, activated factor X, and other enzymes of the coagulation cascade

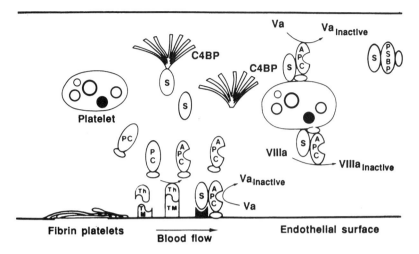

Fig 43.3. Function and formation of activated protein C. Thrombin (Th) formed within the vessel complexes with thrombomodulin (TM) on the endothelial surface. Protein C (PC) is converted to activated protein C (APC) by the TM–Th complex. Protein S (PS) circulates as free PS and as PS reversibly bound to C4b binding protein (C4BP). APC-free PS complex inactivates factors Va and VIIIa. (Reprinted with permission from Esmon (1987). Copyright 1987 American Association for the Advancement of Science.)

(Furie and Furie, 1992; Isaka *et al.*, 1994). Tissue factor pathway inhibitor is a direct inhibitor of factor Xa and produces feedback inhibition of the tissue factor/factor VIIa complex. Tissue factor pathway inhibitor appears to be largely produced by endothelia (Broze, 1995), and its distribution in the brain is not known.

Antithrombin-III is synthesized by the liver and binds to anticoagulantly active heparan sulfate proteoglycans produced by endothelial cells. Anticoagulantly active heparan sulfate proteoglycans, representing no more than 10% of the total heparan sulfate proteoglycans, is concentrated in the extracellular matrix and is present to only a minor extent on the vascular endothelial surface (de Agostini *et al.*, 1990). Antithrombin III immunoreactivity has been demonstrated in human brain capillaries. In brain, antithrombin III appears to have both a luminal and intracytoplasmic localization (Isaka *et al.*, 1994). Antithrombin III protein is produced by human astrocytes *in vivo* (Des-chepper *et al.*, 1991). However, *in vivo* brain antithrombin III appears to be limited to vascular endothelia (Isaka *et al.*, 1994).

Thrombomodulin is an endothelial integral membrane protein that binds the normally procoagulant thrombin; the thrombomodulin–thrombin complex activates protein C (Fig. 43.3), a crucial circulating anticoagulant that has a major role in preventing thrombosis. Both systemic venous and cerebral venous thromboses are linked to resistance to the effects of activated protein C (Svensson and Dahlback, 1994; Martinelli *et al.*, 1996). Circulating activated protein C levels are reduced in patients with ischemic stroke (Macko *et al.*, 1996), and blockade of activated protein C produces impaired cardiac outcome in a large vessel coronary occlusion model (Snow *et al.*, 1991).

A number of investigative groups have studied thrombomodulin expression by the brain. Ishii *et al.* first reported absence of thrombomodulin in human brain microvessels (Ishii *et al.*, 1986). This was a striking observation, given the abundance of thrombomodulin, and the ease of its demonstration, in other vascular beds. Later groups were able to demonstrate presence of thrombomodulin in human brain, albeit with some difficulty (Boffa *et al.*, 1991; Wong *et al.*, 1991; Isaka *et al.*, 1994; Maruno *et al.*, 1994). Taken together, these observations indicate restricted expression of thrombomodulin by human brain microvessels.

Recent work by Tran and colleagues has shed some light on restricted expression of brain thrombomodulin (Tran *et al.*, 1996). Capillary-like

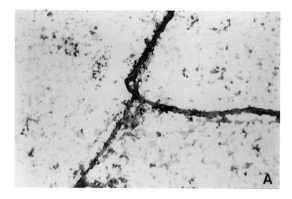

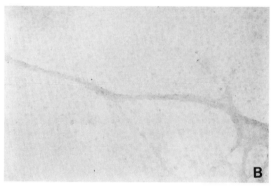

Fig. 43.4. *In situ* hybridization of thrombomodulin mRNA by bovine brain capillary endothelial cells, monolayers and capillary-like structures, *in vitro*. Antisense (A) probe demonstrated thrombomodulin TM mRNA expression, while no thrombomodulin expression was detected using the sense probe (B). (From Tran *et al.* 1996, with permission.)

structures, derived from bovine brain endothelia, demonstrated thrombomodulin mRNA (Fig. 43.4). However, thrombomodulin mRNA concentration was (a) regulated by astrocytes *in vitro*, and

(b) vastly diminished in astrocyte-endothelial co-cultures exhibiting elements of the blood–barrier phenotype. These findings suggest an important role for astrocytes at the blood–brain barrier in the regulation of brain expression of thrombomodulin.

Conclusions

The brain has traditionally been viewed as a passive receptacle for thrombi originating elsewhere. There is growing evidence that this view is overly simplistic, and that the brain has unique hemostatic regulatory capacities residing at the blood–brain barrier. Tissue factor, the primary generator of the coagulation cascade, is expressed by astrocyte foot processes. Expression of brain capillary tissue plasminogen activator, the key fibrinolytic protein, appears to be distinctive in comparison to both systemic endothelia and endothelia of larger vessels in the brain. Thrombomodulin, an important antithrombotic molecule, has restricted brain capillary expression, perhaps due to effects of astrocytes. The importance of the unique hemostasis system of the brain appears to be particularly relevant to the pathophysiology of stroke, a brain disorder in which perturbations of hemostasis pathways are prominent.

Acknowledgments

This work is supported by NIH grants NS20289 and NS31945.

References

Akiyama, H., Ideda, K., Kondo, H. *et al.* (1993). Microglia express the type 2 plasminogen activator inhibitor in the brain of control subjects and patients with Alzheimer's disease. *Neurosci. Lett.*, **164**, 233–5.

Bachman, F. (1987). Fibrinolysis. In *Thrombosis and haemostasis*, ed. M. Verstraete, J., Vermylen, H. R. Lijnen and J. Arnout, pp. 227–65. Leuven: Leuven University Press.

Bachman, F. (1995). The enigma of PAI-2. Gene expression, evolutionary and functional aspects. *Thromb. Haemost.*, **74**, 172–9.

Bevilacqua, M. P., Pober, J. S., Majeau, G. R. *et al.* (1984). Interleukin 1 induces biosynthesis and cell surface expression of procoagulant activity in human vascular endothelial cells. J. Exp. Med., **160**, 618–23.

Bevilacqua, M. P., Pober, J. S., Majeua, G. R. *et al.* (1986). Recombinant tumor necrosis factor induces procoagulant activity in cultured human vascular endothelium: Characterization and comparison with the actions of interleukin 1. *Proc. Natl. Acad. Sci. USA,* **83**, 4533–7.

Boffa, M. C., Jackman, R. W., Peyri, N. *et al.* (1991). Thrombomodulin in the central nervous system. *Nouv. Rev. Fr. Hematol.,* **33**, 423–9.

Broze, G. J. Jr. (1995). Tissue factor pathway inhibitor. *Thromb. Haemost.,* **74**, 90–3.

Colucci, M., Balconi, G., Lorenzet, R. *et al.* (1983). Cultured human endothelial cells generate tissue factor in response to endotoxin. *J. Clin. Invest.,* **71**, 1893–6.

Cunningham, D. D., Pulliam, L. and Vaughan, P. J. (1993). Protease nexin-1 and thrombin: injury-related processes in the brain. *Thromb. Haemost.* **70**, 168–71.

de Agostini, A. I., Watkins, S. C., Slayter, H. S. *et al.* (1990). Localization of anticoagulantly active heparin sulfate proteoglycans in vascular endothelium: antithrombin binding on cultured endothelial cells and perfused rat aorta. *J. Cell Biol.,* **111**, 1293–304.

Deschepper, C. F., Bigornia, V., Bernes, M. E. and Lapointe, M. C. (1991). Production of thrombin and antithrombin III by brain and astroglial cell cultures. *Molec. Brain Res.,* **11**, 355–8.

Drake, T. A., Morrisey, J. H. and Edgington, T. S. (1989). Selective cellular expression of tissue factor in human tissues: implications for disorders of hemostasis and thrombosis. *Am. J. Pathol.,* **134**, 1087–97.

Drake, T. A., Cheng, J., Chang, A. and Taylor, F. B. Jr (1993). Expression of tissue factor, thrombomodulin, and E-selectin in baboons with lethal *Escherichia coli* sepsis. *Am. J. Pathol.,* **142**, 1458–70.

Eddleston, M., de la Torre, J. C., Oldstone, M. B. A. *et al.* (1993). Astrocytes are the primary source of tissue factor in the murine central nervous system: a role for astrocytes in cerebral hemostasis. *J. Clin. Invest.,* **92**, 349–58.

Esmon, C. T. (1987). The regulation of natural anticoagulant pathways. *Science,* **235**, 1348–52.

Fleck, R. A., Rao, L. V. M., Rapaport, S. I. and Varki, N. (1990). Localization of human tissue factor antigen by immunostaining with monospecific, polyclonal anti-human tissue factor antibody. *Thromb. Res.,* **57**, 765–81.

Furie, B. and Furie, B. C. (1992). Molecular and cellular biology of blood coagulation. *N. Engl. J. Med.,* **326**, 800–6.

Ishii, H., Salem, H. H., Bell, C. E. *et al.* (1986). Thrombomodulin, an anticoagulant protein, is absent in the human brain. *Blood,* **67**, 362–5.

Isaka, T., Yoshimine, T., Maruno, M. *et al.* (1994). Altered expression of antithrombotic molecules in human glioma vessels. *Acta Neuropathol.,* **87**, 81–5.

Kalderon, N., Ahonen, K. and Federoff, S. (1990). Developmental transition in plasticity properties of differentiating astrocytes: age-related biochemical profile of plasminogen activators in astroglial cultures. *Glia,* **3**, 413–26.

Kollros, P., Konkle, B. A., Ambarian, A. P. and Henrikson, P. (1994). Plasminogen activator inhibitor-1 expression by brain microvessel endothelial cells is inhibited by elevated glucose. *J. Neurochem.,* **63**, 903–9.

Kittaka, M., Wang, L., Sun, N. *et al.* (1996). Brain capillary tissue plasminogen activator in a diabetes stroke model. *Stroke,* **27**, 712–19.

Levin, E. G. and del Zoppo, G. J. (1994). Localization of tissue plasminogen activator in the endothelium of a limited number of vessels. *Am. J. Pathol.,* **144**, 855–61.

Lijnen, H. R. and Collen, D. (1995). Fibrinolytic agents: mechanisms of activity and pharmacology. *Thromb. Haemost.,* **74**, 387–90.

Loskutoff, D. J., Sawdey, M., Keeton, M. and Schneiderman, J. (1993). Regulation of PAI-1 gene expression *in vivo. Thromb. Haemost.,* **70**, 135–7.

Maragoudakis, M. E., Gullino, P. M. and Leikes, P. I. (eds) (1994). *Angiogenesis: Molecular Biology, Clinical Aspects.* New York: Plenum Press.

National Institute of Neurological Disorders and Stroke t-PA Stroke Study Group (1995). Tissue plasminogen activator for acute ischemic stroke. *N. Engl. J. Med.,* **333**, 1581–7.

Macko, R. F., Ameriso, S. F., Gruber, A. *et al.* (1996). Impairments of the protein C system and fibrinolysis in infection-associated stroke. *Stroke,* **27**, 2304–11.

Martinelli, I., Landi, G., Merati, G. *et al.* (1996). Factor V gene mutation is a risk factor for cerebral venous thrombosis. *Thromb. Haemost.,* **75**, 393–4.

Maruno, M., Yoshimine, T., Isaka, T. *et al.* (1994). Expression of thrombomodulin in astrocytomas of various malignancy and in gliotic and normal brain. *J. Neuro-Oncol.,* **19**, 155–60.

Okada, Y., Copeland, B. R., Fitridge, R. *et al.* (1994). Fibrin contributes to microvascular obstructions and parenchymal changes during early focal cerebral ischemia and reperfusion. *Stroke,* **25**, 1847–54.

Rao, J. S., Sawaya, R., Gokaslan, Z. L. *et al.* (1996). Modulation of serine proteinases and metalloproteinases during morphogenic glial–endothelial interactions. *J. Neurochem.,* **66**, 1657–64.

Shatos, M. A., Orfeo, T., Doherty, J. M. *et al.* (1995). Alpha-thrombin stimulates urokinase production and DNA synthesis in cultured human cerebral microvascular endothelial cells. *Arterioscler. Thromb. Vasc. Biol.,* **15**, 903–11.

Snow, T. R., Deal, M. T., Dickey, D. T. and Esmon, C. T. (1991). Protein C activation following coronary artery occlusion in the in situ porcine heart. *Circulation,* **84**, 293–9.

Svensson, P. J. and Dahlback, B. (1994). Resistance to activated protein C as a basis for venous thrombosis. *N. Engl. J. Med.,* **330**, 517–22.

Tracy, P. B. and Mann, K. G. (1986). A model for assembly of coagulation factor complexes on cell surfaces: prothrombin activation on platelets. In *Biochemistry of Platelets,* ed. D. R. Phillips and M. A. Shuman, pp. 295–318. Orlando, Florida: Academic Press, Inc.,

Tran, N. D., Wong, V. L. Y., Schreiber, S. S. *et al.* (1996). Regulation of brain capillary endothelial thrombomodulin mRNA expression. *Stroke,* **27**, 2304–11.

van Hinsbergh, V. W. M., van den Berg, E. A., Fiers, W. and Dooijewaard, G. (1990). Tumor necrosis factor induces the production of urokinase-type plasminogen activator by human endothelial cells. *Blood,* **75**, 1991–8.

407

van Hinsbergh, V. W. M., Koolwijk, P. and Hanemaaijer, R. (1996). Plasminogen activators in fibrinolysis and pericellular proteolysis. Studies on human endothelial cells in vitro. In *Molecular, Cellular, and Clinical Aspects of Angiogenesis*, ed. M. E. Maragoudakis, 1996, pp. 37–49, New York: Plenum Press.

Wang, L., Kittaka, M., Sun, N. *et al.* (1997). Chronic nicotine treatment enhances focal ischemic brain injury and depletes free pool of brain microvascular tissue plasminogen activator in rats. *J. Cereb. Blood Flow Metab.*, **17**, 136–46.

Wong, V. L. Y., Hofman, F. M., Ishii, H. and Fisher, M. (1991). Regional distribution of thrombomodulin in the human brain. *Brain Res.*, **556**, 1–5.

Yamamoto, M., Sawaya, R., Mohanam, S. *et al.* (1994). Expression and cellular localization of messenger RNA for plasminogen activator inhibitor type 1 in human astrocytomas *in vivo. Cancer Res.*, **54**, 3329–32.

Zlokovic, B. V., Wang, L., Sun, N. *et al.* (1995). Expression of tissue plasminogen activator in cerebral capillaries: possible fibrinolytic function of the blood–brain barrier. *Neurosurgery*, **37**, 955–61.

44 Microvascular pathology in cerebrovascular ischemia

HENRYK M. WISNIEWSKI and ALBERT S. LOSSINSKY

- Introduction
- The normal and injured blood–brain barrier
- Experimental models of global brain ischemia
- Morphological expressions observed in EICD
- Closing remarks and future perspectives

Introduction

The profile of cerebrovascular pathology that is observed in an experimental rat model of global ischemia produced by cardiac arrest with subsequent resuscitation and blood reperfusion shares a commonality with several other types of cerebrovascular injury. Total and immediate hemostasis in this model results in profound morphological, cytochemical and immunological alterations of the microvasculature. These changes include the appearance of a variety of vasospastic events within the vessel wall and individual endothelial cells, increased numbers of endothelial microvillar formations, cellular invaginations, microthrombus formation and a focal and selective increase in vessel permeability to macromolecules and blood cellular components. Adhesion molecule upregulation in these blood vessels reflects a state of immunological preparedness of the affected blood vessel endothelial cells for attaching white blood cells and platelets during and after ischemic events within the CNS that often complicate the recovery state.

This chapter highlights some of the major events that are expressed within the vasculature as a result of cerebral ischemia produced by total blood hemostasis, i.e. global cerebral ischemia. This type of cerebral ischemia is contrasted to regional ischemia, in which the ischemia is produced by the occlusion of a major vascular branch to the brain or spinal cord.

Understanding the pathogenesis of cerebral ischemic events in man has critical import in the clinical arena, since stroke lists third in the number of deaths in males in the United States following heart disease and cancer. It is known that the great majority of ischemic strokes (around 80%) are related to thromboembolic and atherothrombotic processes (del Zoppo, 1995). A key goal for the clinician in this human drama, besides preventing lethal intracranial pressure produced by water influx into the brain parenchyma, is also establishing novel methods of protecting the viability of neurons before, during and after a cerebrovascular accident. Our focus here will be to present a brief description of major pathological events that occur within the microvascular compartment as a consequence of cerebral ischemia. Our perspectives will be a blend of what we know from the historical literature and from our own interests in understanding the pathophysiology of a variety of blood–brain barrier (BBB) injuries including ischemia.

The normal and injured blood–brain barrier

It is a generally accepted view that the mammalian BBB is composed of a uniquely structured arrangement of the endothelial cells, perivascular basement membrane and astroglial cells that collectively impart its special qualities as the gatekeeper between the blood and CNS tissue compartments. A low level of vesicular transport and tightly fastened juxtaposed endothelial cell junctional complexes have been classically demonstrated to be the major structural features responsible for maintaining the normal physiological function of the BBB (Reese and Karnovsky, 1967; Brightman, 1989). The application of the scanning electron microscope assisted transmission electron microscopic studies by presenting the relatively smooth surface of normal endothelial cells of the CNS (Fig. 44.1). If the blood supply is interrupted by an occluding embolus of a major blood vessel such as a middle cerebral artery, the brain tissue no longer receiving crucial oxygen and glucose becomes ischemic. It has been well established in the early structural studies of several animal models of regional ischemia that this type of ischemic deficit produces significant degenerative changes to the neurons and glial cells within the affected neuropil. The reader is referred to several studies that have described neuronal and glial cell alterations, vascular changes, and cerebral blood flow in several animal models of regional ischemia (Garcia and Kamijyo, 1974; Berry *et al.*, 1975; Garcia, 1975; Kalimo *et al.*, 1977; Garcia *et al.*, 1977, 1978; Suzuki *et al.*, 1983 and others). One of the most profound observations noted in the early studies of brain ischemia produced by single artery ligation was the dramatic increase of the permeability of the BBB to intravenously injected protein tracers, including horseradish peroxidase (Westergaard *et al.*, 1976; Garcia *et al.*, 1978; Lossinsky *et al.*, 1979; Pluta *et al.*, 1994*b*). These studies presented ultrastructural evidence for increased vesicular and vesiculo-tubular transport of the tracer and established avenues for a series of subsequent investigations that delved deeper into questions related to the mechanism of transvascular transport of macromolecules across the ischemic BBB. One only has to study the literature to realize the tremendous

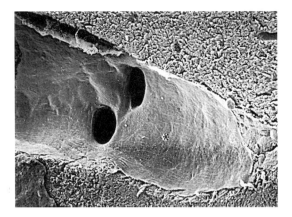

Fig. 44.1. SEM of a control rat microblood vessel. Note the smooth endothelial cell (EC) surface (*). Original magnification ×590.

contributions to our understanding of human brain ischemia and stroke made by the numerous researchers who have developed and studied the various experimental models of regional cerebral ischemia. These efforts have contributed considerably to our understanding of the dynamics of neuronal, glial and vascular changes of the CNS.

Experimental models of global brain ischemia

The desire for neurologists and neuropathologists to develop new models that may mimic more closely the clinical conditions of stroke observed in man in the clinical arena in addition to regional ischemic models resulted in the development of additional models of global or total body ischemia. In models of total body hemostasis, one can not only study brain and spinal cord ischemia, but ischemic changes that occur in other organs as well. One such model of global ischemia introduced by Korpachev *et al.* (1982) and elaborated by Pluta *et al.* (1991), Kawai *et al.* (1992) and Mies *et al.* (1993) encompasses several features that have contributed to our overall understanding of the physiological and anatomical aspects of ischemia in an animal that is rendered totally ischemic for up to 10 minutes followed by resuscitation and blood reperfusion. Some have suggested that this model closely mimics the situation of acute myocardial arrest with rapid resuscitation, that is a model of experimentally induced clinical death (EICD) (Pluta *et al.*, 1991). This methodological approach includes the use of a hook-like probe that is inserted through the chest wall and plural cavity and serves to ligate the entire vascular tree including all afferent and efferent vessels to the heart. Once the vessels are 'hooked', simple finger pressure applied to the sternum for several minutes produces ventricular arrest and consequently, hemostasis throughout the entire circulatory system. It was shown that after clinical death was produced, subsequent resuscitation of the animals after 5 or 10 min time periods enabled study of neuronal or vascular changes that occur within the brain and spinal cord, as well as cellular changes that manifest in other organs of these animals (Pluta *et al.*, 1991).

More recent studies have been performed in this rat model designed to focus on the question of whether or not the neuropathological picture observed in long-term post-resuscitation stages (Zelman and Mossakowski, 1988) differs from that observed in early phases of this pathological process (Mossakowski *et al.*, 1986). The results of such studies suggested that rats who survived 6 months following EICD developed cerebral abnormalities including neuronal degeneration, with or without a glial response. Such a response in these animals was termed post-resuscitation encephalopathy (Zelman and Mossakowski, 1988). Vascular studies by Szumanska *et al.* (1988) demonstrated a gradual loss of both alkaline phosphatase and adenylate cyclase on the luminal aspect of endothelial cells (ECs) with reaction product appearing on the abluminal EC surface. Such an enzymatic shift was observed 24 h after 10 min EICD, but was restored to the normal luminal EC surface localization two days later. These studies also implicated vesiculo-canalicular profiles rather than open EC junctions as the potential mechanism for increased BBB permeability.

Morphological expressions observed in EICD

Experiments conducted on the model of early (acute) stages of EICD in rats questioned the disposition of the blood–brain barrier (BBB), i.e.

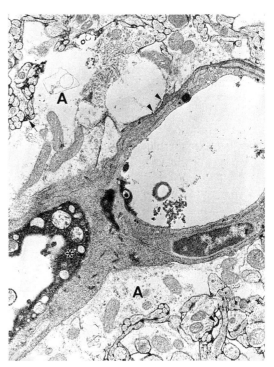

Fig. 44.2. This TEM was taken from a rat that was exposed to about 5 min EICD with 2 min recovery time. HRP was intravenously injected two minutes prior to insult and circulated for a total of seven minutes prior to transcardiac vascular perfusion with buffered aldehydes. Note the HRP reaction product within a damaged EC (*), the basement membrane (arrowheads) and the ECS (arrows). Edematous perivascular astrocytic processes are also noted (A). Original magnification ×8200.

whether or not the barrier was compromised during acute EICD and if permeability using standard horseradish peroxidase (HRP) histochemical techniques could be evaluated. Earlier findings in these rats suggested a focal BBB disturbance was observed throughout the brain in grey matter-associated capillaries and arterioles following 1–6 h of EICD (Pluta *et al.*, 1991; Fig. 44.2). A combination of transmission and scanning electron microscopy has contributed well to our understanding of microvascular abnormalities in EICD. These studies have revealed abnormalities associated with vasospastic changes including ridging of the EC surface, similar to that which has been previously demonstrated (MacDonald *et al.*, 1991; Wisniewski *et al.*, 1995). Vasospastic changes observed in

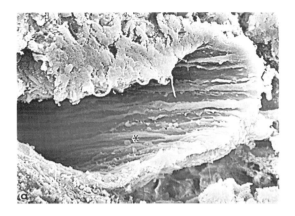

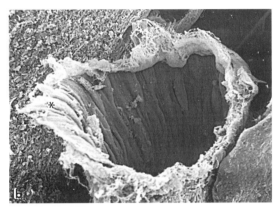

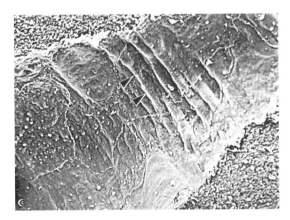

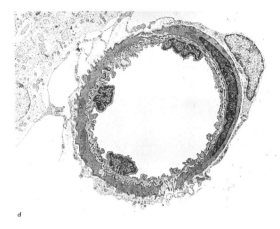

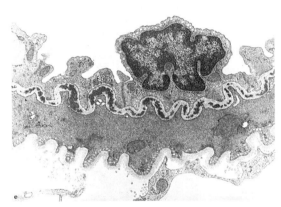

Fig. 44.3. (a)–(c). These SEMs were obtained from rats subjected to 10 min EICD with resuscitation and blood reflow for 24 h total time. Note the EC ridging effect in (a) and (b), (*), probably arterioles, while in (c), the EC ridges are arranged across the vessel (arrowheads), probably a small vein. Original magnifications (a) ×5400; (b) ×1500; (c) ×4000. (d), (e). These TEMs demonstrate the cross-sectional view of a leptomeningeal vessel from a rat subjected to 10 min EICD with 7 days recovery period. This small artery is in the process of vasospasm. In (e), note a high magnification of the EC seemingly in the process of spasm. (d) ×3000; (e) ×12000.

ischemic models have been suggested to vary according to the type of muscle arrangement of the blood vessel. According to the literature, thicker muscular arteries and arterioles constrict circumferentially (Fig. 43.3a, b, d, e), whereas thinner-walled veins and venules constrict by shortening their length due to the longitudinal skeletal muscle arrangement (Fig. 44.3c; Wisniewski et al., 1995). Many substances are known to produce vasospasm in the cerebrovasculature. Although the exact mechanisms are unclear, the causation of the vasospastic response is probably multifactorial and has great clinical interest. Experiments of cerebral ischemia followed by reperfusion have been investigated in vessels within living leptomeningeal (pial) arteries in neonatal piglets (Mirro et al., 1992). These authors observed that normal pial vessels constricted similarly in response to hyperventilation (hypocapnia) both before and after ischemia with reperfusion. A therapeutic strategy used by clinicians to vasoconstrict the cerebral circulation is modulated by manipulating regional blood perfusion by lowering PCO_2, thus attenuating the elevated intracranial pressure caused by cerebral edema (Volpe, 1987). This is of critical importance following stroke in humans, to minimize the increased intracranial pressure by osmotically shifting water back into the vascular compartment, some of which is maintained by constricted cerebral vessels. In the past several years, the vasoconstrictor peptide endothelin (ET-1) has been isolated from the medium of cultured porcine aortic ECs (Yanagisawa *et al.*, 1988). This vasoconstrictor has been suggested to be released from astrocytes following brain infarcts and traumatic injuries (Jiang *et al.*, 1993). Ischemia-induced upregulation of cerebrovascular endothelins has also been demonstrated in the EICD model in rat hippocampus (Gajkowska and Mossakowski, 1995). Thus, the perivascular astroglial response presented here (e.g. Fig. 44.2) may have important implications for understanding mechanisms of vasoconstriction. Besides ET-1, a potent vasoconstrictor of smooth muscle cells, pial arterioles are also known to constrict when exposed to serotonin or arachidonate (Rosenblum and Nelson, 1988).

Prostaglandin enteroperoxides from platelets are also thought to be capable of producing intracerebral vasospasms during cerebral infarction (Hallenbeck and Furlow, 1979). Not only do blood vessels constrict by virtue of smooth muscle component, but vasoconstriction is also aided by constricting ECs. Endothelial cells contain contractile proteins including actin-containing stress fibers associated with proteins such as myosin, tropomyosin and α-actinin, all of which have been shown to contract when dissected by microlaser and stimulated with magnesium ions and adenosine triphosphate (Wong *et al.*, 1983). The morphological features of vasoconstriction of ECs and basement membranes were observed in the EICD model of BBB injury presented here (Fig. 44.3d, e). These changes included severe undulations of the ECs and basement membranes with the increased appearance of EC microfilaments. In some severely damaged ECs that demonstrated obvious rupture of EC membranes, it is reasonable that

during such severe EC injury, levels of substances such as prostacyclin (PGI$_2$) are significantly reduced. Moreover, thromboxane A2 (TXA2), released from platelets, as well as other vasocontractile prostaglandins could play an additional role in cerebrovascular constriction and spasm (Ellis *et al.*, 1977). Normal cerebral vessels are protected from the constrictive action of TXA$_2$ by the simultaneous EC production of PGI$_2$, as well as other vasodilating substances known to be secreted by ECs, including nitric oxide (Durieu-Trautmann *et al.*, 1993). Thus, there appears to exist a balance between vasoconstriction and vasodilation by virtue of a balance of the above-mentioned substances within the vessels or blood plasma that modulates normal physiological vascular function.

Explanation for the observed constricted vessels in these studies probably relates to the dramatic EC damage demonstrated in Fig. 44.2. Such EC injury might be capable of exerting dual influences on the vessel wall as follows: One is the accumulation and aggregation of platelets producing microthrombi attached to the damaged blood vessel wall causing a continuous supply of vasoconstrictors including thromboxane A$_2$, serotonin and/or norepinephrine, etc. The other is the diminution of prostaglandin PGI$_2$ synthesis in the arterial wall, i.e. the vasculature is continuously exposed to the unopposed actions of vasocontractile agents resulting in an extended state of vasoconstriction (Sasaki *et al.*, 1981). An excellent review on vasospasm has also been presented by del Zoppo (1994).

Other observations of EC pathology observed in the EICD rat model included dramatically increased numbers of EC microvilli, enlarged junctional ridging and crater-like pits, usually located in a parajunctional location. Analysis of scanning and high-voltage electron micrographs of blood vessels in chronic relapsing experimental allergic encephalomyelitis suggested increased microvillar projections on the luminal EC surfaces (Lossinsky and Wisniewski, 1987; Lossinsky *et al.*, 1989, 1991; Wisniewski and Lossinsky, 1991), similar to what occurs in cerebral blood vessels following chronic hypertension in the rat (Grady and Blaumanis, 1986), or the deep crater-like openings that appear in the luminal EC surface in other pathological conditions (Kawamura *et al.*, 1974; Nelson *et al.*, 1975; Hughes, 1987). The elongated EC microvilli

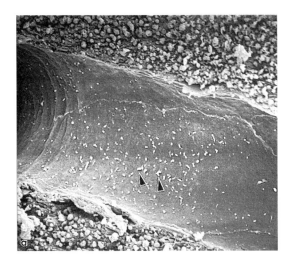

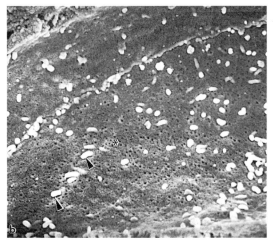

Fig. 44.4. (a), (b). These SEMs demonstrate the increased EC microvilli (arrowheads) observed in the EICD rat model. Time of global ischemia was 10 min with 6 hr recovery period. Note the increased EC pits observed in (b) (*).Original magnifications (a) ×4100; (b) ×14 600.

have been defined ultrastructurally as 'fronds' by Cross and Raine, (1991), who suggested that white blood cells can actually be physically captured by these EC projections as they pass by the target ECs. The microvilli probably serve to 'slow down' the inflammatory cells as they roll along the EC surface just prior to attachment, like a tennis ball rolling over a thick shag carpet (Fig. 44.4; Lossinsky *et al.*, 1989). That there is a commonality in the expression of increased endothelial microvilli observed in several models of CNS

injury is supported by studies of autoinflammatory disease (Lossinsky *et al.*, 1989), in which these increased cellular projections are thought to serve as points of physicochemical attachment via specific membrane-associated adhesion molecules, discussed in greater detail below. These microvilli appear to be expressed on endothelial cells in select blood vessels in both arterial but mostly venous branches. Increased microvilli were primarily remarkable in ECs of venous blood vessels in models of autoimmune disease (Lossinsky *et al.*, 1989), and they were observed in both vascular trees in EICD of rats (Pluta *et al.*, 1991).

Other important and relevant questions related to cerebral ischemic models concern the precise mechanisms of the inflammatory response. Questions related to if and when white blood cells occlude the microvasculature and infiltrate the ischemic brain neuropil have been addressed (del Zoppo *et al.*, 1991; Mori *et al.*, 1991; del Zoppo, 1994; Garcia *et al.*, 1994; 1995; Clark *et al.*, 1995). These investigators studied the nature of neutrophil infiltration in models of regional cerebral ischemia. It is known that several glycoprotein molecules are part and parcel of the normal constituency of normal ECs and some white blood cells, and all tissues. Moreover, when the normal homeostatic environment of the blood vessels is interrupted, some of these glycoproteins, also known as adhesion molecules, are synthesized by the ECs in abundance. Intercellular adhesion molecule-1 (ICAM-1/CD-54) and platelet-endothelial cell adhesion molecule-1 (PECAM-1/CD-31) are two such adhesion molecules of the immunoglobulin supergene family that serve as attachment ligands for leukocytes, tumor cells and, in the case of PECAM-1, for platelets (Rothlein *et al.*, 1986; Marlin and Springer, 1987; DeLisser *et al.*, 1994). The corresponding attachment molecules that serve as ligands on the leukocytes, for example, are the leukocyte function associated molecule-1 (LFA-1, CD11A/18) (Figdor *et al.*, 1990). During ischemic events, it is known that ICAM-1 upregulates before and during neutrophil attachment and invasion (Clark *et al.*, 1995). Other studies of the microvasculature from various human brain tumor biopsies have demonstrated intense ICAM-1 upregulation (Lossinsky *et al.*, 1995).

Our search for understanding of the mecha-

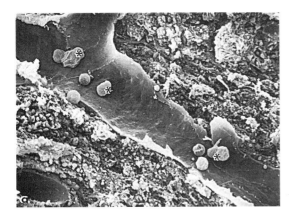

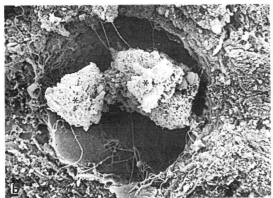

Fig. 44.5. (a), (b). These SEMs demonstrate the appearance of erythrocytes and leukocytes attached to the EC (*) (a), or the appearance of microthrombi (*) (b). These rats were subjected to EICD for 10 min with survival time of 24 h (a) or 3 h (b). Original magnifications (a) ×3700; (b) ×4100.

nisms of microthrombus formation (Pluta *et al.*, 1991) and platelet aggregation in the EICD rat model (Pluta *et al.*, 1994a) presented some features of the ischemic microvasculature. Another excellent review on this topic has been presented by Rosenblum (1986). The ultrastructural images of the numerous EC microvilli observed in Fig. 44.4 add morphological support to our immunocytochemical understanding concerning the intimate relationship between the ischemic ECs and the leukocytes and platelets. Microthrombus formation is focal in nature in the EICD model (Fig. 44.5), and appears to be active in animals with 10 min ischemia and 6 h of blood recirculation viewed by transmission (Pluta *et al.*, 1994a) or scanning electron microscopy (Pluta *et al.*, 1991).

Closing remarks and future perspectives

It is clear that ischemia produced by the obstruction of blood supply to the cerebral cortex may lead to profound consequences for the patient. Present day treatments for stroke include reverse osmotic therapy with hypertonic mannitol (Koc *et al.*, 1994), various drugs including NMDA channel blockers (Lemons *et al.*, 1993; Yang *et al.*, 1994), or enzymes such as streptokinase (Multicenter Acute Stroke Trial, 1996) and other anticoagulant therapy (Rothrock and Hast, 1991). It is clear that all of the various experimental studies have offered clinicians new insights that have been instrumental for the treatment of stroke. Direct administration of clot-dissolving enzymes to the site of the embolic plug or redirecting oxygenated blood from the arterial circulation in a retrograde direction via the venous system directly to the ischemic brain tissue are among the novel strategies that will undoubtedly prove useful to alleviate some of the suffering of this dreaded human affliction. The studies by Clark *et al.*, (1995) point attention to the fact that not all brain ischemia models are similar in light of the variability of results related to leukocyte sticking and plugging. For example, Garcia *et al.* (1994) and del Zoppo *et al.* (1991) presented histological evidence for early granulocyte involvement in models of regional ischemia in monkeys while in the studies of Clark *et al.* (1995), immunocytochemical evidence was found for granulocyte infiltration after 24 h using anti-granulocyte antibodies in a rat model of two-vessel occlusion of transient reversible ischemia. It is clear that future studies applying immunocytochemical techniques to detect the time and location of adhesion molecules in conjunction with ultrastructural methodological approaches (transmission, scanning and high-voltage electron microcopy) will be of critical importance for elucidating this discrepancy. Finally, studies using antibodies against ICAM-1 (Sobel *et al.*, 1990; Clark *et al.*, 1991a, b; Zhang *et al.*, 1994), or PECAM-1 (Rosenblum *et al.*, 1994), have shown that blockage of adhesion molecules and leukocyte adhesion reduces CNS ischemia or platelet attachment respectively. A similar approach using interleukin-1 receptor antagonist also demonstrated attenuation of necrotic neurons following occlusion of the middle artery in rats (Garcia *et al.*, 1995). Such discoveries convince us of the need for additional research efforts in this exciting and important field of study.

Acknowledgments

These studies were supported in part by the New York State Office of Mental Retardation and Developmental Disabilities, Institute for Basic Research in Developmental Disabilities (HMW, ASL) in cooperation with Professors Miroslaw J. Mossakowski and Ryszard Pluta, Department of Neuropathology, Medical Research Center of the Polish Academy of Sciences, Warsaw, Poland.

References

Berry, K., Wisniewski, H. M., Svarzbein, L. and Baez, S. (1975). On the relationship of brain vasculature to production of neurological deficit and morphological changes following acute unilateral common carotid artery ligation in gerbils. *J. Neurol. Sci.*, **25**, 75–92.

Brightman, M. W. (1989). The anatomic basis of the blood–brain barrier. In *Implications of the Blood–Brain Barrier and its Manipulation*, vol. 1, ed. E. A. Neuwelt, pp. 53–83. New York: Plenum Publishing Corporation.

Clark, W., Madden, K., Rothlein, R. and Zivin, J. (1991*a*). Reduction of CNS ischemic injury using leukocyte antibody treatment. *Stroke*, **22**, 877–83.

Clark, W., Madden, K., Rothlein, R., and Zivin, J. (1991*b*). Reduction of central nervous system injury by monoclonal antibody to intercellular adhesion molecule. *J. Neurosurg.*, **75**, 623–27.

Clark, W. M., Lauten, J. D., Lessov *et al.* (1995). Time course of ICAM-1 expression and leukocyte subset infiltration in rat forebrain ischemia. *Mol. Chem. Neuropathol.*, **26**, 213–30.

Cross, A. H. and Raine, C. S. (1991). Central nervous system endothelial cell-polymorphonuclear cell interactions during autoimmune demyelination. *Am. J. Pathol.*, **139**, 1401–9.

DeLisser, H. M., Newman, P. J. and Albelda, S. M. (1994). Molecular and functional aspects of PECAM-1 CD31. *Immunol. Today*, **15**, 490–5.

del Zoppo, G. J. (1994). Microvascular changes during cerebral ischemia and reperfusion. *Cerebrovasc. Brain Metab. Rev.*, **6**, 47–96.

del Zoppo, G. J. (1995). Acute stroke – on the threshold of a therapy? *N. Engl. J. Med.*, **333**, 1632–3.

del Zoppo, G. J., Schmidt-Schönbein, Mori, E. *et al.* (1991). Polymorpho-nuclear leukocytes occlude capillaries following middle cerebral artery occlusion and reperfusion in baboons. *Stroke*, **22**, 1276–83.

Durieu-Trautmann, O., Federici, C., Creminon, N. *et al.* (1993). Nitric oxide and endothelin secretion by brain microvessel endothelial cells: regulation by cyclic nucleotides. *J. Cell Physiol.*, **155**, 104–11.

Ellis, E. F., Nies, A. S. and Oates, J. A. (1977). Cerebral arterial smooth muscle contraction by thromboxane A₂. *Stroke*, **8**, 480–2.

Figdor, C. G., van Kooyk, Y. and Keizer, G. D. (1990). On the mode of action of LFA-1. *Immunol. Today*, **11**, 277–80.

Gajkowska, B. and Mossakowski, M. J. (1995). Localization of endothelin in the blood–brain interphase in rat hippocampus after global cerebral ischemia. *Folia Neuropathol.*, **33**, 221–30.

Garcia, J. H. (1975). The neuropathology of stroke. *Human Pathology*, **6**, 583–98.

Garcia, J. H. and Kamijyo, Y. (1974). Cerebral infarction. Evolution of histopathological changes after occlusion of a middle cerebral artery in primates. *J. Neuropathol. Exp. Neurol.*, **33**, 408–21.

Garcia, J. H., Kalimo, H., Kamijyo, Y. and Trump, B. F. (1977). Cellular events during partial cerebral ischemia. I. Electron microscopy of feline cerebral cortex after middle-cerebral-artery occlusion. *Virchows Arch. B. Cell Pathol.*, **25**, 191–206.

Garcia, J. H., Lossinsky, A. S., Kaufman, F. C. and Conger, K. A. (1978). Neuronal ischemic injury: light microscopy, ultrastructure and biochemistry. *Acta Neuropathol. (Berl.)*, **43**, 85–95.

Garcia, J. H., Liu, K. F., Yoshida, Y. *et al.* (1994). Influx of leukocytes and platelets in an evolving brain infarct (Wistar rats). *Am. J. Pathol.*, **144**, 188–99.

Garcia, J. H., Liu, K. F. and Relton, J. K. (1995). Interleukin-1 receptor antagonist decreases the number of necrotic neurons in rats with middle cerebral artery occlusion. *Am. J. Pathol.*, **147**, 1477–86.

Grady, P. A. and Blaumanis, O. R. (1986). Endothelial cell changes in response to long-term hypertension in the rat. *Soc. Neurosci.*, (Abst.), **12**, 164.

Hallenbeck, J. M. and Furlow, T. W. Jr. (1979). Prostaglandin I₂ and Indomethacin prevent impairment of post-ischemic brain reperfusion in the dog. *Stroke*, **10**, 626–37.

Hughes, J. T. (1987). Endothelial changes in baboon cerebral arteries after experimental arterial spasm: a study using scanning electron microscopy. In *Stroke and Microcirculation*, ed. J. Cervós Navarro and R. Ferszt, pp. 487–94. New York: Raven Press.

Jiang, M. H., Hoog, A., Ma, K. C. *et al.* (1993). Endothelin-1-like immunoreac-tivity is expressed in reactive astrocytes. *Neuroreport*, **7**, 935–37.

Kalimo, H., Garcia, J. H., Kamijyo, Y. *et al.* (1977). The ultrastructure of 'brain death'. II. Electron microscopy of feline cortex after complete ischemia. *Virchows Archiv. B. Cell Pathol.*, **25**, 207–21.

Kawai, K., Nitecka, L., Reutzler, C. A. *et al.* (1992). Global cerebral ischemia associated with cardiac arrest in the rat: dynamics of early neuronal changes. *J. Cereb. Blood Flow and Metab.*, **12**, 238–49.

Kawamura, J., Gertz, S. D., Sunaga, T. *et al.* (1974). Scanning electron microscopic observations on the luminal surface of the rabbit common carotid artery subjected to ischemia by arterial occlusion. *Stroke*, **5**, 765–74.

Korpachev, V. G., Lysenkov, S. P. and Tel, L. Z. (1982). Modeling clinical death and postresuscitation disease in rats. *Patologicheskaia Fizologiia i Eksterimentalnaia Terapiia* (In Russian), **No. 3**, 78–80.

Koc, R. K., Akdemir, H., Kandemir, O. *et al.* (1994). The therapeutic value of naloxone and mannitol in experimental focal cerebral ischemia. *Res. Exp. Med.*, **194**, 277–85.

Lemons, V., Chehrazi, B. B., Kauten, R. *et al.* (1993). The effect of nimodipine on high-energy phosphates and intracellular pH during cerebral ischemia. *J. Neurotrauma*, **10**, 73–81.

Lossinsky, A. S. and Wisniewski, H. M. (1987). Brain endothelial cell gateways for macromolecular and inflammatory cell transport. *Can. J. Neurol. Sci.*, (Abstract), **14**, 342.

Lossinsky, A. S., Garcia, J. H., Iwanowski, L. and Lightfoote, W. E. Jr (1979). New ultrastructural evidence for a protein transport system in endothelial cells of gerbil brains. *Acta Neuropathol. (Berl.)*, **47**, 105–10.

Lossinsky, A. S., Badmajew, V., Robson, J. *et al.* (1989). Sites of egress of inflammatory cells and horseradish peroxidase transport across the blood–brain barrier in a murine model of chronic relapsing experimental allergic encephalomyelitis. *Acta Neuropathol (Berl.)*, **78**, 359–71.

Lossinsky, A. S., Pluta R., Song, M. J. *et al.* (1991). Mechanisms of inflammatory cell attachment in chronic relapsing experimental allergic encephalomyelitis. A scanning and high-voltage electron microscopic study of the injured mouse blood–brain barrier. *Microvasc. Res.*, **41**, 299–310.

Lossinsky, A. S., Mossakowski, M. J., Pluta, R. and Wisniewski, H. M. (1995). Intercellular adhesion molecule-1 (ICAM-1) upregulation in human brain tumors as an expression of increased blood–brain barrier permeability. *Brain Pathol.*, **5**, 339–44.

MacDonald, R. L., Weir, B. K. A., Chen, M. H. and Grace, M. G. A. (1991). Scanning electron microscopy of normal and vasospastic monkey cerebrovascular smooth muscle cells. *Neurosurg.*, **29**, 544–50.

Marlin, S. D. and Springer, T. A. (1987). Purified intercellular adhesion molecule-1 (ICAM-1) is a ligand for lymphocyte function-associated antigen 1 (LFA-1). *Cell*, **51**, 813–19.

Mies, G., Kawai, K., Saito, N. *et al.* (1993). Cardiac arrest-induced complete cerebral ischaemia in the rat: dynamics of postischaemic *in vivo* calcium uptake and protein synthesis. *Neurol. Res.*, **15**, 253–63.

Mirro, R., Lowery-Smith, L., Armstead, W. M. *et al.* (1992). Cerebral vasoconstriction in response to hypocapnia is maintained after ischemia/reperfusion injury in newborn pigs. *Stroke*, **23**, 1613–16.

Mori, E., del Zoppo, G. J., Chambers, J. D. *et al.* (1991). Inhibition of polymorphonuclear leukocyte adherence suppresses no-reflow after focal cerebral ischemia in baboons. *Stroke*, **23**, 712–18.

Mossakowski, M. J., Hilgier, W., Januszewski, S. (1986). Morphological abnormalities in the central nervous system of rats in experimental post resuscitation period. *Neuropatologia Polska*, **24**, 471–84.

The Multicenter Acute Stroke Trial – Europe Study Group (1996). Thrombolytic therapy with streptokinase in acute ischemic stroke. *N. Engl. J. Med.*, **335**, 145–50.

Nelson, E., Sunaga, T., Shimamoto, T. *et al.* (1975). Ischemic carotid endothelium. Scanning electron microscopical studies. *Archiv. Pathol.*, **99**, 125–31.

Pluta, R., Lossinsky, A. S., Mossakowski, M. J. *et al.* (1991). Reassessment of a new model of complete cerebral ischemia in rats. Method of induction of clinical death, pathophysiology and cerebrovascular pathology. *Acta Neuropathol.*, **83**, 1–11.

Pluta, R., Lossinsky, A. S., Walski, M. *et al.* (1994a). Platelet occlusion phenomenon after short- and long-term survival following complete cerebral ischemia in rats produced by cardiac arrest. *J. Brain Res.*, **35**, 463–71.

Pluta, R., Lossinsky, A. S., Wisniewski, H. M. and Mossakowski, M. J. (1994b). Early blood–brain barrier changes in the rat following transient complete cerebral ischemia induced by cardiac arrest. *Brain Res.*, **663**, 41–52.

Reese, T. S. and Karnovsky, M. J. (1967). Fine structural localization of a blood–brain barrier to exogenous peroxidase. *J. Cell Biol.*, **34**, 207–17.

Rosenblum, W. I. (1986). Biology of Disease. Aspects of endothelial malfunction and function in cerebral microvessels. *Lab. Invest.*, **55**, 252–68.

Rosenblum, W. I. and Nelson, G. H. (1988). Endothelium-dependent constriction demonstrated *in vivo* in mouse cerebral arterioles. *Circ. Res.*, **63**, 837–43.

Rosenblum, W. I., Murata, S., Nelson, G. H. *et al.* (1994). Anti-CD31 delays platelet adhesion/aggregation at sites of endothelial injury in mouse cerebral arterioles. *Am. J. Pathol.*, **145**, 33–6.

Rothlein R., Dustin, M., Marlin, S. D. *et al.*, (1986). A human intercellular adhesion molecule (ICAM-1) distinct from LFA-1. *J. Immuno.*, **137**, 1270–4.

Rothrock, J. F. and Hast, R. G. (1991). Antithrombotic therapy in cerebrovascular disease. *Ann. Int. Med.*, **115**, 885–95.

Sasaki, T., Wakai, S., Asano, T. *et al.* (1981). The effect of lipid hydroperoxide of arachidonic acid on the canine basilar artery. An experimental study on cerebral vasospasm. *J. Neurosurg.*, **54**, 357–65.

Sobel, R. A., Mitchell, M. A. and Fondren, G. (1990). Intercellular adhesion molecule-1 (ICAM-1) in cellular immune reactions in the human central nervous system. *Am. J. Pathol.*, **136**, 1309–16.

Suzuki, R., Yamaguchi, T., Kirino, T. *et al.* (1983). The effects of 5-minute ischemia in Mongolian gerbils: I. Blood–brain barrier, cerebral blood flow, and local cerebral glucose utilization changes. *Acta Neuropathol. (Berl.)*, **60**, 207–16.

Szumanska, G., Mossakowski, M. J. and Januszewski, S. (1988). Changes in the activity of alkaline phosphatase and adenylate cyclase in brain vascular network in experimental post resuscitation syndrome. *Neuropatologia Polska*, **26**, 335–57.

Volpe, J. J. (1987). *Neurology of the Newborn*, ed. J. J. Volpe, pp. 264–5. Philadelphia: W. B. Saunders Company.

Westergaard, E., Go, G., Klatzo, I. and Spatz, M. (1976). Increased permeability of cerebral vessels to horseradish peroxidase induced by ischemia in Mongolian gerbils. *Acta Neuropathol. (Berl.)*, **35** 307–25.

Wisniewski, H. M. and Lossinsky, A. S. (1991). Structural and functional aspects of the interaction of inflammatory cells with the blood–brain barrier in experimental brain inflammation. *Brain Pathol.* (Mini-review), **1**, 89–96.

Wisniewski, H. M., Pluta, R., Lossinsky, A. S. and Mossakowski, M. J. (1995). Ultrastructural studies of cerebral vascular spasm after cardiac arrest-related global cerebral ischemia in rats. *Acta Neuropathol.*, **90**, 432–40.

Wong, A. J., Pollard, T. D., and Herman, I. M. (1983). Actin filament stress fibers in vascular endothelial cells *in vivo*. *Science*, **219**, 867–69.

Yanagisawa, M. H., Kurihara, S., Kimura, Y. *et al.* (1988). A novel potent vasoconstrictor peptide produced by vascular endothelia cells. *Nature*, **332**, 411–15.

Yang, G., Chan, P. H., Chen, S. F. *et al.* (1994). Reduction of vasogenic edema and infarction by MK-801 in rats after temporary focal cerebral ischemia. *Neurosurgery*, **34**, 339–45.

Zelman, I. B. and Mossakowski, M. J. (1988). Remote pathological brain changes in rats following experimentally induced clinical death. *Neuropatologia Polska*, **26**, 151–62.

Zhang, R., Chopp, M., Liu, Y. *et al.* (1994). Anti-ICAM-1 antibody reduces ischemic cell damage after transient middle cerebral artery occlusion in the rat. *Neurology*, **44**, 1747–51.

45 HIV infection and the blood–brain barrier

CAROL K. PETITO

- Introduction
- Neuropathology of HIV infection and its relationship to the cerebral vasculature
- The blood–brain barrier in HIV infection
- Mechanisms of enhanced vascular permability in AIDS brains
- Consequences of the vascular leak in AIDS brains

Introduction

The cerebral blood vessels are important targets of disease in patients infected with the human immunodeficiency virus (HIV). Vascular abnormalities include direct infection by HIV or opportunistic organisms, alterations related to inflammation or gliosis in the brain, and changes secondary to abnormal cellular or serum components in the systemic circulation. Cerebral ischemia or hemorrhage are two of the consequences of such vascular changes. Of particular interest, however, are the changes in the blood–brain barrier (BBB) that occur in almost half of the patients with the acquired immunodeficiency syndrome (AIDS). This chapter summarizes the neuropathology and cerebrovascular pathology that occur in patients with AIDS, discusses the abnormalities in the BBB that develop in the absence of any apparent brain pathology, and reviews the potential mechanisms for, and the effects of, this enhanced vascular permeability.

Neuropathology of HIV infection and its relationship to the cerebral vasculature

Brain and spinal cord diseases are frequent in patients with AIDS (Petito *et al.*, 1986; Sharer,

1992). Approximately 30% had HIV encephalitis with microglial nodules and either the multinucleated giant cells that are characteristic of HIV or HIV protein or genomic material at autopsy during the first decade of the HIV epidemic. Subcortical regions, especially the basal ganglia and cerebral white matter, are the major regions of brain affected by HIV encephalitis; cortical involvement is usually associated with more severe forms of this infection and rarely is the sole site of brain involvement. In some cases, HIV infection is concentrated in the white matter where it presents as a HIV leukoencephalitis. Since this infection is associated with HIV infection of monocyte/microglial cells rather than of neuroectodermal cells (Koenig *et al.*, 1986; Wiley *et al.*, 1986), one of the leading hypotheses regarding mechanisms of brain damage in HIV encephalitis is related to the neurotoxic effects of HIV-infected or activated macrophages or monocytes (Price *et al.*, 1988; Chiodi and Fenyo, 1991). Opportunistic infections are the second general category of central nervous system (CNS) diseases in AIDS and include cytomegalovirus (CMV), toxoplasmosis, and Epstein–Barr virus-induced lymphoma. Their incidence varies but is approximately 30%, 14%, and 6% respectively (Petito *et al.*, 1986). A third general category of HIV-related neuropathological abnormalities includes a number of nonspecific changes such as inflammation, neuronal loss or white matter atrophy for which an etiology is either not identified or not known.

Vascular changes were recognized in the earliest descriptions of the neuropathology of AIDS. The inflammatory components of HIV encephalitis are in close proximity to small intraparenchymal blood vessels; a calcific vasculopathy develops in the basal ganglia of children with AIDS; and a number of infectious vasculitides, including those due to HIV, CMV and Varicella-Zoster virus, involve not only extraparenchymal arteries but also intraparenchymal vessels. Capillary changes described include endothelial hypertrophy or hyperplasia (Smith *et al.*, 1990), accumulations of hemosiderin-laden macrophages in perivascular spaces (Gelman *et al.*, 1992) and enhanced expression of basement membrane laminin and hypertrophy of astrocytic foot processes (Taruscio *et al.*, 1991).

An unresolved question is whether HIV directly infects brain endothelium *in vivo*. If present, such an infection could be not only a means by which virus enters the brain but also could be responsible for altered endothelial function, including the integrity of its blood–brain barrier. Evidence for such infection includes the ability to infect primary human brain endothelial cells in culture (Moses *et al.*, 1993; Poland *et al.*, 1995) and the presence of productive endothelial infection in animal retroviral encephalitis, including that caused by simian immunodeficiency virus (SIV) (Pitts *et al.*, 1987; Mankowski *et al.*, 1994; Steffan *et al.*, 1994). However, several facts militate against a significant role of endothelial infection by HIV. HIV infection of cerebral endothelium is absent (see for example Gosztonyi *et al.*, 1994) or rare (Wiley *et al.*, 1986) in HIV encephalitis and has not been detected in brains of HIV-infected preAIDS patients. When HIV or SIV-infected cells are found in the endothelium, there is some evidence that they actually represent infected monocytes traversing the vessel wall rather than endothelial cells infected by HIV or SIV (Smith *et al.*, 1990; Lackner *et al.*, 1991; Falangola *et al.*, 1995).

Vascular cell adhesion molecule (VCAM) expression is selectively elevated on cerebral endothelium in brains with HIV or SIV encephalitis (Sasseville *et al.*, 1994; Nottet *et al.*, 1996) and, with HIV, E-selectin also is increased (Nottet *et al.*, 1996). These ligands are important modulators of monocyte adhesion and migration. Changes in their expression highlight the potential for the BBB to mediate the inflammatory response in AIDS brains as well as to enhance entry of HIV-infected monocytes.

The blood–brain barrier in HIV infection

Evaluations of paired samples of cerebrospinal fluid (CSF) and serum find increases in the normal CSF:serum ratio of albumin in HIV-infected patients (McArthur *et al.*, 1992; Singer *et al.*, 1994). This increase is greater in patients with AIDS when compared to HIV-infected asymptomatic persons prior to the onset of AIDS. In addition, the increased CSF:serum ratio of albumin is greater in AIDS patients with neurological symptoms when compared to AIDS patients without neurological signs and symptoms (Singer *et al.*, 1994). While these studies strongly support the concept of an altered barrier in AIDS, by themselves, they do not identify the cause of the barrier breakdown nor do they distinguish between increased permeability of intraparenchymal capillaries of the BBB and increased permeability of vessels at other sites such as the leptomeninges or choroid plexus. Since these latter sites often display inflammation, infection or immune complex deposition (Sharer,1992; Falangola and Petito, 1993; Falangola *et al.*, 1995), they could give rise to the altered CSF:serum albumin ratio in AIDS patients.

Post-mortem studies, however, have convincingly documented a BBB leak within the brain of AIDS patients. Using the technique of immunohistochemistry to detect serum proteins in post-mortem material as a marker of enhanced vascular permeability in brain (Liu *et al.*, 1989), these studies have identified a BBB leak in the brain parenchyma (Lenhardt and Wiley, 1989; Petito and Cash, 1992; Powers *et al.*, 1993).

Our own study examined the integrity of the BBB in three groups of patients: AIDS patients with normal brains; AIDS patients with HIV encephalitis, and HIV-negative controls (Petito and Cash, 1992). Cases were matched for age and post-mortem interval and those with focal lesions or anoxic-ischemic encephalopathy were excluded. For each case, a section of parasagittal cerebral

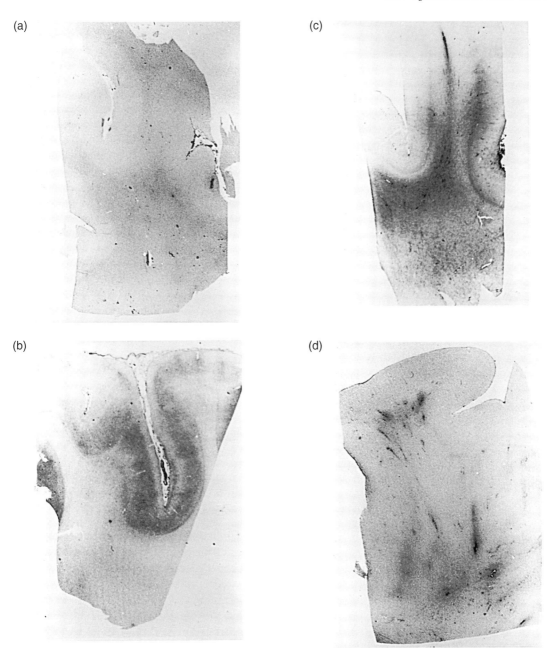

Fig. 45.1. Immunoreactivity for fibrinogen is absent in the brain parenchyma of a HIV-negative control with a normal brain (a). In regions of necrosis, however, a BBB leak is apparent, as depicted in a recent cortical infarct of an HIV-negative patient (b). Two AIDS brains without HIVE display diffuse (c) or perivascular (d) immunoreactivity in the centrum semi-ovale. Hematoxylin, original magnification ×4.5.

cortex and centrum semi-ovale was prepared for immunohistochemistry using primary antibodies directed against fibrinogen and IgG as evidence of barrier leak. The results were as follows.

(1) The two groups of AIDS cases had significant increases in serum proteins in the centrum semi-ovale as compared with the HIV-negative controls (Fig. 45.1). (2) The extravasated serum proteins were present diffusely in the centrum

COMBINED DISTRIBUTION OF POSITIVE IMMUNOREACTIVITY OF FIBRINOGEN AND IgG

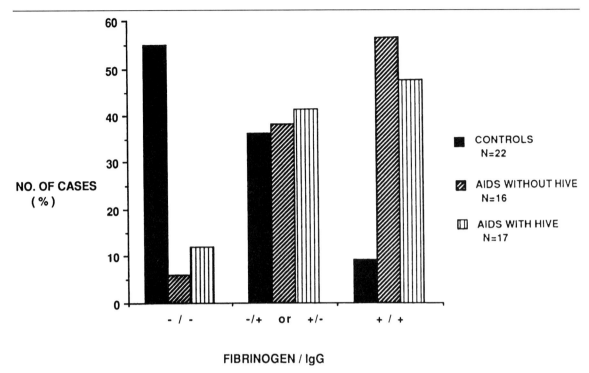

Fig. 45.2. Immunoreactivity to fibrinogen (FIB) and IgG in brain parenchyma, graded as 0, mild (1+), moderate (2+) and severe (3+). The results depicted are expressed as negative (Grades 0 and 1+) or positive (grades 2+ and 3+). They show significant differences between each AIDS group and the HIV-negative controls but no differences between the AIDS groups with or without HIV encephalitis.

semi-ovale or were localized around blood vessels, the size and shape of which suggested venous origins. (3) The presence of a BBB leak occurred with the same 45–50 % incidence in AIDS cases with normal brains as in AIDS cases with HIV encephalitis (Fig. 45.2). (4) A vascular leak was always associated with necrosis, including that accompanying cerebral infarcts (Fig. 45.1B), opportunistic infections and those few inflammatory lesions of HIV encephalitis that were sufficiently severe to cause actual tissue necrosis.

On the basis of the above results, we hypothesized that the BBB breakdown in AIDS patients is caused by systemic rather than local factors since the vascular leak was not dependent on any coexisting brain pathology and since the vascular leak occurred with equal frequency in AIDS brains with HIV encephalitis as in AIDS brains without encephalitis. A subsequent study by Powers *et al.*

(1993), using the same technique of immunoreactivity of serum proteins in post-mortem brain as a marker for an altered BBB, found a similar incidence of BBB leak in AIDS brains, including those cases without pathological lesions.

Mechanisms of enhanced vascular permeability in AIDS brains

Serum cytokines, particularly tumor necrosis factor and interleukin-1, are among the leading candidates that have been proposed as causes of the breakdown of the BBB in AIDS (Petito and Cash, 1992; Powers *et al.*, 1993). Both are increased in the serum of AIDS patients (Lahdevirta *et al.*, 1988; Gallo *et al.*, 1989; Mintz *et al.*, 1989; Grunfeld *et al.*, 1991) and both produce enhanced vascular permeability in the CNS of experimental animals (Saukkonen *et al.*, 1990; Quagliarello *et al.*, 1991). Tumor necrosis factor is directly toxic to cultured brain-derived endothelial cells by inhibiting their DNA synthesis and by inducting loss of contact inhibition (Yoshida *et al.*, 1989). In addition, cytokines have complex interactions with immune cells, astrocytes and microglia and thus could indirectly affect the BBB. For example, cytokines induce alterations on endothelial adhesion molecules (Pober *et al.*, 1986), which could in turn alter endothelial function and barrier properties. Cytokines, including TNF and interleukin-1, also are produced in the brains of AIDS patients, especially when inflammation and HIV encephalitis are present (Tyor *et al.*, 1992). These brain-derived cytokines are another potential cause of BBB changes in HIV infection.

HIV viral proteins – in particular, gp120 and tat – also are good candidates for enhancing vascular permeability in AIDS brains. They are temporarily elevated in serum during the early stages of HIV infection and rise again with, and parallel the severity of, AIDS (Cao *et al.*, 1987). There is good evidence that HIV and HIV proteins can affect cerebral endothelium. Brain-derived endothelial monolayer cultures exhibit enhanced permeability when co-cultured with HIV-infected monocytes (Dhawan *et al.*, 1995). Radiolabeled gp120, or components of this molecule, can cross the BBB and be detected in ventricles and parenchymal homogenates of newborn rat pups 1 h after a subcutaneous injection (Hill *et al.*, 1993). Tat protein does not appear to cross the normal BBB but is taken up by endothelial cells throughout the body, including the brain vasculature (Fawell *et al.*, 1994). When this occurs, tat alters cellular function and indeed does so in all cell systems tested to date (Magnuson *et al.*, 1995). Hofman *et al.* (1994) showed that tat protein activates cerebral endothelial cells *in vitro* and increases their expression of E-selectin, IL-6, and plasminogen activator inhibitor-1.

Intrinsic alterations in the brain itself could be responsible for a BBB leak although this hypothesis is insufficient to explain the vascular leak in brains that display no pathological changes. Brain-derived cytokines, inflammation and alterations in vascular adhesion molecules are potential intrinsic brain-derived stimuli for altering the BBB.

Abnormalities in astrocytes are another potential intrinsic stimulus for altering the BBB in AIDS. These cells play a pivotal role in establishing and maintaining a normal BBB (Abbott *et al.*, 1992) and astrocyte dysfunction or death has the potential to interfere with normal vascular permeability (Krum, 1994). There is ample evidence that HIV infection alters normal astrocyte morphology and function. Reactive astrocytosis with prominent hypertrophy and increased glial fibrillary protein is prominent, even in the absence of obvious neuropathological lesions (Powers *et al.*, 1993; Weis *et al.*, 1993). Astrocyte cell death by apoptotic mechanisms accompanies and parallels the severity of HIV encephalitis (Petito and Roberts, 1995). HIV proteins, particularly gp120, alter normal metabolic properties of astrocytes in culture, interfering with functional properties such as ion transport (Benos *et al.*, 1994), glial fibrillary acidic protein (GFAP) expression (Pulliam *et al.*, 1993), and beta-adrenergic regulation (Levi *et al.*, 1993). Lastly, astrocytes *in vivo* may harbor defective HIV infection, as evidenced by restricted astrocyte expression of certain HIV proteins (Saito *et al.*, 1994; Tornatore *et al.*, 1994).

Consequences of the vascular leak in AIDS brains

Although a BBB leak often results in vasogenic edema with its accompanying increases in brain water content and potential for clinically apparent brain swelling, there is little evidence that this develops with the diffuse barrier leak in AIDS brains, other than those cases with focal brain lesions. Imaging studies, as well as post-mortem examinations of the CNS, show brain atrophy with ventricular dilation and mild expansion of the cortical sulci. However, the presence of extravasated serum proteins, the documentation of an altered CSF:serum albumin ratio throughout the period of AIDS, and the absence of brain swelling suggest that the vascular leak is both mild and chronic.

Clinical and experimental studies support the concept that a chronically opened BBB produces myelin and even axonal loss in cerebral white matter, together with associated increases in reactive astrocytes and activated microglia and macrophages (Feigin and Popoff, 1963; Feigin *et al.*, 1973; Price *et al.*, 1976; Nordborg *et al.*, 1994). In addition, there is good evidence that albumin, a major protein component of serum, is toxic to neurons, axons and myelin following intra-striatal injection *in vivo* (Hassel *et al.*, 1994) and may potentiate glutamate-induced neurotoxicity *in vitro* (Eimerl and Schramm, 1991). It is tempting to speculate, therefore, that a minor BBB leak over a prolonged period of time is responsible for some of the diffuse white matter changes that accompany systemic HIV infection but that are not necessarily associated with HIV encephalitis.

A vascular leak could permit or enhance entry of inflammatory cells, including lymphocytes and monocytes, the principal inflammatory cells in brains of HIV-infected patients in the absence of opportunistic infections. Activated monocytes have the potential to directly damage brain by their release of a variety of neurotoxic substances such as cytokines, free radicals, nitric oxide and glutamate. In addition, activated monocytes have the potential to stimulate astrocyte hypertrophy and possibly hyperplasia which, by itself, could adversely affect the normal function of brain. Finally, since it is likely that HIV gains entry into brain by passage of infected monocytes, increased entry of these cells, if facilitated by a barrier leak, would increase the potential or the severity of developing HIV encephalitis.

An abnormally permeable BBB may be responsible for, or associated with, AIDS-related dementia. This dementing illness develops in approximately one third of all AIDS patients by the time of death and displays a constellation of behavioral and motor symptoms and signs that are in addition to the cognitive decline. McArthur *et al.* (1992) found that enhanced vascular permeability, as measured by the CSF:serum albumin ratio, was significantly increased in HIV-infected demented patients when compared with HIV-infected non-demented patients. The same relationship between BBB leakage and dementia was found by Powers *et al.* (1993) in their study of serum protein extravasation in post-mortem brain. Since AIDS dementia is closely linked to HIV encephalitis (Navia *et al.*, 1986), the link between BBB abnormalities and dementia may be fortuitous if HIV infection is the etiology of both. However, since post-mortem studies have shown that the BBB leak occurs in the absence of HIV encephalitis, it remains possible that a primary breakdown of the BBB could, by itself, cause a dementing illness if the leak is chronic and if it results in diffuse white matter damage.

Acknowledgments

This paper is supported by grants from the National Institutes of Health (1RO1-NS27416 and 1RO1-NS35331).

References

Abbott, N. J., Revest, P. A. and Romero, I. A. (1992). Astrocyte–endothelial interaction: physiology and pathology. *Neuropathol. Appl. Neurobiol.*, **18**, 424–33.

Benos, D. J., Hahn, B. H., Bubien, J. K., Ghosh, S. K., Mashburn, N. A., Chaikin, M. A., Shaw, G. M. and Benveniste, E. N. (1994). Envelope glycoprotein gp120 of human immunodeficiency virus type 1 alters ion transport in astrocytes: implications for AIDS dementia complex. *Proc. Natl. Acad. Sci. USA*, **94**, 494–8.

Cao, Y. Z., Valentine, F., Hojvat, S. *et al.* (1987). Detection of HIV antigen and specific antibodies to HIV core and envelope proteins in sera of patients with HIV infection. *Blood*, **70**, 575–8.

Chiodi, F. and Fenyo, E. M. (1991). Neurotropism of human immunodeficiency virus. *Brain Pathol.*, **1**, 185–91.

Dhawan, S., Weeks, B. S., Soderland, C. *et al.* (1995). HIV-1 infection alters monocyte interactions within human neurovascular endothelial cells. *J. Immunol.*, **134**, 422–32.

Eimerl, S. and Schramm, M. (1991). Acute glutamate toxicity in cultured cerebellar granule cells: agonist potency, effects of pH, Zn^{2+} and the potentiation by serum albumin. *Brain Res.*, **560**, 282–90.

Falangola, M. F. and Petito, C. K. (1993). Choroid plexus infection in cerebral toxoplasmosis in AIDS patients. *Neurology*, **43**, 2035–40.

Falangola, M. F., Castro-Filha, B. G. and Petito, C. K. (1994). Immune complex deposition in the choroid plexus of AIDS patients. *Ann. Neurol.*, **36**, 437–40.

Falangola, M. F., Hanly, A., Galvao-Castro, B. and Petito, C. K. (1995). HIV infection of human choroid plexus: a possible mechanism of viral entry into the CNS. *J. Neuropathol. Exp. Neurol.*, **54**, 499–503.

Fawell, S., Seery, J., Daikh, Y. et al. (1994). Tat-mediated delivery of heterologous proteins into cells. *Proc. Natl. Acad. Sci. USA*, **91**, 664–8.

Feigin, I. and Popoff, N. (1963). Neuropathological changes late in cerebral edema: the relationship of trauma, hypertensive disease and Binswanger's encephalopathy. *J. Neuropathol. Exp. Neurol.*, **22**, 500–11.

Feigin, I., Budzolovich, G., Weinberg, S. and Ogata, J. (1973). Degeneration of white matter in hypoxia, acidosis and edema. *J. Neuropathol. Exp. Neurol.*, **32**, 125–43.

Gallo, P., Frei, K., Rordord, C. et al. (1989). Human immunodeficiency virus type 1 (HIV-1) infection of the central nervous system: an elevation of cytokines in cerebrospinal fluid. *J. Neuroimmunol.*, **23**, 109–16.

Gelman, B. B., Rodriguez-Wolf, M. G., Wen, J. et al. (1992). Siderotic cerebral macrophages in the acquired immunodeficiency syndrome. *Arch. Pathol. Lab. Med.*, **116**, 509–16.

Gosztonyi, G., Artigas, J., Lamperth, L. and Webster, H. F. (1994). Human immunodeficiency virus (HIV) distribution in HIV encephalitis: study of 19 cases with combined use of *in situ* hybridization and immunocytochemistry. *J. Neuropathol. Exp. Neurol.*, **53**, 521–34.

Grunfeld, C., Kotler, D. P., Shigenaga, J. K. et al. (1991). Circulating interferon-alpha levels and hypertriglyceridemia in the acquired immunodeficiency syndrome. *Am. J. Med.*, **90**, 154–62.

Hassel, B., Iversen, E. G. and Fonnum, F. (1994). Neurotoxicity of albumin *in vivo*. *Neurosci. Lett.*, **167**, 29–32.

Hill, J. M., Mervis, R. F., Avidor, R. et al. (1993). HIV envelope protein-induced neuronal damage and retardation of behavioral development in rat neonates. *Brain Res.*, **603**, 222–3.

Hofman, F. M., Dohadwala, M. M., Wright, A. D. et al. (1994). Exogenous tat protein activates cerebral nervous system-derived endothelial cells. *J. Neuroimmunol.*, **54**, 19–29.

Koenig, S., Gendelman, H. E. and Orenstein, J. F. (1986). Detection of AIDS virus in macrophages in brain tissue from AIDS patient with encephalopathy. *Science*, **233**, 1089–93.

Krum, J. M. (1994). Experimental gliopathy in the adult rat. CNS: effect on the blood–spinal cord barrier. *Glia*, **11**, 354–66.

Lackner, A. A., Smith, M. O., Munn, R. J. et al. (1991). Localization of simian immunodeficiency virus in the central nervous system of rhesus monkeys. *Am. J. Pathol.*, **139**(3), 609–21.

Lahdevirta, J., Maury, C. P. J., Teppo, A. M. and Repo, H. (1988). Elevated levels of circulating cachectin/tumor necrosis factor in patients with acquired immunodeficiency syndrome. *Am. J. Med.*, **85**, 289–91.

Lenhardt, T. M. and Wiley, C. A. (1989). Absence of humorally mediated damage within the central nervous system of AIDS patients. *Neurology*, **39**, 278–80.

Levi, G., Patrizio, M., Bernardo, A. et al. (1993). Human immunodeficiency virus coat protein gp120 inhibits the β-adrenergic regulation of astroglial and microglial functions. *Proc. Natl. Acad. Sci. USA*, **90**, 1541–5.

Liu, L. T. M., Atack, J. R. and Rapaport, S. I. (1989). Immunohistochemical localization of intracellular proteins in the human central nervous system. *Acta Neuropathol.*, **78**, 16–21.

Magnuson, D. S. K., Knudsen, B. E., Geiger, J. D. et al. (1995). Human immunodeficiency virus type 1 tat activates non-*N*-methyl-d-aspartate excitatory amino acid receptors and causes neurotoxicity. *Ann.Neurol.*, **37**, 373–80.

Mankowski, J. L., Spelman, J. P., Ressetar, H. G. et al. (1994). Neurovirulent simian immunodeficiency virus replicates productively in endothelial cells of the central nervous system *in vivo* and *in vitro*. *J. Virol.*, **68**, 8202–8.

Marshall, D. W., Brey, R. L., Butzin, C. A. et al. (1991). CSF changes in a longitudinal study of 124 neurologically normal HIV-1-infected United States Air Force personnel. *J. Acquir. Immune Defic. Synd.*, **4**, 777–81.

McArthur, J. C., Nance-Sproson, T. E., Griffin, D. E. et al. (1992). The diagnostic utility of elevation in cerebrospinal fluid beta₂-microglobulin in HIV-1 dementia. *Neurology*, **42**, 1707–12.

Mintz, M., Rapaport, R., Oleske, J. M. et al. (1989). Elevated serum levels of tumor necrosis factor are associated with progressive encephalopathy in children with acquired immunodeficiency syndrome. *Am. J. Dis. Child.*, **143**, 771–4.

Moses, A. V., Bloom, F. E., Pauza, C. D. and Nelson, J. A. (1993). Human immunodeficiency virus infection of human brain capillary endothelial cells occurs via a CD4/ galactosylceramide-independent mechanism. *Proc. Natl. Acad. Sci. USA*, **90**, 10474–8.

Navia, B. A., Cho, E-S., Petito, C. K. and Price, R. W. (1986). The AIDS dementia complex: II. Neuropathology. *Ann. Neurol.*, **19**, 525–35.

Nordborg, C., Sokrab, T. E. O. and Johansson, B. B. (1994). Oedema-related tissue damage after temporary and permanent occlusion of the middle cerebral artery. *Neuropathol. Appl. Neurobiol.*, **20**, 56–65.

Nottet, H. S. L. M., Persidsky, Y., Sasseville, V. G. et al. (1996). Mechanisms for the transendothelial migration of HIV-1-infected monocytes into brain. *J. Immunol.*, **156**, 1284–95.

Petito, C. K. and Cash, K. S. (1992). Blood–brain barrier abnormalities in the acquired immunodeficiency syndrome: immunohistochemical localization of serum proteins in post mortem brain. *Ann. Neuro.*, **32**, 658–66.

Petito, C. K. and Roberts, B. K. (1995). Evidence for apoptotic cell death in HIV encephalitis. *Am. J. Pathol.*, **146**, 1–10.

Petito, C. K., Cho, E-S., Lemann, W. et al. (1986). Neuropathology of acquired immunodeficiency syndrome (AIDS): an autopsy review. *J. Neuropathol. Exp. Neurol.*, **45**, 635–46.

Pitts, O. M., Powers, J. M., Bilello, J. A. and Hoffman, P. M. (1987). Ultrastructural changes associated with retroviral replication in central nervous system capillary endothelial cells. *Lab. Invest.*, **56**, 401–9.

Pober, J. S., Gimbrone, M. A. Jr, Lapierre, L. A. *et al.* (1986). Overlapping patterns of activation of human endothelial cells by interleukin 1, tumor necrosis factor and immune interferon. *J. Immunol.*, **137**, 1893–6.

Poland, S. D., Rice, G. P. A. and Dekaban, G. A. (1995). HIV-1 infection of human brain-derived microvascular endothelial cells *in vitro*. *J. Acquir. Immune Defic. Synd. Hum. Retrovirol.*, **8**, 437–45.

Powers, C., Kong, P. A., Crawford, T. D. *et al.* (1993). Cerebral white matter changes in acquired immunodeficiency syndrome dementia: Alterations of the blood–brain barrier. *Ann. Neurol.*, **34**, 339–50.

Price, D. L., James, A. E. Jr, Sperber, E. and Strecker, E. P. (1976). Communicating hydrocephalus: cisternographic and neuropathologic studies. *Archiv. Neurol.*, **33**, 15–20.

Price, R. W., Brew, B., Sidtis, J. *et al.* (1988). The brain in AIDS: Central nervous system HIV-1 infection and AIDS dementia complex. *Science*, **239**, 586–92.

Pulliam, L., West, D., Haigwood, N. and Swanson, R. A. (1993). HIV-1 envelope gp120 alters astrocytes in human brain cultures. *AIDS Res. Hum. Retrovir.*, **9**, 439–44.

Quagliarello, V. J., Wispelwey, B., Long, W. J. and Scheid, W. M. (1991). Recombinant human interleukin-1 induced meningitis and blood–brain barrier injury in the rat. Characterization and comparison with tumor necrosis factor. *J. Clin. Invest.*, **87**, 1360–1366.

Saito, Y., Sharer, L. R., Epstein, L. G. *et al.* (1994). Overexpression of nef as a marker for restricted HIV-1 infection of astrocytes in postmortem pediatric central nervous tissues. *Neurology*, **44**, 474–80.

Sasseville, V. G., Newman, W., Brodie, S. J. *et al.* (1994). Monocyte adhesion to endothelium in simian immunodeficiency virus-induced AIDS encephalitis is mediated by vascular cell adhesion molecule-1/aβ1 integrin interactions. *Am. J. Pathol.*, **144**, 27–40.

Saukkonen, K., Sande, S., Cioffe, C. *et al.* (1990). The role of cytokines in the generation of inflammation and tissue damage in experimental gram-positive meningitis. *J. Exp. Med.*, **171**, 439–48.

Sharer, L. R. (1992). Pathology of HIV-1 infection of the central nervous system: a review. *J. Neuropathol. Exp. Neurol.*, **51**, 3–11.

Singer, E. J., Syndulko, K., Fahy-Chandon, B. *et al.* (1994). Intrathecal IgG synthesis and albumin leakage are increased in subjects with HIV-1 neurologic disease. *J. Acquir. Imm. Defic. Synd.*, **7**, 265–71.

Smith, T. W., DeGirolami, U., Hénin, D. *et al.* (1990). Human immunodeficiency virus (HIV) leukoencephalopathy and the microcirculation. *J. Neuropathol. Exp. Neurol.*, **49**, 357–70.

Steffan, A. M., Lafon, M. E., Gendrault, J. L. *et al.* (1994). Feline immunodeficiency virus can productively infect cultured endothelial cells from cat brain microvessels. *J. Gen. Virol.*, **75**, 3647–53.

Taruscio, D., Malchiodi Albedi, F., Bagnato, R. *et al.* (1991). Increased reactivity of laminin in the basement membranes of capillary walls in AIDS brain cortex. *Acta Neuropathol.*, **81**, 552–6.

Tornatore, C., Chandra, R., Berger, J. R. and Major, E. O. (1994). HIV-1 infection of subcortical astrocytes in the pediatric central nervous system. *Neurology*, **44**, 481–7.

Tyor, W. R., Glass, J. D., Griffin, J. W. *et al.* (1992). Cytokine expression in the brain during AIDS. *Ann. Neurol.*, **31**, 349–60.

Weis, S., Haug, H. and Budka, H. (1993). Astroglial changes in the cerebral cortex of AIDS brains: a morphometric and immunohistochemical investigation. *Neuropathol. Appl. Neurobiol.*, **19**, 329–35.

Wiley, C. A., Schrier, R. B., Nelson, J. A. *et al.* (1986). Cellular localization of human immunodeficiency virus infection within the brains of acquired immune deficiency syndrome patients. *Proc. Natl. Acad. Sci. USA*, **93**, 7089–93.

Yoshida, S., Minakawa, T., Takai, N. and Tanaka, R. (1989). Effects of cytokines on cultured microvascular endothelial cells derived from gerbil brain. *Neurosurgery*, **25**(3), 373–7.

46 Hypertension

BARBRO B. JOHANSSON

- Introduction
- Acute hypertension
- Chronic hypertension
- Hypertensive encephalopathy
- The possible role of blood–brain barrier dysfunction in vascular dementia
- Concluding remarks

Introduction

This chapter deals with blood–brain barrier dysfunction in acute and chronic hypertension and its role in the development of edematous brain lesions such as white matter changes, glial hypertrophy and morphological brain damage. The clinical relevance of experimental data is also discussed.

Acute hypertension

Blood–brain barrier (BBB) dysfunction can be observed after an acute increase in blood pressure induced by various vasoactive drugs (Johansson et al., 1970, Johansson, 1989) or by compression of the aorta (Johansson and Linder, 1974, Sokrab et al., 1988). There is no fixed level at which this occurs. Factors such as vascular tone, abruptness of the pressure increase and the drugs used all play a role. An increase in systolic pressure exceeding 60 mmHg will result in multifocal opening of the BBB to albumin in most experimental models. A number of studies have shown that the BBB dysfunction is related to vascular distension (Johansson, 1989, Table 46.1) rather than to extensive vasoconstriction – vasospasm – as earlier suggested (Byrom, 1954).

The tension in the vessel wall increases with the pressure and with the diameter of the vessels. Thus, vessels dilated by drugs or hypercapnia will be exposed to a higher stress than constricted vessels and will accordingly be more vulnerable to an increase in blood pressure (Fig. 46.1; Johansson, 1974b; 1989). Likewise, it has been shown that the BBB leakage that occurs during epileptic seizures is a combined effect of the vasodilatation and concomitant hypertension and does not occur if the blood pressure increase is prevented (Petito et al., 1977; Johansson and Nilsson, 1977).

Another evidence for the importance of vascular tone is that a high sympathetic activity (Bill and Linder, 1976) protects the vessels. This should be considered when comparing data from animal studies with the clinical situation. Acute hypertensive episodes in humans are usually – although not always – associated with high sympathetic activity, whereas most drugs as well as aortic compression will activate the baroreflexes and reduce the sympathetic tone. There is evidence that not only the sympathetic nerves but also noradrenergic nerve terminals from the locus coeruleus enable the vessels to stand a high intraluminal pressure (Johansson, 1979; Harik and McGunigal, 1984). Anesthesia, particularly inhalation anesthesia, enhances

Table 46.1. *Evidence indicating that the blood–brain barrier dysfunction in acute hypertension is related to vasodistension and vascular stress and not to ischemia*

1. The permeability increase can be observed within minutes and thus long before the extravasation would be expected if induced by ischemia.
2. The sagittal sinus venous pressure increases concomitantly with the BBB dysfunction indicating an increased blood flow.
3. Blood flow is higher in leaking regions than in areas with an intact BBB.
4. Vasodilatation increases the vulnerability and vasoconstriction reduces the vulnerability.
5. Brain energy metabolites do not differ in intact and leaking areas.
6. Intravital studies on pial arteries do not support the spasm concept.

Sources: Johansson *et al.*, 1970; Häggendal and Johansson 1972*a*; Johansson, 1974*a,b*; Johansson and Siesjö, 1977; MacKenzie *et al.*, 1976; Auer and Johansson, 1980

the risk for hypertensive BBB opening, probably a combined effect on sympathetic activity, vascular tone and on membrane fluidity (Johansson, 1978, 1989).

Extravasation of plasma constituents is predominantly observed in cortical and subcortical structures but also in deep grey matter, particularly when dilated vessels are exposed to high pressure such as during hypercapnia and epileptic seizures (Johansson and Nilsson, 1977). The extravasated substances spread to the white matter particularly in longstanding hypertension or severe acute hyper-

tension. Clustering of extravasated regions may occur in the border zones between the main cerebral arteries, a fact that was taken to support the hypothesis that ischemia was involved in the breakdown of the BBB. However, during an abrupt increase in blood pressure the pressure *increase* is likely to be particularly large in the boundary zones and the change in pressure may be more important than the absolute pressure level (Häggendal and Johansson, 1972*a,b*).

A local intravascular pressure increase caused by intracarotid injection of blood or saline can also open the BBB (Häggendal and Johansson, 1972*b*; Rapoport, 1976). If combined with a rise in blood pressure, an intracarotid injection of nonionic contrast media can markedly potentiate the BBB damage during carotid angiography in rats (Whisson *et al.*, 1994).

Studies on the BBB in acute hypertension have concentrated on substances that normally have little access to the brain. Whether the passage of substances with carrier-mediated entry into the brain is changed has not been elucidated.

After an episode of acute hypertension the BBB opening is rapidly reversible when the pressure normalizes. A short exposure of brain parenchyma to plasma constituents may not lead to morphological changes. However, even after a 5–10 min hypertensive episode induced by compression of the abdominal aorta, excluding drug effects, focal spongy lesions with proliferations of astrocytes, invasion of macrophages and/or selective degener-

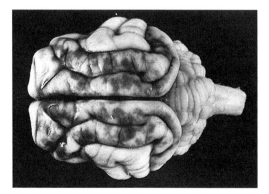

Fig. 46.1. Multifocal confluent areas of extravasation of Evans Blue–albumin complex in the cerebral cortex of a cat after an acute increase in blood pressure. A few minutes before the blood pressure increase the cat was given papaverine to reduce the vascular tone. From Johansson, 1974, with permission from Munksgaard, Copenhagen.

ation of neurons are occasionally observed (Sokrab *et al.*, 1988).

Whether the passage of plasma constituents into the brain in acute hypertension occurs through opened tight junction or across the endothelial cell membrane is debated (Hansson *et al.*, 1975; Nag *et al.*, 1977; Nagy *et al.*, 1979). Using peroxidase as tracer, an apparent increase in pinocytotic activity has been observed in a number of studies. Plasmalemma pits, endothelial balloons and craters have been observed in intracerebral vessels in scanning electron microscopy (Povlishock *et al.*, 1980). However, evidence for opening of tight junctions has also been reported (Nagy *et al.*, 1979) and the significance of pinocytosis and channels in the endothelium is debated (Bundgaard *et al.*, 1979). Drugs that stabilize membranes and/or prevent endocytosis, such as local anesthetics, phenothiazines, anion transport inhibitors and desipramine (Johansson and Linder, 1981; Johansson, 1989) significantly reduce protein extravasation in acute hypertension, an observation that may favor transendothelial passage, however, the same drugs could possibly affect tight junctions. Various sized molecules have been reported to enter to the same extent, a finding that was taken to support the endothelial route by the authors (Mayhan and Heistad, 1985). Flunarizine (Nag, 1991) but not other calcium blockers (Edvinsson *et al.*, 1983; Zumkeller *et al.*, 1991) have been reported to reduce protein leakage; the difference might be related to the effect of dihydropyridine derivatives on the vascular tone. Scanning and transmission electron microscopy of pial arterioles exposed to acute severe hypertension induced by intravenous norepinephrine or angiotensin showed discrete destructive endothelial lesions and abnormalities in a small number of smooth muscle cells, changes that could be inhibited by pretreatment with inhibitors of cyclooxygenase or by topical application on the brain surface of scavengers of free oxygen radicals (Kontos *et al.*, 1981). It has been proposed that nitric oxide might have a role in the disruption of the BBB during hypertension (Mayan, 1995). The increased permeability is associated with a transient reduction or loss of terminal sialic acid groups on the endothelium and of net negative endothelial charge in leaking areas (Nag, 1986).

Chronic hypertension

In hypertension the arterial smooth muscles respond to the enhanced work load by enlarging arterial volume. An enhanced media thickness with or without lumen changes has been observed over a large range of arterial sizes in the intracranial cerebral vascular bed in hypertensive animals (Johansson, 1984; Nordborg *et al.*, 1985; Baumbach and Heistad, 1989). The altered vascular geometry increases the vascular resistance and enables arterial vessels to tolerate a higher intraluminal pressure, protecting the BBB in genetic hypertensive rats, but does not seem to do so in renal hypertensive rats. Adrenergic and neuropeptide Y-containing vasoconstrictory nerve fibers have been reported to be denser in blood vessels from spontaneously hypertensive rats than in normotensive rats (Kawamura and Takebayashi, 1991).

The endothelial cells of intracerebral arterioles and capillaries of genetically hypertensive rats show an increased labeling of endothelial cells with [^{3}H]thymidine and activation of lysosomal enzymes suggesting an accelerated turnover of the cells (Hazama *et al.*, 1979; Yamada *et al.*, 1980).

Renal hypertension is more likely to result in BBB dysfunction and brain edema than genetic hypertension (Johansson and Linder, 1980, 1981; Mueller and Luft, 1982). Whether the increased tendency to brain edema in renal hypertension compared to essential hypertension is due to less efficient structural adaptation to the blood pressure or is related to circulating vascular substances is not known.

The first systematic studies on the BBB and cerebral lesions in experimental hypertension were reported by Byrom (1954), who showed that renal hypertensive rats with severe episodes of acute blood-pressure elevations showed areas of increased permeability in the brain. Through a closed cranial window he inspected pial arteries and observed alternating constriction and dilatation during the episodes of acute rise in blood pressure, often combined with convulsions. He also noted small areas of Trypan Blue extravasation, indicating BBB dysfunction, and suggested that a physiological constrictor response got out of hand resulting in vasospasm, ischemia of the vessel wall and multifocal edema. In a later publication, Byrom (1969) discussed the possibility that extravasation might also take place from the dilated parts of the vessels. A detailed combined permeability and immunohistochemical study on cerebral changes in renal hypertension further stressed the relation between permeability disturbance and morphological changes (Nag, 1984).

In the spontaneously hypertensive rats (SHR) no or little plasma extravasation is observed in the tissue (Fredriksson *et al.*, 1985) and SHR are much more resistant to drug-induced blood pressure elevation than normotensive or renal hypertensive rats (Johansson, 1984). Unless provoked by high salt and low protein diets (Hazama *et al.*, 1975; Fredriksson *et al.*, 1987), even rats of the stroke-prone spontaneously hypertensive strain usually do not develop the typical multifocal BBB dysfunction before the mean arterial pressure exceeds 210–220 mmHg. The first change noted is accumulation of perivascular extravasated plasma proteins. Immunohistochemical and electron-microscopical studies suggest a crucial pathophysiological role for the accumulation of plasma constituents and brain edema in the development of brain lesions (Hazama

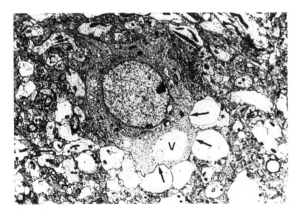

Fig. 46.2. Electronmicroscopic appearance of the central part of an area with plasma extravasation in the caudate-putamen of a stroke-prone spontaneously hypertensive rat. Swollen cell processes bulge into the perikaryon (arrows) of a nerve cell, which shows increased electron lucency and vacuolation (V) of the cytoplasm. Peripherally the cytoplasm appears watery and the cytoplasmic organelles cluster around the well-preserved nucleus. Magnification × 4800. Reproduced by permission from Fredriksson *et al.* (1988*a*), with permission from Springer-Verlag.

et al., 1975; Ogata *et al.*, 1980; Fredriksson *et al.*, 1985). Edema leads to astrocytic proliferation, perivascular spongiosis and edematous loosening of the white matter. The cytoplasm and dendrites are primarily affected whereas the nuclei of neurons within the edematous and spongiotic grey matter may be well preserved (Fig 46.2, Fredriksson *et al.*, 1988*a*,*b*). Cell destruction by cytolysis will ultimately lead to formation of spongy and cystic lesions (Fredriksson *et al.*, 1988*b*). Excitotoxic damage to neurons has been described as an axon-sparing, dendrite-affecting lesion characterized by swelling of the postsynaptic structures (Rothman and Olney, 1987). Interestingly, after opening of the BBB in models with no primary neuronal damage glutamate increases in the extracellular fluid concomitant with the development of edema (Westergren *et al.*, 1994). With time, hyaline degeneration, fibrinoid necrosis and microaneurysms occur in the penetrating arterioles, often surrounded by spongiocystic grey matter lesions (Fredriksson *et al.*, 1988*c*). In the presence of endothelial cell damage, platelet aggregation and other intravascular events are likely to predispose for thrombosis. Lipohyalinosis and fibrinoid necrosis may give rise to small-vessel stenosis and occlusion. However, infarcts and hemorrhages are late phenomena and the edematous lesions described above are the main characteristics in the early phase.

Hypertensive vascular degenerative changes are typically multifocal with marked fibrinoid necrosis alternating with apparently normal cerebral arterial segments (Fredriksson *et al.*, 1988*c*). The multifocal rather than diffuse appearance of BBB disturbance as well as vascular degenerative changes in hypertension suggests an uneven stress on the vasculature.

Hypertensive encephalopathy

Hypertensive encephalopathy is an acute, usually rapidly progressive, syndrome characterized by elevated arterial blood pressure associated with neurological signs and symptoms such as headache, seizures, altered mental status and visual disturbances. Hypertensive encephalopathy is most likely to appear in patients with rapidly developing

The possible role of blood–brain barrier dysfunction in vascular dementia

The pathology behind white matter hyperintensities (WMHI) observed on magnetic resonance imaging on MRI is heterogeneous and includes dilated perivascular spaces, cystic changes, gliosis and demyelination (Chimowitz *et al.*, 1989), i.e. changes described above as probable late effects of focal brain edema. Hypertension is one of the risk factors for WMHI, which may be associated with cognitive changes (Schmidt *et al.*, 1991; van Swieten *et al.*, 1991). WMHI are commonly observed in an elderly non-selected population (Lindgren *et al.*, 1994) but rarely found in normotensive individuals in the absence of neurological disorders below the age of 55 years. When the blood pressure is moderately or markedly increased, however, WMHI are not infrequent in that age group (Johansson, 1994). Prospective studies are needed to evaluate if such changes in young hypertensives predispose for vascular dementia.

or intermittent hypertension such as in eclampsia and pheochromocytoma (Johansson *et al.*, 1974). Severe renal hypertension is another risk group and less commonly it is seen in a malignant phase of chronic essential hypertension. Current antihypertensive treatment has reduced the incidence of hypertensive encephalopathy in patients with known hypertension but new risk groups such as cocaine abusers have been identified (Johansson, 1997). Neuroimaging studies support the hypothesis that BBB disturbances and reversible brain edema play an important role at least in a majority of patients with this syndrome (Rail and Perkin, 1980, Hauser *et al.*, 1988; Schwartz *et al.*, 1992; Weingarten *et al.*, 1994).

There is some discrepancy in the reports as to the involvement of grey and white matter. Usually both are involved and judging from animal studies, where serial studies can more easily be performed, the initial BBB breakdown is usually in the cortex and border zone between white and grey matter. However, like in all other types of vasogenic brain edema, the edema fluid will spread more easily in the white matter even if there is no local BBB disturbance in that region (Fredriksson *et al.*, 1985)

It seems likely that pressure-induced breakdown of the BBB and the resulting edema are the primary events in most cases of hypertensive encephalopathy. Vasoactive substances and rheological factors may contribute. Ischemia may develop but the fact that most imaging studies show a reversible picture speaks against long-standing ischemia at least in the majority of surviving patients.

Concluding remarks

Although it is generally accepted that acute and chronic hypertension can lead to BBB disturbance, the possible consequences of altered passage of nutrients and plasma constituents for long-term glial and neuronal function and the development of morphological changes in the brain have attracted little interest. Current data indicate an important role of focal brain edema and altered extracellular environment for focal brain lesion in hypertension.

References

Auer, L. M. and Johansson, B. B. (1980). Dilatation of pial arterial vessels in hypercapnia and in acute hypertension. *Acta Physiol. Scand.*, **109**, 249–51.

Baumbach, G. L. and Heistad, D. D. (1989). Remodelling of cerebral arterioles in chronic hypertension. *Hypertension*, **13**, 968–72.

Bill. A. and Linder, J. (1976). Sympathetic control of cerebral blood flow in acute arterial hypertension. *Acta Physiol. Scand*, **96**, 114–21.

Bundgaard, M., Frøkjaer-Jansen, J. and Crone, C. (1979). Endothelial plasma-lemmal vesicles as elements in a system of branching invaginations from the cell surface. *Proc. Natl. Acad. Sci. USA*, **76**, 6439–42.

Byrom, F. B. (1954). The pathogenesis of hypertensive encephalopathy and its relation to the malignant phase of hypertension: Experimental evidence from the hypertensive rat. *Lancet*, **2**, 201–11.

Byrom, F. B. (1969). *The Hypertensive Vascular Crisis. An Experimental Study.* London: Heinemann.

Chimowitz, M. I., Awad, I. A. and Furlan, A. J. (1989). Periventricular lesions on MRI. Fact and theories. *Stroke*, **20**, 963–7.

Edvinsson, L., Johansson, B. B., Larsson, B. *et al.* (1983). Calcium antagonists: effects on cerebral blood flow and blood–brain barrier permeability in the rat. *Br. J. Pharmacol.*, **79**, 141–8

Fredriksson, K., Auer, R. N., Kalimo, H. *et al.* (1985). Cerebrovascular lesions in stroke-prone spontaneously hypertensive rats. *Acta Neuropathol. (Berl.)*, **68**, 284–94.

Fredriksson, K., Kalimo, H., Westergren, I. *et al.* (1987). Blood–brain barrier leakage and brain edema in stroke-prone spontaneously hypertensive rats. Effects of chronic sympathectomy and low protein/high salt diet. *Acta Neuropathol. (Berl.)*, **74**, 259–68.

Fredriksson, K., Kalimo, H., Nordborg, C. *et al.* (1988*a*). Nerve cell injury in the brain of stroke-prone spontaneously hypertensive rats, *Acta Neuropathol. (Berl.)*, **76**, 227–37.

Fredriksson, K., Kalimo, H., Nordborg, C. *et al.* (1988*b*). Cyst formation and glial response in the brain lesions of stroke-prone spontaneously hypertensive rats. *Acta Neuropathol. (Berl.)*, **76**, 441–50.

Fredriksson, K., Nordborg, C., Kalimo, H. *et al.* (1988*c*). Cerebral microangiopathy in stroke-prone spontaneously hypertensive rats. *Acta Neuropathol. (Berl.)*, **75**, 241–52.

Häggendal, E. and Johansson, B. (1972*a*). On the pathophysiology of the increased cerebrovascular permeability in acute arterial hypertension in cats. *Acta Neurol. Scand.*, **48**, 265–70.

Häggendal, E., Johansson, B. B. (1972*b*). Effect of increased intravascular pressure on the blood–brain barrier to protein in dogs. *Acta Neurol. Scand.*, **48**, 271–5.

Hansson, H.-A., Johansson, B. B., Blomstrand, C. (1975). Ultrastructural studies on cerebrovascular permeability in acute hypertension. *Acta Neuropathol. (Berl.)*, **32**, 187–98.

Harik, S. I. and McGunigal, T. (1984). The protective influence of the locus ceruleus on the blood–brain barrier. *Ann. Neurol.*, **15**, 568–74.

Hauser, R. A., Lacey, D. M. and Knight, M. R. (1988). Hypertensive encephalopathy. Magnetic resonance imaging demonstration of reversible cortical and white matter lesions. *Arch. Neurol.*, **45,** 1078–83.

Hazama, F., Ozaki, T., Amano, O. (1979). Scanning electron microscopic study of endothelial cells of cerebral arteries from spontaneously hypertensive rats. *Stroke*, **10,** 245–52.

Hazama, F., Ooshima, A., Tanaka, T. *et al.* (1975). Vascular lesions in the various substrains of spontaneously hypertensive rats and the effects of chronic salt ingestion. *Jap. Circulat. J.*, **39**, 7–22.

Johansson, B. B. (1974*a*). Regional cerebral blood flow in acute arterial hypertension. *Acta Neurol. Scand.*, **50**, 366–72.

Johansson, B. B. (1974*b*). Blood–brain barrier dysfunction in acute hypertension after papaverine induced vasodilatation. *Acta Neurol. Scand.*, **50**, 573–80.

Johansson, B. B. (1978). Effect of an acute increase of the intravascular pressure on the blood–brain barrier. A comparison between conscious and anesthetized rats. *Stroke*, **9**, 588–90.

Johansson, B. B. (1979). Neonatal 6-hydroxydopamine treatment increases the vulnerability of the blood–brain barrier to acute hypertension in conscious rats. *Acta Neurol. Scand.*, **60**, 198–203.

Johansson, B. B. (1984). Cerebral vascular bed in hypertension and consequences for the brain. *Hypertension*, **6** (suppl III), 81–6.

Johansson, B. B. (1989). Hypertension and the blood–brain barrier. In *Implications of the blood–brain barrier and its manipulation*, vol. 2, ed. E. A. Neuwell, pp. 389–410. Plenum Press: New York.

Johansson, B. B. (1994). Pathogenesis of vascular dementia: the possible role of hypertension. *Dementia*, **5**, 174–6.

Johansson, B. B. (1997). Hypertensive encephalopathy. In *Primer on Cerebrovascular Diseases*, ed. K. M. A. Welch, C. Caplan, D. Reis, B. Weir , B. Siesjö, pp. 367–70. San Diego: Academic Press.

Johansson, B. B. and Linder, L.-E. (1974). Blood–brain barrier dysfunction in acute hypertension induced by aortic clamping. *Acta Neurol. Scand.*, **50**, 360–5.

Johansson, B. B. and Linder, L.-E. (1980). The blood–brain barrier in renal hypertensive rats. *Clin. Exp. Hypertens. Part A, Theory and Practice*, **2**, 983–993.

Johansson, B. B. and Linder, L.-E. (1981). Hypertension and brain edema. An experimental study on acute and chronic hypertension in the rat. *J. Neurol. Neurosurg. Psychiat.*, **44**, 402–6.

Johansson, B. B. and Nilsson, B. (1977). The pathophysiology of the blood–brain barrier dysfunction induced by severe hypercapnia and by epileptic brain activity. *Acta Neuropathol. (Berl.)*, **38**, 153–8.

Johansson, B. B. and Siesjö, B. (1977). Brain energy metabolism in angiotensin-induced acute hypertension in rats. *Acta Physiol. Scand.*, **100**, 182–6.

Johansson, B. B., Li, C.-L., Olsson, Y. and Klatzo, I. (1970). The effect of acute arterial hypertension on the blood–brain barrier to protein tracers. *Acta Neuropathol. (Berl.)*, **16**; 117–24.

Johansson, B. B., Strandgaard. S, and Lassen, N. A. (1974). On the pathogenesis of hypertensive encephalopathy. *Circ. Res.*, **34** (suppl 1), 167–71.

Johansson, B. B., Auer, L. M. and Linder, L.-E. (1982). Phenothiazine-protection of the blood–brain barrier during acute hypertension: evidence for a modification of the endothelial cell membrane. *Stroke*, **13**, 220–5.

Kawamura, K. and Takebayashi, S. (1991). Perivascular innervation of the cerebral arteries in spontaneously hypertensive rats – an immunohisto-chemical study. *Angiology*, **42**, 123–32.

Kontos, H. A., Wei, E. P., Dietrich, W. D. *et al.* (1981). Mechanisms of cerebral arteriolar abnormalities after acute hypertension. *Am. J. Physiol.*, **240**, H511–27

Lindgren, A., Roijer, A., Rudling, O. *et al.* (1994). Cerebral lesions on magnetic resonance imaging, heart disease, and vascular risk factors in subjects without stroke. A population-based study. *Stroke*, **25**, 929–34.

MacKenzie, E. T., Strandgaard, S., Graham, D. I. *et al.* (1976). Effect of acutely induced hypertension acts on pial arteriolar caliber, local cerebral blood flow and the blood–brain barrier. *Circ. Res.*, **39**, 33–41.

Mayhan, W. G. (1995). Role of nitric oxide in disruption of the blood–brain barrier during acute hypertension. *Brain Res.*, **686**, 99–103.

Mayhan, W. G. and Heistad, D. D. (1985). Permeability of blood–brain barrier to various sized molecules. *Am. J. Physiol.*, **248**, 1712–18.

Mueller, S. M. and Luft, F. C. (1982). The blood–brain barrier in renovascular hypertension. *Stroke*, **13**, 229–34.

Nag, S. (1984). Cerebral changes in chronic hypertension: Combined permeability and immunohistochemical studies. *Acta Neuropathol. (Berl.)*, **62**, 178–84. .

Nag, S. (1986). Cerebral endothelial plasma membrane alterations in acute hypertension. *Acta Neuropathol. (Berl.)*, **70**, 38–43

Nag, S. (1991). Protective effect of flunarizine on blood–brain barrier permeability alterations in acutely hypertensive rats. *Stroke*, **22**, 1265–9.

Nag, S., Robertson, D. and Dinsdale, H. B. (1977). Cerebral cortical changes in acute experimental hypertension, an ultrastructural study. *Lab. Invest.*, **36**, 150–61.

Nagy, Z., Mathieson, G. and Hüttner, I. (1979). Opening of tight junctions in cerebral endothelium. II. Effect of pressure-pulse induced acute arterial hypertension. *J. Comp. Neurol.*, **185**, 579–86.

Nordborg, C., Fredriksson, K. and Johansson, B. B. (1985). The morphometry of consecutive segments in cerebral arteries of normotensive and spontaneously hypertensive rats. *Stroke*, **16**, 313–20.

Ogata, J., Fujishima, M., Tamaki, K. *et al.* (1980). Vascular changes underlying cerebral lesions in stroke-prone spontaneously hypertensive rats. *Acta Neuropathol. (Berl.)*, **54**, 183–8.

Petito, C. K., Schaefer, J. A. and Plum, F. Ultrastructural characteristics of the brain and the blood–brain barrier in experimental seizures. *Brain Res.* **127**, 251–67.

Povlishock, J. T., Kontos, H. A., Rosenblum, W. I. *et al.* (1980). A scanning electronmicroscopic analysis of the intraparenchymal brain vasculature following experimental hypertension. *Acta Neuropathol. (Berl.)*, **51**, 203–13.

Rail, D. L. and Perkin, G. D. (1980). Computerized tomographic appearance of hypertensive encephalopathy. *Archiv. Neurol.*, **37**, 310–11.

Rapoport, S. I. (1976). Opening of the blood–brain barrier by acute hypertension. *Exp. Neurol.*, **52**, 467–79.

Rothman, S. M. and Olney, J. W. (1987). Excitotoxicity and the NMDA receptor. *Trends Neurosci.*, **10**, 299–302.

Schmidt, R., Fazekas, F., Offenbacher, H. *et al.* (1991). Magnetic responance imaging white matter lesions and cognitive impairment in hypertensive individuals. *Archiv. Neurol.*, **48**, 417–420.

Schwartz, R. B., Jones, K. M., Kalina, P. *et al.* (1992). Hypertensive encephalopathy: findings on CT, MR imaging and SPECT imaging in 14 cases. *Am. J. Roentgenol.*, **159**, 379–83.

Sokrab, T.-E. O., Johansson, B. B., Kalimo, H. and Olsson, Y. (1988). A transient hypertensive opening of the blood–brain barrier can lead to brain damage. *Acta Neuropathol. (Berl.)*, **75**, 557–565

van Swieten, Geyskes, G. G., Derix, M. M. A. *et al.* (1991). Hypertension in the elderly is associated with white matter lesion and cognitive decline. *Ann. Neurol.*, **30**, 825–30

Weingarten, K., Barbut, D., Filippi, C. and Zimmerman, R. D. (1994). Findings on spin-echo and gradient-echo MR imaging. *Am. J. Roentgenol.*, **162**, 665–70.

Westergren, I., Nyström, B., Hamberger, A. *et al.* (1994). Concentration of amino acids in extracellular fluid after opening of the blood–brain barrier by intracarotid infusion of protamine sulphate. *J. Neurochem.*, **62**,159–65.

Whisson, C. C., Wilson, A. J., Evill, C. A., Sage, M. R. (1994). The effect of intracarotid nonionic contrast media on the blood–brain barrier. *Am. J. Neuroradiol.*, **15**, 95–100.

Yamada, E., Hazama, F., Amano, S. and Hanakita, J. (1980). Cytochemical investigation on acid phosphatase activity in cerebral arteries in spontaneously hyeprtensive rats. *Jap. Circ. J.*, **44**, 467–75.

Zumkeller, M., Hollerhage, H. G., Reale, E. and Dietz, H. (1991). Ultrastructural changes in the blood–brain barrier after nimodipine treatment and induced hypertension. *Exp. Neurol.*, **113**, 315–21.

47 The blood–brain barrier in brain tumours

P. A. STEWART and D. MIKULIS

- Introduction
- Barrier loss in tumors
- Vascular permeability routes in the normal blood–brain barrier
- Structural changes in tumor vessel walls that underlie barrier loss
- Brain adjacent to tumors
- Pathogenic mechanisms that lead to barrier loss in tumors
- Attempts to further open the blood–tumor barrier to enhance drug delivery

Introduction

Tumors are vascularized by sprouting of capillaries from pre-existing vessels in a process termed angiogenesis (reviewed by Plate and Risau, 1995). The new vessels constitute the tumor vascular bed, or blood–tumor barrier, which, in most cases, is highly abnormal in terms of its angioarchitecture, barrier properties and ultrastructure. The angioarchitecture within most tumors consists of large-diameter, tortuous vessels that are irregularly spaced, leaving variably sized avascular regions (Baish et al., 1996). As a result there are regions of flow-limited transport and the blood flow through the tumor as a whole is reduced, despite the lower resistance that would be expected from the increase in vessel diameter.

Barrier loss in tumors

In all brain tumors, with the exception of low-grade gliomas (Fig. 47.1), the vessels are more permeable than normal brain capillaries (reviewed by Stewart, 1994). Loss of barrier properties has some advantages in that it allows imaging of the tumor using contrast-enhancing agents that do not cross the intact barrier (Fig. 47.1) and it also permits delivery of hydrophilic drugs to the tumor. However, barrier loss also gives rise to cerebral edema, which is a significant cause of morbidity and mortality in the patient. Furthermore, the increased tissue pressure created by the edema, and the mass effect of the tumor within the closed cranium, further limit blood flow to the tumor and surrounding brain.

Evidence from a variety of experimental tumors shows that barrier loss, as measured, for example, by diffusion of intravascular tracers across vessel walls, is heterogeneous (reviewed by Blasberg et al., 1990). Similarly, enhancement of tumors with contrast agents is also variable (Fig. 47.2). In many of the large 'ring-enhancing' tumors, areas of no enhancement represent necrosis within the tumor, however, even when no necrosis is evident (Fig. 47.2A), the permeability of the tumor vasculature to contrast agent is still variable (Fig. 47.2B). It is not certain whether variable enhancement, i.e. passage of the contrast agent across tumor vessel walls, is due to variable barrier breakdown or heterogeneous flow-limited delivery of contrast agent, or both.

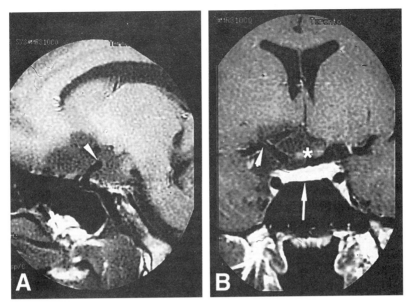

Fig. 47.1. Lack of barrier breakdown in a low-grade astrocytoma. A. T1-weighted spin echo sequence performed before intravenous administration of gadolinium-DTPA showing the distal internal carotid artery (arrowhead) surrounded by tumor that has significantly decreased signal compared to adjacent normal brain. B. The same imaging sequence was repeated in coronal projection following intravenous administration of 10 cm³ 0.1 mM/kg gadolinium–DTPA. The arrow shows intense enhancement of the cavernous sinus and pituitary gland. The asterisk indicates the optic chiasm. The arrowhead shows the distal carotid artery dividing into middle and anterior cerebral branches. The artery is surrounded by non-enhancing tumor. In comparing the pre- and post-contrast images no change in signal intensity could be seen, indicating that the blood–brain barrier is intact. Based on these imaging findings the differential diagnosis included parasellar epidermoid tumor and low-grade astrocytoma. Because the lesion was felt to be in an extra-axial location, epidermoid tumor was thought to be present, however open biopsy revealed a low-grade astrocytoma.

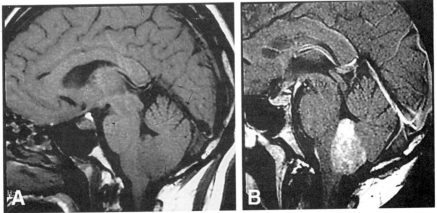

Fig. 47.2. Sagittal T1-weighted spin echo pre-contrast (A) and post-contrast (B) images show variable enhancement within the biopsy-proven cerebellar ependymoma. The pre-contrast image (A) shows no evidence of necrosis within the tumor, therefore the heterogeneous enhancement within tumor (B) is not due to the presence of necrotic tissue.

In addition to the structural properties that restrict diffusion across the intact blood–brain barrier (described below), brain microvessels also express a collection of nutrient transport mechanisms (reviewed by Part II of this volume). Very little is known about the expression of the barrier nutrient transport mechanisms in tumor vessels. The sodium-independent L-system, which transports large neutral amino acids, is preserved within tumor vessels in glioma-bearing rats (Cornford *et al.*, 1992) whereas the glucose transporter is not expressed in human primary and secondary brain tumor vessels (Harik and Roessmann, 1991),

Vascular permeability routes in the normal blood–brain barrier

In non-barrier vessels hydrophilic solutes cross the capillary wall via one or more permeability routes. In all capillary beds except those in neural tissue, the endothelial cells are joined by tight junctions that are discontinuous. Clefts (spaces) between the tight junctions form continuous channels that span the vessel wall (Bundgaard, 1984). The continuous channels constitute the paracellular route by which solutes pass from the lumen to the extravascular space between adjacent endothelial cells. Two types of transcellular pore also allow movement of solutes across capillary walls. These are the vesicular route and fenestrations. Endothelial vesicles are thought to carry solutes across the vessel wall by either 'ferrying' pinocytosed fluids from the lumin to the ablumin (Milici *et al.*, 1987; Villegas and Broadwell, 1993), or by fusing to form transient, open channels (tubulo-vesicular structures) through which solutes diffuse into the perivascular spaces (Frokjaer-Jensen, 1983). A high density of endothelial vesicles is characteristic of skeletal muscle capillaries. Fenestrations are 'windows' in attenuated areas of the endothelial cytoplasm 60–70 nm in diameter that may or may not be closed by a membranous diaphragm. Open fenestrations, for example those in liver and spleen, form large gaps in the capillary walls, whereas fenestrations closed by a diaphragm characteristic of endocrine and exocrine gland vessels have much smaller pores (Bearer *et al.*, 1985).

In blood–brain barrier vessels the endothelial cells are joined by continuous tight junctions that seal the paracellular route, lack fenestrations and have a very low density of endothelial vesicles (Reese and Karnovsky, 1967; Brightman and Reese, 1969). These structural features ensure that most hydrophilic solutes can only gain entry to neural tissue by passing through the endothelial cells via specific transport mechanisms.

Structural changes in tumor vessel walls that underlie barrier loss

For descriptive purposes, brain tumors can be divided into three groups: primary tumors that develop *in situ* and derive their blood supply from neural vessels, secondary tumors that arise elsewhere in the body and metastasize to brain, and also derive their vasculature from neural vessels, and meningiomas, which arise from extra-axial tissue within the cranium or spinal canal and which initially derive their vascular supply from the meninges. Some meningiomas, however, invade neural tissue and eventually derive some of their blood vessels from the neural vasculature. The description that follows is a condensation of a large number of studies in which the ultrastructural features of tumor vasculature in humans and animal models have been described. Representative references only are included.

In general, it is clear that changes in all three permeability routes described above may be responsible for increased permeability in tumor vessels. In addition to structural changes, a proportion of endothelial cells necrose, leaving infrequent, but large gaps in the vessel wall. These large gaps could be responsible for significant fluid extravasation and microhemorrhages within the tumor.

A common finding in all studies is that the interendothelial junctions in tumor vessels are abnormal (Long, 1970; Hirano and Matsui, 1975; Waggener and Beggs, 1976; Dean and Lantos, 1981; Nishio *et al.*, 1983; Yamada *et al.*, 1981; Stewart *et al.*, 1985; Coomber *et al.*, 1988*b*; Roy and Sarkar, 1989; Shibata, 1989). Junctions are described 'shortened' i.e. the area of overlap between adjoining endothelial cells is restricted, suggesting a shorter, more direct paracellular diffusion path, or 'open', suggesting a widened paracellular channel. This suggests that paracellular movement of fluid is a significant cause of blood–brain barrier breakdown and tumor-associated edema.

There is good agreement on the development of fenestrae in tumor vessels. Fenestrae are extremely rare in glial tumor vessels, even in glioblastoma multiforme (Long, 1970; Waggener and Beggs, 1976; Dean and Lantos, 1981; Coomber *et al.*, 1988*b*; Roy and Sarkar, 1989; Shibata, 1989). An interesting radiological study (Schmiedl *et al.*, 1992) showed that barrier breakdown in gliomas was size dependent. Small tracer molecules passed into the tumors faster than medium sized molecules, which, in turn, entered the tumors faster than large molecules. Since fenestrae are thought to represent one form of the large vascular pore, the resistance to large molecules in gliomas could be related to the lack of fenestrae.

Fenestrae have been described in primary nonglial tumor vessels and are common in most, if not all metastatic tumor vessels (Hirano and Matsui, 1975; Waggener and Beggs, 1976; Shibata, 1989; P. A. Stewart *et al.*, unpublished observations). A quantitative study (P. A. Stewart *et al.*, unpublished results) has shown that fenestrae are present in particularly high densities in vessels of meningioma, compared with other metastatic tumors. This is not surprising since normal dural vessels, from which most meningioma vessels are derived, are also fenestrated. In some tumor types, then, fenestrae form a second permeability route for the movement of fluids into the tumor and surrounding brain.

Vesicles have been described as increased or decreased, sometimes within the same tumor type. Because the distribution of vesicles from profile to profile varies widely, and their apparent number per section is affected by the angle of cut relative to the long axis of the vessel, and the section thickness, it is actually very difficult to draw conclusions about their numerical density without careful morphometric studies. Even among the morphometric studies, however, vesicular densities in tumor vessels have been described as increased (Shibata, 1989), decreased (Nishio *et al.*, 1983), or unchanged (Stewart *et al.*, 1985) within experimental glial tumors. Furthermore, since a change in the activity of vesicles or tubulo-vesicular structures could

conceivably occur without any change in vesicle numbers, it is difficult to draw any conclusions about the role of vesicles in barrier breakdown in tumors.

Brain adjacent to tumors

Many tumors grow in the brain both by increasing tumor mass and by infiltrating surrounding normal brain. Since the infiltrated areas appear grossly normal, they are not usually removed during surgery. It is generally assumed that remaining tumor cells in peritumoral brain, if not destroyed by subsequent radio- or chemotherapy, are responsible for tumor recurrence. The barrier is generally intact in peritumoral brain, but ultrastructural abnormalities including junctional changes and increases in the density of endothelial vesicles have been reported in peritumoral vessels that are associated with infiltrating tumor cells (Stewart *et al.*, 1987; Roy and Sarkar, 1989).

Pathogenic mechanisms that lead to barrier loss in tumors

The mechanisms that lead to the formation of abnormal vessels in brain tumors is not well understood, however two factors can be considered.

A. Inductive tissue factors

It is generally accepted that inductive signals from normal brain cells induce and possibly maintain the development of the blood–brain barrier phenotype in central nervous system vessels (Stewart and Wiley, 1981; Ikeda *et al.*, 1996). Astrocytes, which form endfeet ensheathing the abluminal surface of the vessels, are a good candidate for the inducing cell type because of their intriguing structural association with the vessels; however experimental evidence in favour of this hypothesis is controversial (Janzer and Raff, 1987; Holash *et al.*, 1993). Presumably similar kinds of inductive mechanisms determine the differential vessel phenotype in all tissues (reviewed by Risau, 1995).

Circumstantial evidence from a variety of brain tumors is consistent with the hypothesis that tumors fail to elaborate normal inductive factors that are necessary for the development and maintenance of blood–brain barrier features in new vessels. Low-grade astrocytomas are relatively normal in appearance and presumably in metabolic function, and they are associated with relatively normal blood vessels in which the blood–brain barrier is intact (Fig. 47.1). Presumably these cells would be still secreting blood–brain barrier inductive signals that would maintain a relatively normal barrier phenotype in the surrounding blood vessels. Malignant astrocytoma and glioblastoma multiforme are much more abnormal in structure. Presumably these abnormal cells would no longer be producing appropriate inductive signals and the new vessels would fail to develop the blood–brain barrier phenotype completely. Metastatic tumors introduce an entirely different cellular environment into the brain. The cells are not of neural origin and they are malignant, therefore secretion of blood–brain barrier inductive signals would not be expected. Blood vessels in metastatic tumors lack blood–brain barrier features and they differ from vessels in glioblastoma with regard to their expression of fenestrations (see above).

Alternatively, tumor cells may secrete inductive signals that elicit the formation of tumor-appropriate blood vessels. When C6 glioma cell spheroids are transplanted into brain or muscle, the tumor blood vessels are identical in both sites and are different from those of normal brain and of normal muscle (Coomber *et al.*, 1988a). Vessels in peritumoral areas showed a transitional phenotype between normal brain or muscle and tumor.

B. Factors related to angiogenesis

Folkman and his collaborators have proposed that tumor angiogenesis is necessary for tumor growth and that tumor cells induce angiogenesis by secretion of growth factors that act on endothelial cells (Folkman and Shing, 1992). Many of these growth factors also increase vascular permeability either directly or indirectly. It has recently been found that tumors elaborate both angiogenic and anti-angiogenic factors. Folkman suggests that the switch to the angiogenic phenotype that allows tumors to grow beyond millimeter sizes and metastasize, is due to a change in net balance of positive and negative regulators of blood vessel growth. (Folkman, 1995).

Among the positive regulators of blood vessel growth, vascular endothelial growth factor (VEGF) (also know as vascular permeability factor, VPF) is a particularly interesting candidate since its receptors VEGFR-1 and -2 are expressed exclusively in endothelial cells. During embryogenesis VEGF is secreted by ventricular neuroepithelial cells at the time when endothelial cells proliferate rapidly and grow into the brain from the perineural plexus. Expression of VEGF is high in the fetal and newborn brain, when endothelial cells are rapidly proliferating, but is reduced in adult brain, when endothelial cell proliferation has ceased (Breier *et al.*, 1992). When tumors begin to grow within the brain, VEGF expression is again upregulated in the tumor cells and its receptors are upregulated in endothelial cells. In low-grade gliomas expression is slightly upregulated only in some tumor cells but it is significantly upregulated in high-grade gliomas (reviewed by Plate and Risau, 1995). Histological analysis of human glioma biopsies revealed a striking association of VEGF mRNA producer cells with areas of necrosis (Plate *et al.*, 1996). Because hypoxia is a powerful upregulator of VEGF *in vitro*, Risau and his collaborators have proposed that in gliomas, pallisading cells that surround areas of necrosis, and are therefore hypoxic, secrete VEGF that exerts paracrine control of angiogenesis during tumor progression. In support of this hypothesis are their further observations that infection of endothelial cells *in vivo* with a retrovirus encoding a dominant-negative mutant of the Flk-1/VEGF receptor (also known as VEGFR-2) prevents growth of a wide range of solid human tumors transplanted in experimental animals (Millauer *et al.*, 1996a,b).

VEGF was first identified as a vascular permeability factor isolated from ascites fluid that caused marked vascular extravasation following intradermal injection (Senger *et al.*, 1983). It was subsequently found to be related to PDGF, to have endothelial mitogenic properties and to be secreted by a variety of tumor types including gliomas (Weindel *et al.*, 1994; Keck *et al.*, 1989). It is likely, therefore, that VEGF/VPF is responsible, at least in part, for both angiogenesis and the increased vascular permeability in human brain tumors.

Attempts to further open the blood–tumor barrier to enhance drug delivery

It is widely assumed that the blood–brain barrier in tumors, although higher than that in surrounding brain, still limits delivery of chemotherapeutic drugs to the tumor; however it should not be forgotten that tissue pressure within the tumor and drug cytotoxicity are still important factors in treatment outcome (Stewart, 1994). Various strategies are being explored for opening the blood–tumor barrier to increase drug delivery. Opening the blood–brain barrier in the entire cerebral hemisphere in which the tumor resides using intra-arterial infusion of hyperosmotic mannitol increases the permeability of tumor vessels to a variety of molecules (Neuwelt *et al.*, 1987); however other studies have shown that the increase in the tumor itself is quite small, whereas the increase in drug concentration in the brain surrounding tumor and the distant normal cortex is substantial (Warnke and Blasberg, 1987). Increased perme-

ability in the cortex exposes normal brain to neurotoxic drugs. Furthermore, normal endothelial cells within the hemisphere are damaged by the substantial changes in osmolarity (Lossinsky *et al.*, 1995). Nevertheless, treatment of human patients in which osmotic barrier breakdown was combined with the delivery of chemotherapeutic drugs has produced impressive increases in survival in some tumor types, for example, primary CNS lymphoma (Neuwelt and Goldman, 1991; Williams *et al.*, 1995); however the success of this technique in patients with malignant gliomas, that account for the majority of brain tumors, is modest (Neuwelt *et al.*, 1986; Williams *et al.*, 1995). More recently a technique that specifically opens up the blood–tumor barrier without affecting the normal blood–brain barrier, using a bradykinin analog, RMP-7, has been used to increase delivery of carboplatin into experimental glial tumors. This technique resulted in substantial increases in drug delivery to the tumors and prolonged survival in tumor-bearing rats (Matsukado *et al.*, 1996), and may hold some promise for treatment of humans.

References

Baish, J. W., Gazit, Y., Berk, D. A. *et al.* (1996). Role of tumor vascular architecture in nutrient and drug delivery: an invasion percolation-based network model. *Microvasc. Res.*, **51**, 327–46.

Bearer, E. L., Orci, L. and Sors, P. (1985). Endothelial fenestral diaphragms: A quick-freeze, deep-etch study. *Cell Biol.*, **100**, 418–28.

Blasberg, R. G., Groothuis, D. and Molnar, P. (1990). A review of hyperosmotic blood–brain barrier disruption in seven experimental brain tumor models. In *Pathophysiology of the Blood–Brain barrier*, ed. B. B. Johansson, C. Owman and H. Widner, pp. 197–219.

Breier, G., Albrecht, U., Sterrer, S. and Risau, W. (1992). Expression of vascular endothelial growth factor during embryonic angiogensis and endothelial cell differentiation. *Development*, **114**, 521–32.

Brightman, M. W. and Reese, T. S. (1969). Junctions between intimately apposed cell membranes in the vertebrate brain. *J. Cell Biol.*, **40**, 648–77.

Bundgaard, M. (1984). The three-dimensional organization of tight junctions in a capillary endothelium revealed by serial-section electron microscopy. *J. Ultrastruct. Res.*, **88**, 1–17.

Coomber, B. L., Stewart, P. A., Hayakawa, E. M. *et al.* (1988*a*). A quantitative assessment of microvessel ultrastructure in C$_6$ astrocytoma spheroids transplanted to brain and to muscle. *J. Neuropathol. Exp. Neurol.*, **47**, 29–40.

Coomber, B. L., Stewart, P. A., Hayakawa, K. *et al.* (1988*b*). Quantitative morphology of human glioblastoma multiforme microvessels: Structural basis of blood–brain barrier defect. *J. Neuro-Oncol.*, **5**, 299–307.

Cornford, E. M., Young, D., Paxton, J. W. *et al.* (1992). Melphalan penetration of the blood–brain barrier via the neutral amino acid transporter in tumor-bearing brain. *Cancer Res.*, **52**, 138–43.

Dean, B. R. and Lantos, P. L. (1981). The vasculature of experimental brain tumours. Part 2. A quantitative assessment of morphological abnormalities. *J. Neurol. Sci.*, **49**, 67–77.

Folkman, J. (1995). Angiogenesis in cancer, vascular, rheumatoid and other disease. *Nature Medicine*, **1**, 27–31.

Folkman, J. and Shing, Y. (1992). Angiogenesis. *J. Biol. Chem.*, **267**, 10931–4.

Frokjaer-Jensen, J. (1983). The plasmalemmal vesicular system in capillary endothelium. In *Structure and Function of Endothelial Cells. Progress in Applied Microcirculation*, Vol. 1, ed. K. Mebmer and F. Hammersen, pp. 17–34. Basel: Karger.

Harik, S. I. and Roessmann, U. (1991). The erythrocyte-type glucose transporter in blood vessels of primary and metastatic brain tumors. *Ann. Neurol.*, **29**, 487–91.

Hirano, A. and Matsui, T. (1975). Vascular structures in brain tumors. *Human Pathol.*, **6**, 611–21.

Holash, J. A., Noden, D. M. and Stewart, P. A. (1993). Re-evaluating the role of astrocytes in the induction and maintenance of the blood–brain barrier. *Dev. Dynam.*, **197,** 14–25.

Ikeda, E., Flamme, I. and Risau, W. (1996). Developing brain cells produce factors capable of inducing the HT7 antigen, a blood–brain barrier-specific molecule, in chick endothelial cells. *Neurosci. Lett.*, **209,** 1–4.

Janzer, R. C. and Raff, M. C. (1987). Astrocytes induce blood–brain barrier properties in endothelial cells. *Nature*, **325,** 253–7.

Keck, P. J., Hauser, S. D., Krivi, G. *et al.* (1989). Vascular permeability factor, an endothelial cell mitogen related to PDGF. *Science*, **246,** 1309–12.

Long, D. M. (1970). Capillary ultrastructure and the blood–brain barrier in human malignant brain tumors. *J. Neurosurg.*, **32,** 127–44.

Lossinsky, A. S., Vorbrodt, A. W. and Wisniewski, H. M. (1995). Scanning and transmission electron microscopic studies of microvascular pathology in the osmotically impaired blood–brain barrier. *J. Neurocytol.*, **24,** 795–806.

Matsukado, K., Inamura, T., Nakano, S. *et al.* (1996). Enhanced tumor uptake of carboplatin and survival in glioma-bearing rats by intracarotid infusion of bradykinin analog, RMP-7. *Neurosurgery*, **39,** 125–34.

Milici, A. J., Watrous, N. E., Stukenbrok, H. and Palade, G. E. (1987). Transcytosis of albumin in capillary endothelium. *J. Cell Biol.*, **105,** 2603–12.

Millauer, B., Longhi, M. P., Plate, K. H. *et al.* (1996a). Dominant-negative inhibition of FLK-1 suppresses the growth of many tumor types *in vivo. Cancer Res.*, **56,** 1615–20.

Millauer, B., Shawver, L. K., Plate, K. H. *et al.* (1996b). Glioblastoma growth inhibited *in vivo* by a dominant-negative FLK-1 mutant. *Nature*, **367,** 576–9.

Neuwelt, E. A. and Goldman, D. L. (1991). Primary CNS lymphoma treated with osmotic blood–brain barrier disruption: prolonged survival and preservation of cognitive function. *J. Clin. Oncol.*, **9,** 1580–90.

Neuwelt, E. A., Howieson, J., Frenkel, E. P. *et al.* (1986). Therapeutic efficacy of multiagent chemotherapy with drug delivery enhancement by blood–brain barrier modification in glioblastoma. *Neurosurgery*, **19,** 573–82.

Neuwelt, E. A., Specht, H. D., Barnett, P. A. *et al.* (1987). Increased delivery of tumor-specific monoclonal antibodies to brain after osmotic blood–brain barrier modification in patients with melanoma metastatic to the central nervous system. *Neurosurgery*, **20,** 885–95.

Nishio, S., Ohta, M., Abe, M. and Kitamura, K. (1983). Microvascular abnormalities in ethylnitrosourea (ENU)-induced rat brain tumors: structural basis for altered blood–brain barrier function. *Acta Neuropathol.*, **59,** 1–10.

Plate, K. H. and Risau, W. (1995). Angiogenesis in malignant gliomas. *Glia*, **15,** 339–47.

Plate, K. H., Breier, G., Weich, H. A. and Risau, W. (1996). Vascular endothelial growth factor is a potential tumour angiogenesis factor in human gliomas *in vivo. Nature*, **359,** 845–8.

Reese, T. S. and Karnovsky, M. J. (1967). Fine structural localization of a blood–brain barrier to exogenous peroxidase. *J. Cell Biol.*, **34,** 207–17.

Risau, W. (1995). Differentiation of endothelium. *FASEB J*, **9,** 926–33.

Roy, S. and Sarkar, C. (1989). Ultrastructural study of micro-blood vessels in human brain tumours and peritumoural tissue. *J. Neuro-Oncol.*, **7,** 283–94.

Schmiedl, U. P., Kenney, J. and Maravilla, K. R. (1992). Kinetics of pathologic blood–brain barrier permeability in an astrocytic glioma using contrast-enhanced MR. *Am. J. Neuroradiol.*, **13,** 5–14.

Senger, D. R., Galli, S. J., Dvorak, A. M. *et al.* (1983). Tumor cells secrete a vascular permeability factor that promotes accumulation of ascites fluid. *Science*, **219,** 983–5.

Shibata, S. (1989). Ultrastructure of capillary walls in human brain tumors. *Acta Neuropathol.*, **78,** 561–71.

Stewart, D. J. (1994). A critique of the role of the blood–brain barrier in the chemotherapy of human brain tumors. *J. Neuro-Oncol.*, **20,** 121–39.

Stewart, P. A. and Wiley, M. J. (1981). Developing nervous tissue induces formation of blood–brain barrier characteristics in invading endothelial cells: A study using quail-chick transplantation chimeras. *Dev. Biol.*, **84,** 183–92.

Stewart, P. A., Hayakawa, K., Hayakawa, E. M. *et al.* (1985). A quantitative study of blood–brain barrier permeability ultrastructure in a new rat glioma model. *Acta Neuropathol.*, **67,** 96–102.

Stewart, P. A., Hayakawa, K., Farrell, C. L. and Del Maestro, R. F. (1987). Quantitative study of microvessel ultrastructure in human peritumoral brain tissue. Evidence for a blood–brain barrier defect. *J. Neurosurg.*, **67,** 697–705.

Villegas, J. C. and Broadwell, R. D. (1993). Transcytosis of protein through the mammalian cerebral epithelium and endothelium. II. Adsorptive transcytosis of WGA-HRP and the blood–brain and brain–blood barriers. *J. Neurocytol.*, **22,** 67–80.

Waggener, J. D., Beggs, J. L. (1976). Vasculature of neural neoplasms. In *Neoplasia in the Central Nervous System*, ed. R. A. Thompson and J. R. Green. pp. 27–49. New York: Raven Press.

Warnke, P. C. and Blasberg, R. G. (1987). The effect of hyperosmotic blood–brain barrier disruption on blood to tissue transport in ENU-induced gliomas. *Ann. Neurol.*, **22-3,** 300–5.

Weindel, K., Moringlane, J. R., Marmé, D. and Weich, H. A. (1994). Detection and quantification of vascular endothelial growth factor/vascular permeability factor in brain tumor tissue and cyst fluid: The key to angiogenesis? *Neurosurgery*, **35,** 439–49.

Williams, P. C., Henner, W. D., Roman-Goldstein, S. *et al.* (1995). Toxicity and efficacy of carboplatin and etoposide in conjunction with disruption of the blood–brain tumor barrier in the treatment of intracranial neoplasms. *Neurosurgery*, **37,** 17–28.

Yamada, K., Hayakawa, T., Ushio, Y. *et al.* (1981). Regional blood flow and capillary permeability in the ethylnitrosourea-induced rat glioma. *J. Neurosurg.*, **55,** 922–8.

48 The pathophysiology of blood–brain barrier dysfunction due to traumatic brain injury

JOHN T. POVLISHOCK

- Introduction
- Evidence for traumatically induced disruption of the blood–brain barrier
- Cellular and subcellular substrates of the passage of large molecular weight species through the BBB following traumatic brain injury
- Mediators of traumatically induced macromolecular passage through the BBB
- Alterations in nutrient transport in the BBB following traumatic brain injury
- Summary and conclusions

Introduction

Over the past 20 years, our appreciation of the pathobiology of traumatic brain injury has increased significantly. Prior to that time, it was unknown whether the morbidity associated with traumatic brain injury was a direct result of traumatically induced vascular failure or alternatively the direct disruption of brain parenchyma and its neural connections. We now appreciate that the traumatic episode involves a progression and possible interaction of brain parenchymal and vascular changes across the full spectrum of traumatic brain injury, ranging from mild through severe. In relation to the brain parenchyma, it is now understood that brain injuries of varying severity are capable of releasing a surge of neurotransmitters that participate in abnormal agonist–receptor interactions causing altered postsynaptic signal transduction correlated with behavioral abnormalities (Hayes *et al.*, 1988, 1992; McIntosh *et al.*, 1989*a*; Katayama *et al.*, 1990). Importantly, these same neuroexcitatory surges have also been linked to post-traumatic glucose hypermetabolism (Hayes *et al.*, 1984; Yoshino *et al.*, 1991; Hovda, 1996) that can have catastrophic consequences if an uncoupling of flow and metabolism occurs. In addition to these neuroexcitatory-mediated changes, it is known that the shear and tensile forces of injury also stretch axons throughout the neuraxis, resulting in focal alterations of axoplasmic transport that lead to axonal swelling and detachment (Povlishock *et al.*, 1983; Povlishock, 1992; Povlishock and Jenkins, 1995). With this process, the downstream detached axonal appendages and their terminals undergo Wallerian change and participate in target deafferentation, some of which sets the stage for both adaptive and maladaptive neuroplastic re-arrangements (Erb and Povlishock, 1991, Povlishock *et al.*, 1992; Phillips *et al.*, 1994; Povlishock and Christman, 1995). Further, these neuroexcitatory and axotomy-mediated events can also contribute to neuronal cell loss, involving either chromatolytic or apoptotic mechanisms.

Accompanying these changes in the brain parenchyma, various vascular abnormalities have been identified. In patients sustaining severe traumatic injury, ultra-early ischemia has been recognized, together with evidence of impaired autoregulation and vascular reponsiveness (Bouma *et al.*, 1991). In severe forms of injury, hemorrhage has been described in contusional foci, with hematoma formation in various brain sites, including the basal ganglion and brain stem (Adams, 1992).

In addition to these overt vascular abnormalities, mild, moderate, and severe head injury can also evoke change in the blood–brain barrier permeability to circulating macromolecules, such as endogeous serum proteins and/or exogenously applied tracers. To date, most of our knowledge of the traumatic disruption of the blood–brain barrier has been derived from such studies of macromolecular passage, with virtually no consideration as to whether the traumatic episode can perturb nutrient transport. This emphasis on macromolecular passage has stemmed, in part, from the widespread belief that the passage of macromolecules correlates with the formation of brain edema, i.e. an increase of brain water, which, in turn, translates into increased intracranial pressure with catastrophic consequences for the patient.

Because, to date, most investigators have focused on macromolecular extravasation following traumatic brain injury, this chapter, by necessity, will consider information gleaned primarily through the study of these macromolecular events. The causal factors involved in such macromolecular permeability change will be considered and, where possible, the implications of these perturbations for nutrient transport will be discussed.

Evidence for traumatically induced disruption of the blood–brain barrier

As alluded to above, there is extensive evidence to support the premise that traumatic injury is capable of evoking change in the blood–brain barrier, at least to circulating proteins and/or large molecular weight species. In animals, this fact has long been recognized through the use of Evans Blue, a dye that binds to serum proteins. Using Evans Blue dye in a fluid-percussion model of traumatic brain injury in rabbit and an impact acceleration model in subhuman primates respectively, Lindgren and Olson (1968) and Ommaya and colleagues (1963) demonstrated the extravasation of the Evans Blue dye into the interstices of the brain parenchyma following traumatic brain injury. Using

fluid-percussion brain injury in cats, we also identified in the passage of the exogenous tracer, horseradish peroxidase, from the blood to brain front following the traumatic episode (Povlishock et al., 1978). These findings have been confirmed by multiple investigators using various models of traumatic brain injury and other exogenous and endogenous tracers, including various serum proteins and immunoglobulins visualized through the use of antibodies. Through the use of horseradish peroxidase, sometimes interfaced with antibodies targeted to serum albumin and/or circulating immunoglobulins, various investigators have consistently confirmed the opening of the blood–brain barrier to serum proteins, following various forms of mechanical brain injury involving fluid percussion injury (McIntosh et al., 1987, 1989; Cortez et al., 1989; Tanno et al., 1992a,b; Aihara et al., 1994; Dietrich et al., 1994; Fukuda et al., 1995; Schmidt and Grady, 1993), cortical impaction (Shapira et al., 1993; Mathew et al., 1994, 1996; Duvdevani et al., 1995; Baldwin et al., 1996) and impact acceleration injury (van den Brink, 1994). As one would anticipate, such opening of the blood–brain barrier was typically seen at the site of direct mechanical loading. Since most models invariably elicit direct or indirect contact with the cortical surface most injuries evoke forms of cortical contusional change associated with petechial hemorrhage seen either at the grey-white interface in gliding contusions or as a petechial hemorrhage scattered throughout the gray as associated with surface contusions (Povlishock et al., 1994).

In addition these local barrier changes seen with focal mechanical loading, more diffuse or generalized opening of the barrier to serum proteins has also been observed in various models. With central fluid percussion injury, opening of the barrier to exogenous horseradish peroxidase has been observed bilaterally in the neocortex, hippocampus, and thalamus, with striking abnormalities seen in the midline of the brainstem, involving the cervicomedullary junction (Schmidt and Grady, 1993). Interestingly, with parasagittal or lateral fluid-percussion injuries, the overall distribution of the peroxidase extravasation was changed in that the tracer passage was now confined ipsilateral to the injury unlike the bilateral distribution seen with midline injury (Schmidt and

Grady, 1993). Collectively, these findings speak in the fact that placement of the mechanical forces and their movement relative to the brain play a role in the anatomical localization of the sites of barrier failure to macromolecules, a point which will be expanded upon later.

In general, these relatively overt barrier changes to serum proteins and large molecular weight exogenous tracers have been observed within minutes of the traumatic episode, becoming maximal within the first 1–2 h post-injury, with evidence of closure of the barrier several hours later (Fukuda *et al.*, 1995; Povlishock *et al.*, 1978; Shapira *et al.*, 1993; Tanno *et al.*, 1992a). Evidence of this temporal profile of barrier opening has been obtained primarily in animal models through the use of delayed administration of various exogenous tracers, allowing the investigators to discern specific sites and temporal profiles of barrier breakdown (Fukuda *et al.*, 1995; Tanno *et al.*, 1992a). In addition to the acute changes in the barrier permeability to serum proteins, limited evidence suggests a secondary 'reopening' of the blood–brain barrier to macromolecules following the traumatic episode (Baldwin *et al.*, 1996; Fukuda *et al.*, 1995; Mathew *et al.*, 1994). Such delayed or secondary opening of the blood–brain barrier to macromolecules may have its basis in varied factors; yet, it would seem most likely that the recruitment of inflammatory cells and the vasoactive agents which they release could explain, in part, this delayed opening.

In addition to evidence for traumatic opening of the blood–brain barrier to macromolecules in animals, similar barrier alterations have been described in brain-injured humans. In humans, as one would imagine, the evidence for the traumatic opening in the blood–brain barrier is more limited and obviously the accrual of such evidence is restricted by the nature of the investigative studies that one can perform in brain-injured patients. Despite these limitations, however, evidence exists that traumatized patients do show opening of the blood–brain barrier at least to circulating agents normally excluded by the intact barrier (Lang *et al.*, 1991; Kushi *et al.*, 1994; Todd and Graham, 1990). Most of our information regarding the traumatic opening of the blood–brain barrier has been derived through studies utilizing intravascular gadolinium coupled with MR imaging. As gadolinium is normally excluded by the intact blood–brain barrier, its presence in the injured brain indicates a compromise of barrier function. Using this approach, Kushi and colleagues (1994) have elegantly shown that the traumatic brain injury can evoke the passage of gadolinium from the blood to the brain within the first days post-injury. Typically, this gadolinium passage appears most conspicuous in sites showing contusional change, involving foci of petechial hemorrhage dispersed within a normal vascular tree. As with animals, this opening of the blood–brain barrier appears relatively transient, with closure of the barrier within days of the injury.

Cellular and subcellular substrates of the passage of large molecular weight species through the BBB following traumatic brain injury

As alluded to above, traumatic brain injury consistently has been linked with the opening of the blood–brain barrier to large molecular weight species including exogenously administered tracers as well as endogenous immunoglobulins and serum proteins visualized through the use of antibodies. Clearly, in the foci of direct mechanical loading and contusion, microvascular rending and/or petechial hemorrhage are the major conduits through which thcsc cxtracellular tracers and/or serum proteins reach the brain front, although this point has not been universally acknowledged. Despite the finding of direct microvascular rending, however, there is also ample evidence that the traumatic episode can involve more subtle perturbations of the blood–brain barrier rather than direct endothelial rending. Such subtle microvascular perturbations have been posited to involve transient disruption of the interendothelial tight junctions, creation of tubular–vesicular channels from the luminal to the abluminal endothelial surface, and/or the activation of the dramatic endothelial pit-vesicular activity purportedly involved in the sequestration and movement of the macromolelcules from the blood-to-brain front.

Evidence in support of tight junctional disruption in traumatic brain injury is relatively modest, with most evidence for junctional cleaving inferred from related studies using hypertension or hyperosmotic opening of the blood–brain barrier (Nagy et al., 1979a,b,c). More information, however, does not exist on the involvement of tubular-vesicular channels and/or increased pit-vesicular activity in the sequestration and transendothelial passage of various serum proteins and extracellular tracers from the blood-to-brain front (Povlishock and Dietrich, 1992). Following relatively mild traumatic brain injury, the presence of numerous endothelial segments within capillaries, arterioles, and venules has been demonstrated that shows evidence of dramatic pit-vesicular activity (Povlishock et al., 1978). Typically, using exogenous tracers such as horseradish peroxidase, within minutes of the traumatic episode, numerous endothelial pits and vesicles are observed containing this tracer. In these studies, luminal endothelial pits are assumed to achieve confluence with endothelial vesicles that, in turn, apparently fuse with abluminal pits to discharge the protein tracer into the underlying basal lamina from where it is free to diffuse into the extracellular space of the brain parenchyma (Povlishock et al., 1978).

In addition to these pit-vesicular transport mechanisms, high voltage electron microscopy has demonstrated the presence of tubular-vesicular profiles extending from the luminal to abluminal front (Lossinksy et al., 1989). In general, it was believed that these tubular-vesicular profiles represented a coalescence of the luminal and abluminal pits with endothelial vesicles, thereby creating an open conduit from the blood-to-brain front.

Based upon the above passages, there is good evidence that traumatic brain injury evokes generalized endothelial activation, which suggests the sequestration and movement of serum proteins and/or exogenous tracers from the blood-to-tissue front. Although both the identification of tubular-vesicular profiles and endothelial vesicles and pits suggests that these subcellular structures are involved in the breakdown of the blood–brain barrier to macromolecules, critical evaluation of these findings suggest that these assumptions may be over simplistic and perhaps compromised by the limitations inherent in inferring biological processes from static fixed morphological images.

In this regard, it is now known that the nature of the primary aldehyde fixation may influence the overall number of endothelial vesicles and pits and therefore skew the overall interpretations derived therefrom. Further, there is now evidence from our laboratory as well as others that the pit and vesicle-laden segments, in themselves, are not necessarily correlated with the finding of tracer in the related brain tissue (Povlishock et al., 1980). Moreover, there is a more direct criticism that the pit and vesicles themselves do not directly participate in the transport of materials from the blood-to-brain front (Balin et al., 1987; Broadwell, 1989). Thus, although it appears that the endothelial vesicles and pits are routinely found, they may reflect a generalized form of endothelial activation rather than constituting the actual substrates of the blood–brain barrier perturbation to macromolecules. Precisely how the barrier is subtly broached in the case of traumatic brain injury is, as yet, unknown, but it is quite possible that the endothelial membrane itself is perturbed, allowing for direct diffusion of macromolecules down a concentration gradient from the blood-to-brain front. This concept is somewhat controversial, and it is complicated by the fact that the electron microscopic methods used to follow these purported changes in the blood–brain barrier do not necessarily impart a complete picture of the endothelial cell in vivo. Unfortunately, the membrane and cytoplasmic details seen at the ultrastructural level are the results of the protein and amino acid cross-linking achieved through fixation and do not necessarily picture the dynamic fluid phases of the membrane in the living state.

The complexity of the issues associated with fixation and the interpretations derived from ultrastructural analysis are clearly illustrated from a set of experiments conducted some time ago to gain a better impression of the correlations that existed between in vivo processes and any visualized ultrastructural change in the blood–brain barrier (Povlishock et al., 1983). To appreciate this relationship, animals were subjected to traumatic brain injury after they had received systematic injections of horseradish peroxidase. As anticipated from the data presented above, the traumatic episode resulted in opening of the blood–brain barrier to the circulating exogenous tracer. When these sites were examined by ultrastructural means, the tracer

could be recognized throughout the interstices of the brain parenchyma. In relation to the vascular endothelium, the tracer was present in numerous endothelial vesicles and abluminal pits, suggesting that these pits and vesicles had participated in a metabolically active process of sequestration and transendothelial transport of the extracellular peroxidase tracer.

Moving on the premise that these ultrastructural images confirmed the presence of a metabolically active process or transcytosis, these studies were repeated in a paradigm that would deactivate any metabolically dependent processes prior to the infusion of peroxidase. Simply stated, in this paradigm, the animals were injured and then subjected to aldehyde fixation, followed by the infusion of intravascular exogenous horseradish peroxidase. It was assumed that if the transfer of peroxidase was either directly or indirectly dependent upon a metabolically active process, no peroxidase passage would occur in the fixed 'dead' endothelium. To our surprise, however, microscopic examination of the brain tissue revealed peroxidase passage, despite the fact that the tracer was administered when the animal was dead and the tissues were fixed. When these sites showing peroxidase passage were examined at the ultrastructural level, an equally surprising series of changes were found. In those animals that had received the tracer following fixation, pits and vesicles could again be identified in the endothelia localized within these sites manifesting peroxidase passage into the brain parenchyma. Now, however, in contrast to the *in vivo* situation, no peroxidase could be found within any of the vesicles or pits. Rather, now the tracer was confined to the cytosol of endothelium, suggesting that the tracer had diffused directly through the luminal and abluminal endothelial membranes to reach the underlying basal lamina. Based upon this data, it would appear that peroxidase transfer seen in these studies was not dependent upon any metabolically dependent process. Rather, it would seem that the horseradish peroxidase passage was dependent upon its direct diffusion through altered endothelial cell membrane. Collectively, these findings illustrate the difficulties associated with making functional assessments through routine ultrastructural analysis and explain, in part, why we still do not have a complete under-

standing of the actual extracellular pathways by which macromolecules move through the blood-to-brain front in traumatic brain injury.

Mediators of traumatically induced macromolecular passage through the BBB

Mechanical factors

As alluded to above, there can be no doubt that mechanical factors play a role in the generation of traumatically induced macromolecules through the blood–brain barrier. As elegantly shown by Schmidt and Grady (1993), placement of the injury pulse in a central versus a paracentral position results in a differential pattern of CNS exogenous horseradish peroxidase extravasation following traumatic brain injury. As noted, injuries applied in the parasagittal position result in protein extravasation, primarily within the cortex and brainstem unilateral to the site of injury whereas placement of the injury pulse in the central position consistently results in a bilateral distribution of the extravasated tracer, indicating that the placement of mechanical force is, in itself, determining the location of the altered vascular permeability. While the mechanical factors can clearly influence the vascular permeability, the key question is precisely how they do so.

It is noteworthy in the above-described experiments that the vast majority of brain sites analyzed showed no evidence of petechial hemorrhage or direct endothelial rending, suggesting that the mechanical forces in themselves were capable of altering the endothelial cells directly, perhaps through some of the mechanisms previously described. That mechanical forces can directly affect endothelial structure and function without direct rending has been alluded to by several authors, who have shown that mechanical loading, particularly that involving rapid deformation of the endothelial cell, can result in endothelial cell dysfunction and failure. Using isolated endothelial cells in culture, Ellis and colleagues (1996) subjected these cells to rapid mechanical loading and discovered that the endothelial cells demonstrated an increased uptake of propidium iodide, an agent normally excluded by the intact endothelium. Interestingly, the injury required to perturb the endothelial cells was significantly higher than that required to perturb either neurons or glia, suggesting that the thresholds for injury are higher in endothelium than any other brain parenchymal cell type. Despite this differential response to injury, however, the fact remains that endothelial cells can be injured by mechanical loading, and that, as such, mechanical factors are likely to be involved in the brain microvascular response to injury.

Systematic factors

Although it is well appreciated that the traumatic episode itself can evoke alterations in the blood–brain barrier to circulating macromolecules, it is also appreciated that other traumatically induced systematic changes can contribute to the overall duration of any observed altered vascular permeability. It is well known that many traumatic brain injuries result in a transient rise in systematic blood pressure contributing a post-injury hypertensive phase. Therefore, it is reasonable to assume that such post-traumatic hypertension can increase the driving forces of transmural bulk flow. The correctness of this assumption has been shown by van den Brink and colleagues (1994), who assessed the passage of radiolabeled albumin in two different models of traumatic brain injury, one involving trauma with post-traumatic hypertension and the other involving trauma not complicated by a significant post-traumatic hypertensive surge. Through this approach, van den Brink and colleagues (1994) recognized that both injuries were capable of opening the barrier to the normally excluded serum albumin; yet, importantly, they also observed that those injuries complicated by post-traumatic hypertension, showed an increased permeability index in contrast to those not sustaining post-traumatic hypertension. Similar observations were also reported by Nawashiro and colleagues (1994, 1995), indicating that post-traumatic hypertension may be a major player in influencing the overall magnitude of the post-traumatic barrier change.

Vasoactive factors and other mediators

In the previous passages, it has been shown that the mechanical and systematic factors can play a role in contributing to the traumatically induced passage of macromolecules through the blood–brain barrier following traumatic brain injury. Additionally, there is now compelling evidence that other vasoactive factors may also play a role in this process. In the following passages, an attempt will be made to address the major vasoactive substances purported to be involved in this process and present the experimental evidence to support their role in traumatic brain injury.

Evidence for the involvement of oxygen radicals

Perhaps one of the most intensively investigated areas regarding vascular compromise with traumatic brain injury centers on the potential damaging consequences of free oxygen radicals. It has long been recognized that with traumatic injury oxygen radicals play a major role in contributing to the impaired vascular responses seens following the traumatic episode. It is well known that, following injury, pial arterioles show sustained vascular dilation and fail to respond to normal physiological challenges such as hypocapnia (Kontos, 1989; Povlishock and Kontos, 1985, 1992; Wei et al., 1980, 1981). Detailed studies of these events have shown that this sustained vascular dilation and lack of physiological responsiveness are directly linked to the accelerated metabolism of arachidonate through both the cyclooxygenase and lipoxygenase pathways, with the resulting production of oxygen radicals as a byproduct (Povlishock and Kontos, 1992; Wei et al., 1981). Typically, in the conversion of the PGG2 to the PGH2 via prostaglandin hydroperoxidases in the cyclooxygenase pathway, superoxide anions are released, and these have been directly linked to various vasoactive processes. Evidence for the involvement of the superoxide anion has been found in studies using various radical scavengers, which provide considerable protection when given prior to injury (Kontos, 1989; Wei et al., 1981). More direct evidence of superoxide anion formation and involvement has been obtained through the use of the water-soluble dye Nitroblue Tetrazolium applied into a cranial window overlying the CSF compartment and pial vessels revealing traumatically induced vascular change. This approach was based on the premise that the post-traumatic generation of oxygen radicals would result in the reduction of the Nitroblue Tetrazolium to an insoluble dye which could then be measured spectrophotometrically. Further, it was assumed that the addition of superoxide dismutase would allow for a determination of the proportion of Nitroblue Tetrazolium reduction attributable to the superoxide anion. Through this approach, it was observed that the traumatic event was associated with significant Nitroblue Tetrazolium reduction of which a significant portion was associated with superoxide dismutase inhibition, indicating the presence of the superoxide anion (Kontos and Wei, 1986; Povlishock and Kontos, 1992). Interestingly, in these studies, the Nitroblue Tetrazolium was found to be generated over one hour post-injury, indicating a relatively long production of this radical species (Povlishock and Kontos, 1992). That these radicals are involved in the barrier changes associated with traumatic brain injury has also been shown through several lines of evidence. Our laboratories have shown that the topical applicaiton of arachidonic acid, which leads to the production of oxygen radicals, can cause dramatic opening of the blood–brain barrier to exogenous horseradish peroxidase, particularly within the intraparenchmal vessels incident to the site of topical arachidonatic acid application (Wei *et al.*, 1986). Interestingly, these vessels showing increased peroxidase passage demonstrated the same ultrastructural features described after traumatic brain injury; namely, the preservation of interendothelial tight junctions, with a concomitant increase in endothelial pits and vesicles, most likely reflecting a generalized endothelial activation (Wei *et al.*, 1986).

That these alterations in vascular permeability, triggered by the application of arachidonate, have their basis in the generation of oxygen radical, was convincingly shown by the use of radical scavengers. Specifically, when these same vascular permeability responses were assessed in the presence of superoxide dismutase and catalase, there was a significant attenuation of peroxidase passage from the blood-to-brain front, indicating that the superoxide anion and/or other radical species were directly responsible for the observed peroxidase extravasation.

Further evidence that oxygen radical-mediated events are responsible for the extravasation of macromolecules following traumatic brain injury has been convincingly shown by Smith and colleagues (1994), who demonstrated a direct correlation between the production of hydroxyl radicals and peroxidation and the subsequent blood–brain barrier disruption, following cortical impact in the rat. In this study, the hydroxyl radical was assessed via salicylate trapping method, while lipid peroxidation was assessed through the analysis of phosphatidylcholine hydroperoxide levels via a HPLC-chemiluminescence technique. Alteration of the blood–brain barrier to macromolecules was assessed by the direct measurement of the extravasation of Evans Blue dye bound to serum proteins. Through this approach, Smith and colleagues (1994) demonstrated that the traumatic episode resulted in a rapid burst of hydroxyl radicals, which became maximal within minutes of the traumatic episode and faded within the first hour post-injury. Additionally, they demonstrated that the lipid peroxidation evoked by this radical surge was more delayed, evolving over 30 and 60 minutes post-injury in the same time frame paralleling the passage of the Evans Blue dye into the brain parenchyma. These studies indicate that free radicals, specifically the hydroxyl radical, are involved in macromolecular extravasation following traumatic brain injury. Importantly, they show that hydroxyl radicals mediate their effects via lipid peroxidation, which alters endothelial membrane characteristics to allow for the direct diffusion of macromolecules from the blood-to-brain front. Further evidence that this radical-mediated lipid peroxidation is pivotal was provided by the finding that these processes could be inhibited by the use of a lipid peroxidation inhibitor such as Tirilazad mesylate, which significantly blunted lipid peroxidation and Evans Blue dye extravasation (Smith *et al.*, 1994).

Cytokines

In addition to the potential role of free oxygen radicals in the pathobiology of traumatically induced brain–barrier change, considerable attention has focused on the potential role and interaction of cytokines in the process of both immediate and delayed blood–brain barrier perturbation. Evidence for such cytokine involvement is derived from multiple approaches examining either closed head-injury models, i.e. those models in which there is no overt penetration of the brain parenchyma, or penetrating brain-injury models in which a stab wound is introduced into the brain. Using closed head-injury models, Goss and colleagues (1995) demonstrated a rapid and significant increase in IL-1β RNA within 6 h of traumatic brain injury. Similar elevations of the cytokines IL-1β, interleukin 6 (IL-6) and tumor necrosis factor (TNF) have been reported following penetrating injury (Aloisi et al., 1992; Berman, 1987; Guilian et al., 1986, 1988; Hofman, 1989; Nieto-Sampedro and Bermen, 1987). It is well recognized that IL-1β is an important initiator of inflammatory reaction, and it is of interest that this cytokine is significantly elevated in CSF fluids from patients who have sustained severe head injury (DeKosky et al., 1994; McClain et al., 1987; Ott et al., 1994; Young et al., 1988). Further, many of the vascular abnormalities associated with traumatic brain injury can be elicited by the direct infusion of IL-1β into the ventricular compartment, and IL-1β has been linked to increased endothelial permeability (Bevilacqua et al., 1985; Mantovani and Dejana, 1987; Pober et al., 1986). Although some controversy surrounds the initial sites of cytokine production, most now believe that the cytokines can be derived from resident glial cell populations as well as macrophages.

While the overall temporal expression of these cytokines can vary among various animal models, there is little doubt that these cytokines are elevated in the first hours post-injury. Using a weight drop model of cortical injury, Shohami and colleagues (1994) demonstrated that TNFα levels increased 2 h post-injury and peeked at 4 h, while the levels of IL-6 lagged behind those of TNFα, peaking by 8 h post-injury. Despite this temporal delay, the fact that these cytokines are expressed relatively early in the post-traumatic period is consistent with the premise that they originate from brain parenchymal elements rather than being recruited from monocytes and macrophages, whose temporal appearance would significantly lag behind the observed cytokine expression.

Evidence that some of these cytokines can, in part, contribute to some of the increased macromolecular passage seen following traumatic brain injury is suggested by multiple studies, perhaps the most compelling of which show the attenuation of the increased blood–brain barrier permeability to macromolecules following treatment with various cytokine antagonists. Specifically, using a weight-drop model of head injury, Shohami and colleagues (1994) have shown that the use of tumor necrosis factor binding protein, a physiological inhibitor of tumor necrosis factor, significantly protects against blood–brain barrier disruption to serum proteins following traumatic brain injury. Thus, there is evidence that cytokines may also be players in the process of traumatically induced altered permeability.

Bradykinin

Another potential mediator of traumatically induced blood–brain barrier disruption to macromolecules is bradykinin. Although the evidence for this is less than compelling, it is known that bradykinin is a potent vasodilator of pial arterioles when applied by perivascular application (Wahl, 1982; Wahl et al., 1983; Whalley and Wahl, 1983) or by topical CSF applicaiton (Kontos et al., 1986; Unterberg et al., 1986). Similarly, bradykinin can also dilate intraparenchymal arteries (Dacey et al., 1988), suggesting that it could be a factor in many of the pial and intraparenchymal vascular responses observed following traumatic brain injury. While there is little direct evidence that the kallikrein–kinin system is directly involved in traumatic opening of the blood–brain barrier, there is evidence for the role of bradykinin in brain edema, suggesting that it may have some role in the altered vascular permeability associated with trauma. Following cryogenic lesioning, kallikrein inhibitors have been shown to exert a protective effect on the genesis of brain edema (Unterberg et al., 1986). Similarly, following traumatic brain injury, the subsequent rise in brain bradykinin concentration and the parallel cerebral arteriolar vasodilation could be attenuated by pretreatment with a β$_2$-kininergic receptor antagonist (Ellis et al., 1988). Thus, although there is evidence that bradykinin may contribute to some of the vascular abnormalities associated with traumatic brain injury, its overall role in the genesis of increased vascular permeability to macromolecules remains to be ascertained.

Polyamines

As with other vasoactive factors, the role of the polyamines in the breakdown of the blood–brain barrier following traumatic brain injury is not well understood. Interest in the polyamines has stemmed primarily from the findings in the field of cerebral ischemia (Schmidz *et al.*, 1993) as well as radiation-induced brain injury (Fike *et al.*, 1994), where it has been shown that polyamine inhibitors exert a protective effect, ranging from a reduction of cerebral edema to the attenuation of the passage of macromolecules through the blood–brain barrier.

In the case of traumatic brain injury, it has been recognized by two groups (Baskaya *et al.*, 1996; Shohami *et al.*, 1992) that the traumatic episode can result in the activation of polyamine biosynthesis. Despite this finding, however, it is unclear if this rise in polyamines actually contributes to brain edema and/or the alteration of blood–brain barrier to macromolecules. Not only is the data on edema formation somewhat inconsistent (Shohami *et al.*, 1992; Baskaya *et al.*, 1996), but also in the one study addressing this issue, Shohami and colleagues (1992) failed to demonstrate that polyamine inhibitors could blunt the generation of traumatically induced vasogenic edema and the related passage of macromolecules across the blood–brain barrier. Therefore, although the literature is limited, it would not appear that polyamines are major players in the pathogenesis of altered blood–brain barrier status following traumatic brain injury.

Alterations in nutrient transport in the BBB following traumatic brain injury

As alluded to in the Introduction, studies on perturbation of the blood–brain barrier following traumatic brain injury have focused on the passage of macromolecules with little consideration of nutrient transport. The only possible exception to this macromolecular focus is found in a recent communication by Cornford and colleagues (1996) who examined the GLUT1 glucose transporter following traumatic brain injury. In this study, Cornford and colleagues harvested tissue from two patients including the site of missile injury as well

as a focus of cortical contusion. Light microscopic immunocytochemistry, complemented by parallel immunogold immunocytochemistry, targeting the GLUT1 glucose transporter in microvascular endothelial cells were employed. These approaches were also interfaced with parallel immunogold strategies for assessing the passage of macromolecules (albumin) through the blood–brain barrier. Admittedly assessing a small sample size, Cornford and colleagues observed that within the foci of overt hemorrhage, GLUT1 immunoreactivity was absent. However, in the surrounding pericontusional domains, perhaps analogous to the ischemic penumbra, Cornford and colleagues observed microvessels showing reduced density.

Quantitative immunogold analyses of these microvascular segments demonstrated that the transporter was predominantly localized to the luminal and abluminal endothelial membranes, with the number of immunoreactive sites per unit area dramatically increased in those endothelial segments showing heightened immunoreactivity. Conversely, in those sites showing reduced immunoreactivity, there were proportionally fewer GLUT1 immunoreactive sites per unit area. Interestingly, this upregulation of the GLUT1 transporter occurred in foci showing extravasation of albumin into the brain parenchyma, suggesting that there was a direct correlation between these high GLUT1 densities and the observed flux of macromolecules. While any interpretations derived from this study must be made with caution, these findings are intriguing. They suggest the fact that foci showing increased macromolecular flux into the brain paranchyma contain microvacular endothelial cells with increased glucose transporter density, which obviously could influence the flux of glucose into the brain parenchyma. If the related brain foci, as posited by some, are hypermetabolic, these changes may be consistent and, as such, adaptive; however, the overall implications of these findings require further detailed analyses.

Summary and conclusions

As explicated in the above passages, there is no doubt that traumatic brain injury can evoke dramatic changes in the blood–brain barrier's permeability to macromolecules that may enter the brain both at the site of direct mechanical loading and at other microvascular foci remote from the site of primary injury. The precise subcellular and biochemical mechanisms associated with macromolecular passage remain to be fully elucidated, but it is clear that mechanical forces of injury and any subsequent post-traumatic hypertensive surge and/or release of various vasoactive factors can play a role in the traumatic perturbation of the blood–brain barrier. As experimental and limited clinical evidence point to a rapid post-traumatic opening of the blood–brain barrier, followed by a delayed closure, with some evidence of reopening, it would appear that multiple factors are at work in influencing the barrier change at various times post-injury. Obviously, these spatial/temporal barrier changes must be carefully dissected out, for without a precise spatial temporal understanding of the barrier perturbation and the factors related thereto, it will be impossible to design potential therapies for blunting these alterations.

While there can be no doubt that traumatic brain injury is a major player in perturbing the blood–brain barrier, it is somewhat remarkable that the overall implications of this barrier change have not been fully developed in the scientific literature. It is widely stated that the opening of the blood–brain barrier to macromolecules contributes to the subsequent development of brain edema, which may lead to increased intracranial pressure. The precise interlinkage of these events, however, has not been carefully studied. Further, the potential that these traumatically induced alterations of the blood–brain barrier may allow for the influx of nomally excluded damaging agents has received little consideration. This has contributed to a relatively incomplete appreciation of the significance of traumatically induced blood–brain barrier perturbation.

Lastly, in this vein, it is somewhat disquieting that in all the assessments of traumatic perturbation of the blood–brain barrier, virually no consideration has been given to the central issue of nutrient transport and what relation, if any, it shares with ongoing pathobiology associated with traumatic brain injury. As it is now becoming clear that the traumatic episode may trigger a host of intraparenchymal changes that may lead to disordered metabolism, this issue is of more than mere academic interest and requires continued investigation.

Acknowledgments

This work was supported, in part, by NIH grant NS20193 and The Commonwealth Center for the Study of Brain Injury.

References

Adams, J. H. (1992). Head Injury. In *Greenfield's Neuropathology*, ed. J. H. Adams and L. W. Duchen, pp. 106–52; New York: Oxford University Press.

Aihara, N., Tanno, H., Hall, J. J. *et al.* (1994). Immunocytochemical localization of immunoglobulins in the rat brain: relationship to the blood–brain barrier. *J. Comp. Neurol.*, **342**, 481–96.

Aloisi, R., Care, M., Borsellino, G. *et al.* (1992). Production of hemolymphopoietic cytokines (IL6, IL-8, colony-stimulating factors) by normal human astrocytes in response to IL-1beta and tumor necrosis factor-alpha. *J. Immunol.*, **149**, 2358–66.

Baldwin, S. A., Fagaccia, I., Brown, D. R. *et al.* (1996). Blood brain barrier breach following cortical contusion in the rat. *J. Neurosurg.*, **85**, 476–81.

Balin, B. J., Broadwill, R. D. and Salcman, M. (1987). Tubular profiles do not form tranendothelial channels through the blood–brain barrier. *J. Neurocytol.*, **16**, 721–35.

Baskaya, M. K., Rao, M., Puckett, L. *et al.* (1996). Effect of difuoromethylornithine treatment on regional ornithine decarboxylase activity and edema formation after experimental brain injury.

Bevilacqua, M. P., Pobert, J. S., Wheeler, M. E. *et al.* (1985). Interleukin 1 acts on cultured human vascular endothelium to increase the adhesion of polymorponuclear leukocytes, monocytes, and related leukocyte cell lines. *J. Clin. Invest.*, **76**, 2003–11.

Bouma, G. J., Muizelaar, J. P., Choi, S. C. *et al.* (1991). Cerebral circulation and metabolism after severe traumatic brain injury; the elusive role of ischemia. *J. Neurosurg.*, **75**, 685–93.

Broadwell, R. D. (1989). Transcytosis of macromolecules through the blood–brain barrier: a cell biological perspective and critical appraisal. *Acta Neuropathol.*, **79**, 117–28.

Cornford, E. M., Hyman, S., Cornford, M. E. and Caron, M. J. (1996). Glut1 glucose transporter activity in human brain injury. *J. Neurotrauma*, **13**, 523–36.

Cortez, S. C., McIntosh, T. K. and Noble, L. J. (1989). Experimental fluid–percussion brain injury: vascular disruption and neuronal and glial alterations. *Brain Res.*, **482**, 271–82.

Dacey, R. G., Bassett, J. E. and Takayasu, M. (1988). Vasomotor responses of rat intracerebral arterioles to vasoactive intestinal peptide substance P. Neuropeptide Y and bradykinin. *J. Cereb. Blood Flow Metab.*, **8**, 254–61.

DeKosky, S. T., Miller, P. D., Styren, S. *et al.* (1994). Interleukin-1β elevation in CSF following head injury in humans is attenuated by hypotheria. *J. Neurotrauma*, **11**, 177–81.

Dietrich, W. D., Alonso, O. and Halley, M. (1994). Early microvascular and neuronal consequences of traumatic brain injury: a light and electron microscopic study in rats. *J. Neurotrauma*, **11**(3), 289–301.

Duvdevani, R., Roof, R. L., Fulop, Z. *et al.* (1995). Blood–brain barrier breakdown and edema formation following frontal cortical contusion: does hormonal status play a role? *J. Neurotrauma.* **12**(1), 65–75.

Ellis, E. F., Holt, S. A., Wei, E. P. and Kontos, H. A. (1988). Kinins induce abnormal vascular reactivity. *Am. J. Physiol.*, **255**, H397–H400.

Erb, D. E. and Povlishock, J. T. (1991). Neuroplasticity in cat following traumatic brain injury: an immunocyto-chemical study of terminal loss and recovery. *Exp. Brain Res.*, **83**, 253–67.

Fike, J. R., Gobbel, G. T., Marton, L. J. and Seilhan, T. M. (1994). Radiation brain injury is reduced by the polyamine inhibitor α-difluoromethylornithine. *Rad. Res.*, **138**, 99–106.

Fujisawa, H., Maxwell, W. L., Graham, D. I. *et al.* (1994). Focal microvascular occlusion after acute subdural haematoma in the rat: a mechanism for ischaemic damage and brain swelling. *Acta Neurochirurg.*, **60**, 193–6.

Fukuda, K., Tanno, H., Okimura, Y. *et al.* (1995). The blood–brain barrier disruption to circulating proteins in the early period after fluid percussion brain injury in rats. *J. Neurotrauma*, **12**(3), 315–24.

Goss, J. R., Styren, S. D., Miller, P. D. *et al.* (1995). Hypothermia attenuates the normal increase in interleukin 1β RNA and nerve growth factor following traumatic brain injury in the rat. *J. Neurotrauma*, **12**, 159–67.

Guilian, D. and Lahman, L. B. (1985). Interleukin1 stimulation of astroglial proliferation after brain injury. *Science*, **228**, 497–9.

Hayes, R. L., Pechura, C. M., Katayama, Y. *et al.* (1984). Activation of pontine cholinergic sites implicated in unconsciousness following cerebral concussion in the cat. *Science*, **223**, 301–3.

Hayes, R. L., Jenkins, L. W., Lyeth, B. G. *et al.* (1988*a*). Pretreatment with phenycyclidine, an *N*-methyl-D-aspartate-receptor antagonist, attenuates long-term behavioural deficits in the rat produced by traumatic brain injury. *J. Neurotrauma*, **5**, 259–74.

Hayes, R. L., Katayama, Y., Jenkins, L. W. *et al.* (1988*b*). Regional rates in glucose utilization in the cat following concussive head injury. *J. Neurotrauma*, **5**, 121–37.

Hayes, R. L., Jenkins, L. W. and Lyeth, B. G. (1992). Neurotransmitter-mediated mechanisms of traumatic brain injury: acetylcholine and excitatory amino acids. *J. Neurotrauma*, **9**, S173–187.

Hofman, F. M. (1989). Cytokines in central nervous system disease. In *Neuroimmune Networks: Physiology and Diseases*, pp. 65–71. New York: Alan R. Liss.

Holmin, S., Mathiesen, T. and Biberfeld, P. (1995). Inracerebral inflammatory response to experimental brain contusion. *Acta Neurochirurg.*, **132**, 110–19.

Hovda, D. A. (1996). Metabolic Dysfunction. In *Neurotrauma*, ed. R. K. Narayan, J. E. Wilberger and J. T. Povlishock, pp. 1459–78. McGraw-Hill.

Katayama, Y., Becker, D. P., Tamura, T. and Hovda, D. A. (1990). Massive increases in extracellular potassium and the indiscriminate release of glutamate following concussive brain injury. *J. Neurosurg.*, **73**, 889–900.

Kontos, H. (1989). Oxygen radicals in CNS damage. *Chem. Biol. Interact.*, **72**, 229–55.

Kontos, H. and Wei, E. (1986). Superoxide production in experimental brain injury. *J. Neurosurg.*, **64**, 803–7.

Kontos, H., Wei, E., Povlishock, J. *et al.* (1980). Cerebral arteriolar damage by arachidonic acid and prostaglandin G_2. *Science*, **209**, 1242.

Kushi, H., Katayama, Y., Shibuya, T. *et al.* (1994). Gadolinium DTPA-enhanced magnetic resonance imaging of cerebral contusions. *Acta neurochirurg.*, **60**, 471–4.

Lang, D. A., Hadley, D. M., Teasdale, G. M. *et al.* (1991). Gadolinium DTPA enhanced magnetic resonance imaging in acute head injury. *Acta Neurochirurg.*, **109**, 5–11.

Lossinsky, A. S., Song, M. J. and Wisniewski, H. M. (1989). High voltage electron microscopic studies of endothelial cell tubular structures in the mouse blood–brain barrier following brain trauma. *Acta Neuropathol.*, **77**, 480–8.

Mantovani, A. and Dejana, E. (1987). Modulation of endothelial function by interleukin 1; a novel target for pharmacological intervention? *Biochem. Pharmacol.*, **36**, 301–5.

Mathew, P., Graham, D. I., Bullock, R. *et al.* (1994). Focal brain injury: histological evidence of delayed inflammatory response in a new rodent model of focal cortical injury. *Acta Neurochirurg.*, **60**, 428–30.

Mathew, P., Bullock, R., Teasdale, G. and McCulloch, J. (1996). Changes in local microvascular permeability and in the effect of intervention with 21-aminosteroid (Tirilazad) in a new experimental model of focal cortical injury in the rat. *J. Neurotrauma*, **13**, 465–72.

McClain, C. M., Cohen, D., Ott, L. and Dinarello, C. A. (1987). Ventricular fluid interleukin 1 activity in patients with head injury. *J. Lab. Clin. Med.*, **110**, 48–54.

McIntosh, T. K., Nobel, L., Andrews, B. and Faden, A. I. (1987). Traumatic brain injury in the rat: characterization of a midline fluid-percussion model. *CNS Trauma*, **4**, 119–34.

McIntosh, T. K., Vink, R., Soares, H. *et al.* (1989*a*). Effects of the *N*-methyl-D-aspartate receptor blocker MK-801 on neurologic function after experimental brain injury. *J. Neurotrauma*, **6**, 247–59.

McIntosh, T. K., Vink, R., Nobel, L. *et al.* (1989*b*). Traumatic brain injury in the rat: characterization of a lateral fluid-percussion model. *Neuroscience*, **28**, 233–44.

McKinney, J. S., Willoughby, K. A., Liang, S. and Ellis, E. F. (1996). Stretch-induced injury of cultured neuronal glial and endothelial cells. Effect of polyethylene glycol-conjugated superoxide dismutase. *Stroke*, **27**, 934–40.

Nagy, Z., Mathieson, G and Huttner, I. (1979*a*). Blood–brain barrier opening to horseradish peoxidase in acute arterial hypertension. *Acta Neuropathol.*, **48**, 45–53.

Nagy, Z., Mathieson, G and Huttner, I. (1979*b*). Opening of tight junctions in cerebral endothelium. II. Effect of pressure-pulse induced acute arterial hypertension. *J. Comp.Neurol.*, **185**, 579–86.

Nagy, Z., Pappius, H. M., Mathieson, G and Huttner, I. (1979*c*). Opening of tight junctions in cerebral endothelium. I. Effect of hyperosmolar mannitol infused through the internal carotid artery. *J. Comp. Neurol.*, **185**, 569–78.

Nawashiro, H., Shima, K. and Chigasaki, H. (1994). Blood–brain barrier, cerebral blood flow, and cerebral plasma volume immediately after head injury in the rat. *Acta Neurochirurg.*, **60**, 440–2.

Nawashiro, H., Shima, K. and Chigasaki, H. (1995). Immediate cerebrovascular responses to closed head injury in the rat. *J. Neurotrauma*, **12**, 189–97.

Nieto-Sampedro, M. and Berman, M. A. (1987). Interleukin 1-like activity in rat brain: sources, targets, and effect of injury. *J. Neurosci.*, **17**, 214–19.

Ommaya, A. K., Rockoff, S. D. and Baldwin, M. (1963). Experimental concussion. A first report. *J. Neurosurg.*, **21**, 249–65.

Ott, L., McClain, C. J., Gillespie, M. and Young, B. (1994). Cytokines and metabolic dysfunction after severe head injury. *J. Neurotrauma*, **11**, 447–72.

Pardridge, W. M. (1985). Cerebral vascular permeability status in brain injury. In *Central Nervous System Trauma Status Report*, ed. D. P. Becker and J. T. Povlishock, pp. 503–512.

Phillips, L. L., Lyeth, B. G., Hamm, R. J. and Povlishock, J. T. (1994). Combined fluid percussion brain injury and entorhinal cortical lesion: a model for assessing the interaction between neuroexcitation and deafferentation. *J. Neurotrama*, **11**, 631–56.

Pober, J. S., Gimbrone, M. A., Lapierre, L. A. *et al.* (1986). Overlapping patterns of activation of human endothelial cells by interleukin 1, tumor necrosis factor, and immune interferon. *J. Immunol.*, **137**, 1893–6.

Povlishock, J. T. (1992). Traumatically induced axonal injury: pathogenesis and pathobiological implications. *Brain Path.*, **2**, 1–12.

Povlishock, J. T. and Christman, C. W. (1995). Diffuse axonal injury. In *The Axon*, ed. S. G. Waxman, J. D. Kocsis and P. K. Stys, pp. 504–29. New York: Oxford University Press.

Povlishock, J. T. and Dietrich, W. T. (1992). The blood–brain barrier in brain injury: an overview. In *The Role of Neurotransmitters in Brain Injury*, ed. M. Globus and W. D. Dietrich, pp. 265–9. New York: Plenum Press.

Povlishock, J. T. and Jenkins, L. W. (1995). Are the pathobiological changes evoked by traumatic brain injury immediate and irreversible? *Brain Pathol.*, **5**, 415–26.

Povlishock, J. T. and Kontos, H. A. (1982). The pathophysiology of pial and intraparenchymal vascular dysfunction. In *Head Injury: Basic and Clinical Aspects*, ed. R. G. Grossman and P. L. Gildenberg, pp. 15–29. New York: Raven Press.

Povlishock, J. T. and Kontos, H. (1985). Continuing axonal and vascular change following experimental brain trauma. *CNS Trauma*, **2**, 285–98.

Povlishock, J. T. and Kontos, H. A. (1992). The role of oxygen radicals in the pathobiology of traumatic brain injury. *Human Cell*, **5**, 345–53.

Povlishock, J. T., Becker, D. P., Sullivan, H. G. and Miller, J. D. (1978). Vascular permeability alterations to horseradish peroxidase in experimental brain injury. *Brain Res.*, **153**, 223–39.

Povlishock, J. T., Kontos, H. A., Rosenblum, W. I. *et al.* (1980). A scanning electron-microscopic analysis of the intraparenchmal brain vasculature following experimental hypertension. *Acta Neuropathol.*, **51**, 203–13.

Povlishock, J. T., Kontos, H. A., DeWitt, D. S. and Wei, E. P. (1981). Effects of mechanical brain injury and acute hypertension upon the cerebral vasculature: morphophysiological consideration of those factors involved in the genesis of cerebrovascular dysfunction. In *Cerebral Microcirculation and Metabolism*, ed. J. Cervos-Navarro and E. Fritschka, pp. 67–75. New York: Raven Press.

Povlishock, J. T., Becker, D. P., Cheng, C. L. Y. and Vaughan, G. W. (1983). Axonal change in minor head injury. *J. Neuropathol. Exp. Neurol.*, **42**, 225–42.

Povlishock, J. T., Erb, D. E. and Astruc, J. (1992). Axonal response to traumatic brain injury: reactive axonal change, deafferentation, and neuroplasticity. *J. Neurotrauma*, **11**, 723–32.

Povlishock, J. T., Hayes, R. L. Michel, M. E. and McIntosh, T. K. (1994). Workshop on animal models of traumatic brain injury. *J. Neurotrauma*, **11**, 723–32.

Rinder, L. and Olsson, Y. (1968). Studies on vascular permeability changes in experimental brain concussion. I. Distribution of circulating fluorescent indicators in brain and cervical cord after sudden mechanical loading of the brain. *Acta Neuropathol.*, **11**, 183–200.

Rosenstein, J. M. and More, N. S. (1994). Immunocytochemical expression of the blood–brain barrier glucose transporter (GLUT-1) in neural transplants and brain wounds. *J. Comp. Neurol.*, **350**, 229–40.

Schmidt, R. H. and Grady, M. S. (1993). Regional patterns of blood–brain barrier breakdown following central and lateral fluid percussion injury in rodents. *J. Neurotrauma*, **10**, 415–30.

Schmitz, M. P., Combs, D. J. and Dempsey, R. J. (1993). Difluoromethylornithine decreases postischemic brain edema and blood–brain barrier breakdown. *Neurosurgery*, **33**, 882–8.

Schoettle, R. J., Kochanek, P. M., Margargee, M. J. *et al.* (1990). Early polymorphonuclear leukocyte accumulation correlates with the development of posttraumatic cerebral edema in rats. *J. Neurotrauma*, **7**, 207–17.

Shapira, Y., Setton, D., Artru, A. A. and Shohami, E. (1993). Blood–brain barrier permeability, cerebral edema, and neurological function after closed head injury in rats. *Neurosurg. Anesth.*, **77**, 141–8.

Shohami, E. Nates, J. L., Glanta, L. *et al.* (1992). Changes in brain polyamine levels following head injury. *Exp. Neurol.*, **117**, 189–95.

Shohami, E., Novikov, M., Bass, R., *et al.* (1994). Closed head injury triggers early production of TNFα and IL-6 by brain tissue. *J. Cereb. Blood Flow Metab.*, **14**, 615–19.

Shohami, E., Bass, R., Wallach, D. *et al.* (1996). Inhibition of tumor necrosis factor alpha (TNFα) activity in rat brain associated with cerebroprotection after closed head injury. *J. Cereb. Blood Flow Metab.*, **16**, 378–84.

Smith, S. L. and Hall, E. D. (1996). Mild pre- and posttraumatic hypothermia attenuates blood–brain barrier damage following controlled cortical impact injury in the rat. *J. Neurotrauma*, **9**, 21–32.

Smith, S. L., Andrus, P. K., Zhang, A. J.-R. and Hall, E. D. (1994). Direct measurement of hydroxyl radicals, lipid peroxidation, and blood–brain barrier disruption following unilateral cortical impact head injury in the rat. *J. Neurotrauma*, **11**, 393–404.

Tanno, H., Nockels, R. P., Pitts, L. H. and Noble, L. J. (1992*a*). Breakdown of the blood–brain barrier after fluid percussion injury in the rat. Part 1: Distribution and time course of protein extravasation. *J. Neurotrauma*, **9**, 21–32.

Tanno, H., Nockels, R. P., Pitts, L. H. and Noble, L. J. (1992*b*). Breakdown of the blood–brain barrier after fluid percussion injury in the rat. Part 2: Effect of hypoxia on permeability to plasma proteins. *J. Neurotrauma*, **9**, 335–47.

Tanno, H., Nockels, R. P., Pitts, L. H. and Noble, L. J. (1993). Immunolocalization of heat shock protein after fluid percussive brain injury and relationship to breakdown of the blood–brain barrier. *J. Cereb. Blood Flow Metab.*, **13**, 116–24.

Todd. N. V. and Graham, D. I. (1990). Blood–brain barrier damage in traumatic brain contusion. *Acta Neurochirurg.*, **51**, 296–9.

Unterberg, A., Dautermann, C., Baethmann, A. and Muller-Esterl, W. (1986). The kallikrein–kinin system as mediator in vasogenic brain edema. *J. Neurosurg.*, **64**, 269–76,

van den Brink, W. A., Santos, B. O., Marmarou, A. and Avezaat, C. J. J. (1994). Quantitive analysis of blood–brain barrier damage in two models of experimental head injury in the rat. *Acta Neurochirurg.*, **60**, 456–8.

Wahl, M., Young, A. R., Edvinsson, K. and Wagner, F. (1983). Effects of bradykinin on pial arteries and arterioles *in vivo* and *in situ*. *J. Cereb. Blood Flow Metab.*, **3**, 231–7.

Wahl, M., Unterberg, A. and Baethmann, A. (1985). Intravital fluorescence microscopy for the study of blood–brain barrier function. *J. Microcirc. Clin. Exp.*, **4**, 3–18.

Wahl, M., Unterberg, A., Whalley, E. T. *et al.* (1986). Cerebrovascular effects of bradykinin. In *Neural Regulation of Brain Circulation*, ed. C. Owman and S. E. Hardebo, pp. 419–30. New York: Elsevier.

Wahl, M., Unterberg, A., Whalley, E. T. *et al.* (1987). Effect of bradykinin on cerebral hemodynamics and blood–brain barrier function. In *Peptidergic Mechanisms in the Cerebral Circulation*, ed. L. Edvinsson and J. McCulloch, pp. 166–90. Chichester: Horwood.

Wahl, M. Schilling, L., Unterberg, A. and Baethman, A. (1993). Mediators of vascular and parenchymal mechanisms in secondary brain damage. *Acta Neurochirurg.*, **57**, 64–72.

Wei, E., Kontos, H., Dietrich, D. *et al.* (1981). Inhibition by free radical scavengers and by cyclooxygenase inhibitors of pial arteriolar abnormalities from concussive brain injury in cats. *Circ. Res.*, **48**, 95.

Wei, E. P., Ellison, M. D., Kontos, H. A. and Povlishock, J. T. (1986). O$_2$ radicals in arachidonate-induced increased blood–brain barrier permeability to proteins. *Am. J. Physiol.*, **251**, H693–H699.

Wei, E., Dietrich, D., Povlishock, J. *et al.* (1980). Functional morphological and metabolic abnormalities of the cerebral microcirculation after concussive brain injury in cats. *Circ. Res.*, **46**, 37–47.

Whalley, E. T. and Whal, M. (1983). Analysis of bradykinin receptor mediating relaxation of cat cerebral arteries *in vivo* and *in vitro*. *Naunyn-Schmiedeberg Arch. Pharmacol.*, **323**, 66–71.

Yoshino, A., Hovda, D. A. Kamamata, T. *et al.* (1991). Dynamic changes in local cerebral glucose utilization following cerebral conclusion in rats: evidence of a hyper- and subsequent hypometabolic state. *Brain Res.*, **561**, 106–19.

Young, A. B., Ott, L. G., Beard, D. *et al.* (1988). The acute phase response of the brain-injured patient. *J. Neurosurg.*, **69**, 375–380.

49 Cerebral malaria and the brain microvasculature

GARETH TURNER

- Introduction: the clinical syndrome of cerebral malaria
- The pathophysiology of cerebral malaria
- Endothelial cell adhesion molecules in cerebral malaria
- Morphological and functional changes in the blood–brain barrier during cerebral malaria
- Conclusion

Introduction: the clinical syndrome of cerebral malaria

Examining the pathophysiology of disease in an organ often provides insight into its normal function. In the case of the central nervous system, infections that primarily affect the brain have yielded valuable information about cellular immune responses in the CNS, as in bacterial meningitis, and the potential mechanisms for cellular traffic across the blood–brain barrier, as in HIV encephalitis. Human malaria is another infection that can affect the brain, but in contrast to the viral encephalitides the pathogen remains exclusively within the vascular space of the brain, binding to cerebral endothelial cells and not entering the brain parenchyma.

Human malaria is caused by four *Plasmodium* parasites, of which *P. falciparum* is the commonest and most serious pathogen. Infection can be asymptomatic or lead to a mild febrile illness, but a small minority of patients suffer severe complications affecting a number of organs. In particular one of the most serious complications of severe disease is cerebral malaria. Using strict criteria cerebral malaria (CM) is defined as an acute, diffuse and potentially reversible encephalopathy with a decreased level of consciousness in the presence of proven infection with *P. falciparum* and in the absence of hypoglycemia or other CNS infection (WHO, 1990). The degree of neurological deficit can vary from confusion and stupor to deep coma. Localizing neurological signs are occasionally present but by no means common, although global signs of extensor posturing, areflexia and pupil changes are poor prognostic signs. A striking clinical finding is the apparently rapid reversibility of cerebral symptoms. A child in a deep coma may be fully conscious and alert a matter of hours later. However over 10% of patients recovering from the illness suffer permanent neurological manifestations. Severe malaria is uncommon compared to mild or asymptomatic malaria infection. However its prevalence in Africa, Asia and South America, and the high mortality rate from cerebral malaria (estimates vary between 15–30% in different populations) ensures that it remains a major health problem.

The pathophysiology of cerebral malaria

Severe malaria caused by *P. falciparum* infection is characterized by the process of sequestration. Host

454

erythrocytes infected with the late maturing stages of the parasite disappear from the peripheral circulation (causing a decrease in the observed peripheral blood parasitemia) and become sequestered in the deep vascular beds of various organs (White and Ho, 1992). The first pathological studies of fatal malaria demonstrated that this process occurred preferentially in the brain in cases of cerebral malaria, and first suggested the theory that sequestration of parasitized erythrocytes in the cerebral microvasculature is associated with cerebral malaria (Marchiafava and Bignami, 1894).

Subsequently a debate arose as to the specificity of this finding, and the link between sequestration and the incidence of coma. Quantitative studies of sequestration in different organs from fatal cases confirmed that sequestration of parasitized red blood cells (PRBC) in the cerebral microvasculature was significantly associated with clinical cerebral malaria (MacPherson *et al.*, 1985; Pongparatn *et al.*, 1991). Sequestration in the brain was higher in these patients than in other organs, thus the clinical syndrome of cerebral malaria appeared to be associated with cerebral sequestration. The question of whether sequestration in the brain is specific to cerebral cases, and absent in non-cerebral malaria (NCM), has been a thorny issue. Some authors have reported high levels of sequestration in the brains of fatal non-cerebral cases, and others have found a confusing variability in both pathology and sequestration levels within the two separate groups. A recent study of 50 adult Vietnamese patients has helped clarify this issue (G. Turner *et al.*, in preparation). In well-defined groups of cerebral and non-cerebral cases there was definite evidence for PRBC sequestration in some non-cerebral cases and all cerebral cases, who died soon after admission to hospital (and thus after a shorter duration of illness and treatment). Late deaths in both groups showed no observed sequestration in either group due to temporally related clearance of parasites. Quantitatively in time-to-death matched pairs of CM and NCM there was significantly more sequestration in the brains of cerebral than non-cerebral cases. Thus it seems that sequestration of PRBC is necessary for but not solely sufficient to cause cerebral malaria, whereas coma does not occur without sequestration.

If cerebral coma does not always follow PRBC sequestration in the brain, what other factors determine whether a particular host develops coma in the presence of sequestration? Early pathological studies envisaged that the physical consequences of sequestration (the presence of parasites in the microvasculature of the brain) would cause 'sludging' and 'stagnation', e.g. physical obstruction of blood vessels and slowing of blood flow. As well as binding to endothelial cells, PRBC can bind to uninfected erythrocytes, the phenomenon of rosetting (Wahlgren *et al.*, 1994). A parasite line that can bind uninfected cells at a high frequency might be expected to form micro-aggregates of cells *in vivo*, which could contribute to the blockage of vessels in combination with sequestration, and thus increase the chances of coma developing. The concept that coma might be due to global or diffusely focal hypoxia has lost ground given the relatively low degree of permanent neurological complications in survivors and the lack of widespread pathological evidence for severe ischemia in postmortem brain samples. However another consequence of the presence of large numbers of highly metabolically active parasites in the cerebral vasculature is the possibility of metabolic competition, either for vital energy substrates such as glucose or amino acids necessary for neurotransmitter synthesis.

Along with the theory that parasite sequestration in the brain directly causes disease an alternative theory of the pathogenesis of severe disease has developed. Some earlier pathological studies had noted that levels of sequestration in other organs were insufficient to account for their dysfunction (such as renal failure). This proposes that a soluble parasite derived 'toxin' may be the cause of other complications of the disease, and some felt that this may also be the cause of cerebral symptoms in cases where no sequestration was seen in patients dying of cerebral malaria (Clark and Rockett, 1994). It may also be the case that sequestration of parasites allows release of high concentrations of such a toxin to act locally rather than in the circulation. Attempts to isolate a toxin from *P. falciparum* have recently been successful, with the purification of a phospholipid moiety that induces activation and TNFα secretion by human monocytes (Jakobsen *et al.*, 1995).

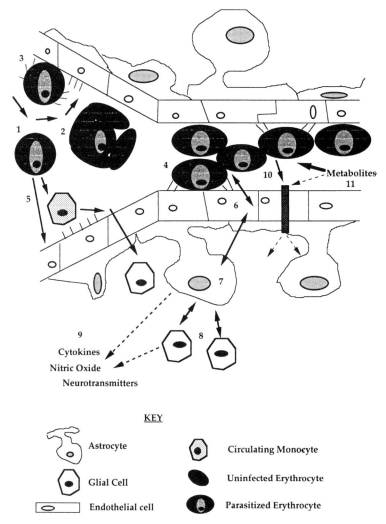

KEY

Astrocyte	Circulating Monocyte
Glial Cell	Uninfected Erythrocyte
Endothelial cell	Parasitized Erythrocyte

Fig. 49.1. A schematic diagram of possible pathophysiological mechanisms in cerebral malaria. *P. falciparum*-infected erythrocytes (1) and rosettes (2) in the cerebral microcirculation can interact with cerebral endothelial cells either by 'rolling' (3) or firm adhesion (4) to host adhesion molecules. Activation of the endothelial cells by parasites or their products (5) could also allow localization and transmigration of host leukocytes such as circulating monocytes. Signalling through the blood–brain barrier from bound PRBC to endothelial cells (6) or astrocytes (7) could also allow interaction with parenchymal glial cells (8), allowing production and release of soluble mediators, which could affect neuronal function (9). There may also be direct effects on specific blood–brain barrier functions (10) and competition for key metabolites (11).

Another attractive theory to account for the symptoms of coma is the release of host mediators that could affect the brain. A host mediator that could have pathological or physiological effects, with a short half-life and area of action determined by diffusion, might explain the acute onset, reversibility and lack of permanent tissue damage that partly characterizes the coma of cerebral malaria. There have been successive candidates for such a mediator since the 1970s, including by-products of iron metabolism caused by parasite-induced breakdown of hemoglobin, reactive oxygen intermediates and free radicals, soluble cytokines and, most recently, nitric oxide (Clark *et al.*, 1991).

Most research has been done on the role of tumour necrosis factor. TNFα acts as a pyrogen during malaria infection, but seems also to have a protective role in controlling the levels of parasitemia. Levels of TNFα are raised in severe disease and are significantly higher in children with cerebral, compared to non-cerebral malaria (Kwiatkowski *et al.*, 1990). Polymorphism in the upstream promoter region of the TNF gene has been shown to be present in African populations in malaria endemic areas, implying a possible relationship between the host ability to produce TNF in response to a given infection and the development of cerebral malaria (McGuire *et al.*, 1994).

Nitric oxide has been proposed as a possible short-lived, diffusable mediator which, when released from monocytes, endothelial cells or brain cells may interfere with neurotransmitter release (such as glutamate via calcium dependent mechanisms) and thus induce generalized unconsciousness (in an anesthetic-like manner). Measurement of nitric oxide is difficult due to its short half-life and diffusibility, thus the levels of circulating nitrates are often taken as a surrogate. These have been shown to be raised in malaria, although controversy still exists as to whether this is associated with the incidence of cerebral malaria as some studies have found an apparently protective effect in severe disease. As yet no immunohistochemical or *in situ* hybridization data is available to confirm the presence of these mediators in brain samples from fatal cerebral malaria cases.

Thus several different factors have been suggested to account for the action of malaria parasites on the brain in cerebral malaria. A schematic representation of how these factors might act at the level of the blood–brain barrier to influence neuronal function is shown in Fig. 49.1.

Endothelial cell adhesion molecules in cerebral malaria

The process of sequestration has been modelled *in vitro* using cultured parasite lines that demonstrate cytoadherence to endothelial and other cell lines. This adhesion process has been shown to be mediated by specific host sequestration receptors that have been identified and characterized using a variety of techniques (Berendt *et al.*, 1994; Pasloske and Howard, 1994). The putative receptors include thrombospondin (Roberts *et al.*, 1985), CD36 (Barnwell *et al.*, 1989; Ockenhouse *et al.*, 1989; Oquendo *et al.*, 1989), ICAM-1 (Berendt *et al.*, 1989), E-selectin and VCAM-1 (Ockenhouse *et al.*, 1992) and chondroitin-6-sulphate (Rogerson *et al.*, 1995; Chairoj *et al.*, 1996). The characteristics of these receptors are shown in Table 49.1.

These molecules have all been shown to support the adhesion of cultured parasite lines *in vitro*. Immunohistochemical studies of the distribution of the putative sequestration receptors on cerebral microvascular endothelial cells have shown their expression in cerebral malaria and simian models of CM (Aikawa *et al.*, 1992; Ockenhouse *et al.*, 1992). ICAM-1, E-selectin and VCAM-1 expression is increased on cerebral vessels during cerebral malaria, whereas CD36 and TSP expression was scattered and low in controls and did not increase during disease. By quantitative estimation of the numbers of vessels expressing receptors and showing sequestration, there was a significant correlation between the expression of all the sequestration receptors and the localization of PRBC in cerebral microvessels (Turner *et al.*, 1994). This result implied that expression of receptors identified as supporting cytoadherence *in vitro* may be involved in sequestration *in vivo*.

Morphological and functional changes in the blood–brain barrier during cerebral malaria

What effects do parasites and their products have on the blood–brain barrier? This has been examined at both pathological and physiological levels in the human, and in the two main animal models of human cerebral malaria, the murine and simian hosts. Evan's Blue dye extravasation and focal petechial hemorrhages in the brain parenchyma were observed in mice who succumbed to a neurological syndrome with some similarities to human cerebral malaria (Chan-Ling *et al.*, 1992). Hemorrhages and fluorescent dye extravasation were also observed in the retinal model, used as a way of examining the function of the retinal blood barrier. These findings imply that the blood–brain

Table 49.1. *Host receptors for parasitized erythrocytes*

Receptor	Summary	Expression
Thrombospondin	Trimeric glycoprotein ~420 kDa. Cell matrix adhesion molecule. PRBC bind to purified protein, polyclonal antisera inhibit binding	Secreted by endothelial cells, platelets and monocytes. Only focally expressed by the BBB in human cerebral malaria
CD36	Glycoprotein ~88 kDa. Cell surface receptor for matrix proteins including TSP. PRBC bind to protein purified from platelets, and recombinant protein on cell lines. Monoclonal antibodies and peptide analogs inhibit adhesion to nascent molecule	Expressed by mature monocytes, platelets and widespread endothelial marker but very sparsely expressed in brain. Binds nearly all field isolates of parasites
ICAM-1	80–110 kDa adhesion molecule, member of Ig superfamily. PRBC bind to purified and recombinant protein, and cell lines expressing or transfected with recombinant ICAM-1	Cytokine-inducible expression on endothelial cells. Expressed basally on human and simian cerebral endothelium. Expression up-regulated in human cerebral malaria, and co-localizes with sites of parasite sequestration. Inducible expression noted in the brains of murine and simian models of cerebral malaria
VCAM-1	Ig superfamily ~110 kDa. Adherence of selected parasite lines to recombinant proteins can be inhibited by antisera	Very little basal expression in human or simian brain. Expressed inducibly on endothelium. Increased expression in human and simian cerebral malaria
E-selectin	Cell surface adhesion molecule of the Selectin family with complex domain structure. Few parasite field isolates show significant levels of binding to this molecule.	Expression restricted to activated endothelial cells. Increased expression in human and simian brain in cerebral malaria
Chondroitin sulphate A	Poly-sulphated matrix protein, possibly expressed on several molecules on endothelial and other cell surfaces	Expression in the brain in human CM unknown, but is expressed on simian brain endothelial cell lines

barrier is compromised in the mouse model, although an important difference exists between this and the human disease, namely the sequestered cells, which are host leukocytes rather than infected erythrocytes.

Pathological studies in human cerebral malaria also show several different types of hemorrhage in the brain parenchyma. These include simple petechial hemorrhages, which are not a specific feature of malaria but occur in other conditions such as hypoxia, barotrauma and poisoning. There are also two other specific types of hemorrhages, ring hemorrhages and Dürck's granulomas. The former is a central vessel surrounded by a zone of uninfected erythrocytes and an outer ring of infected erythrocytes and monocytes (Fig. 49.2). The latter consists of a patchy gliotic reaction surrounding a central necrosed vessel, with a collection of host monocytes and lymphocytes extravasated into the brain parenchyma. The frequent co-existence of these lesions with ring hemorrhages and their morphological background of gliosis and resolving hemorrhage suggests that they may represent a later stage of the ring hemorrhage lesion

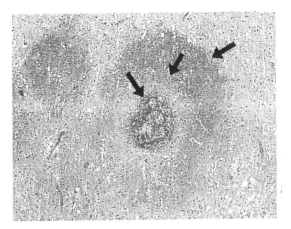

Fig. 49.2. A ring hemorrhage in the brain of a fatal case of cerebral malaria. The arrows show the areas of demarcation between concentric zones of parasitized erythrocytes (outermost ring), host leukocytes, uninfected erythrocytes, and gliosis (inner rings) surrounding a central necrosed vessel.

as host leukocytes clear infected RBC debris from the brain parenchyma, although this is not known.

The endothelial cells of the blood–brain barrier exhibit important structural and phenotypic variation in malaria. Electron microscopic studies of cerebral malaria have shown the ruffling and blebbing of endothelial cells, and the formation of pseudopodia that interact with PRBC and corresponding structures on activated monocytes. Microscopically they also appear to phagocytose pigment granules left from ghosted erythrocytes following schizogony. These findings have been confirmed in cultured brain endothelial cells from a simian model of cerebral malaria (Robert *et al.*, 1996). Endothelial cells cultured and different PRBC lines derived from the monkeys bind to each other intimately at electron-dense knobs, and endothelial pseudopodia engulf some PRBC to the extent that phagocytosis of the entire red cell occurs.

There remain few ways to examine the function of the blood–brain barrier during malaria. A single study of radioactive albumin traffic showed no clear breakdown of BBB permeability during CM, although its role in regulating transfer of molecules smaller than this is unknown (Warrell, 1989). A number of radiological studies, including CT and MRI series, have been done in adult Asian and childhood African patients. Radiologically and

pathologically it seems that the majority of patients, even those who die, do not have a significant degree of edema. However, on the basis of radiography, intracranial pressure monitoring and some pathological data, a subset of patients suffer extremely bad edema which can be associated with brainstem herniation and death, or if survived, is associated with permanent neurological deficit after recovery (Looaresuwan *et al.*, 1983, 1996). Intracranial pressure monitoring in African children has confirmed rises in association with cerebral malaria that are associated with prognosis. Although treatment with mannitol helped reduce intracranial pressure in some of these patients the effects were not long-lasting and the rises were difficult to control (Newton *et al.*, 1994). A study of the efficacy of corticosteroid treatment in adult Thai groups of cerebral and non-cerebral malaria found them to be deleterious in cerebral malaria (Warrell *et al.*, 1982), in contrast to its protective role in childhood meningitis for instance. Thus although most patients seem to be able to survive cerebral malaria without developing cerebral edema, a subset do develop this complication in a very aggressive form.

We thus know more about pathological changes at the blood–brain barrier, from animal models and autopsy data from fatal malaria cases, than we know about the physiological function of the BBB during malaria infection *in vivo*. Examination of the effects of the parasitized erythrocyte on cerebral endothelial cells *in vitro* may provide the link between these two very different areas.

Conclusion

Cerebral malaria gives us a fascinating insight into the functional importance of the blood–brain barrier in brain function. Many patients may undergo cerebral sequestration during malaria without suffering coma or even severe disease, and identifying susceptibility factors in the subset who go on to cerebral involvement is an important goal. The majority of research to date has focused on the mechanisms by which the parasitized erythrocyte adheres to the cerebral endothelial cell and interest is developing around the mechanisms by which parasite and host factors interact at the boundary of the cerebral vasculature to cause coma. Complex interactions can be envisaged between the parasitized erythrocyte and host leukocyte in the vascular space, endothelial cells and astrocytes of the blood–brain barrier and microglia and neurons of the brain parenchyma. As yet, however, these relationships are poorly understood. The reward of understanding cerebral malaria promises to be delineating the role of the blood–brain barrier as a gateway to the brain, and how its dysfunction can alter consciousness.

Acknowledgment

I would like to thank all my colleagues in the Oxford Tropical Centre and The Wellcome Trust Research Unit in Viet Nam for their help and discussions, which have contributed to the ideas presented here, especially Dr Tony Berendt, Professor Nick White, Dr Chris Newbold, Dr Nick Day and Dr David Ferguson.

References

Aikawa, M., Pongparatn, E., Tegoshi, T. *et al.* (1992). A study on the pathogenesis of human cerebral malaria and cerebral babesiosis. *Mem. Inst. Oswaldo. Cruz.*, **87**, 297–301.

Barnwell, J., Asch, A., Nachman, R. *et al.* (1989). A human 88 kDa membrane glycoprotein (CD36) functions in vitro as a receptor for a cytoadherence ligand on *Plasmodium falciparum*-infected erythrocytes. *J. Clin. Inv.*, **84**, 1054–61.

Berendt, A., Simmons, D., Tansey, J. *et al.* (1989). Intercellular adhesion molecule-1 is an endothelial cell adhesion receptor for *Plasmodium falciparum*. *Nature*, **341**, 57–9.

Berendt, A., Ferguson, D., Gardner, J. *et al.* (1994). Molecular mechanisms of sequestration in malaria. *Parasitology*, **108**, 19–28.

Chairoj, S., Angkasekiwinai, P., Buranakiti, A. *et al.* (1996). Cytoadherence characeristics of *Plasmodium falciparum* isolates from Thailand: evidence for chondroitin sulphate A as a cytoadherence receptor. *Am. J. Trop. Med. Hyg.*, **55**(1), 76–80.

Chan-Ling, T., Neill, A. and Hunt, N. (1992). Early microvascular changes in murine cerebral malaria detected in retinal wholemounts. *Am. J. Pathol.*, **140**, 1121–30.

Clark, I. and Rockett, K. (1994). The cytokine theory of human cerebral malaria. *Parasitol. Today* **10**, 410–12.

Clark, I., Rockett, K. and Cowden, W. (1991). Proposed link between cytokines, nitric oxide and human cerebral malaria. *Parasitol. Today.*, **7**, 205–7.

Jakobsen, P., Bate, C., Taverne, J. and Playfair, J. (1995). Malaria: toxins, cytokines and disease. *Parasite Immunol.*, **17**, 223–31.

Kwiatkowski, D., Hill, A., Sambou, I. *et al.* (1990). TNF concentration in fatal cerebral, non-fatal cerebral and uncomplicated *Plasmodium falciparum* malaria. *Lancet*, **336**, 1201–4.

Looaresuwan, S., Warrell, D., White, N. *et al.* (1983). Do patients with cerebral malaria have cerebral oedema? – a computed tomography study. *The Lancet*, **I**, 434–7.

Looaresuwan, S., Wilairantana, P., Krishna, S. *et al.* (1996). Magnetic resonance imaging of the brain in cerebral malaria. *Clin. Inf. Dis.*, **21**, 300–9.

Macpherson, G., Warrell, M., White, N. *et al.* (1985). Human cerebral malaria - a quantitative ultrastructural analysis of parasitised erythrocyte sequestration. *Am. J. Pathol.*, **119**, 385–401.

Marchiafava, E. and Bignami, A. (1894). On summer-autumnal malaria fevers. in *Malaria and the Parasites of Malaria Fevers*, vol 150, pp. 1–234. London: The New Sydenham Society.

McGuire, W., Hill, A., Allsop, C. *et al.* (1994). Variation in the TNF-alpha promoter region associated with susceptibility to cerebral malaria. *Nature*, **371**, 508–11.

Newton, C., Peshu, N., Kendall, B. *et al.* (1994). Brain swelling and ischemia in Kenyans with cerebral malaria. *Arch. Dis. Child.*, **70**, 281–7.

Ockenhouse, C., Tandon, N., Magowan, C. *et al.* (1989). Identification of a platelet membrane glycoprotein as a falciparum malaria sequestration receptor. *Science*, **243**, 1469–71.

Ockenhouse, C., Tegoshi, T., Maeno, Y. *et al.* (1992). Human vascular endothelial cell adhesion receptors for plasmodium falciparum-infected erythrocytes: roles for endothelial leukocyte adhesion molecule 1 and vascular cell adhesion molecule 1. *J. Exp. Med.*, **176**, 1183–9.

Oquendo, P., Hundt, E., Lawler, J. and Seed, B. (1989). CD36 directly mediates cytoadherence of *Plasmodium falciparum* parasitised erythrocytes. *Cell*, **58**, 95–101.

Pasloske, B. and Howard, R. (1994). Malaria, the red cell, and the endothelium. *Ann. Rev. Med.*, **45**, 283–95.

Pongparatn, E., Riganti, M., Punpoowong, B. and Aikawa M. (1991). Microvascular sequestration of parasitised erythrocytes in human falciparum malaria. *Am. J. Trop. Med. Hyg.*, **44**, 168–75.

Robert, C., Peyrol, S., Pouvelle, B. *et al.* (1996). Ultrastructural aspects of *Plasmodium falciparum*-infected erythrocyte adherence to endothelial cells of *Saimiri* brain microvascular cultures. *Am. J. Trop. Med. Hyg.*, **54**(2), 169–77.

Roberts, D., Sherwood, J., Spitalnik, S. *et al.* (1985). Thrombospondin binds falciparum parasitised erythrocytes and may mediate cytoadherence. *Nature*, **318**, 64–6.

Rogerson, S., Chaiyaroj, S., Ng, K. *et al.* (1995). Chondroitin sulphate A is a cell surface receptor for *Plasmodium falcipairum* infected erythrocytes. *J. Exp. Med.*, **182**, 15–20.

Turner, G., Morrison, H., Jones, M. *et al.* (1994). An Immunohistochemical study of the Pathology of Fatal Malaria. *Am. J. Pathol.*, **145**(5), 1057–69.

Wahlgren, M., Fernandez, V., Scholander, C. and Carlson, J. (1994). Rosetting. *Parasitol. Today*, **10**, 73–9.

Warrell, D. (1989). Cerebral malaria. *Q. J. Med.*, **265**, 369–71.

Warrell, D., Looaresuwan, S. and Warrell, M. (1982). Dexamethasone proves deleterious in cerebral malaria: a double-blind trial in 100 comatose patients. *N. Engl. J. Med.*, **306**, 313–19.

White, N. and Ho, M. (1992). The pathophysiology of malaria. *Adv. Parasitol.*, **31**, 83–173.

WHO (Division of Control of Tropical Diseases) (1990). Severe and complicated malaria. *Trans. Roy. Soc. Trop. Med. Hyg.*, **84**, 1–65.

50 Molecular basis of tissue tropism of bacterial meningitis

JAAKKO PARKKINEN

- Introduction
- Bacterial virulence factors in circulation
- Site of bacterial invasion into the subarachnoid space
- Binding sites in the brain for *E. coli* S fimbriae
- Binding specificities of other bacteria causing meningitis
- Proteolytic mechanisms in bacterial invasion
- Concluding remarks

Introduction

Bacterial meningitis continues to be a serious health threat with high morbidity and mortality. Despite the availability of potent bactericidal antibiotics, bacterial infection of the subarachnoid space often leads to serious complications. The most common etiologic agents in adults and children after the neonatal period are *Haemophilus influenzae*, *Neisseria meningitidis*, and *Streptococcus pneumoniae*. During the neonatal period, when the disease is more common than at any later time of life, the most common causative organisms are *Streptococcus agalactiae* and *Escherichia coli*.

Bacterial meningitis is generally a hematogenous infection (Tunkel and Scheld, 1993). It is typically preceded by colonization of host nasopharynx by the causative organism. Colonization is followed by bacterial invasion through the mucosal epithelium and bacteremia. Subsequently, blood-borne bacteria invade the subarachnoid space. The release of bacterial components in the cerebrospinal fluid (CSF) induces the secretion of inflammatory cytokines, which contribute to increased permeability of the blood–brain barrier (BBB) and generation of an intense subarachnoid inflammation. Further complications include increased intracranial pressure, alterations in cerebral blood flow, and cerebral edema.

The pathophysiology of bacterial meningitis is only partially known at present. Studies with nasopharyngeal organ culture have illustrated the different events following colonization of the nasopharyngeal epithelium with meningococci and *H. influenzae* type b (Stephens and Farley, 1991). These events include bacterial adhesion to nonciliated cells, multiplication and invasion through the epithelium. Mucosal invasion by meningococci and *H. influenzae* appears to occur via different mechanisms; meningococci utilize parasite-directed endocytosis and transcytosis through the epithelial cells, whereas the adhesion of *H. influenzae* leads to separation of epithelial cell tight junctions, followed by intercellular invasion by bacteria. The pathophysiology of the inflammatory reactions following intracisternal inoculation of bacteria or bacterial components have been addressed in several studies (Tunkel and Scheld, 1993). The advances reached in these studies have contributed to the development of adjunctive treatment strategies for bacterial meningitis.

One of the open questions in the pathogenesis

Table 50.1. *Microbial–host interactions of bacteria causing meningitis and their possible pathogenic function during bacterial invasion into the subarachnoid space*

Microbial–host interaction	Possible pathogenic function	Refs.
Bacterial adhesion to brain vascular endothelial cells	Enrichment of bacteria to the brain vasculature	(1), (2)
Bacterial adhesion to basement membrane proteins	Targeting of bacteria to the basement membrane in the fenestrated endothelium of the choroid plexus	(3), (4)
Binding of plasminogen and t-PA to the bacteria and generation of bacterium-bound plasmin	Degradation of noncollagenous basement membrane proteins, traversal of bacteria across the basement membrane	(4), (5), (6)
Bacterial binding to the basolateral surface of choroidal ependymal cells	Promotion of bacterial traversal through the ependymal cell layer	(1), (7)
Adhesion to the apical surface of the ependymal cells	Resistance of the rinsing effect of CSF flow	(1), (7)

References: (1) Parkkinen *et al.*, 1987; (2) Stins *et al.*, 1994; (3) Virkola *et al.*, 1993; (4) Virkola *et al.*, 1996; (5) Parkkinen *et al.*, 1991; (6) Ullberg *et al.*, 1994; (7) Sterk *et al.*, 1991.

of bacterial meningitis has been the site and mechanisms of the entry of blood-borne bacteria in the subarachnoid space. Most of the data obtained in animal models have suggested that bacteria invade the subarachnoid space via the choroid plexus. There is also evidence on the molecular level of how this tissue tropism of bacterial invasion site may be determined. These and other tentative bacteria–host interactions during early invasion of blood-borne bacteria into the CSF compartment are the focus of this presentation (Table 50.1). The later events in meningitis, which follow bacterial entry to the CSF and result in enhanced permeability of the BBB and subarachnoid space inflammation, may also provide additional routes for bacterial traversal across the BBB. These inflammatory events have been reviewed by Tunkel and Scheld.

Bacterial virulence factors in circulation

The ability of bacteria to survive in circulation is a prerequisite for the hematogenous spread of bacteria into the subarachnoid space. The capsular polysaccharides of pathogenic bacteria are important virulence factors that inhibit neutrophil phagocytosis and resist classical complement-mediated bactericidal activity (Kasper, 1986). In the absence of specific host antibodies against the capsular polysaccharide, bacteria are profoundly resistant to phagocytosis.

Bacterial polysaccharides may also be poor immunogens, allowing the bacteria to escape host immune response. The capsular polysialic acid, which consists of $\alpha2$–8 linked sialic acids and occurs in the majority of *E. coli* strains, causing meningitis in newborn infants and group B meningococci, has been shown to be structurally identical with the polysialic acid glycans occuring in developing mammalian brain (Finne *et al.*, 1983). This structural identity is thought to result in host immunological tolerance to the capsular polysialic acid, which hampers its use as a vaccine. As polysialic acid occurs in the neural cell adhesion molecule (N-CAM) in the developing brain (Finne, 1987), the existence of the same glycan structure in bacteria causing meningitis might suggest that the bacterial polysialic acid could interact with adhesion molecules in the host brain. However, polysialic acid is thought to have merely anti-adhesive properties in N-CAM (Finne, 1987), and no polysialic acid binding lectin-like proteins have been identified in host tissues.

The capsular polysaccharide of group B streptococci, another common causative agent in newborn meningitis, contains other types of sialyloligosac-charide structures that are also closely similar to those occurring in mammalian glycoconjugates. However, unlike the capsular polysialic acid which is immunologically cross-reactive with brain poly-sialic acid, antibodies to group B capsular polysac-charide do not cross-react with host glycan struc-tures (Häyrinen *et al.*, 1989).

Besides the polysaccharide capsule, pathogenic bacteria have other virulence factors that enhance their survival in blood. These include proteins that enable the bacteria to utilize transferrin and heme-bound iron (Otto *et al.*, 1992). The same bacterial properties should enhance their survival in the CSF as well. On the other hand, since some bacte-ria commonly found in septicemia very rarely cause meningitis, there are evidently other bacterial prop-erties that promote bacterial invasion from circula-tion to the subarachnoid space.

Site of bacterial invasion into the subarachnoid space

Studies on the pathogenesis of *H. influenzae* menin-gitis in the infant rat model have indicated that the first site of inflammation in the cranial vault is the choroid plexus, and that bacterial densities early in disease are higher in the lateral ventricles than in the cisterna magna or in the subarachnoid space (Smith *et al.*, 1982). These results suggested that bacteria enter the CSF compartment via the chor-oid plexus. In experimental meningococcal menin-gitis in the same animal model, bacteria were found associated with choroidal cells and the lumi-nal pole of arachnoidal capillaries, which suggested that meningococci might traverse the BBB either through choroid plexus or arachnoidal capillaries (Nassif and So, 1995). On the other hand, the first pathological lesions observed after intravenous injection of *Streptococcus suis*, a common causative organism of meningitis in pigs, were found in the choroid plexus (Williams and Blakemore, 1990). The consideration of choroid plexus as the first site of bacterial entry in the CSF is supported by the exceptionally high blood flow in this organ (ca. 200 ml/g/min), which should lead to the delivery of more blood-borne organisms to this site than to other anatomic locations within the brain.

The choroid plexuses constitute a richly vascu-larized secretory epithelium protruding in a leaflike fashion from the roof of the ventricles into the CSF. Their major function is to produce CSF by active secretion. The central core consists of capillary endothelium that is surrounded by a single layer of ependymal cells. The vessels in the capillary bed are fenestrated, and the BBB in this region is formed by the intercellular tight junctions between the choroidal ependymal cells.

The first indication of the existence of specific interactions between bacteria causing meningitis and choroidal cells came from studies on *E. coli* strains causing neonatal meningitis. About one-third of the *E. coli* strains isolated from verified meningi-tis carry a specific type of fimbriae, designated as S fimbriae. Fimbriae are filamentous surface pro-teins of gram-negative bacteria typically mediating bacterial attachment to host mucosal epithelial cells. S fimbriae have a sialyloligosaccharide-spe-cific binding activity, which has specific binding sites in the choroid plexus (Parkkinen *et al.*, 1987).

Binding sites in the brain for *E. coli* S fimbriae

There is both epidemiological and experimental evidence which suggests that *E. coli* S fimbriae have a pathogenetic role in neonatal meningitis. S fimbria antigen has been shown to be associated with *E. coli* strains isolated from newborn sepsis (16%) and meningitis (36%) as opposed to strains isolated from feces of healthy children (3%). Due to phase variation of S fimbriae, the frequency of genes encoding them may be higher than sug-gested by the frequency of fimbrial antigen. Notably, S fimbriae occurred in 8 of 11 strains with the serotype O18:K1:H7, which is the most common serotype among the strains isolated from septic neonatal infections and probably represents a single virulent clone. The O18:K1:H7 strains also carry type 1 fimbriae, a mannose-specific lectin, but apparently no other adhesin or hemolysin (Korhonen *et al.*, 1985).

In experimental meningitis in the infant rat model, fimbrial phase variation of the O18:K1:H7 *E. coli* to the S-fimbriated form was observed in blood and cerebrospinal fluid after inoculation of nonfimbriated or type 1-fimbriated subpopulations (Saukkonen *et al.*, 1988). Inoculation of an S-fimbriated subpopulation resulted in higher frequency of meningitis and higher bacterial counts in blood and CSF than did inoculae with nonfimbriated or type 1-fimbriated subpopulations. This suggested a virulence role for S fimbriae during the invasive phase of meningitis.

S fimbriae were originally found on the basis of their ability to recognize sialyl galactoside structures[1] on human erythrocytes. The binding sites of S fimbriae on the human erythrocytes were identified as the highly clustered O-linked NeuAcα2–3Galβ1–3GalNAc chains of glycophorin A (Parkkinen *et al.*, 1986). Recently, S fimbriae were shown to bind with higher affinity NeuGc-containing than NeuAc-containing oligosaccharides and also bind gangliosides (Hanisch *et al.*, 1993). It is noteworthy that NeuGc does not occur in man, and its preferential binding by S fimbriae may indicate that S fimbriae have evolved in primates or other species in which NeuGc is a regular constituent of glycoconjugates. The low affinity of S fimbriae to human erythrocytes at 37 °C suggests that S fimbria-mediated hemagglutination does not take place in circulation, and that the binding sites in the target structures in the brain (see below) are structurally different from the erythrocyte receptors.

S fimbriae are morphologically similar to other *E. coli* fimbriae, being about 1–2 μm long and 5–7 nm thick. They consist of a major protein subunit SfaA with a molecular weight of 17 kD, and of three minor proteins SfaH, SfaG, and SfaS (Schmoll *et al.*, 1989). The SfaS subunit, a 34 kD protein, is the adhesin subunit that possesses the sialyl galactoside-specific binding activity (Moch *et al.*, 1987). Additionally, SfaA has been shown to have a binding activity for sulfated glycolipids (Prasadarao *et al.*, 1993).

The target tissues of S fimbriae have been studied by incubating purified S fimbriae on tissue sections of different organs of the newborn rat, which rapidly develops meningitis after intraperitoneal inoculation of S-fimbriated bacteria (Parkkinen *et*

al., 1987). The specificity of binding was controlled by inhibition with the receptor analog sialyllactose (NeuAcα2–3Galβ1–4Glc), and by preceding neuraminidase treatment of the sections. As a further control, binding of a fluorochrome-labeled S-fimbriated recombinant strain and the nonfimbriated recipient strain to the tissue sections was studied. Of the different organs of the newborn rat studied, only brain and kidney revealed intense binding of S fimbriae. The binding sites in the brain are located on the vascular endothelium and on the epithelium lining the choroid plexuses and brain ventricles (Fig. 50.1). In the kidney, S fimbriae bind to vascular endothelium and glomeruli. Vascular endothelium and alveolar epithelium in the lung showed weak binding of S fimbriae, whereas no binding was observed to liver and spleen sections.

The presence of binding sites for S fimbriae on vascular endothelial cells has been demonstrated also by using primary cultures of human umbilical cord endothelial cells (Parkkinen *et al.*, 1989) and bovine brain cortical microvascular cells (Stins *et al.*, 1994). Most of the binding of S fimbriae to the endothelial cells was mediated by the sialyloligosaccharide-specific lectin activity of the SfaS subunit. Another binding activity mediated by the SfaA subunit was identified, which was specific for sulfated glycolipids on the bovine brain endothelial cells (Prasadarao *et al.*, 1993). Serum inhibited the binding of S fimbriae to endothelial cells only partially, irrespective whether obtained from patients with acute inflammation or from newborn infants, and highly sialylated serum glycoproteins, such as α1-acid glycoprotein, were ineffective inhibitors at physiological concentrations (Parkkinen *et al.*, 1989). This suggested that S fimbria-mediated binding of bacteria to vascular endothelium may take place in circulation. According to the binding studies with tissue sections, S fimbriae bind clearly more intensively to vascular endothelium in brain and kidney than in several other organs of the newborn rat. This suggests that organ-specific expression of highly sialylated glycoproteins or glycolipids on vascular endothelial cells may contribute to the organ specificity in the secondary organ colonization by blood-borne bacteria.

Besides endothelial cell binding, the binding of S fimbriae to the choroidal ependymal cells may

---

[1] Sialic acid is a generic name of different neuraminic acid derivatives including *N*-acetyl (NeuAc) and *N*-glycolyl (NeuGc) neuraminic acids

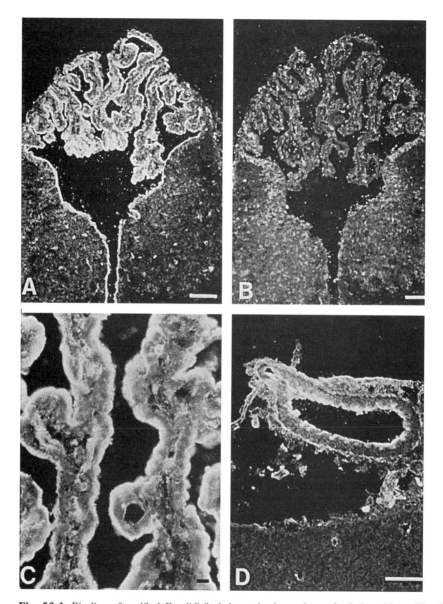

Fig. 50.1. Binding of purified *E. coli* S fimbriae to brain sections of a 3-day-old rat. The fimbriae bound to the luminal surface of the epithelial cells lining the choroid plexus (A,C) and ventricles (A), and the binding was completely inhibited in the presence of 20 mM NeuAcα2–3Galβ1–4Glc (B). (D) Binding of S fimbriae to the endothelium of a subarachnoid blood vessel (top) and of small cortical blood vessels (below). Scale bar indicates 100 μm (A,B,D) or 10 μm (C). Reprinted from Parkkinen *et al.*, 1987, by copyright permission of The American Society for Clinical Investigation.

also be important in the pathogenesis of meningitis. In the choroid plexus, bacteria should gain access to the ependymal cells through the intercellular gaps of the fenestrated endothelium, provided that they penetrate the subendothelial basement membrane (see below). Traversal across the choroidal ependymal cell layer would require either bacterial transcytosis or disruption of the intercellular tight junctions. The mechanism may vary for different bacteria as meningococci have been shown to employ transcytosis and *H. influenzae* the disruption of intercellular tight junctions during the penetration of the nasopharyngeal epithelium (Stephens and Farley, 1991). In both cases, close association of the bacteria with the ependymal cells should promote the penetration, and the presence of specific binding sites for bacteria on the choroidal ependymal cells may therefore be of pathogenic importance.

There is a constant flow of CSF from the ventricles to the subarachnoid space, where it is cleared back to the circulation, and a total exchange of CSF occurs every 3–4 h. Studies with animal meningitis models have suggested that meningitis is a dynamic process with bacteria entering from blood and being constantly cleared back to circulation with the CSF flow through arachnoid villi (Scheld *et al.*, 1979; Smith *et al.*, 1982). In this respect, the observed intense binding of S fimbriae to the apical surfaces of the choroidal and ventricular ependymal cells may be important also in resisting the clearance of bacteria by the CSF flow, similarly as bacterial adhesion is a prerequisite in the colonization of mucosal epithelia rinsed by flowing secretions.

Binding specificities of other bacteria causing meningitis

Tissue tropism of the binding of *H. influenzae* type b has been studied by using different cell lines. Fimbriated bacteria bind to several cell types including ciliated columnar epithelial cells, ependymal cells, and endothelial cells (Sterk *et al.*, 1991). Since the fimbriated bacteria also bound to blood cells it was suggested that a shift to non-fimbriated form is required for bacteria in the bloodstream to escape clearance mechanisms mediated by blood cells. Interestingly, the binding of fimbriated *H. influenzae* was inhibited with gangliosides containing the NeuAcα2–3Gal sequence but not with corresponding asialo glycolipids (van Alphen *et al.*, 1991).

S. suis, a common causative organism of meningitis in pigs, has also a sialyl galactoside-specific binding activity. However, the specificity of *S. suis* to the rest of the oligosaccharide structure differs from *E. coli* S fimbriae as the binding sites for *S. suis* on human erythrocytes are sialylated poly-*N*-lactosamine chains (Liukkonen *et al.*, 1992).

Proteolytic mechanisms in bacterial invasion

After adhesion to vascular endothelium, the next step during CSF invasion by bacteria is the traversal across the endothelium. In the fenestrated endothelium of the choroid plexus, where the basement membrane is accessible, e.g. for circulating antibodies (Levine *et al.*, 1987), bacteria may interact with the basement membrane directly. In other parts of the brain, bacteria would need to disrupt the tight junctions between the endothelial cells or traverse the endothelial cells by transcytosis. Considering the interactions of the bacteria with basement membranes, it is interesting that many bacteria bind basement membrane components, e.g. the S-fimbriated *E. coli* binds laminin (Virkola *et al.*, 1993) and *H. influenzae* laminin and type IV collagen (Virkola *et al.*, 1996).

Basement membranes are composed of a network of type IV collagen that is filled by laminin, heparan sulfate proteoglycan, and some minor glycoproteins (Yurchenco and Schnitty, 1990). Penetration of this structure by bacteria evidently requires a proteolytic mechanism. However, only a few gram-negative bacteria have been described to produce significant amounts of proteases that could degrade host extracellular matrices. On the other hand, there are some clues suggesting that bacteria may employ plasmin for extracellular matrix degradation.

Some gram-positive (Reddy and Markus, 1972) and gram-negative (Sodeinde *et al.*, 1992) bacteria produce plasminogen activators, and recent findings indicate that various bacteria expose binding sites for plasmin (Lottenberg *et al.*, 1987) and plasminogen (Parkkinen and Korhonen, 1989; Ullberg *et al.*, 1989, 1990; Kuusela and Saksela, 1990). Plasmin is a serine protease that is present as the inactive zymogen form, plasminogen, at relatively high concentrations in plasma and extracellular fluids. The relatively unspecific proteolytic activity of plasmin is under physiological settings directed to target proteins by lysine binding sites that reside in the five kringle structures at the N-terminal portion of plasmin(ogen) (Wiman *et al.*, 1979). Besides localizing plasmin activity, the binding of plasminogen remarkably enhances its activation by tissue plasminogen activator (t-PA), and also protects plasmin from its main inhibitor, α_2-antiplasmin.

Besides fibrin, plasmin effectively degrades non-collageneous components of basement membranes, and pericellular plasminogen activation has been shown to be an important factor in the penentration of extracellular matrices by invasive animal cells, such as monocyte/macrophages and cancer cells (Danø *et al.*, 1985). Studies with a mouse model of plague have provided evidence of the importance of plasmin also in bacterial spreading through tissue barriers (Sodeinde *et al.*, 1992). The high virulence of the causative organism of plague, *Yersinia pestis*, has been shown to depend on a small plasmid that differentiates it from the other much less virulent *Yersinia* species. The plasmid encodes three proteins, one of which is an outer membrane protein that activates plasminogen by cleaving the same Ile–Val peptide bond as urokinase and t-PA. The *Pla* gene was shown to increase the lethality of bacteria millionfold when inoculated subcutaneously but had little effect when the bacteria were inoculated intravenously (Sodeinde *et al.*, 1992). This indicated that the Pla protein was required for bacterial invasion into the circulation.

Since bacteria causing meningitis have not been found to have endogenous plasminogen activator activity, the question arises of whether they could employ a host-derived plasminogen activator. Interestingly, it has been shown that during endotoxemia there is a rapid increase in plasma t-PA concentration that precedes the increase in its inhibitor, plasminogen activator inhibitor-1 (PAI-1) (Suffredini *et al.*, 1989). The excess of t-PA over PAI-1 in the early phase of endotoxemia suggests that bacterium-bound plasminogen might be activated by t-PA during septicemia. This might be particularly important for bacteria causing meningitis, since the vascular endothelial cells in brain and especially the choroid plexuses are rich in plasminogen activator activity (Soreq and Miskin, 1981).

The possibility that bacteria causing meningitis might employ plasminogen and t-PA for the generation of bacterium-bound plasmin has been studied with the S-fimbriated O18:K1:H7 *E. coli* (Parkkinen *et al.*, 1991). Purified S fimbriae bound both t-PA and plasminogen in a lysine-sensitive manner, and this resulted in several-fold acceleration of plasminogen activation. A similar accelerat-

ing effect was also observed with S-fimbriated wild-type and recombinant strains but not with nonfimbriated bacteria. The accelerating effect was about 10-fold with S-fimbriated bacteria, whereas CNBr-fragmented fibrinogen, a potent promoter of t-PA-catalyzed plasminogen activation, caused about 50-fold acceleration under similar conditions. The generated plasmin remained bacterium-bound and the enhancement of plasminogen activation and generation of bacterium-bound plasmin were inhibited by ε-aminocaproic acid, indicating that the interactions were mediated by lysine-binding sites of plasminogen.

It was recently shown that meningococci and *H. influenzae* type b also bind t-PA (Ullberg *et al.*, 1994). Furthermore, it was recently demonstrated that *H. influenzae* penetrated a reconstituted Matrigel basement membrane in the presence of t-PA and plasminogen and that bacterium-bound plasmin degraded laminin (Virkola *et al.*, 1996). It may thus be that the ability to utilize t-PA for efficient generation of bacterium-bound plasmin activity is distinctive for bacteria causing meningitis. However, further studies are required to clarify whether this takes place also in a plasma mileu in the presence of physiological protease inhibitors and t-PA concentrations occurring in blood.

Concluding remarks

There are several lines of evidence suggesting that the invasion of blood-borne bacteria into the subarachnoid space takes place in the choroid plexuses. A common property for bacteria causing meningitis appears to be the ability to bind to sialic acid containing glycoconjugates. Studies with *E. coli* S fimbriae suggest that brain vascular endothelial cells and the choroidal ependymal cells have specific sialylated glycoconjugates that mediate tissue-specific adhesion of bacteria. To clarify the importance of these binding activities as a possible determinant of subarachnoid space colonization, bacterial mutants deficient of specific adhesion proteins should be studied in animal models.

Further pathogenic interactions may include bacterial adhesion to basement membrane components exposed in the fenestrated endothelium of the choroid plexus. The binding of t-PA and plasminogen to the bacterial surface and the generation of bacterium-bound plasmin may lead to proteolytic degradation of noncollagenous basement membrane proteins and facilitate bacterial penetration through the basement membrane. These interactions have been demonstrated *in vitro* but they should be tested under conditions more closely mimicking physiological conditions, e.g. in terms of protease inhibitors. Transgenic mice with loss of gene function of t-PA and plasminogen (Carmeliet and Collen, 1995) may provide an animal model for the testing of the importance of these interactions *in vivo*.

References

Carmeliet, P. and Collen, D. (1995). Gene targeting and gene transfer studies on the plasminogen/plasmin system: implications in thrombosis, hemostasis, neointima formation and atherosclerosis. *FASEB J.* **9**, 934–8.

Danø, K., Andreasen, P. A., Grøndahl-Hansen, J. *et al.* (1985). Plasminogen activators, tissue degradation, and cancer. *Adv. Cancer Res.*, **44**, 140–266.

Finne, J. (1987). Polysialic acid – a glycoprotein carbohydrate involved in neural adhesion and bacterial meningitis. *Trends Biochem. Sci.*, **10**, 129.

Finne, J., Leinonen, M. and Mäkelä, P. (1983). Antigenic similarities between brain components and bacteria causing meningitis. Implications for vaccine development and pathogenesis. *Lancet*, **ii**, 355–7.

Hanisch, F.-G., Hacker, J. and Schroten, H. (1993). Specificity of S fimbriae on recombinant *Escherichia coli*: preferential binding to gangliosides expressing NeuGcα(2–3)Gal and NeuAca(2–8)NeuAc. *Infect. Immun.*, **61**, 2108–15.

Häyrinen, J., Pelkonen, S. and Finne, J. (1989). Structural similarity of the type-specific group B streptococcal polysaccharides and the carbohydrate units of tissue glycoproteins: evaluation of possible cross-reactivity. *Vaccine*, **7**, 217–24.

Kasper, D. L. (1986). Bacterial capsule - old dogmas and new tricks. *J. Infect. Dis.*, **153**, 409.

Korhonen, T. K., Valtonen, M. V., Parkkinen, J. *et al.* (1985). Serotypes, hemolysin production, and receptor recognition of *Escherichia coli* strains associated with neonatal sepsis and meningitis. *Infect. Immun.*, **48**, 486–91.

Kuusela, P. and Saksela, O. (1990). Binding and activation of plasminogen on the surface of *Staphylococcus aureus*. *Eur. J. Biochem.*, **193**, 759–65.

Levine, S. (1987). Choroid plexus: target for systemic disease and pathway to the brain. *Lab. Invest.*, **56**, 231–3.

Liukkonen, J., Haataja, S., Tikkanen, K. *et al.* (1992). Identification of *N*-acetylneuraminyl α2–3 poly-*N*-acetyllactosamine glycans as the receptors of sialic acid-binding *Streptococcus suis* strains. *J. Biol. Chem.*, **267**, 21105–11.

Lottenberg, R., Broder, C. C. and Boyle, M. D. P. (1987). Identification of a specific receptor for plasmin on a group A streptococcus. *Infect. Immun.*, **55**, 1914–18.

Moch, T., Hoschützkü, H., Hacker, J. *et al.* (1987). Isolation and characterization of the α-sialyl-2,3-galactosyl-specific adhesin from fimbriated *Escherichia coli*. *Proc. Natl. Acad. Sci. USA*, **84**, 3462–6.

Nassif, X., and So., M. (1995). Interactions of pathogenic *Neisseriae* with nonphagocytic cells. *Clin. Microbiol. Rev.*, **8**, 376–88.

Otto, B. R., Verweij van Vught, A. M. and MacLaren, D. M. (1992). Transferrins and heme-compounds as iron sources for pathogenic bacteria. *Crit. Rev. Microbiol.*, **18**, 217–23.

Parkkinen, J., and Korhonen, T. K. (1989). Binding of plasminogen to *Escherichia coli* adhesion proteins. *FEBS Lett.*, **250**, 437–40.

Parkkinen, J., Rogers, G. N., Korhonen, T. K. *et al.* (1986). Identification of the *O*-linked sialyloligosaccharides of glycophorin A as the erythrocyte receptors of S-fimbriated *Escherichia coli*. *Infect. Immun.*, **54**, 37–42.

Parkkinen, J., Korhonen, T. K., Pere, A. *et al.* (1987). Binding sites in the rat brain for *Escherichia coli* S fimbriae associated with neonatal meningitis. *J. Clin. Invest.*, **81**, 860–5.

Parkkinen, J., Ristimäki, A. and Westerlund, B. (1989). Binding of *Escherichia coli* S fimbriae to cultured human endothelial cells. *Infect. Immun.*, **57**, 2256–9.

Parkkinen, J., Hacker, J. and Korhonen, T. K. (1991). Enhancement of tissue plasminogen activator-catalyzed plasminogen activation by *Escherichia coli* S fimbriae associated with neonatal septicaemia and meningitis. *Thromb. Haemost.*, **65**, 483–6.

Prasadarao, N. V., Wass, C. A., Hacker, J. *et al.* (1993). Adhesion of S-fimbriated *E. coli* to brain glycolipids mediated by the sfaA gene encoded protein of S fimbriae. *J. Biol. Chem.*, **268**, 10356–63.

Reddy, K. N. N., and Markus, G. (1972). Mechanism of activation of human plasminogen by streptokinase. *J. Biol. Chem.*, **247**, 1683.

Saukkonen, K. M. J., Nowicki, B. and Leinonen, M. (1988). Role of type 1 and S fimbriae in the pathogenesis of *Escherichia coli*, O18:K1 bacteremia and meningitis in the infant rat. *Infect. Immun.*, **56**, 892–7.

Scheld, W. M., Park, T.-S. Dacey, R. G. *et al.* (1979). Clearance of bacteria from cerebrospinal fluid to blood in experimental meningitis. *Infect. Immun.*, **24**, 102–5.

Schmoll, T., Hoschützky, H., Morschhäuser, J. *et al.* (1989). Analysis of genes for the sialic acid-binding adhesin and two other minor fimbrial subunits of the S-fimbrial adhesin determinant of *Escherichia coli*. *Mol. Microbiol.*, **3**, 1735–44.

469

Smith, A. L., Daum, R. S., Scheifele, D. *et al.* (1982). Pathogenesis of *Haemophilus influenzae* meningitis. In *Haemophilus influenzae, Epidemiology, Immunology, and Prevention of Disease*, ed. S. H. Sell and P. F. Wright, pp. 89–109. New York: Elsevier Science Publishing Co.

Sodeinde, O. A., Subrahmanyam, Y. V. B. K, Stark, K. *et al.* (1992). A surface protease and the invasive character of plague. *Science*, **258**, 1004–7.

Soreq, H. and Miskin, R. (1981). Plasminogen activator in the rodent brain. *Brain Res.*, **216**, 361–74.

Stephens, D. S., and Farley, M. M. (1991). Pathogenic events during infection of the human nasopharynx with *Neisseria meningitidis* and *Haemophilus influenzae*. *Rev. Infect. Dis.*, **13**, 22–33.

Sterk, L. M., van Alphen, L., Geelen van den Broek, L. *et al.* (1991). Differential binding of *Haemophilus influenzae* to human tissues by fimbriae. *J. Med. Microbiol.*, **35**, 129–38.

Stins, M. F., Prasadarao, N. V., Ibric, L. *et al.* (1994). Binding characteristics of S fimbriated *Escherichia coli* to isolated brain microvascular endothelial cells. *Am. J. Pathol.*, **145**, 1228–36.

Suffredini, A. F., Harpel, P. C. and Parrillo, J. E. (1989). Promotion and subsequent inhibition of plasminogen activation after administration of intravenous endotoxin to normal subjects. *N. Engl. J. Med.*, **320**, 1165–72.

Tunkel A. R., and Scheld, W. M. (1993). Pathogenesis and pathophysiology of bacterial meningitis. *Ann. Rev. Med.*, **44**, 103–20.

Ullberg, M., Kronvall, G. and Wiman, B. (1989). New receptor for human plasminogen on gram positive cocci. *Acta Pathol. Microbiol. Immunol. Scand.*, **97**, 996–1002.

Ullberg, M., Kronvall, G., Karlsson, I., and B. Wiman. (1990). Receptors for human plasminogen on gram-negative bacteria. *Infect. Immun.*, **58**, 21–5.

Ullberg, M., Wiman, B. and Kronvall, G.. (1994). Binding of tissue type plasminogen activator (t-PA) to *Neisseria meningitidis* and *Haemophilus influenzae*. *FEMS Immunol Med. Microbiol.*, **9**, 171–7.

van Alphen, L., Geelen van den Broek, L., Blaas, L. *et al.* (1991). Blocking of fimbria-mediated adherence of *Haemophilus influezae* by sialyl gangliosides. *Infect. Immun.*, **59**, 4473–7.

Virkola, R., Parkkinen, J., Hacker, J. and Korhonen, T. K. (1993). Sialyloligosaccharide chains of laminin as an extracellular matrix target for S fimbriae of *Escherichia coli*. *Infect. Immun.*, **61**, 4480–4.

Virkola, R., Lähteenmäki, K., Eberhard, T. *et al.* (1996). Interactions of *Haemophilus influezae* with the mammalian extracellular matrix. *J. Infect. Dis.*, **173**, 1137–47.

Williams, A. E. and Blakemore, W. F. (1990). Pathogenesis of meningitis caused by *Streptococcuc suis* type 2. *J. Infect. Dis.*, **162**, 474–81.

Wiman, B., Linjen, H. R. and Collen, D. (1979). On the specific interaction between the lysine- binding sites in plasmin and complementary sites in alpha2-antiplasmin and fibrinogen. *Biochem. Biophys. Acta*, **579**, 142.

Yurchenco, P. D. and Schnitty, J. C. (1990). Molecular architecture of basement membranes. *FASEB J.*, **4**, 1577–90.

Index

Page numbers in *italics* refer to figures and tables